Cardiology
1982

Cardiology: 1982

Printed in the United States of America

First Edition

International Standard Book Number: 0-914316-27-3

International Standard Serial Number: 0275-0066

Cardiology 1982

WILLIAM C. ROBERTS, MD
Chief, Pathology Branch
National Heart, Lung, and Blood Institute
National Institutes of Health, Bethesda, Maryland, and
Clinical Professor of Pathology and Medicine (Cardiology)
Georgetown University, Washington, D.C.

DEAN T. MASON, MD
Professor of Medicine and Physiology
Chief, Cardiovascular Medicine
University of California, Davis
School of Medicine and University Medical Center
Davis and Sacramento, California

MARY ALLEN ENGLE, MD
Stavros S. Niarchos Professor of Pediatric Cardiology
Director, Pediatric Cardiology
The New York Hospital–Cornell University Medical Center, New York

LAWRENCE H. COHN, MD
Professor of Surgery
Harvard Medical School
Department of Surgery
Division of Thoracic and Cardiac Surgery
Brigham and Women's Hospital, Boston

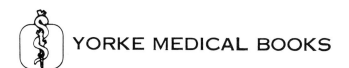

YORKE MEDICAL BOOKS

Contents

7. Congenital Heart Disease 315

Preface

We were pleased with the response to our first book, CARDIOLOGY 1981. This year's edition contains 665 summaries, a 47% increase over last year's book. To allow the reader to determine better which author summarized a particular article, the number of articles summarized in each of the 9 chapters by each of the 4 authors is shown below. The summaries were edited and organized into the various chapters by WCR.

CARDIOLOGY 1982

| AUTHOR | CHAPTER NUMBER | | | | | | | | | TOTALS |
	1	2	3	4	5	6	7	8	9	
WCR	106	53	37	44	76	44	9	14	66	449*
DTM	24	26	15	3	2	0	0	13	4	87**
MAE	0	0	2	1	0	0	45	0	2	50
LHC	13	6	6	0	29	1	37	0	13	105
TOTALS	143	85	60	48	107	45	91	27	85	691

* Includes 12 references that were not summarized.
** Includes 14 references that were not summarized.

We owe special thanks to several people who worked nights and weekends to complete this book, especially Mary McMahon, Marcia McManus, Teresa Roginski, Leslie Silvernail, Jeanne Macaluso, Joan-Ellen Macredis, Barbara Hebert, Dana Crim, Brenda Mayes, and Margaret Moore.

Gay C. Morgulas, Director of Yorke Medical Books, deserves particular thanks for orchestrating publication of the book rapidly and with dedication and care.

WILLIAM C. ROBERTS, MD
DEAN T. MASON, MD
MARY ALLEN ENGLE, MD
LAWRENCE H. COHN, MD

Coronary Heart Disease: General Aspects

DETECTION AND DIAGNOSIS

Coronary heart disease in Rochester, Minnesota, 1950–1975

A total of 3,080 residents of Rochester, Minnesota, had a diagnosis of CAD made during the 26 years between January 1, 1950, and December 31, 1975.[1,2] No patient had had a diagnosis of CAD before inclusion in this study, nor any clinical evidence of CHF or other significant noncoronary heart disease. Of the 3,080 patients, the initial manifestation of CAD was *AMI* in 1,321 (43%), *angina pectoris* in 1,215 (39%), and *sudden unexpected death* in 544 (18%). The incidence of diagnosis of CAD decreased approximately 10 years earlier than did the decline in mortality, and changed little thereafter. The age-adjusted case fatality rate for the incidence of AMI decreased from 19% in 1965–1969 to 9% in 1970–1975. The death rate during the 5 years after diagnosis of angina pectoris also decreased by almost 50% and the AMI patients dismissed from the hospital showed little change in subsequent survival.

Significance of exercise-induced ST-segment elevation

DeFeyter and associates[3] from Amsterdam, the Netherlands, examined the relation between ECG ST elevation during treadmill exercise (≥ 1 mm, using the conventional 12 leads), the severity of CAD, and LV wall motion abnormalities in 680 patients. They divided the patients into 3 groups: 1) 218 without clinically significant CAD; 2) 178 with clinically significant CAD but without previous AMI, and 3) 284 with clinically significant CAD with previous AMI. ST elevation during exercise (predominantly in lead V_2) occurred in 2 patients (1%) in group 1, 3 patients (2%) in group 2, and 147 patients (52%) in group 3. CAD (number of vessels involved and severity of stenoses) was comparable in groups 2 and 3. All patients in group 1 had a normal LV contraction pattern; 64% of the patients in group 2 had wall motion abnormalities (predominantly hypokinesia), and 95% of group 3 had wall motion abnormalities (mainly akinesia, dyskinesia, or aneurysm). A strongly positive correlation occurred between ST elevation and LV dysfunction in patients in group 3 (Fig. 1-1). The overall sensitivity and specificity of the stress test in detecting wall motion abnormalities were 55% and 100%, respectively. The sensitivity increased with deterioration in LV function, reaching 81% and 90% in patients with dyskinesia and aneurysm, respectively. Maximal ST elevation (≥ 3 mm) was confined to patients with dyskinesia or aneurysm. The

Fig. 1-1. Relation between height of ST-segment elevation and severity of LV wall motion abnormalities. Reproduced with permission from DeFeyter et al.[3]

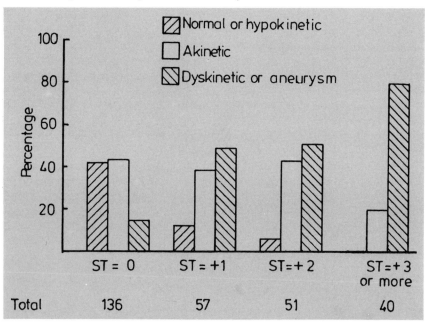

frequency of ST elevation during exercise also was related to the location of previous AMI, with a positive response in 85% of patients with anterior AMI and in only 33% of patients with "inferior" AMI. Thus, ST-segment elevation during exercise in patients with previous AMI is a sensitive and specific indicator of advanced LV asynergy.

Regional left ventricular wall motion abnormalities in CAD detected by echo

The reliability and sensitivity of echo in finding wall motion abnormalities and the relationship of abnormalities to the location and extent of coronary narrowing have not been established. Corya and associates[4] from Indianapolis, Indiana, evaluated prospectively by M-mode echo LV wall motion in 503 patients who had all undergone selective coronary angiography and LV angiography because of chest pain or dyspnea or to determine the feasibility of operative therapy. Patients with complete left BBB, previous cardiac surgery, a recognized cardiomyopathy, or inadequate angiographic or echo study were excluded. Of the 319 patients with angiographically narrowed coronary arteries, 212 (66%) had abnormal M-mode echoes. Of the CAD patients, 34% had normal wall motion on M-mode echo. More abnormalities were detected when patients were examined by both M-mode and 2-D echo because M-mode was more sensitive in detecting anterior wall abnormalities and 2-D in detecting posterior wall abnormalities. Both M-mode and 2-D echo showed a low incidence of false positive diagnoses (<2%) for patients with normal findings at cardiac catheterization. Abnormal echo motion was found by M-mode in 89% of patients with ECG Q waves of myocardial infarction and in 61% of patients with CAD without Q waves.

Diagnosing proximal LAD coronary narrowing by septal myocardial perfusion imaging

Significant narrowing of the proximal LAD places a large area of myocardium in jeopardy. Because an aggressive surgical approach has been recommended in this condition, a noninvasive means to diagnose proximal LAD disease would be clinically important. Since the blood supply to the septum is derived primarily from the LAD, LAD stenosis might be expected to cause abnormalities in septal perfusion. Attempts to diagnose proximal LAD disease by abnormal septal wall motion on echo have yielded conflicting results. Myocardial perfusion imaging (MPI) with thallium-201 has been extensively used to document and localize both transient ischemia and AMI. Pichard and associates[5] from New York City assessed the usefulness of MPI to identify proximal LAD obstruction before the first septal perforator in 60 CAD patients. Perfusion of the septum and anteroapical areas with thallium-201 injected during exercise was compared with results of coronary arteriography. Septal MPI defect was found in 92% of patients with obstruction of the proximal LAD, in 28% of patients with LAD obstruction distal to the first septal perforator, in no patients with obstructions involving right or LC arteries, and in 11% of patients without CAD. Anteroapical MPI defects were found with similar frequency in the 3 groups with obstructive CAD. Septal MPI defect had a sensitivity of 92% and a specificity of 85% in the diagnosis of proximal LAD disease. Normal septal perfusion with thallium-201 virtually excluded significant proximal LAD narrowing.

Comparison of upright and supine bicycle exercise in detection of CAD by RNA

Assessment of LV performance by RNA during both supine and upright bicycle exercise has been reported useful for detection of CAD. Since there are important physiologic differences between supine and upright exercise, the 2 procedures may differ in sensitivity and specificity for detection of CAD, and different criteria for interpretation of test results as abnormal may be required. These 2 exercise scintigraphic techniques have not been directly compared in patients with and without CAD. Freeman and associates[6] from Los Angeles, California, performed upright and supine multigated cardiac blood pool scintigraphy at rest and during maximum exercise in 37 patients, 15 with normal coronary arteriograms, 12 with CAD without prior AMI, and 10 with CAD and remote AMI. Heart rate and systolic BP were similar during upright and supine exercise in normal patients, but were significantly lower during supine exercise in both CAD groups. LV EF, RV EF, and LV segmental wall motion were similar in the upright and supine positions at rest or during maximum exercise within each group and showed high concordance of exercise responses. Although LV end-diastolic volume increased in all 3 groups during upright exercise and in both CAD groups during supine exercise, it did not change during supine exercise in patients without CAD. The fall of LV end-systolic volume in normals was greater during supine exercise than during upright exercise. LV end-systolic volume rose in the CAD patients in both positions. Therefore, although LV EF, RV EF, and LV segmental wall motion responses are similar in the upright and supine positions, LV end-systolic and LV end-diastolic volume changes are not. For detecting and evaluating CAD by RNA, the 2 different positions of exercise appear to have similar diagnostic significance.

Stress thallium-201 myocardial scintigraphy and exercise technetium ventriculography in detecting and locating CAD

The ability of visually interpreted stress thallium scintigraphy and 45° left anterior oblique (LAO) exercise RNA, alone or in combination, to assess the extent and location of CAD was evaluated by Elkayam and associates[7] from Los Angeles, California, in 64 patients, 56 of whom had CAD (multivessel in 46, and 1-vessel in 10) and 8 had normal coronary arteries. The LAD was involved in 51 patients, the LC in 40, and the right in 39. The overall accuracy for predicting CAD was 96% for thallium scintigraphy, 89% for exercise RNA, and 98% for both tests in combination; the specificity for the exclusion of CAD was 75% for both tests, alone or in combination. From 130 diseased coronary arteries in these patients, thallium scintigraphy correctly detected 49%, exercise RNA detected 58%, and the combined tests detected 71%. The absence of narrowing in individual arteries was correctly predicted by thallium scintigraphy in 85%, by RNA in 77%, and by the test combination in 71%.

The sensitivity of both tests was clearly related to the severity of CAD. Performance of the 2 tests in combination detected 80% of severe (90−100% diameter narrowing), 77% of moderately severe (75−89% diameter narrowing), and only 53% of mildly stenotic (50−74% diameter narrowing) lesions. For individual LAD disease, exercise RNA was more sensitive (80%) than thallium scintigraphy (55%), and the tests in combination had a sensitivity of 84%; the respective specificities were 69%, 92%, and 69%. For individual LC narrowing, the sensitivity of stress-thallium was 40%, of stress-RNA 58%, and of the combined tests, 65%; the respective specificities were 100%, 83%, and 83%. The following sensitivity values were found for individual right narrowing: thallium scintigraphy 51%, RNA 31%, and the tests in combination 59%; the specificity was 72%, 76%, and 60%, respectively. Narrowing in the posterior circulation (LC and/or right) was detected by stress-thallium in 60%, by stress-technetium RNA in 62%, and by the tests in combination in 77%; the specificity was 100%, 82%, and 82%, respectively. Thallium scintigraphy and technetium RNA correctly detected the presence of multivessel CAD in 43% and 57% of patients, respectively. The combination detected significantly more patients with multivessel CAD (70%) than either test alone; the specificity was 88% for thallium, 76% for technetium, and 76% for the combined tests. Thus, the combination of visually interpreted stress redistribution thallium scintigraphy and exercise RNA provides more diagnostic information than either test alone, and combined testing provides an effective means for noninvasive evaluation of the extent and location of the CAD. In the future, application of quantitative thallium analysis and 2-view exercise RNA should further improve the diagnostic yield of these combined noninvasive tests.

Probabilistic analysis of scintigraphic rest and exercise left ventricular ejection fractions for CAD detection

Interpretation of a diagnostic modality requires consideration of the entire distribution of potential responses in both the normal and diseased population to extract the maximum available information from the test. Diamond and Forrester[8] from Los Angeles, California, delineated a probabilistic format for interpretation of scintigraphic LV EF to diagnose CAD. The format is distinguished: 1) by accurate assessment of CAD likelihood based upon age, sex, and symptom classification using a logistical regression model, and 2) by consideration of LV EF as a continuous probabilistic variable that obeys beta frequency distribution. This format allows assessment of the probability of CAD in an individual patient, according to Bayes' theorem of conditional probability of disease, given combinations of LV EF at rest and/or with exercise, and thereby is designed to provide more information than conventional categorical classifications of "normal" or "abnormal" test observations.

2-D echo evaluation of exercise-induced right and left ventricular asynergy and correlation with thallium scanning in CAD

Maurer and Nanda[9] from Rochester, New York, prospectively obtained adequate real time 2-D echoes before and immediately after graded treadmill exercise testing in 41 of 48 patients who subsequently underwent cardiac catheterization for suspected CAD. The findings were correlated with thallium perfusion scans performed 5–10 minutes and 3 hours after the same exercise test. Exercise-induced wall motion abnormalities were detected in 19 of 23 patients with significant CAD and no prior AMI, and in all 5 patients with known previous AMI. Three patients with CAD experienced new isolated RV asynergy with exercise that would have been missed if only the left ventricle had been evaluated. Exercise-induced thallium perfusion defects correlated well with exercise-induced asynergy as detected with echo. 2-D echo performed immediately after treadmill stress testing is a feasible and rewarding technique in the evaluation of patients suspected of having CAD.

Relation of thallium-201 myocardial perfusion pattern to regional and global left ventricular function with exercise

Graded exercise testing with ECG monitoring has been the standard noninvasive method for over 10 years for detecting clinically significant CAD. Recently, 2 nuclear cardiologic techniques, myocardial imaging with thallium-201 (TMI) and RNA with exercise, have improved the sensitivity of the exercise ECG alone. These 2 radionuclide imaging techniques, while affording enhanced sensitivity in the detection of CAD, can also provide complementary information. TMI provides a measure of myocardial perfusion inequalities, whereas RNA examines the results of changes in LV function. Kirshenbaum and associates[10] from Boston and Worcester, Massachusetts, utilized thallium-201 redistribution pattern after exercise to determine by RNA measured rest and exercise LV regional and global function in 61 patients, 50 with CAD. Sixteen patients had exclusively transient thallium defects, suggesting ischemia, and their mean LV EF was 65% at rest and 58% during exercise. Eight patients had exclusively persistent thallium defects, suggesting scar, and their LV EF was unchanged during exercise, 58%–59%. LV EF increased during exercise in the 17 patients without exercise thallium defects, 7 with CAD: 66%–73%. Individual LV wall segments that exhibited transient or persistent thallium defects contracted abnormally both at rest and during exercise, as compared with LV segments without exercise thallium defects. Thus, 1) only transient thallium defects reliably predict worsening LV global function during exercise; 2) both transient and persistent thallium defects can be associated with resting dysynergy, and 3) in some CAD patients, apparent hypoperfusion does not necessarily predict LV dysfunction during exercise.

PROGNOSIS AFTER EXERCISE TESTING WITH ST-SEGMENT ELEVATION >2 mm

In patients with symptomatic CAD, the occurrence of ST-segment depression >2 mm provoked by exercise is associated with angiographically demonstrable, severe, multivessel coronary narrowing. Podrid and associates[11] from Boston, Massachusetts, analyzed 212 men with CAD in whom ST-segment depression >2 mm could be reproduced with exercise. Of 142 patients who had no other type of heart disease and were not receiving digitalis, the mean ST-segment depression was 2.9 mm. Follow-up, an average of 59

Fig. 1-2. Survival among 142 patients with CAD. Solid line represents survival when death alone is considered; dashed line denotes survival when either death or CABG is considered to be the end point. Reproduced with permission from Podrid.[11]

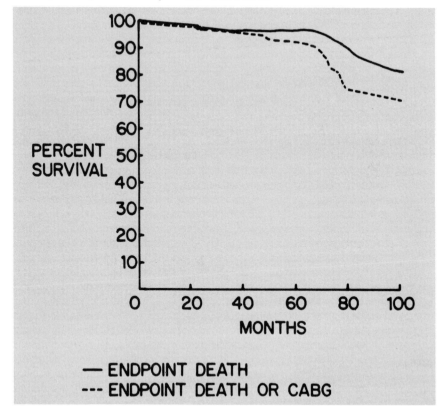

months, disclosed that 11 patients had died and 9 had had coronary artery bypass grafting (CABG). Survival correlated with exercise tolerance, but not with the degree of ST depression, peak heart rate, or peak BP during exercise (Fig. 1-2). Thus, profound ST-segment depression during exercise testing in patients with CAD is not associated with a poor prognosis, and medical management is usually highly successful and associated with a low mortality.

PROGNOSIS AFTER CORONARY ANGIOGRAM

Prognosis in 1,000 women under age 50 years studied by coronary angiography

Proudfit and associates[12] from Cleveland, Ohio, determined the course after coronary angiography of 1,000 women < 50 years of age suspected of having CAD and who were followed for at least 5 years (mean, 8.4). The survival rate at 5 years for 761 patients who had < 50% diameter reduction of any major coronary artery was 97%. Of 727 women who had normal arteries or < 30% diameter reduction of any artery, 7 had coronary events (death, AMI, or CABG), and of 34 women who had 30% to almost 50% diameter reduction of at least 1 coronary artery, 6 had coronary events. Survival for 236 women who had severe narrowing of 1 or more coronary arteries at 5 years was 74%, but many of these patients were withdrawn from study because of CABG.

Follow-up of 121 patients with normal or near normal coronary arteriograms

Isner and associates[13] from Boston, Massachusetts, reviewed long-term outcome in 121 patients (72 women, 49 men; aged 18–77 years [mean, 49]) with normal (90%) or nearly normal (10%) coronary angiograms performed between January 1969 and September 1979 at their medical center. No patient had an associated noncoronary form of heart disease. The follow-up of 121 patients ranged from 1–11 years (mean, 4.3). During this period, 3 patients (2.5%) died suddenly and unexpectedly and 4 others (3%) had AMI. Of 7 patients who underwent a second coronary angiogram, 3 had narrowings in excess of that observed at the initial study. Of the 118 surviving patients, 24 (20%) had resolution of chest discomfort. The remaining 94 (80%) continued to have chest discomfort similar to that which brought them to coronary angiography; the pain was unchanged in 70 (59%), worse in 12 (10%), and diminished in 12 (10%). Thus, in most patients the nature, frequency, and intensity of their chest pain were unaffected by the information that their coronary arteriograms were normal. The finding of normal or nearly normal coronary arteriograms implies a highly favorable prognosis, but it does not establish immunity from fatal or nonfatal coronary events. The likely basis for these subsequent events is progression of the coronary narrowing, rather than coronary spasm or underestimation of the extent of coronary narrowing by angiography.

ANGIOGRAPHIC PROGRESSION OF CAD

To determine whether risk factors or angiographic features could be correlated with progression of CAD, Shub and associates[14] from Rochester, Minnesota, independently analyzed serial coronary angiograms in 65 symptomatic CAD patients for progression without knowledge of their respective risk factors. An important design feature of this study was that observer variability of coronary lesion assessment was objectively evaluated and taken into account in defining progression of CAD. The reproducibility of lesion assessment varied with the severity of stenosis; moderate stenoses had the greatest intraobserver and interobserver variability. At initial study, 337 partial and 68 complete occlusions were identified. Of the 337 partial occlusions at risk of progression, 73 (22%) progressed; 13 (4%) of the initial lesions regressed. In the 65 patients with persistent or increasing angina, progression occurred in 51 (78%) over a mean period of 24 months. Apart from the tendency of high-grade stenoses ($\geq 98\%$) to progress to complete occlusion, no measured clinical, laboratory, or angiographic variable showed any significant effect on progression of CAD. Therefore, although certain risk factors may predispose to CAD, in this selected group of symptomatic patients these same risk factors did not predict its progression. Thus, definitions of progression should incorporate the factor of observer variability, and therapeutic measures designed to influence progression of CAD should take into account this apparently unpredictable progression. It is of interest, however, that only a tenth of their patients had total serum cholesterols <200 mg/dl at both initial and follow-up studies and 6 of them demonstrated progression. What number of those 10 have or were <160 mg/dl (probably the really normal value) is unclear.

Kimbiris and Segal[15] from Philadelphia, Pennsylvania, summarized their views on CAD progression: 1) Coronary atherosclerosis is a progressive disease and is expected to progress in more than half of symptomatic patients in 1–2 years. 2) Patients with chest pain resembling angina pectoris who have normal coronary arteriograms have considerable likelihood of remaining normal for long periods of time. 3) It is not possible to predict which patients will have stable or progressive CAD. 4) Individual risk factors for CAD do not appear to affect progression in a 2–3 year follow-up period, but combinations of more than 1 risk factor increase the rate of CAD progression. 5) Coronary artery bypass grafting (CABG) accelerates CAD progression of stenosis proximal to the vein anastomosis more frequently in arteries with patent grafts. Nongrafted vessels are not affected by surgery and progress as in patients without surgery. 6) Since new trials probably will be done to modify risk factors for prevention, arrest, or regression of CAD and more patients will undergo well-accepted modes of CABG therapy, it can be expected that more patients with angina pectoris will eventually be restudied with repeat coronary arteriograms.

For the reasons outlined above, cardiac catheterization laboratories that perform coronary arteriography, particularly those with large numbers of patients, should develop standardized techniques, recording the degree of obliquity of each projection and the use or nonuse of nitroglycerin before coronary arteriography, so that repeat coronary arteriograms can be performed under almost identical conditions for optimal comparison. Sagittal views should be obtained routinely in every patient for more accurate interpretation of coronary arterial anatomy. Improved methodology for more accurate interpretation of coronary arteriograms requires continued development.

LIPIDS

General topics

LIPOPROTEINS, CARDIOVASCULAR DISEASE, AND DEATH (FRAMINGHAM STUDY)

Gordon and associates[16] from Framingham, Massachusetts, from a 6-year follow-up of men and women aged 49–82 years, found that a low density lipoprotein (LDL) cholesterol concentration was associated with a low frequency of CAD, but with a statistically significant excess of stroke in women and of deaths from non-CAD causes in both sexes. An inverse relation of high density lipoprotein (HDL) cholesterol level with CAD and its major consequences, death and CHF, was observed. Triglyceride determinations added little information regarding cardiovascular risk to that elicited from HDL and LDL cholesterol and other known cardiovascular risk factors. Although the relation of HDL and LDL cholesterol to CAD risk has been well documented, their relationship to other cardiovascular diseases, as well as to noncardiovascular diseases and death, is largely unexplored. This report presents the first systematic view of these non-CAD relationships in the Framingham Study. The data reiterate the finding from earlier Framingham Study reports that higher levels of HDL cholesterol are associated with lower CAD risk, even in persons aged 49–82 years, the age group included in this study. The more detailed earlier analysis of this relation found that although the association was evident over the full age range for men, it seemed to be true for women only younger than 70 years. It is, therefore, not surprising that the relationship over the age range 49–82 years is weaker for women than for men.

INTERMEDIATE DENSITY LIPOPROTEIN AND CHOLESTEROL-RICH VERY LOW DENSITY LIPOPROTEIN IN ANGIOGRAPHICALLY DETERMINED CAD

Tatami and associates[17] from Kanazawa, Japan, studied the relation between the concentrations of intermediate density lipoprotein (IDL) and other lipoproteins and the extent of CAD in 182 consecutive patients evaluated by selective coronary angiography. The extent of CAD correlated significantly and positively with very low density lipoprotein (VLDL) cholesterol, IDL cholesterol, and LDL cholesterol, and negatively with HDL cholesterol. Analysis of 4 subgroups divided by IDL cholesterol and LDL cholesterol levels indicated that moderately increased levels of IDL cholesterol were closely associated with a high frequency of CAD. Moreover, a multivariate regression analysis demonstrated that IDL cholesterol for men, LDL cholesterol for men and women, and HDL cholesterol for men were significant variables in the final weighing procedure. IDL cholesterol was closely associated with cholesterol-rich VLDL. This study shows that IDL and cholesterol-rich VLDL combine to contribute to the development of CAD.

CHOLESTEROL LEVELS INCLUDING APOLIPOPROTEIN-B IN PATIENTS WITH AND WITHOUT CORONARY NARROWING DETERMINED BY ANGIOGRAM

Whayne and associates[18] from Oklahoma City, Oklahoma, performed serum lipid studies in 161 men with angiographically documented CAD and in 72 men with angiographically normal arteries. Age, plasma total cholesterol, triglyceride, and VLDL and LDL cholesterol were significantly greater in the patients with CAD than in those with normal coronary arteries. In contrast, no difference was observed in the mean levels of HDL cholesterol between the 2 groups, although patients with HDL cholesterol <40 mg/dl had a higher rate of CAD than those with HDL cholesterol >40 mg/dl. Multivariant analysis showed that *age* and *total plasma cholesterol* were the 2 variables most significantly related to the presence of CAD. In a subgroup of patients with plasma total cholesterol <265 mg/dl, however, the most reliable variable was plasma apolipoprotein-B (APOB). For patients <50 years of age, APOB and LDL cholesterol were the most significant variables, whereas for patients ≥50 years of age VLDL cholesterol was the most significant variable. Thus, measurement of APOB may have important predictive value for CAD, especially at lower levels of plasma cholesterol.

LIPIDS AND LIPOPROTEINS IN BLACK ADULTS

To provide population data on levels of plasma cholesterol, triglycerides, and HDL and LDL cholesterol, Morrison and associates[19] from Cincinnati, Ohio, studied 627 black adults aged 20–59 years (206 men and 421 women). Comparisons were made with 2,493 white adults, aged 20–59 years (1,111 men and 1,382 women) from the Princeton School Study. Black men had total plasma cholesterol levels that were comparable to those in white men; plasma cholesterol levels were higher in black women than in white women. Black men had lower levels of plasma triglycerides, higher HDL cholesterol levels, and lower LDL cholesterol levels than did white men. Black women not taking exogenous sex steroid hormones had higher total cholesterol and HDL cholesterol levels, and lower triglyceride and LDL cholesterol levels than did white women not taking exogenous sex steroid hormones. Black women taking exogenous sex steroid hormones had lower plasma cholesterol and triglyceride levels and slightly higher HDL and lower LDL cholesterol levels than did white women taking exogenous sex steroid hormones. These differences not only require the use of race-specific lipoprotein distribution tables for characterization of individual subjects, but are consistent with putatively reduced risk for CAD in blacks as compared with whites.

ASSOCIATIONS OF CHOLESTEROL LEVELS AND CARDIOVASCULAR AND
NONCARDIOVASCULAR MORTALITY INCLUDING CANCER

Raised serum cholesterol is a powerful predictor of CAD morbidity and
mortality. The risk of CAD increases with serum cholesterol concentration.
Efforts have been made to reduce cholesterol level by drugs or diet. However,
unlike systemic hypertension and cigarette smoking, whose effects on total
mortality can be countered by preventive measures, some workers have
found a lack of association, or even an inverse association, between cholesterol levels and total mortality and cancer incidence. The Honolulu Heart
Program reported a quadratic relation between serum cholesterol concentrations and total mortality. High total cholesterol concentrations were associated with high mortality rates (mainly due to CAD) and low total cholesterol concentrations also were associated with high mortality rates (mainly
due to malignancies). Yaari and associates[20] from Tel Aviv, Israel, examined
the relation between cholesterol concentration and mortality (from total or
specific causes) in the Israeli Ischemic Heart Disease Study (IIHD) to determine the association of HDL cholesterol and total cholesterol with mortality
from CAD and with total mortality. They examined 10,059 civil servants and

Fig. 1-3.   Age-adjusted 7-year mortality rates by cholesterol concentrations. Reproduced with
permission from Yaari et al.[20]

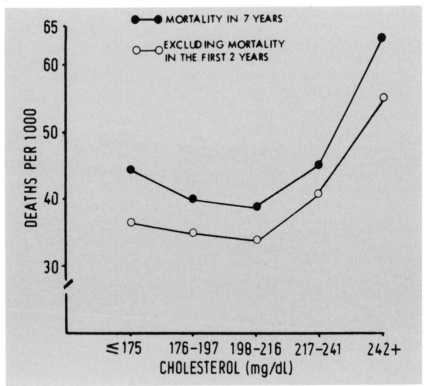

municipal employees, aged 40–65 years. Of them, 475 (5%) died during a 7-year follow-up. High density lipoprotein (HDL) cholesterol levels were determined in the last 6,562 men entering the study, and 305 (5%) of them died. CAD accounted for 37% of the total deaths. A "J"-shaped relation, which persisted after the removal of data on early mortality (first 2 years), was observed between total cholesterol and total mortality (Fig. 1-3). An inverse relation was observed between HDL cholesterol and total mortality. Multivariate analysis of the data to adjust for possible confounding effects of additional mortality risk factors demonstrated that total cholesterol made no independent contribution to total mortality, but that the contribution of low HDL to mortality persisted after adjustment. CAD mortality consistently increased with rising concentrations of total cholesterol. CAD mortality rates decreased markedly with increasing HDL cholesterol concentrations. After adjustment for age and other risk factors, the relation of coronary mortality to HDL cholesterol emerged as the dominant one. There was no clear-cut association between total or HDL cholesterol and cancer mortality (Fig. 1-4). These results indicate that, particularly in older age groups, measures designed to increase HDL cholesterol may prove as valuable in preventing CAD as those designed to reduce LDL cholesterol.

Fig. 1-4. Age-adjusted 7-year cancer mortality rates by cholesterol concentrations. Reproduced with permission from Yaari et al.[20]

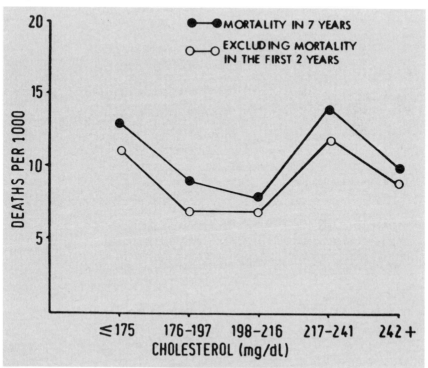

In a recent clinical trial of clofibrate for hypercholesterolemia, a significant excess of noncardiovascular mortality was observed in treated subjects as compared with hypercholesterolemic control subjects. As a group, cancer comprised the most common contribution to noncardiovascular mortality. Additionally, it has been suggested that both cancer of the colon and of the breast are causally related to fat intake. One report of cancer mortality indicated that BP level also was a strong predictor of cancer risk for all sites and for specific major cancer sites. To test these hypotheses, Williams and associates[21] from Framingham, Massachusetts, studied 5,209 subjects for 24 years; 691 of them developed cancer (with histologic confirmation in 94%). Predetermined personal characteristics were tested by multiple logistic regression for associations with subsequent occurrence of cancer at specific sites. Significant associations of various cancer sites with cigarette smoking, alcohol consumption, education, height, weight, and parity agreed with the findings of other studies. Serum cholesterol level was inversely associated with frequency of cancer of the colon and of other sites only in men; these inverse associa-

Fig. 1-5. *Top left:* Age-adjusted incidence of colon and lung cancer by level of cigarette smoking at examination 4 followed-up through examination 13. *Top right:* Age-adjusted cancer incidence by level of serum cholesterol at examination 4. Men aged 35–69 years, followed-up through examination 13. *Bottom:* Age-adjusted cancer incidence by level of serum cholesterol at examination 4. Women aged 35–69 years, followed-up through examination 13. Reproduced with permission from Williams et al.[21]

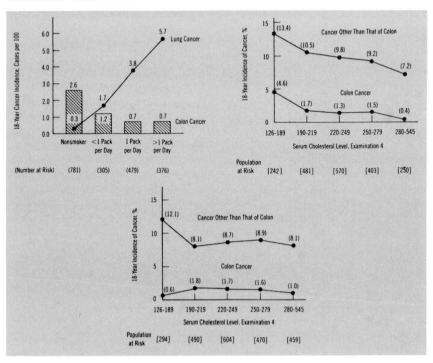

tions were statistically significant after adjustment for age, alcohol consumption, cigarette smoking, education, systolic BP, and relative weight (Fig. 1-5).

HYPOCHOLESTEROLEMIA IN MYELOPROLIFERATIVE DISORDERS

Reduced plasma total cholesterol levels have been reported in patients with polycythemia vera and agnogenic myeloid metaplasia. Gilbert and associates[22] from New York City confirmed the presence of hypocholesterolemia in patients with polycythemia vera and agnogenic myeloid metaplasia. Not only was the total cholesterol decreased, but the LDL and HDL cholesterol also was decreased in comparison with age- and sex-matched patients from the Framingham, Massachusetts population. Men with myeloproliferative disease also had significantly lower total and LDL cholesterol levels than did those with relative or secondary polycythemia. LDL and HDL cholesterol were correlated significantly, suggesting a generalized disturbance of cholesterol metabolism, unexplained by nutritional status. Evaluation of the relation among hematic cell proliferation, degree of myeloid metaplasia, and hypocholesterolemia by multiple regression analysis revealed that splenic size was the variable of most significance in explaining the variation in plasma total, LDL, and HDL cholesterol levels. Uncontrolled disease activity was accompanied by a decline in LDL cholesterol levels. Splenectomy or control of proliferation with chemotherapy or splenic irradiation reversed this abnormality. Thus, levels of plasma total and lipoprotein cholesterol provide information that may be of value in diagnosis and assessment of myeloproliferative disease activity.

SERUM LIPID AND LIPOPROTEIN CONCENTRATIONS IN QUADRIPLEGIC AND RENAL TRANSPLANT PATIENTS

There is a direct relation between low serum level of HDL cholesterol and morbidity due to CAD. The HDL cholesterol fraction has a protective effect against CAD, possibly due to its ability to remove cholesterol from peripheral tissues and to inhibit the uptake of LDL by cells. Physical activity is one factor known to affect serum HDL cholesterol levels. The opposite of physical activity, of course, is represented by the quadriplegic patient. Heldenberg and associates[23] from Tel Aviv, Israel, investigated serum lipids and lipoproteins in 10 young quadriplegic comatose males who had been injured in automobile accidents. All had been in good health before the accident. Their ages ranged from 15–31 years (mean, 21) and the mean duration of coma ranged from 3–60 months (mean, 22). They were all intermittently fed, via a nasogastric tube, an identical formula providing 2,900 calories/day, with a polyunsaturated/saturated fatty acids ratio of 1.1:1. Their mean body weight was 70% of ideal body weight. The results were compared with those from a control group consisting of 10 healthy male students and personnel who volunteered; their ages ranged from 20–35 years (mean, 25). No control subject habitually participated in vigorous physical activity or sports. The diet of this group provided 2,600 calories/day and the ratio of polyunsaturated/saturated fatty acids was 0.9:1. Their mean body weight was 95% of ideal body weight. The HDL cholesterol was significantly lower in the quadriplegic patients, as compared with the control group. The mean LDL cholesterol in the 10 patients was 151 mg/dl and 130 mg/dl in the controls. The mean HDL cholesterol was 40 mg/dl in the patients and 62 mg/dl in the 10 controls. Total serum cholesterol values in both groups were identical (205 mg/dl), as were the triglyceride values (69 mg/dl). These data suggest that quadriplegic patients may have an increased tendency to develop atherosclerosis.

In contrast to the diminished level of HDL in quadriplegic patients, Somer and associates[24] from Little Bay, Australia, found increased HDL cholesterol levels and triglyceride levels in renal transplant recipients. These authors also found that the pre-transplant type of renal disease and the sex of transplant recipient also affected their serum lipid levels.

SERUM TRIGLYCERIDES AS A RISK FACTOR TO PREMATURE CAD

In 1980, Hulley and associates (*N Engl J Med* 302:1383, 1980), from a logistic analysis of a 8.5-year follow-up study, concluded that serum cholesterol was clearly an independent risk factor to CAD, but that serum triglyceride was not. Carlson and Bottiger[25] from Stockholm, Sweden, from data collected in their Stockholm Prospective Study (SPS) concluded the opposite, namely, that elevated serum triglyceride levels were a risk factor to premature CAD. Indeed, the SPS study, which is nearly a 15-year follow-up study of 3,486 men, found plasma triglycerides but not plasma cholesterol to be an independent risk factor for CAD.

Morphologic studies

QUANTIFICATION OF CORONARY NARROWING IN TYPES II, III AND IV HYPERLIPOPROTEINEMIA AND IN KNOWN NORMAL LIPOPROTEIN PATTERNS

Surprisingly few morphologic studies on the coronary arteries of patients with known hyperlipoproteinemia (HLP) have been reported. A study by Roberts and associates in 1973 examined the number of 4 major coronary arteries narrowed 76%–100% in cross-sectional area by atherosclerotic plaques in 40 necropsy patients with type II or IV HLP or with normal lipoprotein patterns, 26 of whom had symptomatic CAD. That study, purely a quantitative one, showed no differences in the number of coronary arteries severely narrowed among the 3 groups of patients analyzed. Cabin and Roberts[26] from Bethesda, Maryland, extended the previous study by examining the entire lengths of each of the 4 major coronary arteries (an average of 26 cm per patient) in 38 necropsy patients with type II or IV HLP or with normal lipoprotein patterns, all of whom had symptomatic CAD. They determined the amount of cross-sectional area narrowing by atherosclerotic plaques in each 5 mm segment of the LM, LAD, LC, and right coronary arteries in 15 patients with type II, in 13 with type IV, and in 10 with known normal lipoprotein patterns. Of the 2,593 segments examined histologically, narrowing of 76%–100% in cross-sectional area was as follows: type II, 39%; type IV, 67%; normal lipoprotein pattern, 35% (controls, 4%) (Fig. 1-6). Utilizing a scoring system of 1–4 for the 4 categories of narrowing (0%–25%; 26%–50%; 51%–75%; 76%–100%), the mean score per 5 mm segment for the patients with type IV HLP was significantly higher (3.5) than that for the patients with type II HLP (3.0), normal lipoprotein patterns (3.0), and the controls (2.3). Thus, the patients with type II HLP and those with normal lipoprotein patterns had similar amounts of severe coronary narrowing and significantly less severe coronary narrowing than the patients with type IV HLP.

Although type III HLP has been recognized to predispose to premature atherosclerosis, no systemic analysis of the status of epicardial coronary arteries in this relatively rare form of HLP has been described. Cabin and associates[27] from Bethesda, Maryland, determined the amount of cross-sectional area narrowing in each 5 mm segment of each of the 4 major epicardial coronary arteries in each of 5 patients with type III HLP and symptomatic, fatal atherosclerotic CAD. Four had angina pectoris; 2 had AMI that healed, and 2 died suddenly. Of the 4 major epicardial coronary arteries, all 4 were nar-

Fig. 1-6.   Mean percent of 5 mm segments of right, LAD, and LC coronary arteries narrowed 76%–100% in cross-sectional area by atherosclerotic plaques in proximal and distal halves of each artery in 15 patients with type II HLP, 13 with type IV HLP, and 10 with normal lipoprotein patterns and symptomatic CAD. Reproduced with permission from Cabin and Roberts.[26]

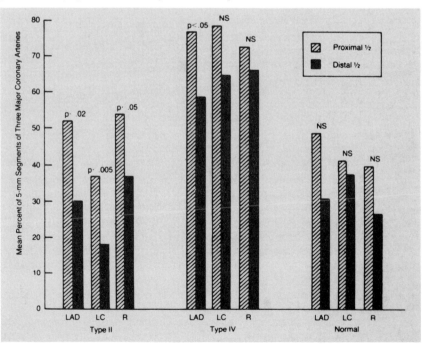

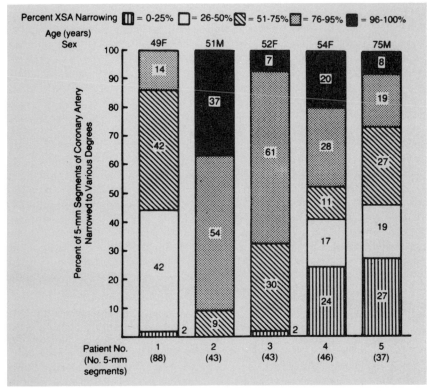

Fig. 1-7. Percent of 5 mm segments of the 4 major epicardial coronary arteries with 5 categories of cross-sectional area (XSA) narrowing by atherosclerotic plaques in each of 5 patients with type III hyperlipoproteinemia. Reproduced with permission from Cabin and Roberts.[26]

rowed 76%–100% in cross-sectional area by atherosclerotic plaques in 2 patients, 3 were narrowed to this degree in 2 patients, and 2 were so narrowed in 1 patient. Three patients had severe narrowing of the LM coronary artery. The percent of 5 mm segments of coronary artery narrowed to various degrees was as follows: 96%–100%, 0–37 (mean, 14); 76%–95%, 14–61 (mean, 35); 51%–75%, 9–41 (mean, 24); 26%–50%, 0–42 (mean, 16), and 0%–25%, 0–27 (mean, 11) (Fig. 1-7). Utilizing a scoring system of 1–4 for the 4 categories of narrowing, scores per 5 mm segment for each patient ranged from 2.5–3.9 (mean, 3.1). Thus, these 5 type III HLP patients had severe diffuse coronary narrowing by atherosclerotic plaques.

Diet and cholesterol

The effect of dietary saturated and polyunsaturated fatty acids and cholesterol on levels of serum cholesterol in humans under controlled isocaloric conditions has been well established through elaboration from cross-cultural comparisons, diet-intervention programs, investigations of subcultural groups with special dietary practices, and studies in non-humans. Several epidemiologic investigations, however, have not found statistically significant correlations cross-sectionally between these nutritional variables and serum cholesterol in individual persons. Some investigators have interpreted this lack of correlation to mean that diet has a lesser role in determining the serum cholesterol level in persons eating freely than is suggested by studies conducted in metabolic wards. This lack of correlation also has been used as a reason for not recommending reduction in dietary cholesterol to adults in the general population. Failure to observe the expected correlations, however, could have been due to methodologic problems, e.g., large intraindividual variation from day to day in lipid composition of the diet, relatively small, stable differences in diet between individual members of a population as compared with cross-cultural differences, inaccuracies in the procedures for measuring diet in populations eating freely, nondietary factors that affect serum cholesterol levels, and selective changes in diet among persons after they have learned that they have hypercholesterolemia.

Shekelle and associates[28] from Chicago, Illinois, investigated the associations of dietary saturated and polyunsaturated fatty acids and cholesterol with serum cholesterol level and risk of death from CAD among participants in the Western Electric Study, selected in 1957 through random sampling of 5,397 men aged 40–55 years. The distributions of serum cholesterol concentration, body mass index, and the dietary variables in the 1,900 middle-aged men examined were similar at the initial examination and at the second examination 1 year later, except that the mean values for energy intake, saturated fatty acids, dietary cholesterol, both dietary scores, and serum cholesterol level were slightly lower (down 3.3%–4.7% from the mean value at initial examination) and the mean value for polyunsaturated fatty acids was slightly higher (up 2.6%). The dietary data collected at the first 2 examinations were averaged for each participant to provide baseline estimates for intake of saturated and polyunsaturated fatty acids and dietary cholesterol, individually and as summarized by the formulas of Keys and Hegsted. The risk of death from CAD during the next 19 years was positively related to the baseline levels of both dietary scores after adjustment for age, body-mass index, systolic BP, cigarette smoking, serum cholesterol, monthly alcohol intake, and 3 other variables. When the risk of death from CAD was analyzed in terms of the component dietary variables, it was inversely related to intake of polyunsaturated fatty acids and positively related to intake of dietary cholesterol. The amount of saturated fatty acids in the diet was not significantly associated with the risk of death from CAD. Other baseline variables significantly related to risk of death from CAD in this multivariate analysis were age, systolic BP, cigarette smoking, and serum cholesterol concentration. This analysis also indicated that the dietary variables were not significantly related to risk of death from competing causes in 2 broad categories: from all types of cancer and from all other causes grouped together. These results support the conclusion that lipid composition of the diet affects serum cholesterol concentration and risk of CAD in middle-aged American men.

The 10-year experience in the 7 Countries Study amplified the 5-year finding that the 16 cohorts of men aged 40–59 at entry differed strikingly in mortality from CAD. This ranged from 1 CAD death in 686 men on the island of Crete to 78 among 817 men in east Finland. No significant part of that variability among the cohorts was explained by age, relative body weight, body fatness (skinfold thickness), cigarette smoking habits, or habitual physical activity, although some variables were important when individuals within cohorts were compared. Mean values for serum cholesterol and arterial BP accounted for two-thirds of the variance of CAD mortality. The average level of serum cholesterol of the cohorts correlated with the average percentage of calories from saturated fatty acids in the diet, and the 10-year CAD death rate correlated highly with the average percentage of diet calories from saturated fatty acids.

In evaluating the importance of fats in the diet, it is necessary to consider the all-causes death rate and the other fatty acids in the diet. Thus, Keys and associates[29] from Minneapolis, Minnesota, analyzed 1,512 patients who died in 10 years among 12,763 men aged 0−59 years at entry. Of the 1,512 deaths, 413 were from CAD. The 16 cohorts differed in all-causes as well as in CAD death rate. Those differences were not related to cohort differences in age, relative weight, activity, cigarette smoking habits, or percent calories from total proteins or fats in the diet, but were related to differences in BP, serum cholesterol, and percentage calories from saturated fatty acids. The correlation with saturates was $r = 0.47$ for all-causes, $r = 0.84$ for CAD death rate. The all-causes death rate was correlated with saturates even when other dietary variables were controlled in multiple regression. Noncoronary death rate was not significantly related to the diet. Both mean BP and serum cholesterol correlated with diet saturates, but the correlation of BP with saturates was explained by intercorrelation between BP and cholesterol. The findings do not prove that saturates in the diet cause increased mortality, but they are consistent with the hypothesis that risk of early death is increased by diet saturates in populations in which CAD is a major cause of death. There is no support for the suggestion that the advantage for CAD of a diet restricted in saturated fats may be offset by increased non-CAD mortality.

It is known that the mean level of plasma cholesterol is low and the ratio of total to HDL cholesterol is low in vegetarian groups living in industrialized societies. Surprisingly few data are available on the relation of meat ingestion to plasma lipid levels and BP levels. Sacks and associates[30] of Boston, Massachusetts, studied 21 strict vegetarians prospectively for 8 weeks: a 2-week control period of the usual vegetarian diet, followed by 4 weeks during which 250 g beef was added isocalorically to the daily vegetarian diet, and then by 2 weeks of the control diet. Plasma HDL cholesterol did not change during the study, whereas plasma total cholesterol rose significantly by 19% at the end of the meat-eating period. Systolic BP increased significantly during the meat eating by 3% over control values, whereas diastolic BP showed no major changes. Plasma renin activity, prostaglandin A and E levels, and urinary kallikrein, norepinephrine, and epinephrine were within normal limits and did not change notably throughout the trial. This study demonstrates an adverse effect of consumption of beef on plasma lipid and BP levels.

Familial hypercholesterolemia

TREATMENT WITH COLESTIPOL AND WITH NIACIN OR CLOFIBRATE

In persons with familial hypercholesterolemia (FH), an autosomal-dominant disorder in which levels of LDL are 2 to 3 times normal and high affinity receptors for LDL on cell membranes are deficient, the risk of CAD is 5 times that in the normolipidemic population. Persons with heterozygous FH can be distinguished from those with other states having elevated levels of LDL by their very high levels of serum cholesterol (300–500 mg/dl), relative resistance to dietary influences, high penetrance (approximately 50% of first-degree relatives are affected), and the frequent occurrence of tendinous xanthomas. Although LDL is believed to be the immediate causative agent in the development of atheromas, this hypothesis has not been tested because of inability of drugs to normalize circulating LDL levels. Thus far, perhaps, the

Fig. 1-8.   Effect on serum lipids of addition of clofibrate (2.0 g per day) to regimen of diet and colestipol (30 g per day) in 18 patients with heterozygous familial hypercholesterolemia. In each panel, points at left denote means of 3 monthly levels with diet alone, points in center denote means of 12 monthly measurements with both diet and colestipol (20 g per day), and points at right the means of 12 monthly measurements with diet, colestipol (30 g per day), and clofibrate. Circles and broken lines denote women, squares and solid lines men, and figures at bottom means ± SD. To convert milligrams of cholesterol per deciliter to millimoles per liter, multiply by 0.02586; to convert milligrams of triglycerides per deciliter to grams per liter, multiply by 0.01. Reproduced with permission from Kane et al.[31]

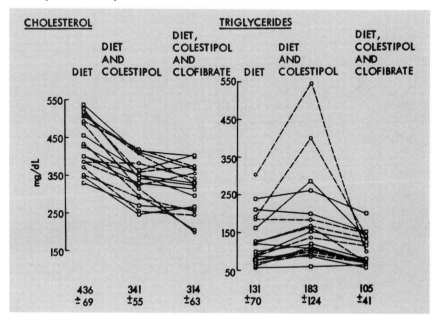

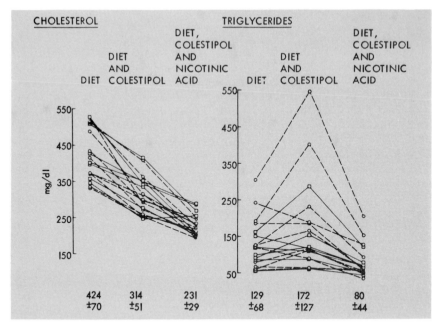

Fig. 1-9. Effect on serum lipids of the addition of niacin (nicotinic acid) to regimen of diet and colestipol in 18 patients. In each panel, points at left denote means of 3 monthly measurements with diet alone, points in center the means of 12 monthly measurements with both diet and 20 g colestipol per day, and points at right the means of monthly measurements with diet, 30 g colestipol per day, and up to 7.5 g nicotinic acid per day. Circles and broken lines denote women, squares and solid lines men, and figures at bottom means ± SD. To convert milligrams of cholesterol per deciliter to millimoles per liter, multiply by 0.02586; to convert milligrams of triglycerides per deciliter to grams per liter, multiply by 0.01. Reproduced with permission from Kane et al.[31]

most effective treatments have been partial ileal bypass and the combination of neomycin and cholestyramine, which reduced serum cholesterol levels by 33% and 38%, respectively. Kane and associates[31] from San Francisco, California, evaluated the effectiveness of a bile acid-binding resin, colestipol, in 50 patients who met rigorous clinical criteria for heterozygous FH and compared the effects of 2 combinations: colestipol with clofibrate (Fig. 1-8) and colestipol with niacin (Fig. 1-9). Complete and sustained normalization of LDL levels occurred in patients receiving the combination of colestipol and niacin and, additionally, the size of the tendinous xanthomas decreased. With colestipol alone, the mean total cholesterol levels in serum decreased 16%–25%. The addition of clofibrate produced a total mean decrease of only 28%. In contrast, serum cholesterol levels fell 45% when colestipol was combined with niacin. LDL cholesterol decreased 55% with colestipol and niacin, whereas HDL cholesterol increased. Thus, colestipol plus niacin is useful in treatment of patients with high levels of LDL.

TREATMENT WITH 3-HYDROXY-3 METHYLGLUTARYL COENZYME A
REDUCTASE (ML-236B)

Mabuchi and associates[32] from Kanazawa, Japan, studied the effects of
ML-236B, a competitive inhibitor of 3-hydroxy-3-methylglutaryl coenzyme A
(HMG-CoA) reductase, on serum levels of lipoproteins and ubiquinone-10 in
7 heterozygous patients with familial hypercholesterolemia (FH). ML-236B
was given at doses of 30–60 mg per day for 24 weeks. Serum cholesterol decreased from 390 ± 9 to 303 ± 8 mg/dl (10.1 ± 0.2 to 7.88 ± 0.2
mmol/liter, $p < 0.001$), and serum triglyceride decreased from 137 ± 18 to
87 ± 9 mg/dl (1.55 ± 0.2 to 0.98 ± 0.1 mmol/liter; $p < 0.05$) (Fig. 1-10).
Intermediate density lipoprotein (IDL) cholesterol, IDL triglyceride, LDL
cholesterol, and LDL triglyceride decreased significantly ($p < 0.01$,
$p < 0.02$, $p < 0.001$, and $p < 0.001$, respectively). No significant changes
occurred in VLDL cholesterol and triglyceride or HDL cholesterol. Serum ubi-
quinone-10 levels did not change, and LDL levels of ubiquinone-10 decreased
by 50% (0.39 ± 0.07 to 0.20 ± 0.01 μg/ml [$p < 0.05$]). No adverse effects
were observed. The authors concluded that ML-236B is effective in lowering
serum cholesterol without lowering serum ubiquinone-10 in heterozygous
patients with FH.

Fig. 1-10.   Effects of ML-236B on serum cholesterol (panel A) and triglyceride (panel B) levels
in heterozygous patients with familial hypercholesterolemia. To convert cholesterol and triglyceride values to millimoles per liter, multiply by 0.026 and 0.01129, respectively. Reproduced
with permission from Mabuchi et al.[32]

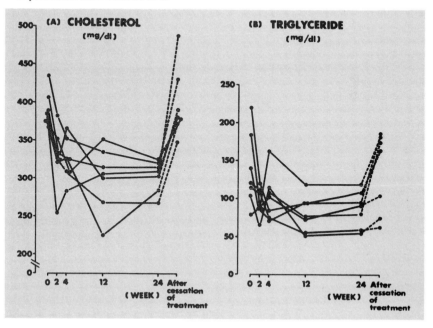

The authors used extremely low doses of ML-236B (compactin), <10% the amount used in previous dog studies. Yet they observed a dramatic 29% reduction in plasma LDL levels without change in plasma HDL levels. The important lesson from this study and from previous experience with compactin, mevinolin, and bile acid-binding resins is that normal regulatory mechanisms can be exploited to lower plasma LDL. The liver responds to cholesterol deprivation by increasing LDL receptors. Therefore, plasma LDL levels fall, but cholesterol delivery continues and crucial body stores of cholesterol are not depleted. In view of previous experience with animals and human beings, it seems likely that the fall in plasma LDL will delay the development of atherosclerosis. The availability of compactin would allow direct tests of this hypothesis. In addition to helping patients with FH, compactin may offer hope to large numbers of patients whose plasma LDL levels are in the upper range for the population and who are predisposed to atherosclerosis, yet do not have FH. Even though such persons eat a high cholesterol diet, their bodies still synthesize 3 times more cholesterol than is absorbed from the intestine. Inhibition of cholesterol synthesis with compactin, with or without a bile acid-binding resin, should stimulate the production of LDL receptors and reduce LDL levels of such patients despite continued consumption of a diet rich in cholesterol.

TREATMENT WITH PLASMA EXCHANGE

It has been almost 10 years since Turnberg and associates successfully treated the xanthomatous neuropathy of a patient with primary biliary cirrhosis by using a cell separator to exchange her plasma with fresh frozen plasma at monthly intervals. Since then, several reports have appeared of other hypercholesterolemic patients treated with plasma exchange. The commonest disorder for which plasma exchange has been used is homozygous familial hypercholesterolemia (FH), followed in frequency by heterozygous FH and, least often, primary biliary cirrhosis. Deposition of cholesterol in tissues is common to all 3 forms of hypercholesterolemia; the object of plasma exchange is, of course, to oppose this trend by repeated removal of lipoproteins from plasma, thus creating a reverse gradient of cholesterol between the extravascular and intravascular compartments. Thompson[33] from London, England, did repeated plasma exchange with a cell separator at weekly to monthly intervals for periods of up to 5 years in 22 patients with severe hypercholesterolemia: 20 with familial hypercholesterolemia (11 homozygotes and 9 heterozygotes), and 2 with primary biliary cirrhosis. The overall results were good, suggesting that exchanging plasma with 2–4 liters of plasma protein fraction at intervals of 1–2 weeks can safely and effectively control hypercholesterolemia in such patients, induce regression of xanthomata, and arrest or retard progression of atherosclerosis.

In 1979 Stoffel and associates demonstrated that apolipoprotein-B-containing lipoproteins (LDL and VLDL) could be removed specifically and efficiently in vitro and in vivo from pig blood by a combination of extracorporeal plasma separation and LDL immunoadsorption. Stoffel and associates[34] applied this technique to 3 patients with FH. The technique consisted of separation of plasma from the blood cells by a blood separation centrifuge, followed by the selective adsorption of LDL from the plasma on anti-LDL "Sepharose." The LDL-free plasma effluent, from which HDL and other plasma proteins were not removed, was returned to the patient with the blood cells. Their 3 patients were treated repeatedly during a 9-month period. No undesirable side effects or changes in clinical, chemical, hematological, or immunological parameters were observed. The new procedure is noninvasive, more specific, and less costly and lowers LDL to greater degrees than do previous treatments of FH.

TREATMENT WITH ILEAL BYPASS

Spengel and associates[35] from London, England, studied LDL turnover on 3 occasions in each of 6 patients with heterozygous familial hypercholesterolemia—on diet, after 1 month on cholestyramine (16 g/day), and 2 months after partial ileal bypass. Partial ileal bypass lowered total and LDL cholesterol levels and increased the fractional catabolic rate of LDL to a greater extent than did cholestyramine; this difference presumably reflects the greater increase in bile acid excretion induced by the surgical procedure. Studies in 2 other heterozygotes showed that partial ileal bypass specifically enhanced receptor-mediated catabolism of LDL. The findings support the concept that therapeutic stimulation of bile acid synthesis increases the rate of receptor-mediated uptake and degradation of LDL by the liver.

High density lipoproteins

RELATION TO CAD

An elevated serum level of LDL is a risk factor, of course, for the development of CAD, whereas elevated levels of HDL appear to have a protective effect. Determination of the total cholesterol to HDL ratio has been suggested as an improved method for assessing risk. Swanson and associates[36] from Minneapolis, Minnesota, determined cholesterol, HDL, and triglycerides in 189 patients undergoing diagnostic cardiac catheterization because of suspected CAD and they assessed the severity of the CAD by the number of major coronary arteries narrowed, equal to, or >70% in diameter. HDL was higher in the group with no vessels narrowed (54 ± 2.3 mg/dl) than in those with 1, 2, or 3 arteries narrowed (43 ± 2, 43 ± 2 and 51 ± 1 mg/dl, respectively), and the cholesterol to HDL ratio was lower in the group with no vessels narrowed (4.1 ± 0.2, as compared with 6.1 ± 0.3, 5.7 ± 0.2, and 6.4 ± 0.3 in the groups with 1, 2, and 3 vessels narrowed). As determined by analysis of variance, patients with no vessels narrowed differed from those with CAD in HDL ($p < 0.005$), triglycerides ($p < 0.01$), cholesterol ($p < 0.005$), and cholesterol to HDL ($p < 0.005$), but no significant differences were found between patients with CAD and a different number of arteries narrowed. There were no significant differences between the groups in age, and although the group with no vessel disease contained more females than did the others, there were no differences in cholesterol, HDL, cholesterol to HDL ratio, or triglycerides between male and female patients without CAD. Thus, the cholesterol to HDL ratio correlates with the presence of, but not with the severity of, CAD.

The well-established inverse relation of HDL cholesterol and the risk of CAD was tested by Uhl and associates[37] from Brooks Air Force Base, Texas, in a cross-sectional group of 572 asymptomatic aircrew members who were being screened for risk of CAD. Tests performed included determinations of fasting serum cholesterol, HDL cholesterol and triglycerides, and performance of a maximal symptom-limited exercise tolerance test. Of the 572 patients, 132 also had an abnormal ST-segment response to exercise testing or were otherwise believed to have an increased risk of organic heart disease and subsequently underwent coronary angiography. Significant CAD was found in 16 men and minimal or subcritical CAD was found in 14; coronary angiograms were normal in the remaining 102 men. The remaining 440 men, who were believed to have a 1% chance of having CAD by sequential testing of risk factors and treadmill testing, had a mean cholesterol level of 213 mg/dl, a mean HDL cholesterol of 51 mg/dl, and a mean cholesterol/HDL ratio of 4.4. The mean values for cholesterol, HDL cholesterol, and cholesterol/HDL cholesterol did not differ significantly in men with normal angiographic findings and those with subcritical CAD. However, 14 of 16 men with CAD had a cholesterol/HDL ratio ≥ 6.0, whereas only 4 men with normal coronary arteries had a ratio of 6.0 or more. Of the classic coronary risk factors evaluated, the cholesterol/HDL ratio of 6.0 or more had the highest odds ratio (172:1). Determination of HDL cholesterol level appears to help identify asymptomatic persons with a greater risk of having CAD.

RELATION TO PLASMA TESTOSTERONE AND OTHER LIPOPROTEIN FRACTIONS

HDL cholesterol levels are strongly related to risk of CAD. Identification of determinants of HDL cholesterol may provide important information concerning the cause of CAD. The relation between 1 possible determinant, testosterone, and HDL cholesterol and other lipoprotein fractions was evaluated in 247 middle-aged men by Gutai and associates[38] from Pittsburgh, Pennsylvania. They found that levels of testosterone (both free and total) correlated positively with HDL cholesterol and negatively with triglycerides and VLDL cholesterol. The association between testosterone and HDL cholesterol could not be explained by intake of alcohol, obesity, age, smoking, or physical activity. Furthermore, the relation of testosterone to HDL cholesterol was independent of the relation of testosterone to VLDL cholesterol or triglycerides.

RELATION TO GALLBLADDER DISEASE

Petitti and associates[39] from Oakland, California, found 65 women (7.5%) among 868 adult female twins examined with a history of gallbladder disease. The percentage with gallbladder disease decreased with an increasing concentration of HDL cholesterol; in contrast, the percentage increased with increasing concentrations of LDL cholesterol, VLDL cholesterol, total cholesterol, and triglyceride. Additionally, the concentration of HDL cholesterol, the Quetelet index of obesity, age, cigarette smoking, and estrogen use were significantly related to a history of gallbladder disease after controlling for all other variables. The relative risk of gallbladder disease increased with increasing age, increasing Quetelet index, current cigarette smoking and estrogen use, whereas the relative risk of gallbladder disease decreased with an increasing concentration of HDL cholesterol.

RELATION TO ALCOHOLISM

In 26 male alcoholics, Devenyi and associates[40] from Toronto, Canada, demonstrated that a subgroup without severe hepatic disease had significantly elevated HDL cholesterol in the immediate post-intoxication period. HDL levels decreased to control levels after 1–2 weeks of abstinence. Those patients with advanced hepatic disease did not have this ethanol-induced rise in HDL. Thus, ethanol consumption in alcoholics is associated with an increase in HDL levels that is offset by the development of alcoholic liver disease.

RELATION TO WEIGHT REDUCTION IN OBESITY

Brownell and Stunkard[41] from Philadelphia, Pennsylvania, measured levels of HDL cholesterol and other lipoproteins in 73 obese men and women before and after a 16-week weight reduction program. There were significant differences between men and women. Men, with a mean 11 kg weight loss, had a 5% increase in HDL, a 16% decrease in LDL, and a 30% decrease in HDL:LDL ratio. Women, with a mean 9 kg weight loss, had a 3% decrease in HDL, a 5% decrease in LDL, and no change in HDL:LDL ratio. These differences suggest that weight reduction may be an important means of improving plasma lipoprotein patterns in men, but of more limited value in women.

RELATION TO EXERCISE TRAINING IN CAD PATIENTS

Studies evaluating the effect of exercise training on HDL cholesterol in healthy men have yielded conflicting results. Therefore, Hartung and associates[42] from Houston, Texas, determined the effect of endurance exercise training on HDL cholesterol in 18 male CAD patients in whom the mean HDL cholesterol was normal before study. The chronic exercise training program consisted of aerobic activities utilizing approximately 70% of maximum oxygen uptake (VO_2max) for 20–40 min 3 times weekly for 3 months. Significant increases in the VO_2max HDL cholesterol/total cholesterol ratio, and a decrease in percent body fat were documented after exercise training. No significant changes were found in total cholesterol, triglycerides, body weight, or LDL cholesterol. Thus, vigorous physical training can contribute to increases in HDL cholesterol in CAD patients without changes in total cholesterol or body weight.

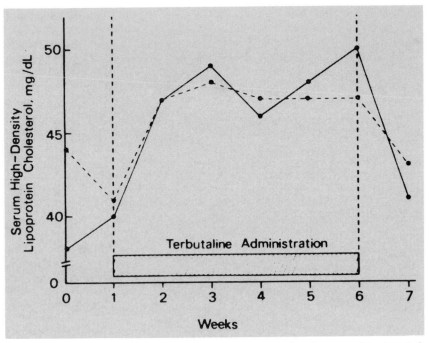

Fig. 1-11. Serial HDL-cholesterol levels in 2 subjects receiving terbutaline over a 5-week period. To convert values to millimoles per liter, multiply by 0.02586. Reproduced with permission from Hooper et al.[43]

EFFECT OF TERBUTALINE

High levels of HDL are associated with a low risk of CAD and low levels with a high risk. HDL appears to be the cholesterol "scavenger" of the body: it removes cholesterol from cells and carries it to the liver for excretion. Because factors associated with protection from CAD (exercise, alcohol consumption, estrogen, thinness, and genetics) are also associated with high HDL-cholesterol levels, it has been proposed that elevated serum HDL, particularly the HDL-2 subfraction, may bring about the protection. In fact, HDL has been called the "antiatherogenic lipoprotein." Although modulation of HDL levels appears to be linked to the turnover of LDL and VLDL, exactly what modulates HDL levels is unknown. It is known that beta adrenergic blockers (e.g., propranolol, metoprolol, atenolol, and sotalol) lower HDL levels. Hooper and associates[43] from Albuquerque, New Mexico, demonstrated that the HDL-cholesterol concentration rose after 2 weeks of terbutaline administration in 15 subjects. After 1 week of terbutaline administration, the HDL concentration had increased significantly and, by the second week, it had risen 10% from the baseline value (Fig. 1-11). One week after terbutaline administration was stopped, HDL-cholesterol values returned to near baseline values. Total cholesterol, triglyceride, and LDL-cholesterol levels did not change significantly throughout the study. Thus, terbutaline, a beta adrenergic agonist, is associated with a significant rise in HDL-cholesterol values. The magnitude of the increase is comparable to that of the rise in HDL cholesterol seen in men who have joined a cardiac rehabilitation program. The mechanism of this rise is unclear.

MISCELLANEOUS RISK FACTORS

Cigarette smoking

Kannel[44] from Framingham, Massachusetts, reviewed the evidence incriminating cigarette smoking in the development of atherosclerosis in general and of CAD in particular as determined from the 20-year follow-up of men and women aged 45–74 years in the Framingham Study. Heavy smoking almost doubled cardiovascular and overall mortality under age 65 years, but beyond age 65 neither a significant nor a substantial gradient could be demonstrated in either sex for cardiovascular mortality. Sudden death was strongly related to cigarette smoking. The proportion of CAD deaths that are sudden increased progressively with the number of cigarettes smoked daily. Not only were cardiovascular events likely to terminate fatally more often in cigarette smokers, but such attacks occurred more commonly than in nonsmokers. Atherosclerotic cardiovascular disease incidents in general and each of its clinical manifestations were related to cigarette smoking. A significant excess of cigarette smokers was found in patients with severe diabetic retinopathy with proliferative changes. In women taking oral contraceptives containing estrogen, cigarette smoking predisposed to cardiovascular disease. Thus, cigarette smoking is particularly hazardous in women over age 35 who have been using oral contraceptives for extended periods. Women who smoked were at increased risk of thromboembolic disease and this risk increased considerably if they also took estrogens.

The exact mechanism whereby cigarette smoking produces cardiac disease is unclear, but several mechanisms seem reasonable. Cigarette smoking transiently increases the adhesiveness of platelets, accelerates the heart rate, and makes the myocardium more vulnerable to ventricular fibrillation. At the same time, oxygen-carrying capacity of the blood is reduced because of the buildup of carboxyhemoglobin and tissue utilization of oxygen is impaired at the myoglobin level. When these effects, plus acute rises in catecholamines and fatty acids, are provoked 20 or more times a day with each inhaled cigarette, it is little wonder that eventually AMI or sudden coronary death is precipitated in smokers with narrowed coronary arteries. In addition to these acute effects, there also may be a long-term chronic atherogenic effect of cigarette smoking.

The major epidemiologic prospective studies not only point to increasing CAD death rates as the amount of cigarette smoking increases but also have shown that those who stopped smoking achieve lower death rates than those who continue to smoke. The exact amount of time required for the CAD mortality rate to return to that of the nonsmoker after cessation of smoking is unclear, but it is possible that 5–10 years of nonsmoking may be required to achieve the same CAD mortality rate as for the never-smoker. Of the 3 major cardiovascular risk factors, cigarette smoking is so powerful a contributor, so highly prevalent, and so potentially correctable that it deserves the highest priority among preventive measures to control cardiovascular disease.

The health benefits of quitting cigarette smoking have usually been inferred from the differences in morbidity and mortality experienced by smokers and ex-smokers. When formal observation of these groups begins, the ex-smokers have quit smoking at various times in the past; thus, it is not usually possible to assess their health-related characteristics at a time when they were smoking. Consequently, it is difficult to be certain that quitting itself and not some other difference or differences between quitters and persistent smokers has been responsible for the apparently better health outcome. Friedman and associates[45] from Oakland, California, compared mortality rates of quitters and persistent cigarette smokers according to major cause of death, with a detailed analysis of death from CAD. After adjustment for major baseline differences in risk characteristics, the relative risk of dying from CAD among persistent smokers was 2.2 times that among quitters. Thus, the apparent benefits of quitting cigarette smoking in reducing mortality from CAD are not attributable to differences in baseline risk status. After a similar adjustment, the risk of death from any cause in the persistent smokers was 1.6 times that in the quitters.

McNamara[46] from Houston, Texas, described in detail how he stopped smoking after receiving advice from T. Joseph Reeves. The method essentially consisted of gradually diminishing the intake of tar per cigarette over a period of several months. As shown in Table 1-1, a carton of cigarettes was smoked, beginning with cigarettes containing either 23 mg tar per cigarette or the level in cigarettes presently smoked, if <23 mg, and going on to 5 more cartons of cigarettes, representing successive phases. If the initial carton contained cigarettes in phase I (23 mg/cigarette), subsequent cartons of cigarettes should contain 16, 8, 5, 4, and finally 3 mg tar per cigarette. If the smoker is already smoking cigarettes containing <23 mg tar/cigarette, fewer phases will be required to reach the goal. The smoker should never backtrack. McNamara presents this method of Reeves in an entertaining and scientific fashion. Because there are 200 cigarettes per carton, the method required smoking 1,200 cigarettes to complete, but the method of Reeves is hardly recommended by McNamara. As far as cardiovascular health is concerned, controlling BP, lowering of cholesterol level, and abstinence from cigarette smoking are essential.

Castelli and associates[47] from Framingham, Massachusetts, tested the hypothesis that those who smoke filter cigarettes are less likely to get clinical manifestations of CAD than those who smoke non-filter cigarettes. Men were classified at the seventh biennial examination (1963–64) according to whether they smoked filter or non-filter cigarettes. Of the cigarette-smoking men under age 55 years at this examination, 58% smoked filter cigarettes; these men had slightly lower prior smoking exposure than did smokers of

TABLE 1-1. *Phases I through X.*

PHASE	BRAND	TAR*/ CIGARETTE
I	Camel, Chesterfield (regular, unfiltered), Macho (regular, box)	23
II	Marlboro, Winston	16
III	Vantage, More, Golden Lights, Northwest King	8
IV	True, Vantage Ultra-lights, Doral II	5
V	Cambridge 100's (soft pack)	4
VI	Kent III, Triumph, Barclay 100's (soft pack), Lady Go-Diva-Go (box)	3
VII	Now 100's (soft pack), Super-Pacifier 100's	2
VIII	Cambridge 85's (soft pack), Barclay 80's (box), Barclay 85's (soft pack), Carlton 100's (box), Carlton 85's (soft pack), Now 85's (soft pack), All-Day-Sucker 120's (box)	1
IX	Cambridge 80's (box)	0.1
X	Now 80's (box), Carlton 80's (box)	<0.01

* The tar content of 187 brands of cigarettes can be found in the Federal Trade Commission "Report of Tar, Nicotine, Carbon Monoxide of the Smoke of 187 Varieties of Cigarettes," March 1981.

non-filter cigarettes. Despite what seemed to be a favorable cigarette-smoking history, the filter-cigarette smokers did not have lower CAD incidence rates than non-filter smokers. This finding was unchanged even after multivariate logistic regression analysis to adjust for the slight differences in age, systolic BP, and serum cholesterol levels between the 2 groups.

Wald and associates[48] from Oxford, England, studied serum levels of cotinine (a principal metabolite of nicotine) in 28 men who did not smoke, and in 276 men who smoked cigarettes only (150 men), cigars only (70 men) and pipes only (56 men). The mean cotinine level for pipe smokers was 389 ng/ml, significantly higher than the mean level for the cigarette and cigar smokers (306 and 121 ng/ml, respectively); no cotinine was detected in the serum from any non-smoker. Large prospective studies have shown that pipe smokers have no material excess risk of CAD, but cigarette smokers do, so that the authors' observations indicate that nicotine is unlikely to be the major cause of the excess CAD mortality in cigarette smokers.

Oral contraceptives and menopausal estrogen therapy

The introduction of oral contraceptives in 1960 has had a profound social, economic, religious, and political impact. The efficacy and ease of use of oral contraceptives has led to their widespread use throughout most of the world. It is estimated that 50–60 million women are current users of oral contraceptives and that 150 million women have used oral contraceptives at some time. In some western populations, it is estimated that up to 25% of all women of childbearing age use oral contraceptives. The safety of oral contraceptives has been a matter of medical and public concern since their introduction.

Dalen and Hickler[49] from Worcester, Massachusetts, examined the relation between oral contraceptive use and various thromboembolic complications, including AMI, pulmonary embolism, subarachnoid hemorrhage, thrombotic stroke, and systemic hypertension. These authors concluded that although the actual incidence of each of the cardiovascular complications of oral contraceptives is small, in their aggregate they assume major importance. The excess mortality attributable to oral contraceptives is about 20 per 100,000 users/year. In contrast, the total mortality of women of childbearing age per year is about 70 per 100,000. With 50 million women using oral contraceptives, the total excess mortality due to the use of oral contraceptives is estimated to be 10,000 deaths per year. These risks, therefore, far exceed the risks of childbirth, which are estimated to be 1/100,000 women of childbearing age per year. Most of the excess deaths attributable to oral contraceptives are due to cerebrovascular accidents and AMI. Most of these excess deaths occur in women over age 35, or in those who smoke or have systemic hypertension, and very likely these deaths could be prevented if oral contraceptives were not used by these women.

Stadel[50] from Bethesda, Maryland, reviewed the evidence that oral contraceptives cause an increased susceptibility to cardiovascular thrombosis and/or atherosclerosis. Most of the risk of serious, potentially fatal cardiovascular disease that is attributable to oral contraceptives is concentrated among women 35 years of age or older and among smokers. Among women who do not smoke cigarettes, the annual risk of death associated with current use of oral contraceptives increases from about 1/100,000 among women aged 15–19 years to about 3/100,000 among those aged 40–44. In women <35 years, these figures are one-fourth or less of the risk of death associated with complications of pregnancy among women using no method of contraception, and they are similar to the risk of death associated with current use of other methods of contraception. As age increases beyond 35, however, the risk of death associated with current use of oral contraceptives among nonsmokers begins to approach the risk of death associated with complications of pregnancy among women using no method of contraception (in women 35 years of age or older, this figure is about 21 deaths/100,000 women per year). It is considerably greater than the risk of death associated with current use of other methods of contraception (in women 35 or older, this figure is about 2–5 deaths/100,000 users per year, regardless of smoking habit).

Among women who smoke cigarettes, the annual risk of death associated with current use of oral contraceptives increases from about 2/100,000 among women 15–19 years old to about 12/100,000 among women 30–34 and around 61/100,000 among women 40–44. In women <35, these figures are only somewhat lower than the risk of death associated with complications of pregnancy among women using no method of contraception, and they are considerably greater than the risk of death associated with current use of other methods (in women <35, this risk is about 1–3 deaths/100,000 users per year). Furthermore, as age increases beyond 35 years, the risk of death associated with current use of oral contraceptives among smokers increasingly exceeds the risk of death associated with complications of pregnancy among women using no method of contraception (about 21 deaths/100,000 women per year) and dramatically exceeds the risk of death associated with other methods (about 2–5 deaths/100,000 users per year).

Although the oral contraceptives that have been widely used in Great Britain, the USA, and similar countries over the past 2 decades appear to cause a substantial increase in the risk of cardiovascular disease among certain groups of women, it is probable that this risk can be reduced while the benefits of oral contraceptives can be retained. First, it seems clear that the risk of cardiovascular disease among current users is directly related to both the estrogen and progestogen content (at least for some progestogens) of the oral contraceptives being used. Thus, the increasing use of "very low dose" oral contraceptives (e.g., 0.5 mg norethindrone with 35 μg ethinyl estradiol) since the mid-1970s may already have begun to reduce the risk of cardiovascular disease that is attributable to oral contraceptives. Second, some evidence suggests that the effects of different oral contraceptive formulations on the risk of cardiovascular disease can be at least partially predicted by their effects on physiologic indicators of the risk of cardiovascular disease (such as antithrombin III activity, BP, and HDL cholesterol). It may be feasible to monitor these variables to identify individual users who seem more likely than others to develop cardiovascular disease as a consequence of oral contraceptive use, and to identify specific oral contraceptive formulations that seem less likely than others to increase the risk of cardiovascular disease.

Evidence that the risk of cardiovascular disease among users varies according to the progestogen and estrogen content of the oral contraceptives employed also suggests another possibility for future research: evaluation of the extent to which women vary in the absorption, distribution, and elimination of contraceptive steroids. If such variation is substantial, an oral contraceptive formulation that is appropriate for some women may be inappropriate for others, and it may, therefore, be desirable to develop procedures for titrating the steroid dosage to achieve similar plasma levels in women with different patterns of absorption, distribution, or elimination.

The use of unopposed estrogen therapy in postmenopausal women is known to increase the risk of endometrial carcinoma. Some evidence suggests that combined therapy with both estrogen and progestogen decreases this risk. Two main groups of progestogens have been used: derivatives of 19-nortestosterone that possess some androgenic activity; and alkylated or halogenated acetoxyprogesterone derivatives regarded as "pure" progestogens because they have neither estrogenic nor androgenic properties, e.g., medroxyprogesterone acetate. Estrogens increase HDL cholesterol and decrease LDL cholesterol, whereas androgens have the opposite effect. Treatment of hypercholesterolemic postmenopausal women with estradiol valerate (2 mg per day for 12 months) decreases the LDL cholesterol concentration by 22% and increases that of HDL cholesterol by 21%. Conversely, the ethisterone derivative danazol and the progestogen lynestrenol, which are used in the treatment of endometriosis, decrease HDL cholesterol by 30%–50%.

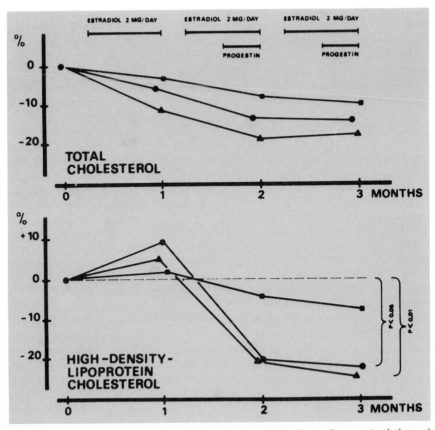

Fig. 1-12. Percentage of change in total cholesterol and high density lipoprotein cholesterol during treatment with estradiol valerate alone for 1 month and after addition of various progestins for 2 months. Solid circles denote group A, given norethindrone acetate; solid squares group B, given medroxyprogesterone acetate; and solid triangles group C, given norgestrel. Reproduced with permission from Hirvonen et al.[51]

Hirvonen and associates[51] from Helsinki, Finland, treated 3 groups of postmenopausal women (6 subjects each) for 3 weeks with estradiol valerate (2 mg per day) and continued the treatment with different sequential estradiol-progestogen regimens as follows (Fig. 1-12): group A received norethindrone acetate (10 mg per day) from day 15 to day 24 of the cycle; group B, medroxyprogesterone acetate (10 mg per day), and group C, norgestrel (0.5 mg per day). These regimens were followed for 2 consecutive cycles. Total cholesterol decreased in all groups by 10%–18% from the baseline values (p < 0.05). HDL cholesterol decreased by 20% from the baseline level during treatment with both the estradiol-norethindrone acetate (p < 0.05) and estradiol-norgestrel (p < 0.01) regimens, whereas estradiol with medroxyprogesterone acetate was not associated with a significant change in HDL cholesterol. These results suggest that the androgenic progestogens of the

19-nortestosterone series reverse the beneficial effect of postmenopausal estrogen treatment on HDL cholesterol, whereas the hydroxyprogesterone derivative medroxyprogesterone acetate has no such effect.

Heredity

CAD IN TWINS

Separating the relative importance of environmental and hereditary components in causation of CAD is obviously difficult. Study of twins affords an opportunity to isolate these components. Holmes and associates[52] from Rochester, Minnesota, described clinical courses and coronary arterial anatomy by angiogram in 2 monozygotic male twin pairs, both of whom had similarly located coronary narrowings. The patients had striking similarities also in clinical courses and in responses to exercise. In 1 twin pair, the onset of clinical evidence of myocardial ischemia occurred at 32 and 33 years, respectively; in the second twin pair, the onset of clinical evidence of myocardial ischemia was at 47 and 48 years, respectively. All 4 patients had type IV HLP. The twin pairs reported by Holmes and associates were identical, as shown by physical appearance, blood groups, and chromosomal polymorphisms. In each pair, the onset of symptoms occurred at nearly the same age and similar risk factors were present in each, including identical environment, smoking, and hyperlipidemia. Similarities in the baseline ECG and in exercise testing, specific workload, angina threshold, ECG changes, and rapid recovery were striking, reflecting similar cardiovascular responses to exercise and limitation by CAD. Similarities in coronary anatomy by coronary angiogram were striking within each pair (Figs. 1-13 and 1-14).

HLA TYPES IN PREMATURE CAD

The mechanism by which heredity exerts an influence on the incidence of CAD has been questioned for years. CAD often affects families, and it has

Fig. 1-13.   Schematic representation of coronary anatomy in first twin pair. *Left:* case 1. *Right:* case 2. Reproduced with permission from Holmes.[52]

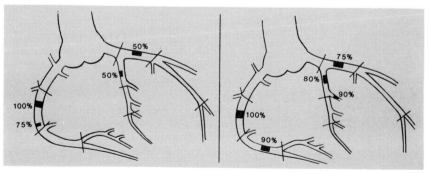

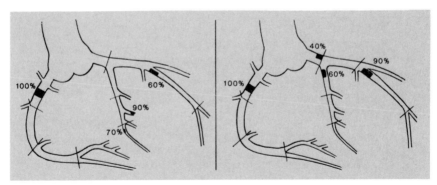

Fig. 1-14. Schematic representation of coronary anatomy in second twin pair. *Left:* case 3. *Right:* case 4. Reproduced with permission from Holmes.[52]

been reported that first-degree relatives of CAD patients have a 2–7-fold increase in the risk of CAD death. Yet this familial aggregation of CAD appears most frequently to be related to the familial aggregation of the known risk factors, such as hypercholesterolemia, systemic hypertension, diabetes mellitus, and obesity. The influence of independent genetic variables in the absence of coexisting known risk factors has not been previously investigated. In the Framingham study, for example, a family history of CAD was not considered an independent risk factor in the cardiovascular risk profile. The few studies investigating how genetic influences in the form of HLA tissue antigens relate to the presence of CAD have not indicated a clear association.

Stone and associates[53] from San Francisco, California, investigated whether isolated genetic factors, controlled by genes in the HLA chromosomal region, could be indicted as independent contributing influences in the genesis of premature CAD. Nineteen patients with fixed obstructive CAD documented by coronary angiography had no CAD risk factors with respect to age, levels of serum cholesterol, fasting triglycerides, and blood glucose, BP, obesity, history of diabetes mellitus or systemic hypertension, and cigarette-smoking history. Sixteen patients had a family history of CAD. HLA typing was restricted to antigens of the A and B loci. Control subjects (n, 1,157) were normal. At the A locus, no antigens demonstrated an observed frequency significantly higher than that expected from the control population. At the B locus, BW 38 had a statistically significant greater frequency (p < 0.01) in the study group with CAD (21%) than in the control population (4%). The association between BW 38 and premature CAD lost its statistical significance when conservatively corrected for the number of HLA antigens tested by the Bonferroni adjustment. The relative risk for CAD if a patient had antigen BW 38 was 6.2. These data suggest a trend toward significance in the relationship of HLA BW 38 and premature CAD. Whether the HLA tissue antigens are involved directly in the pathogenesis of CAD, act as markers for immune response genes, or serve as markers of other, yet undefined, genetic factors is unclear.

Social class

In his textbook of medicine published in 1941, Frederick Price wrote "Angina Pectoris . . . is much more common in those classes of society who are subject to excessive mental or emotional stress or strain, being relatively uncommon in those whose occupation is of a manual character." From London, England, in 1981, however, comes a study by Rose and Marmot[54] that shows clearly how the situation has changed regarding social class and CAD in the past 40 years. The mortality trend for men in social classes 4 and 5 (lower end of the social scale) has risen progressively at least up to 1971 (the latest year for which occupationally related rates were available). For men in social classes 1 in 2 (executive type), the position from 1951–1971 was unchanged, the exception being the considerable decline in the rate of CAD among British doctors.

These authors also surveyed 17,530 London civil servants aged 40–64 years (the Whitehall Study), comparing men in the lowest employment grade with those in the top (administrative) grade. They found the age-adjusted prevalence rate to be 53% higher for angina, 7% higher for ischemic type ECG abnormalities, and 75% higher for ECG abnormalities among men with angina in the lower employment grade than in the top employment grade. Furthermore, at a nearly 8-year follow-up, the CAD mortality was 3.6 times higher in the lower grade group than in the top grade group. This social class difference was partly explained by known CAD risk factors: men in the lower grade smoked more and exercised less, they were shorter and more overweight, and they had a higher BP and lower levels of glucose tolerance. These findings are in contrast to the USA Chicago utility company study by Stamler, which disclosed similar prevalence and incidence rates for CAD in both manual labor and administrative type personnel. A striking finding in the England and Wales study was the size of the social class effect, namely that a person's employment status was a stronger predictor of his risk of dying from CAD than was any of the more familiar risk factors. Death from CAD, in at least 1 reasonably affluent section of the community, namely the administrative grade of the civil service, is, if not rare, at least uncommon by Western standards. One factor that the authors consider possibly responsible for their fortunate position is the relatively low frequency of cigarette smoking.

Hematocrit

In 1962, Burch and DePasquale (*Am J Med* 32:161, 1962) suggested that elevation of the hematocrit and its consequence, increased blood viscosity, may be an important factor in the pathogenesis of CAD. Subsequently, conflicting clinical and epidemiologic evidence for a relation between hematocrit and CAD has appeared. To reevaluate the relation between hematocrit and CAD, Sorlie and associates[55] from Bethesda, Maryland, and San Juan, Puerto Rico, determined hematocrit levels in 2,555 rural and 6,151 urban men aged 45–64 years who were participating in the Puerto Rico Heart Health Program. During the subsequent 8 years these patients were examined 3 additional times. Within the Puerto Rican cohort, the hematocrit was slightly lower in the older aged groups and slightly lower in the rural than in the urban patients. In the rural areas 5% and in the urban areas 3% had hematocrit values <40%. A higher hematocrit level was associated with cigarette smoking, higher relative body weight, higher BP, and higher total serum cholesterol. For urban men, an elevated hematocrit also was associated with an increased risk of AMI, coronary insufficiency, and CAD death. The frequency of AMI, coronary insufficiency, or CAD death was more than doubled in the patients with hematocrit >49%, as compared with the patients with hematocrit <42%. This relation remained statistically significant after adjustment for other "risk factors." Thus, an elevated hematocrit may be an independent risk factor to CAD.

Platelets and prostaglandins

PLATELET ACTIVATION IN CAD

Current concepts of atherosclerosis, based on animal models, suggest a role for platelets in the development of atherosclerotic plaques, possibly through the release of alpha granule constituents. Platelets also may contribute to the development of vascular spasm through production of thromboxane A_2. Platelet activation in the coronary circulation in patients with CAD should occur if these hypotheses apply clinically. Rubenstein and associates[56] from Stanford, California, measured aortic and coronary sinus plasma levels of the platelet alpha granule constituent beta-thromboglobulin (βTG) and thromboxane B_2 (TxB_2) by radioimmunoassay in 15 patients with severe CAD, 7 with angiographically normal coronary arteries and 5 undergoing evaluation for coronary artery spasm. Compared with controls, the CAD patients had significantly greater transmyocardial release of βTG (11 ng/ml -vs-62 ng/ml); TxB_2 gradients had a similar trend, but the difference was not significant. Three of the 5 patients studied developed coronary spasm that was associated with acute elevation in coronary sinus TxB_2; the 2 non-spasm patients with drug provocation had undetectable coronary sinus TxB_2. The investigators concluded that abnormal platelet activation takes place in the coronary circulation of CAD patients, and that production of acute myocardial ischemia by coronary spasm occurs with increased coronary sinus TxB_2.

IN VIVO PLATELET RELEASE REACTION AND MALONDIALDEHYDE FORMATION IN HYPERLIPOPROTEINEMIA

Platelet function is abnormal in many patients with hyperlipidemia, but measurements of abnormal platelet function have been confined to in vitro determinations of platelet aggregation, PF4 activity, plasma anti-heparin activity, and a bleeding time test. Zahavi and associates[57] from London, England, measured platelet function in vivo by measuring plasma β-thromboglobulin (βTG) and platelet factor 4 (PF4), which are specific platelet proteins, in 69 patients with 3 types of primary hyperlipoproteinemia (HLP)

(IIA, IIB, IV) and compared the findings with those in age- and sex-matched healthy controls and in 57 patients with established atherosclerosis and peripheral vascular disease. They found that βTG was significantly increased in the patients with HLP and peripheral vascular disease, as compared with controls, and was significantly higher in the patients with HLP than in those with peripheral vascular disease. PF4 and malondialdehyde (MDA) formation also were increased in patients with HLP. Their results indicate that in vivo platelet "release reaction" and MDA formation are both increased in HLP patients, and that the release reaction is more enhanced in those with HLP than in those with peripheral vascular disease. The authors suggest that abnormal platelet function is related to the elevated levels of serum lipids and lipoproteins in the hyperlipidemic patients and not to the atherosclerotic changes associated with hyperlipidemia.

EFFECT OF PLATELET SUPPRESSANT THERAPY (DIPYRIDAMOLE AND ASPIRIN) ON EXERCISE PERFORMANCE AND PLATELET SURVIVAL TIME IN CAD

It is well known that platelets may contribute to the pathogenesis of atherosclerotic CAD and that platelet reactivity may be activated by exercise. Steele and associates[58] from Denver, Colorado, examined whether platelet suppressant therapy with aspirin (ASA) and dipyridamole (DPY) improved exercise performance in 14 men with CAD. The ASA therapy increased platelet survival time (autologous labelling with chromium-51), but had no effect on either the duration of angina-limited treadmill exercise or the heart rate-systolic BP product ($\times 10^{-2}$) at peak exercise. Combination DPY-ASA therapy had a greater effect on platelet survival, but did not substantially increase the duration of exercise. Administration of DPY alone at a higher dosage increased the exercise duration and had a similar effect on platelet survival. At the time that control exercise was completed with the higher dosage of DPY, the rate-pressure product was decreased. These results suggest that DPY and ASA favorably alter platelet survival in men with CAD and that DPY, but not ASA, favorably alters exercise performance. Although ASA and ASA-DPY may alter platelet response to exercise, the effect is not evident in hemodynamic measurements during exercise.

RELEASE OF PROSTAGLANDINS AND THROMBOXANE IN CAD

There has been recent speculation about the role of prostaglandins and thromboxanes in CAD. These naturally occurring compounds are potent modulators of vascular smooth muscle tone and platelet aggregability. Prostaglandin I_2 (PGI_2)—a powerful vasodilator and inhibitor of platelet aggregation—is the predominant prostaglandin synthesized by the heart. Prostaglandin E_2 (PGE_2), also synthesized in the heart, dilates the coronary vascular smooth muscle in vivo, but simultaneously promotes platelet aggregation. In contrast, thromboxane A_2 (TxA_2) is a potent vasoconstrictor released by platelets that, in turn, causes further aggregation of circulating platelets. Both PGI_2 and TxA_2 are unstable and spontaneously convert to the inactive metabolites 6-keto-prostaglandin $F_{1\alpha}$) (6-keto-$PGF_{1\alpha}$) and thromboxane B_2 (TxB_2), respectively. Several investigators have suggested that prostaglandins and thromboxanes may counterbalance one another in the normal regulation of coronary blood flow. Derangements of platelet function and alterations in prostaglandin and thromboxane production and release have been reported in association with many risk factors related to CAD.

Hirsh and associates[59] from Dallas, Texas, assessed the release of prostaglandins and thromboxanes into the coronary circulation in patients with unstable and stable angina pectoris, nonischemic chest pain syndromes, and various nonischemic cardiac disease. Simultaneous coronary sinus (CS) and ascending aortic (AO) blood samples were obtained from 60 patients for measurement of 6-keto-$PGF_{1\alpha}$ and of TxB_2. Samples from 45 patients also were tested for prostaglandin E_2 (PGE_2) and lactate. Patients with unstable angina pectoris with chest pain within 24 hours of study had higher TxB_2 CS/AO ratios (5.8 ± 2.8) than patients whose most recent anginal pain was >96 hours before study (1.3 ± 0.6), than those with nonischemic chest pain (1.2 ± 0.4), or with valvular or congenital nonischemic heart disease (1.2 ± 0.6). Those whose most recent anginal pain occurred 24−96 hours before study were distributed bimodally: the majority had low TxB_2 CS/AO ratios (range, 0.5−2) like the patients in the 3 aforementioned groups, whereas a few had markedly elevated values (range, 10−47). The 6-keto-$PGF_{1\alpha}$ and PGE_2 CS/AO ratios and myocardial lactate extraction were similar among the 5 groups. These data suggest that local thromboxane release is associated with recent episodes of angina in patients with unstable angina pectoris, but whether this release is a cause or an effect is not known.

PROSTACYCLIN: HEMODYNAMIC AND METABOLIC EFFECTS IN CAD

The precise physiological role of prostacyclin (PGI_2) is unclear, although its greatest effects are inhibition of platelet aggregation and vasodilation. It is synthesized predominantly in vascular endothelium but, unlike other prostaglandins, it has the properties of a circulating hormone. The beneficial effects of prostacyclin administration have been reported in ischemia secondary to severe peripheral vascular disease and in experimental CAD, and reduced prostacyclin production has been demonstrated in atherosclerotic plaques. Bergman and associates[60] from London, England, evaluated the therapeutic potential of prostacyclin in 10 patients with angina pectoris and angiographically proven CAD. Platelet aggregation and coronary and systemic hemodynamic effects were evaluated before and after intravenous infusions of prostacyclin. The ADP concentration required to induce 50% of maximum platelet aggregation increased about 2.5 times with infusion of prostacyclin. Heart rate and cardiac index rose from 77 to 93 beats/min and from 2.5 to 3.5 liters/min/M^2, respectively. Mean BP and systemic and pulmonary resistances fell from 107 to 92 mmHg, and from 1,704 to 1,048, and 80 to 45 dynes cm^{-5}, respectively. Cardiovascular resistance also fell. Mean atrial pacing time to angina rose from 142 to 241 s, while lactate production during rapid atrial pacing was decreased. These coronary and systemic vasodilator effects and the prolongation of pacing time to angina indicate an acute beneficial effect of prostacyclin on angina. Since prostacyclin prevents platelet accumulation and progression to total occlusion in animals with experimental coronary stenoses, the observed inhibition of platelet aggregation suggests that prostacyclin may be useful in unstable angina.

FIBRINOPEPTIDE A AND THROMBOXANE PRODUCTION IN CAD

Interest in the study of blood clotting and platelet function of CAD patients has been stimulated in recent years by knowledge that coronary thrombosis frequently accompanies CAD. This interest has been further increased by the discovery that platelets play a contributory role in the pathogenesis of atherosclerosis and that, when aggregated, platelets produce and release thromboxane A_2, a potent constrictor of coronary arteries. Thus, increased platelet aggregation could be an important additional stimulus for coronary spasm, and a possible cause of angina and AMI. Enhanced blood coagulation and increased platelet aggregation frequently have been reported in patients with CAD. The behavior of blood clotting and platelets has not been investigated in relation to either the frequency of anginal attacks or to the severity of CAD and coronary risk factors.

Serneri and associates[61] from Florence and Pisa, Italy, investigated the occurrence of blood clotting changes and increased platelet biologic activity in 98 CAD patients. The fibrinopeptide A (FPA) level in plasma (an index of in vivo thrombin production), beta-thromboglobulin (βTG) plasma level, and thromboxane B_2 formation by platelets were measured. In the CAD patients (independent of their clinical status, e.g., previous AMI, spontaneous angina, or effort angina), a hypercoagulable state (indicated by significant elevation of FPA plasma level) and increased platelet biologic activity were present. Moreover, plasma FPA concentration and platelet aggregation were markedly higher in patients with frequently occurring spontaneous clinical manifestations (active CAD) than in CAD patients with relatively quiescent symptoms. Abnormalities of blood clotting and platelet changes were not significantly altered by the presence or severity of coronary angiographic fixed obstruction. Multiple regression analysis indicated that hypercoagulability and increased platelet biologic activity were not a consequence of differences in coronary risk patterns in CAD patients, as compared with controls.

Exercise

EFFECT OF MODERATE EXERCISE IN MONKEYS ON AN ATHEROGENIC DIET

Although it is believed by many that exercise protects against CAD, the evidence for this belief is circumstantial, and conclusive evidence is difficult to obtain in human beings. Kramsch and associates[62] from Boston, Massachusetts, studied the effects of moderate conditioning with treadmill exercise on developing CAD in monkeys on an atherogenic diet. They studied 27 young adult male monkeys from Malaysia (macaques) and divided them into 3 groups of 9 animals each. One group, studied for 36 months, received a controlled diet of monkey chow blended with banana mash during the entire period; a second group received this diet for 12 months, then was fed an atherogenic diet for another 24 months. The physical activity in each of these 2 groups was limited to that permitted by housing one animal in a single cage. These 2 groups, therefore, were designated the "sedentary normal control group" and the "sedentary atherogenic control group." The third group consumed the control diet for 18 months but, during this period, the monkeys were gradually conditioned by exercise on a treadmill within the first 12 months and then kept in the physically trained state for an additional 6 months. Thereafter, the animals were given the atherogenic diet for 24 more months during which the exercise program was continued. This group was referred to as the "exercise group." All animals were trained to operate a motorless treadmill wheel especially designed for primates until they were capable of running at a speed of 2.5 km/hour. After training, the 2 sedentary groups were taken to the treadmill only for periodic exercise tests, but the exercising group was trained further until speeds of 2.0–3.5 km/hour could be sustained for 1 hour. The exercise group then continued running at that speed for 1 hour 3 times a week. Good physical training was demonstrated by slow heart rates. The serum total cholesterol was the same (approximately 600 mg/dl) in exercising and nonexercising monkeys, with significantly higher HDL cholesterol and much lower LDL plus VLDL triglyceride in the exercise group. The mean serum total cholesterol rose from 102 mg/dl in the sedentary normal controls to about 620 mg/dl in both sedentary and exercise-conditioned groups on the atherogenic diet. Systolic and diastolic BP was comparable in all monkeys irrespective of diet or exercise. ECG abnormalities suggesting myocardial ischemia at rest or exercise were observed only in monkeys on the atherogenic diet that had not been conditioned by exercise. One sedentary monkey that consumed the atherogenic diet for 23 months died suddenly. Narrowed coronary arteries were demonstrated by angiogram at the end of the study in 3 nonconditioned animals on the atherogenic diet, including the animal that died suddenly at 23 months. In contrast, angiograms of all exercise-conditioned monkeys showed coronary arteries that were strikingly wider than the normal arteries of sedentary animals, i.e., with no detectable narrowings. At necropsy, the hearts of the exercise-conditioned monkeys were considerably larger than those of the sedentary animals on the atherogenic diet or of sedentary normal controls. In sedentary monkeys receiving the prolonged atherogenic diet, grossly visible coronary atherosclerotic plaques were striking. In contrast, the coronary arteries of exercise-conditioned monkeys had fewer plaques and coronary arteries were of considerably larger caliber even at sites of plaques. Histologic study of the atherosclerotic plaques observed disclosed that those in the sedentary monkeys were frequently fibrotic, whereas those in the exercise-conditioned animals contained little if any morphologically detectable collagen and consisted predominantly of lipid-laden foam cells. In addition, the intimal thickenings were smaller in the exercise-conditioned monkeys than in sedentary animals on the atherogenic diet. These data suggest that moderate exercise may prevent or retard CAD in primates, even in the presence of severe hypercholesterolemia.

LEFT MAIN CORONARY NARROWING OR "EQUIVALENT"

Accuracy of angiographic determination of left main narrowing: angiographic-histologic correlative analysis

Accurate identification of the degree of LM coronary artery narrowing is of paramount importance because significant narrowing of this artery generally is considered an indication for coronary bypass operation, regardless of the symptomatic status of the patient. Although coronary angiography is the most reliable means for identifying patients with significant LM stenosis, the accuracy of this technique has not been subjected to critical analysis. Accordingly, Isner and associates[63] from Bethesda, Maryland, evaluated the accuracy of coronary angiography in identifying severe LM narrowing by comparing the degree of narrowing observed by angiography with that observed at necropsy in 28 patients with symptomatic CAD in whom angiography had been performed within 40 days of death. The angiograms were evaluated independently by 3 experienced angiographers. In 20 (71%) of the 28 patients, the degree of LM narrowing was either underestimated (13 patients) or overestimated (10 patients) by 2 or all 3 angiographers; of 84 angiographic judgments made by the 3 angiographers in the 28 patients, 54 (64%) were underestimates (33 judgments, 39%) or overestimates (21 judgments, 25%) of the degree of LM narrowing. Of 12 LM coronary arteries narrowed 76%–100% in cross-sectional area at necropsy, 6 had been underestimated at preoperative angiography by 2 or all 3 angiographers; of 12 LM arteries narrowed 51%–75% in cross-sectional area at necropsy, all 12 had been either under- or over-estimated angiographically by 2 or all 3 angiographers; of 4 LM arteries narrowed 26%–50% in cross-sectional area at necropsy, 2 had been overestimated by 2 or 3 angiographers. Thus, angiographic determination of degrees of LM narrowing during life is subject to considerable error. The angiographic errors appear to have resulted primarily from the presence of atherosclerotic plaque in the LM coronary artery and, possibly, from an insufficient number of angiographic projections.

Risks of coronary arteriography and of coronary bypass surgery with severe stenosis of the left main coronary artery

At one time, it was believed that the risk of coronary angiography and of coronary bypass grafting was considerably increased in patients with severe narrowing of the LM coronary artery, unlike the situation in patients without severe narrowing of the LM coronary artery but with severe narrowing of 1 or more other major coronary arteries. Miller and associates[64] from Seattle, Washington, found 83 patients to have severe ("severe" not defined) narrowing of the LM coronary artery among 1,060 patients undergoing coronary angiography during a 3-year period. Of the 83 patients, 3 died during the cardiac catheterization procedure. Of 74 patients, however, with severe narrowing of the LM coronary artery who underwent coronary bypass grafting, none died in the hospital. The risk of coronary bypass surgery now among patients with severe narrowing of the LM coronary artery appears to be similar to that in patients undergoing bypass operations who show narrowing of the major coronary arteries excluding the LM. Miller and associates believe that preoperative stability was the key to low risk in their LM patients but, of course, intraoperative myocardial protection has been improved greatly in recent years, as emphasized by Loop.[65] To achieve stability, the intraaortic balloon pump was used preoperatively in 14 of their 74 patients.

Fig. 1-15. Cumulative survival (actuarial) data. The 5-year survival of patients with left main equivalent disease treated surgically (LME-SURGICAL) is significantly better than that of patients with left main coronary artery disease treated surgically (LMCA-SURGICAL) or LME medical patients. TVD = 3-vessel disease. Reproduced with permission from Tyras.[66]

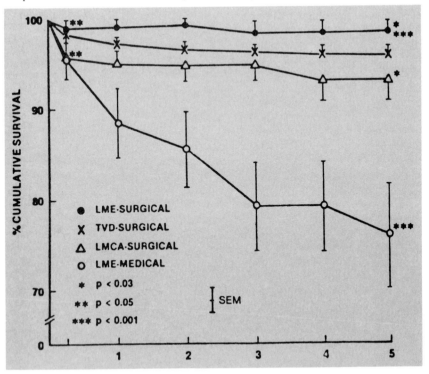

Although some may consider this usage excessive, stability was assured and the results obviously speak for themselves.

Left main "equivalent": results of medical and surgical therapy

Many studies have shown increased survival of patients with LM coronary stenosis after coronary artery bypass grafting (CABG), as compared with those not treated surgically. The finding of severe LM narrowing virtually makes CABG imperative. Some investigators have considered angiographic evidence of a 50% diameter reduction of both LAD and LC coronary arteries proximal to any major branches as *equivalent* to severe LM narrowing. Using this definition of "LM equivalent," Tyras and associates[66] from St. Louis, Missouri, studied 189 such patients, performing CABG in 119 and no bypass in 70. During a similar 4-year period, 203 patients with significant LM coronary narrowing and 742 patients with 3-vessel disease without LM coronary narrowing or "LM equivalent" underwent CABG. The operative mortality in the LM group (4%) was higher than in the "LM equivalent" group (0.8%) ($p < 0.05$); 5-year survival was better in the "LM equivalent" with CABG group (98% ± 1%) than in the "LM equivalent" without CABG group (76% ± 6% [$p < 0.001$]) or in LM patients with CABG (93% ± 2% [$p < 0.03$]) (Fig. 1-15). All groups with CABG had a significantly lower frequency of AMI than did "LM equivalent" without CABG patients. Relief of angina also was significantly better in the CABG group than in the "LM equivalent" without CABG group ($p < 0.005$). Thus, although "LM equivalent" stenosis is not truly equivalent to LM stenosis, such patients without CABG had a significantly higher frequency of cardiac death and AMI than did those with CABG.

ANGINA PECTORIS

Fatal cardiac arrest during cardiac catheterization for angina pectoris

Death during catheterization is rare and the opportunity to study at necropsy a patient who died during this procedure is even rarer. During an 11-year period, Cabin and Roberts[67] from Bethesda, Maryland, studied at necropsy 10 patients with angina pectoris who died during cardiac catheterization performed at 8 hospitals. Nine patients died during attempted coronary angiography and the remaining patient during right-sided cardiac catheterization. At least 3 of the 4 major epicardial coronary arteries were narrowed 76%–100% in cross-sectional area by atherosclerotic plaques in all 10 patients, 7 of whom had this degree of narrowing of the LMCA by plaque, and 2 additional patients had severe (>75%) LMCA narrowing by thromboembolic material superimposed on small atherosclerotic plaques. Among 354 segments of the LM, LAD, LC and right coronary arteries in 8 patients, the narrowing in cross-sectional area by atherosclerotic plaques was 96%–100% in 9 segments, 76%–95% in 49, 51%–75% in 23, 26%–50% in 13, and 0–25% in 6. With use of the following scoring system for the amount of narrowing in each 5 mm segment (1 = 0–25%, 2 = 26%–50%, 3 = 51%–75%, and 4 = 76%–100%), the mean score per segment for the group was 3.34. The investigators concluded that patients with angina pectoris who die during cardiac catheterization have particularly severe and diffuse coronary atherosclerosis and, usually, severe narrowing of the LMCA.

In a patient with angina pectoris who cannot be resuscitated from cardiac arrest during cardiac catheterization, emergency CABG appears warranted. This study suggests that, in such patients, the surgeon can assume that at least 3 and usually all 4 major epicardial coronary arteries are narrowed 76%–100% in cross-sectional area. Furthermore, although the atherosclerotic process is diffuse, the amount of severe luminal narrowing is usually greater in the proximal than in the distal halves of the major coronary arteries and, therefore, each usually would be suitable for grafting.

RNA-obtained ejection fraction and regional wall motion abnormalities during atrial pacing in stable angina pectoris

The approach to the evaluation of myocardial ischemia in the setting of CAD has become increasingly multifaceted. Changes in lactate metabolism, in systemic hemodynamics, and in contrast ventriculographic parameters of EF and regional wall motion induced by atrial pacing have contributed greatly to the detection of myocardial ischemia, and have value for the assessment of the effects of therapeutic interventions. Recent work has suggested that RNA during atrial pacing may combine the advantages of the controlled stress of pacing with the important noninvasive RNA parameters previously obtained only with the stress of exercise. Hecht and associates[68] from Los Angeles, California, evaluated the use of RNA during atrial pacing from the coronary sinus in 12 patients with stable angina pectoris and compared changes in LV EF and regional wall motion with alterations in transmyocardial lactate gradients and hemodynamics. EF declined from 0.60 during control state to 0.51 during submaximal pacing (submax P), with 10 of 12 having decreased EF, 6 developing new regional wall motion abnormalities, and 5 experiencing mild chest pain. During maximal pacing (max P), EF declined further to 0.47, with all patients having decreased EF and experiencing moderate-to-severe chest pain, and 9 developing new regional wall motion abnormalities. Percentage lactate extraction (Ex) decreased from +28.3% to +17.4% during submax P, with only 1 patient producing lactate. During max P, percentage lactate Ex decreased to −0.1%, with 8 patients producing lactate. Significant increases in PA capillary wedge pressure and systemic vascular resistance occurred during max P, and in mean PA pressure and mean systemic arterial BP during both submax and max P. Significant decreases in stroke volume index and stroke work index occurred during both pacing levels and cardiac index did not change with pacing. Thus, RNA can be used to establish decreases in EF and regional wall motion abnormalities that occur in response to incremental atrial pacing in patients with stable CAD, and these changes are more consistent and appear earlier than the metabolic consequences of myocardial ischemia induced by pacing stress.

Effects of intravenous nitroglycerin on ischemic myocardium when given intraoperatively during coronary artery bypass

The precise mechanism of action of the nitrates in the relief of myocardial ischemic pain in CAD patients has been a subject of considerable debate. It has been proposed that the nitrates improve the imbalance between diminished coronary blood flow and the oxygen requirements of the heart by direct dilating action on the diseased coronary arteries, or that they reduce the oxygen requirement of the myocardium by decreasing the external work of the heart. The conventional concept is that the salutary antianginal effects of the nitrates predominantly stem from their action of systemic venodilation, which results in pooling of blood and decrease of heart size (preload reduction), thereby diminishing systolic wall tension (afterload) and oxygen consumption of the ischemic LV. The possibility remains that the nitrates may improve lowered myocardial perfusion in areas of LV ischemia by dilating even diseased vessels and/or by enhancing blood flow through the collateral network. Klein and associates[69] from Davis and Sacramento, California, administered nitroglycerin (NTG) intravenously during coronary artery bypass operations in 24 patients and measured antegrade blood flow through 56 separate intact saphenous vein bypass grafts to analyze NTG perfusion response in the obstructed native coronary artery. In 30 bypassed coronary arteries with proximal luminal diameter narrowing of 50%–90%, NTG significantly reduced graft flow 82 to 63 ml/min, indicating that NTG dilated proximal stenoses with resultant increased coronary artery flow. In 11 bypassed coronary arteries obstructed 90%–100% with well-developed collaterals distally, NTG significantly decreased graft flow 64 to 53 ml/min, thus indicating enhanced collateral flow. In contrast, in 11 bypassed coronary artery obstructions of 90%–100% without collaterals, NTG significantly increased graft flow 91–100 ml/min, indicating nonresponsiveness of the severely narrowed coronary arteries to NTG. Thus, systemic NTG improved perfusion to ischemic myocardium subserved by narrowed coronary arteries with <90% stenosis or by >90% obstructed vessels with substantial collaterals distally. These results indicate the ability of NTG to augment lowered myocardial blood flow in ischemic myocardium in certain coronary subsets, thus supporting the view that the antianginal efficacy of the nitrates in many CAD patients is at least partially due to pharmacologic revascularization, in addition to the action of these agents in reducing cardiac oxygen demands.

Treatment by new beta blocking agents (atenolol and nadolol)

The beneficial effect of beta adrenergic blocking agents in the treatment of angina pectoris, systemic hypertension, and cardiac arrhythmias is well established. Generalized beta blockade, however, is often accompanied by undesired effects. A number of these compounds have been designed to minimize their unwanted properties, and the effectiveness and safety of each new beta receptor antagonist must be specifically established for each therapeutic indication. *Atenolol* is a relative cardioselective beta blocker that possesses potent antianginal and antihypertensive effects when given once daily. Previous studies have been of relatively short duration and the long-term efficacy and potential side effects of the agent have not been evaluated. Schwartz and associates[70] from Stanford, California, evaluated the value of atenolol during a 1-year period of administration and compared these long-term observations with prior short-term observations of the agent in the same patients with chronic stable angina pectoris. After a placebo-controlled, single-blind, dose-ranging trial with 2-week drug periods involving 25, 50, 100, and 200 mg, 9 patients with chronic stable angina were continued on 100 or 200 mg daily for 1 year. Treadmill exercise tests (ET) were performed at times of peak and trough serum atenolol concentrations, and 24-hour ECG ambulatory recordings were obtained after placebo, after 2 weeks of 100 and 200 mg atenolol, and after 3, 6, 9 and 12 months of 100 or 200 mg atenolol. During early and chronic atenolol therapy, anginal frequency and NTG consumption decreased. Twenty-four-hour ECG and ET showed sustained heart rate suppression. Exercise duration until onset of angina was prolonged during all periods of atenolol administration. Maximum improvement in exercise tolerance and relief of angina was not reached until after 3 months of atenolol therapy, despite stable serum drug concentrations. Thus, atenolol 100 or 200 mg given once daily, provided well-tolerated and potent anti-ischemic myocardial actions that were effectively maintained during chronic therapy of angina pectoris.

Shapiro and associates[71] from Washington, D.C., studied 37 patients with stable angina pectoris who had 5 or more episodes of pain per week and also a 1 mm or greater ST-segment depression 80 ms past the J point during a Bruce protocol treadmill test. An 8-week placebo-controlled run-in period preceded double-blind randomization to *nadolol* administration once per day (17 patients) or to identical appearing placebo for 4 weeks (20 patients), after which an exercise test was done. Nadolol is a new nonselective β_1 and β_2 adrenergic blocking agent with a plasma half-life of $17-23$ hours. Diaries for pain episodes and NTG consumption were kept. Exercise tests were performed 24 hours after the last dose of nadolol or placebo. Episodes of pain per week were reduced 60% after nadolol and 28% after placebo ($p < 0.01$). NTG consumption was reduced 67% after nadolol and 36% after placebo, ($p < 0.05$). Resting and peak heart rates and peak rate-pressure products showed typical reductions due to beta blockade 24 hours after nadolol, as compared with the stability of these parameters during placebo, ($p < 0.001$). Exercise time after nadolol increased 42%, which was more than the 14% increase after placebo ($p < 0.05$). Exercise work after nadolol increased 65%, as compared with a 22% increase after placebo ($p < 0.05$). Mean ST-segment depression at end of exercise was little changed before and after treatment in both groups, reflecting consistency of effort. Improvement in symptoms and work capacity associated with nadolol significantly exceeded the placebo group responses. Unlike other available agents of this class, a single daily dose of nadolol produced therapeutically effective 24-hour blockade in patients with disabling angina pectoris.

Comparison of beta blocking agent (atenolol) with anticoagulant (heparin) in preventing acute myocardial infarction in unstable angina pectoris

Several uncontrolled or inadequately controlled studies have suggested that anticoagulation may improve the prognosis in unstable angina pectoris, but anticoagulants have been utilized less frequently since the introduction of beta adrenergic blocking drugs, the benefits of which are well accepted in stable angina. Telford and Wilson[72] from Antrim, Northern Ireland, designed a trial to assess the effect of anticoagulation and/or beta adrenergic blockade in unstable angina pectoris. They conducted a randomized, double-blind, placebo-controlled study of morbidity and mortality, using heparin, atenolol, and a combination of both drugs in 214 patients. During the trial period, transmural AMI developed in 9 (17%) of 54 patients on placebo, in 8 (13%) of 60 on atenolol, in 1 (2%) of 51 on heparin, and in 2 (4%) of 49 on heparin and atenolol combined ($p = 0.02$). The improved prognosis in the heparin-treated patients was maintained at follow-up. All 5 deaths occurred among patients who did not receive heparin. These results show that intravenous heparin therapy was of benefit in preventing AMI in patients with unstable angina pectoris.

Comparison of propranolol and verapamil in stable angina pectoris

To determine the effectiveness of oral verapamil, alone and combined with propranolol, in patients with chronic angina pectoris, Leon and associates[73] from Bethesda, Maryland, performed upright bicycle exercise testing in 11 inpatients in a single-blind, cross-over study. As compared with placebo, which resulted in a mean exercise time of 5.1 ± 0.7 minutes, verapamil (480 mg/day) improved exercise time in all patients (mean increment, 3.4 ± 0.7 minutes, $p < 0.001$) and was more effective than propranolol (160–320 mg/day) (mean increment, 1.3 ± 0.6 minutes, $p < 0.005$). Verapamil plus propranolol further increased exercise time (mean increment, 4.7 ± 0.7 minutes, $p < 0.001$ -vs- verapamil alone) and 9 of 11 patients were pain-free during exercise (in contrast to 2 of 11 with propranolol and 1 of 11 with verapamil). Time to 1 mm ST-segment depression was increased by both verapamil ($p < 0.005$) and verapamil plus propranolol ($p < 0.05$) compared with placebo. At the work load causing angina during the placebo study, verapamil decreased heart rate (from 112 ± 3 to 104 ± 3 beats/min, $p < 0.05$) and insignificantly decreased pressure-rate product (from $18.3 \pm 0.8 \times 10^3$ to $15.9 \pm 0.9 \times 10^3$). Verapamil plus propranolol further decreased heart rate (to 76 ± 3, $p < 0.001$) and pressure-rate product (to $9.7 \pm 0.5 \times 10^3$, $p < 0.001$). Adverse effects from verapamil, alone or with propranolol, included P-R interval prolongation in most patients, transient AV nodal Wenckebach block in 1 patient, and exertional dyspnea, orthostatic dizziness, or pedal edema in 3 others. Thus, in these patients with stable angina 1) verapamil was a more effective antianginal agent than propranolol and 2) verapamil plus propranolol provided more improvement in exercise capacity than either drug alone.

Johnson and associates[74] from Dallas, Texas, compared the relative efficacies of propranolol and verapamil in 18 patients (mean age, 58 years; 16 men, 2 women) with stable angina pectoris. The results of low- (40 mg every 6 hours) and high-dose (80 mg every 6 hours) propranolol and high-dose (120 mg every 6 hours) verapamil therapy were evaluated in a double-blind, randomized, placebo-controlled study that lasted 8 weeks: 2 weeks of placebo therapy, 2 weeks of propranolol or verapamil (1 week low-dose, 1 week high-dose) therapy, 3 days of down-titration followed by 1 week of placebo therapy, 2 weeks of propranolol or verapamil therapy (whichever had not been given earlier in the trial) (1 week low-dose, 1 week high-dose) and 3 days of down-titration. During each period the following were quantitated: 1) chest pain/week; 2) NTG used/week; 3) transient ischemic ST segment deviations and highest grade of ventricular ectopic activity on 2-channel Holter monitor; 4) ST-segment deviations during supine bicycle exercise; 5) LV volumes and EF at rest and during exercise (assessed by equilibrium-gated blood pool scintigraphy); and 6) pulmonary function studies. Propranolol and high-dose verapamil therapy significantly reduced the frequency of angina, and high-dose verapamil therapy diminished both the need for NTG and the frequency of transient ischemic ST segment deviations on Holter monitor. Neither agent exerted a clinically important deleterious influence on LV volumes or the EF. Forced vital capacity and forced expiratory volume were worsened by propranolol, but not by verapamil. Thus, in stable angina pectoris, verapamil is a satisfactory therapeutic alternative to propranolol.

Comparison of calcium antagonists (verapamil and nifedipine) in stable angina pectoris

Dawson and associates[75] from Uxbridge, England, examined the relative efficacy of 2 calcium antagonist drugs, verapamil (120 mg, t.i.d.) and nifedipine (20 mg, t.i.d.) in a double-blind randomized trial. Patients were assessed at the end of 4-week periods by a maximal treadmill exercise test, the frequency of anginal attacks, NTG consumption, and side effects. Sixteen-point precordial maps were recorded at rest, immediately after exercise, and at 1-minute intervals for 10 minutes. Total ST segment depression was used as a measure of myocardial ischemia. Both verapamil and nifedipine increased maximal work capacity, but ST at the termination of the test remained constant. Both drugs reduced the frequency of anginal attacks and NTG consumption. Systolic BP at rest and on exercise was reduced by either drug. Verapamil and nifedipine were equally effective in treating angina, but side effects were more common with nifedipine.

Treatment with nifedipine

Corbalan and associates[76] from Santiago, Chile, studied the effect of nifedipine on exercise tolerance in 30 patients with stable angina pectoris and positive graded exercise testing. Treadmill exercise testing was performed on each of 5 consecutive days. Placebo or nifedipine (10 mg sublingually) was given 30 minutes before exercise on the third day. The following day the intervention was reversed in a double-blind manner. Angina was abolished by nifedipine, but not by placebo, in 12 patients. The time to onset of angina in the remaining patients increased from 4.1 ± 0.4 to 6.7 ± 0.6 min ($p < 0.001$). Time to ST depression ≥ 2 mm increased from 4.0 ± 0.3 to 5.4 ± 0.5 min, while duration of exercise increased from 6.3 ± 0.3 to 8.2 ± 0.4 min ($p < 0.001$). The maximum heart rate was 145 ± 3.3 beats/min with nifedipine and 122 ± 3.8 beats/min with placebo ($p < 0.01$). Resting systolic BP decreased 30 min after nifedipine administration from 131 ± 3.4 to 106 ± 2.9 mmHg ($p < 0.01$). Maximal systolic BP during exercise was lower with nifedipine (127 ± 4.8 mmHg) than with placebo (155 ± 5.6 mmHg, $p < 0.01$). Thus, nifedipine appears to improve exercise tolerance significantly in stable angina pectoris by decreasing peripheral vascular resistance and myocardial oxygen demand.

A 57-page symposium on nifedipine and angina pectoris appeared in the October 1981 issue of The American Journal of Medicine.[77-83] As stated by Sobel[77] from St. Louis, Missouri, the papers presented reflect progress in research on the role of calcium in basic cardiovascular physiology and pathophysiology, as well as in the rapidly expanding clinical research and experience with calcium flux blockade. The recognition that coronary spasm may play an important role in many syndromes associated with CAD has added impetus to such research. Angina is presently viewed as resulting not only from classic, fixed obstruction, but also from contributions of inappropriate or excessive coronary artery vasoconstriction or frank spasm, alone or superimposed on fixed lesions. Accordingly, the rationale for potential utility of calcium channel blocking agents in the treatment of angina depends on several considerations, including the properties of these agents that may counter effects of a fixed obstruction by reducing myocardial oxygen demands secondary to peripheral vasoconstriction, as well as the properties that blunt coronary vasoconstriction or facilitate coronary vasodilation. Thus, these agents offer the promise of increasing oxygen supply to the heart while reducing oxygen demand, in contrast to conventionally available agents, such as nitrates and beta blocking agents, that act primarily by reducing oxygen demand.

Treatment with diltiazem

Hossack and associates[84] from Seattle, Washington, compared the effects of diltiazem, a calcium antagonist drug, with those of placebo on exercise performance during a series of symptom-limited upright exercise tests. Ten patients with chronic stable angina were studied over 7 weeks. The drug was administered in a random, double-blind fashion and was evaluated at increasing dose levels of 120, 180, and 240 mg/day. Diltiazem was effective in increasing the total duration of exercise ($p < 0.001$) and the time to the first onset of angina ($p < 0.02$) and to the first appearance of 1 mm of ST depression ($p < 0.02$). These effects were most marked at the highest dose level of diltiazem. Heart rate was reduced at rest ($p < 0.05$) and during submaximal exercise (p < 0.001). There was a reduction in diastolic BP during submaximal exercise (p < 0.04), but no change in systolic BP. Pressure-rate product was significantly reduced at submaximal (p < 0.001), but not at maximal, exercise. The reduction in pressure-rate product is postulated as the mechanism by which diltiazem enhances duration of exercise. There was no reduction in ECG evidence of myocardial ischemia at peak exercise, either by clinical observation or by computer analysis of spatial ECG variables. Five of 6 patients who continued to take the drug maintained or improved their exercise performance on follow-up study 8 to 10 months later.

Low and associates[85] from Davis and Sacramento, California, compared the effects of diltiazem and placebo in 12 patients with chronic effort angina and catheterization-documented fixed CAD. The 8-week total protocol consisted of a 1-week baseline period followed by the double-blind, randomized, cross-over alternate 1-week administration of placebo and diltiazem in doses of 120, 180, and 240 mg. Maximal exercise tests (MET) were performed at the end of each 1-week period; rest RNA was obtained during 240 mg diltiazem and corresponding cross-over placebo. Resting heart rate decreased from baseline with initial placebo and at diltiazem doses of 60 and 240 mg, but not from placebo during cross-over period. No changes were observed at any dose of diltiazem, either at rest or during MET, in systolic BP or in heart rate times BP double product of myocardial oxygen consumption. Diltiazem at 240 mg, but not at lower doses, increased MET duration (437 s -vs- 490 s) and time to angina (383 s -vs- 441 s). LV EF by RNA was greater with diltiazem than with placebo (0.54 -vs- 0.50). Thus, these data indicate that calcium blockade with diltiazem provides antianginal efficacy by reducing myocardial oxygen demand, and increases exercise tolerance without depression of myocardial performance in effort angina patients with fixed chronic CAD.

Medical -vs- surgical therapy for unstable angina pectoris

Brown and associates[86] from Boston, Massachusetts, analyzed 190 patients who presented with unstable angina pectoris between 1972 and 1976. Coronary angiography, performed in 166 patients, disclosed that 83 patients (50%) were not eligible for randomization because of obstruction in the LM coronary artery (4%), inoperable diffuse coronary narrowing (11%), failure of initial medical therapy (20%), minimal coronary narrowing (13%), or other reasons (2%). The other 83 patients (50%) were eligible for randomization: 39 received medical therapy and 44 underwent urgent coronary artery bypass grafting (CABG). The medical and surgical patients were comparable in terms of clinical characteristics and extent of coronary narrowing. In-hospital (3% medical and 2% surgical) and late (5% medical and 5% surgical) mortalities were similar over a mean follow-up period of 46 months. AMI rate was statistically similar in-hospital (5% medical and 11% surgical) and during chronic evaluation (5% medical and 14% surgical). However, late severe angina (New York Heart Association class III or IV) occurred in a significantly higher percentage of medical patients (28% medical -vs- 9% surgical), and 9 of the 39 medical patients (23%) required late elective CABG for relief of persistent angina. This experience supports the view that acute management of unstable angina pectoris may begin with intensive medical treatment, to be followed by elective CABG for those patients with persistent angina despite medical therapy.

From the prospective randomized study comparing medical with surgical management for patients with unstable angina pectoris in 9 cooperating medical centers under the auspices of the National Heart, Lung, and Blood Institute between 1971 and 1976, 202 of 288 (70%) patients had ≥70% fixed narrowing of the LAD coronary artery, either alone or in association with other coronary narrowings of ≥50%: 102 patients were assigned to the medical group and 100 to the surgical group.[87] The in-hospital mortality rates were 2% in the medical group and 9% in the surgical group: that of patients with distal LAD disease was 3% in the medical group and 2% in the surgical group (p = ns). Non-fatal AMI occurred in 9% of the medical patients and in 23% of the surgically treated patients with severe proximal narrowing. No significant difference was observed in the in-hospital or late mortality or in the frequency of non-fatal AMI in those treated medically or surgically over a mean follow-up period of 4 years after randomization. Severe angina was significantly more common in the medically treated than in the surgically treated groups after 1 year of follow-up (p < 0.002). Thus, most patients with unstable angina respond well to intensive medical therapy. Elective coronary catheterization and elective or semi-elective CABG can usually be done later. Myocardial preservation, not employed in the patients in this study, may improve the operative results.

VARIANT ANGINA AND/OR CORONARY SPASM

Variant angina, migraine and Raynaud's phenomenon: is each a manifestation of a generalized vasospastic disorder?

Although altered adrenergic activity has been proposed as the cause of coronary spasm, and high circulating thromboxane levels are found in patients with variant angina, the true cause of the syndrome is unknown. Likewise, the prodromal phase of migraine is caused by inappropriate vasoconstriction of cranial arteries, and enzymatic markers of cerebral ischemia can be detected in the cerebrospinal fluid after an attack. As in variant angina, abnormal platelet function has been described in migraine. In spite of a variety of known triggering factors, however, the cause of migraine also is unclear. Arterial vasospasm also accounts for the clinical manifestations of Raynaud's phenomenon. In these patients, capillary blood flow in the fingers is lower than normal and decreases abnormally with the sympathetic stimulus of body cooling. Clinical improvement with adrenergic blocking agents, sympathectomy, or beta adrenergic stimulation, and clinical worsening with β blockade further suggest that the sympathetic nervous system has an important role in the pathogenesis of Raynaud's phenomenon. The frequency with which variant angina, migraine, and Raynaud's phenomenon occur together has not been defined, but may be important in the development of a single pathogenetic explanation for the 3 disorders.

Miller and associates[88] from Montreal, Canada, compared the prevalences of migraine and Raynaud's phenomenon in 62 patients with variant angina (chest pain at rest associated with transient ST-segment elevation, rapidly relieved by nitroglycerin and without evidence of myocardial necrosis) with those in 2 control groups: 1 matched for age, sex, and extent of CAD, and a second group without known heart disease. Migraine was diagnosed in 26% of the patients with variant angina, as compared with 6% and 10% in the respective control groups. Raynaud's phenomenon occurred in 24% of the patients with variant angina, as compared with 5% and 3% in controls. Thus, the prevalence of migraine in patients with variant angina was 16 of 62, as compared with 4 of 62 in the coronary control group and 6 of 62 among the noncoronary controls. The prevalence of Raynaud's phenomenon in the patients with variant angina was 15 of 62, as compared with 3 of 62 coronary controls and 2 of 62 noncoronary controls. Seven patients with variant angina, but no controls, had both migraine and Raynaud's phenomenon, and 24 patients with variant angina had at least 1 of the 2 conditions. The high prevalence of migraine and Raynaud's phenomenon in variant angina raises the possibility that a common underlying defect or mechanism may partially account for all 3 conditions. Should this prove to be so, the single clinical syndrome of generalized arterial vasospasm could be diagnosed and possibly treated with a single agent to correct the underlying abnormality. The clinical observation that attacks in different arterial beds usually occur at different times and usually have different triggering mechanisms suggests that local factors also may play a part in the pathogenesis of these disorders.

Endothelial cell damage and thrombus formation after partial arterial constriction: relevance to spasm

In this book, we generally avoid articles having to do entirely with animals. The subject of coronary artery spasm, thrombosis, and platelet aggregation, however, is so important that a paper by Gertz and associates[89] from Jerusalem, Israel, has particular importance, since this type study is not likely to be done in humans. These authors narrowed the LAD coronary artery of 4 dogs and the right common carotid artery in 15 rabbits to about 50% reduction in transluminal diameter for 1 hour by partial ligation with suture thread. Scanning electron microscopic examination of the luminal surface of these arteries revealed endothelial craters and balloons, fragmentation and desquamation on the proximal slope of the constriction. Platelet attachment to exposed subendothelial tissues was evident, and microthrombi were present at the point of maximum constriction. Blood flow, as measured by electromagnetic flow probe, was virtually unchanged upon partial ligation. In control studies, where a second ligature was placed proximal to and before the first to reduce blood flow to the distal constriction site substantially or totally, endothelial desquamation was observed in only 1 of

14 animals, and the number of craters and balloons was significantly reduced. The authors suggest that endothelial damage and thrombus formation may occur at the site of focal arterial constriction, even when the reduction in transluminal diameter is insufficient to alter substantially the rate of flow.

This article was followed by an editorial by Ganz[90] from Los Angeles, California, that made the point that the pendulum may be swinging too far in the direction of spasm and too far away from the direction of anatomic narrowing of coronary arteries in patients with CAD.

Thromboxane A₂ in vasotonic angina pectoris

Thromboxane A_2 (TxA$_2$), an arachidonic acid metabolite causing vasoconstriction and platelet aggregation, is a putative mediator of coronary artery vasospasm. To determine whether platelet-released TxA$_2$ causes coronary arterial vasospasm, Robertson and associates[90] from Nashville, Tennessee, measured plasma thromboxane B_2 (TxB$_2$), the inactive hydration product of TxA$_2$, in the radial artery and coronary sinus blood of 7 patients and performed therapeutic trials of antiplatelet agents in 9. Although coronary sinus TxB$_2$ levels rose from the baseline approximately 5-fold with spontaneous ischemia, samples drawn early in ischemia showed no rise over baseline values. Although 150 mg aspirin reduced urinary TxB$_2$ levels by $\geq 75\%$, it had no effect on the course of the chronic recurrent form of angina pectoris due to vasospasm ("vasotonic angina"). Similarly, indomethacin had no effect on the frequency or duration of ischemia. TxA$_2$ is unlikely to cause vasotonic angina, but it may be released during coronary vasospasm.

Observations linking coronary spasm to coronary atherosclerosis

Brown[91] from Los Angeles, California, reviewed evidence suggesting that coronary arterial spasm is a contributing feature not only in Prinzmetal's variant angina but also in classical angina pectoris, AMI, and sudden coronary death. By use of quantitative angiography and 2 modes of alpha adrenergic stimulation in patients with spontaneous rest angina, vasomotor hyperreactivity was shown to be localized only to the region of a preexisting coronary narrowing by atherosclerotic plaques (Fig. 1-16). These observations support the hypothesis that a dynamic interaction between the histopathologic features of coronary atherosclerosis and normal amounts of coronary smooth muscle shortening accounts for the clinical features in most patients with CAD (Fig. 1-17).

Long-term transtelephonic ECG monitoring in detecting variant angina

To facilitate the outpatient diagnosis of variant angina by documenting transient ST-segment elevation during chest pain, Ginsburg and associates[92]

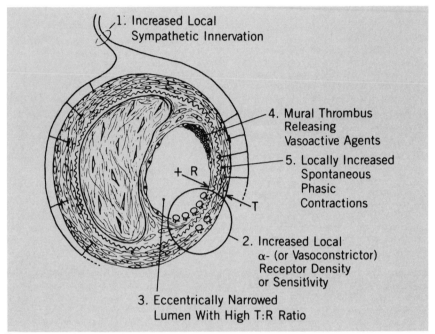

Fig. 1-16. Mechanisms whereby observed hyperreactivity of certain coronary segments in patients with rest angina may be explained. None of these possibilities has been fully confirmed or satisfactorily excluded in terms of their contribution to clinical symptoms. T represents wall thickness; and R, lumen radius from center (+). Reproduced with permission from Brown.[91]

Fig. 1-17. Morphologic spectrum of normal and diseased coronary artery cross-sections. In regions where smooth muscle viability and flexibility are retained, 10% isovolumetric outer circumferential shortening causes dramatic changes in lumen caliber. Size of resting and constricted lumen in each section determines associated anginal syndrome. Reproduced with permission from Brown.[91]

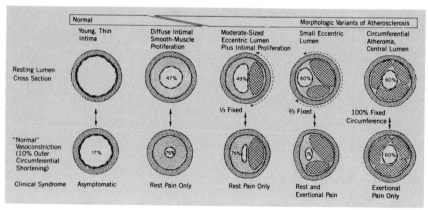

from Stanford, California, evaluated the feasibility of transtelephonic ECG monitoring during angina episodes. Eight patients with known coronary artery spasm underwent simultaneous ambulatory and transtelephonic ECG monitoring during a 24-hour period. Five patients had transient diagnostic ST-segment shifts on both continuous ambulatory and transtelephonic monitoring. Another 8 patients with coronary spasm underwent 24-hour continuous ambulatory monitoring and a separate 14-day period of transtelephonic monitoring. The addition of this longer monitoring period provided diagnostic ST-segment shifts in 3 patients. Thus, transtelephonic monitoring in patients with suspected coronary artery spasm can provide important additional diagnostic information to continuous ambulatory monitoring, particularly in the patient with infrequent or unpredictable chest pain.

Coronary hemodynamic findings during spontaneous angina and variant angina

To define more completely regional coronary hemodynamic changes occurring during spontaneous angina pectoris in patients with variant angina, Feldman and associates[93] from Gainesville, Florida, measured coronary sinus and great vein blood flow (CSF and GCVF) and aortic and LV pressures before and during spontaneous angina in 6 patients with variant angina. During spontaneous angina, ECG in 4 patients showed evidence of transient anterior regional ischemia (ST-T wave changes in I, aV_L, V_{1-6}) and in 2 patients showed evidence of transient posterior regional ischemia (ST-T wave changes in II, III, aV_F). During spontaneous angina, CSF decreased in 5 of 6 patients (27 ± 10 ml/min, $p < 0.05$), as compared with measurements made during a pain-free interval. In all 4 patients with anterior ischemia, GCVF decreased 34 ± 13 ml/min ($p < 0.05$). In the 2 patients with inferior ischemia, GCVF was unchanged, but the difference between CSF and GCVF, an index of posterior regional blood flow, decreased 36 ± 20 ml/min during ischemia. Heart rate was not significantly different during angina, and mean aortic pressure decreased in 3 patients, increased in 2, and was unchanged in 1. LV end-diastolic pressure increased 10 ± 2 mmHg during spontaneous angina ($p < 0.01$). These data provide direct evidence that blood flow to the ischemic region during spontaneous angina is decreased in patients with variant angina, and support the concept that a functionally important decrease in regional myocardial oxygen delivery occurs in certain patients with variant angina coincident with angina and ST-segment and T-wave changes.

Coronary spasm during exercise and effect of verapamil

Exercise-induced angina is usually caused by an imbalance between increased myocardial oxygen demand and blood supply to the myocardium caused by fixed coronary narrowing. Rarely, exertional angina may result from a transient decrease in coronary blood flow due to an increase in coronary vasomotor tone resulting in spasm. Verapamil is effective in preventing spontaneous attacks of angina at rest in patients with coronary artery spasm. Freedman and associates[94] from Sydney, Australia, described 6 patients with coronary spasm documented by angiogram and with fixed coronary narrowings >50% diameter reduction. Each developed angina and ST-segment elevation on exercise testing. Oral verapamil (160–480 mg/day) prevented exercise ischemia in all patients and increased maximal work capacity from 611 ± 250 kpm to 808 ± 160 kpm (p < 0.02). In 2 patients, a relation between the prevention of exercise-provoked ischemia and the plasma concentration of verapamil was demonstrated and, in 1, the relation had a diurnal pattern. Thus, patients with variant angina may develop coronary spasm on effort and they often respond to verapamil.

Clinical course of variant angina with angiographic demonstration of coronary spasm

Coronary artery spasm (CAS) has been demonstrated by coronary angiography with increasing frequency in recent years. Little is known, however, about the clinical course of patients with CAS demonstrated by coronary angiography. Prognosis of patients with variant angina pectoris has been reported as being variable, with a high frequency of serious cardiac complications. Cipriano and associates[95] from Stanford, California, evaluated 25 patients with variant angina not treated with calcium antagonists and followed an average of 2.7 years after angiographic demonstration of spasm: 17 received medical treatment after the demonstration of spasm and 6 underwent coronary artery bypass grafting (CABG). Follow-up indicated that 23 patients are living and 2 have died. Of the 23 survivors, 21 had either no chest pain or markedly reduced symptoms. The demonstration of spasm by angiography was associated with a high frequency of subsequent cardiac complications: AMI (4 patients), cardiac arrest (4 patients), and death (2 patients). Thus, following demonstration of coronary spasm by angiography, major cardiac complications were frequent (11 of 25 patients, 44%); most patients who had an uncomplicated course (11 of 14) had either <50% fixed coronary artery luminal diameter narrowing or CABG; most patients with <50% fixed coronary narrowing (8 of 11) had no major cardiac complications, AMI, or death.

Huckell and associates[96] from Toronto, Canada, studied 18 patients (mean age, 46 years; 12 men, 6 women) with Prinzmetal's angina and followed them an average of 27 months. The mean duration of symptoms before clinical diagnosis was 4 weeks. Four had had a previous AMI and 6 had spontaneous cardiac arrest within 48 hours of diagnosis and hospitalization. At coronary angiography, 10 of the 18 patients had significant CAD, and spasm was demonstrated in 2 of the 10; the remaining 8 patients had angiographically normal coronary arteries and each had spasm demonstrated angiographically. MVP was observed in 8 patients by LV angiography and 7 of them had ST-segment elevation with pain. Of the 10 patients with significant CAD, 6 underwent CABG with good results. Of the remaining patients, 10 were treated with oral isosorbide dinitrate alone or in combination with propranolol, nifedipine, or perhexiline and their symptoms were controlled. Thus, Prinzmetal's angina, with few exceptions, responds well to therapy.

Ergonovine provocative testing for coronary spasm and usefulness in assessing treatment with nifedipine, diltiazem and verapamil

Several studies have demonstrated that administration of ergonovine maleate induces vasoconstriction of 12%–25% in most coronary arteries, and this agent has been used to identify patients with variant angina. Magder and associates[97] from Toronto, Canada, utilized the ergonovine provocative test in 40 patients with chest pain believed to be angina pectoris and in 1 patient with an AMI and angiographically normal coronary arteries. Of the 41 patients, 29 had normal coronary arteries and 12 had mild-to-moderate fixed narrowings. Ergonovine maleate was administered incrementally in total cumulative doses of 0.25 to 1.2 mg. The effect of ergonovine on coronary arterial caliber was determined by comparing the arterial diameter from the angiogram obtained after administration of ergonovine with that from the control. Measurements were made at the same preselected points in both films and also at points of greatest response. Excluding the 3 patients with complete occlusion, the mean reduction in coronary arterial diameter at preselected points was 12 ± 15%. When the points of greatest response were examined, the maximum reduction in coronary arterial diameter was <25% in 13 patients, 25%–50% in 20 patients, and >50% in 8 patients. The patterns of response included complete occlusion in the 3 patients with variant angina, diffuse narrowing in 16, diffuse and focal narrowing in 6, and spasm at the catheter tip in 3. All patients with maximum reductions of >50% in coronary arterial diameter and 6 of those with maximum reductions of 25%–50% had chest pain, but only the 3 with complete occlusion had associated ST-segment changes. Thus, the response in patients with variant angina represents one end of a spectrum of responses to administration of ergonovine. In addition, many patients may have ergonovine-induced chest pain without ECG changes and with only an intermediate degree of coronary arterial spasm.

The administration of ergonovine maleate during coronary arteriography or in the Coronary Care Unit has been considered to be a relatively sensitive diagnostic test for variant angina pectoris due to coronary artery spasm. Ergonovine almost always induces angina with ST-segment elevation and, when this occurs, coronary spasm is invariably found by arteriography. Because the hallmark of coronary spasm is ST-segment elevation on the standard 12-lead ECG, direct visualization of coronary spasm may not be necessary during provocative testing. Ginsburg and associates[98] from Stanford, California, analyzed the results of 61 consecutive outpatient ergonovine provocation tests to determine its safety and efficacy in detecting coronary spasm. Criteria for outpatient testing included: clinical history suggestive of variant angina, noncritical CAD documented by coronary arteriography, normal exercise treadmill test, no symptomatic arrhythmias, and no history of recent AMI. All antianginal medications were gradually discontinued. Ergonovine was given by intravenous bolus at 3-minute intervals in consecutive doses of 0.05, 0.10, and 0.25 mg. A positive test was defined as chest pain accompanied by >0.1 mV ST-segment elevation on standard 12-lead ECG. If pain and ST-segment elevation occurred, intravenous and sublingual NTG were immediately administered for relief of myocardial ischemia. Of the 61 patients studied, 10 had positive tests; there were no complications. Follow-up of the 51 patients with negative test results did not reveal a cardiac etiology for their chest pain. Thus, outpatient ergonovine testing under carefully controlled conditions appears to be a safe and acurate diagnostic test for identifying variant angina pectoris due to coronary spasm in a highly selected population of patients.

Waters and associates[99] from Montreal, Canada studied 27 patients with typical variant angina to evaluate the efficacy of nifedipine, diltiazem, and verapamil in blocking ergonovine-induced episodes of variant angina and to determine if the results of incremental ergonovine testing during treatment correlated with the clinical response. The ergonovine test result was positive (ST segments elevated) in all 27 patients during a control period without medication. During a subsequent treatment period with *nifedipine* (20 mg, every 6 h), the test result converted to negative at the maximal ergonovine dose of 1.4 mg in 11 patients, remained positive at 2 or more ergonovine dose levels higher than those used during the control test in 11 patients, and was unimproved in 5 others. Identical results occurred when ergonovine tests were repeated during treatment with *diltiazem* (120 mg, every 8 h). During treatment with *verapamil* (160 mg, every 8 h), the test result was negative in 8 patients, positive at 2 or more ergonovine dose levels higher than those used during the control test in 10 patients, and positive at a dose similar to that of the control test in the remaining 9.

Variant anginal attacks did not occur during any of the 30 drug treatment periods associated with negative ergonovine tests, occurred during only 1 of the 24 treatment periods associated with a positive test at high ergonovine dose levels (0.2–0.4 mg), and during 12 of the 27 treatment periods with a positive test at 0.1 mg or less ergonovine ($p < 0.001$). During the 7-month (range, 1–15) follow-up period, 14 of 15 patients treated with a drug that had converted the ergonovine test response to negative remained angina free, as compared with only 4 of 12 treated with a drug associated with a persistently positive test ($p < 0.01$).

Thus, nifedipine, diltiazem and verapamil can partially or totally block ergonovine-induced angina and ST elevation in most patients with variant angina. The results of ergonovine testing during treatment with these drugs correlated with the clinical response to therapy.

Histamine provocative testing for coronary spasm

Current hypotheses regarding the pathophysiology of coronary vaso-spasm include abnormalities in sympathetic or parasympathetic neural control, local metabolite abnormalities, and excessive responsiveness to circulatory vasoactive substances, or some combination of these factors. It has been reported that histamine is a potent vasoconstrictor in isolated human coronary arteries. Ginsburg and associates[100] from Stanford, California, gave histamine to 12 patients with nonexertional chest pain and nonobstructive fixed coronary narrowing (<50% luminal diameter narrowing of at least 1 major coronary artery) to investigate its potential role (coronary artery H_1 receptor agonist) in provoking coronary vasospasm. Histamine, at an intravenous dose of 0.5 to 1.0 μg/kg/min, provoked coronary spasm in 4 patients; in 6 patients neither histamine nor ergonovine provoked spasm, and these patients were considered by chronic follow-up evaluation to have a noncardiac etiology of their chest pain. In 1 patient, coronary spasm was provoked with ergonovine, but not by histamine, and 1 ergonovine-positive patient had an equivocally positive histamine result. Pretreatment with *cimetidine* (H_2 receptor antagonist) was necessary to avoid unpleasant side effects of histamine. Thus, histamine should be included among the specific agents capable of inducing coronary vasospasm and it introduces another possible mechanism for the variant angina pectoris syndrome.

Spontaneous remission of variant angina

The chest pain in patients with Prinzmetal's angina is highly variable in intensity and frequency and its course is variable. Girotti and associates[101] from Buenos Aires, Argentina, described 4 patients with variant angina in whom total remission of the anginal pain was documented during follow-up for 7 months, 4 years, 5 years, and 15 years, respectively. Thus, spontaneous and complete recovery may occur in variant angina.

Effect of diltiazem

Pepine and associates[102] from Gainesville, Florida, studied the effects of diltiazem on the frequency of angina and nitroglycerin (NTG) consumption in 12 patients with variant angina (rest pain with ST-segment elevation). Either diltiazem in 2 dosage schedules (120 mg/day and 240 mg/day), or placebo was administered in a randomized, double-blind program over 10 weeks. Significant decreases in anginal frequency and NTG consumption were observed when diltiazem treatment periods were compared with placebo periods. Furthermore, when placebo periods following diltiazem were compared with placebo periods following placebo, significant "carry-over" effect with respect to reduced anginal frequency was observed. No patient had an increase in anginal frequency or in NTG consumption on diltiazem, as compared with placebo. No "rebound effects" or changes in BP or heart rate were observed. One patient complained of dry mouth on diltiazem. These findings, although based on a limited number of patients, suggest that diltiazem is effective in decreasing anginal frequency and NTG consumption in patients with variant angina. These encouraging results warrant evaluation of diltiazem in a larger patient population over a longer period of time.

Effect of verapamil

To assess the efficacy and safety of verapamil in variant angina pectoris, Johnson and associates[103] from Dallas, Texas, studied 16 patients in a double-blind, randomized trial of 9 months' duration. During treatment with verapamil, the frequency of angina fell substantially (13 ± 26 chest pains per week with placebo, 2 ± 3 pains per week with verapamil, mean ± S.D.; $p < 0.01$), as did the use of nitroglycerin tablets (14 ± 34 tablets per week with placebo, 2 ± 3 tablets per week with verapamil; p < 0.05). The number of hospitalizations for clinical instability was significantly lower with verapamil (p < 0.01). The number of episodes of transient ST-segment deviation during treatment with verapamil was reduced (33 ± 39 deviations per week with placebo, 8 ± 12 deviations per week with verapamil; p < 0.01). Verapamil caused no side effects that necessitated either a reduction in dosage or a discontinuation. Ambulatory ECG monitoring assessed objectively the response to verapamil in 6 patients[104] (Fig. 1-18). Thus, verapamil is safe and effective in patients with variant angina.

Freeman and associates[105] from Los Angeles, California, studied the clinical effects of verapamil in 7 patients with recurrent rest angina from vasospasm. All 7 patients had rapid (within 24 hours) and complete (without recurrence of chest pain) chronic salutary response to oral verapamil therapy.

To determine the efficacy and safety of oral verapamil in patients with rest angina pectoris admitted to a coronary care unit, Mehta and associates[106] from Gainesville, Florida, performed a double-blind, placebo-controlled trial in 15 patients who had at least 2 episodes of chest pain associated with ST-T changes per 24 hours during a single-blind, placebo phase (day 1). Patients were then randomized to receive either placebo or verapamil (80 mg, every 6 h) on day 2. The protocol was designed so that those who did not respond to the placebo (nonresponders) received verapamil (80 mg, every 6 h), whereas verapamil nonresponders received increased doses (120

Fig. 1-18. *Left:* Number of episodes of chest pain per 24 h. *Right:* Number of episodes of ST-segment deviation per 24 h before and after institution of verapamil administration in 6 patients. Each line represents data obtained from 1 patient; mean ± SD depicted on either side of lines. Note both number of pains per 24 h and number of episodes of ST-segment deviation per 24 h were reduced sharply by verapamil administration. Reproduced with permission from Johnson et al.[104]

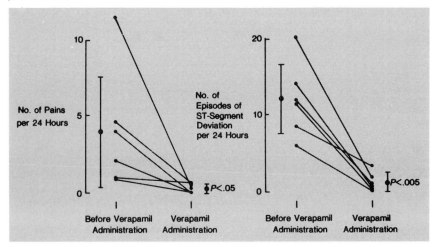

mg, every 6 h) on day 3. Those who did respond (responders) continued to receive their medication. Similar action was taken on day 4, depending on chest pain frequency and clinical evaluation. The study drug was unblinded on day 4. At the end of the 4-day period, 13 patients were receiving verapamil (9 patients, 80 mg every 6 h, and 4 patients, 120 mg every 6 h) and all but 1 were responders. One patient received placebo all through the period of the study and also was considered to be a responder. In the remaining 1 patient, evidence of myocardial necrosis developed after he received a single dose of verapamil (80 mg on day 2). Except for a prolongation of P-R interval in 2 patients while taking verapamil, no side effects were observed. Oral verapamil reduces episodes of myocardial ischemia in most patients with rest angina.

Effect of nifedipine

To determine whether calcium-flux blockade with nifedipine blunts coronary vasospasm, Tiefenbrunn and associates[107] from St. Louis, Missouri, evaluated 4 patients with angiographically demonstrable coronary arterial spasm in the absence of significant fixed coronary arterial stenosis before and after treatment with nifedipine. After initial coronary arteriography, ergonovine was administered in successive doses of 0.05, 0.1, and (when necessary) 0.2 mg intravenously at 3-minute intervals. Three patients had symptomatic high-grade focal coronary arterial spasm with ECG changes, and the fourth exhibited asymptomatic 60% constriction of the LAD. A maximal ergonovine challenge was repeated 30 minutes later, after each patient had been pretreated with 20 mg nifedipine sublingually. Under these conditions, no patient had chest pain or ECG changes. Furthermore, neither focal nor diffuse coronary arterial spasm was demonstrable angiographically after the second challenge. Thus, in each patient, a single dose of nifedipine precluded the angiographic expression of ergonovine-provoked coronary arterial spasm.

Nifedipine also is highly beneficial in rest angina due to *fixed*, severe (14 patients) coronary arterial narrowing, as demonstrated by Moses and associates[108] from Philadelphia, Pennsylvania, who gave this drug to 19 patients with chest discomfort refractory to propranolol and to oral or topical nitrates given to tolerance. The addition of nifedipine (30–120 mg daily) abolished rest angina in 14 patients, decreased its frequency in 2, and had no effect in 3 patients. Five of 7 patients on long-term nifedipine (mean, 6 ± 3 months) remained free of rest pain. Of 7 patients who had the nifedipine dose decreased or discontinued, 5 had recurrent rest angina.

Coronary artery bypass grafting for variant angina pectoris (without obstructive CAD)

Patients with variant angina pectoris refractory to medical therapy pose a difficult management problem. Sussman and associates[109] from Philadelphia, Pennsylvania, described 2 patients with variant angina who had focal spasm in the coronary arteries with fixed obstructions of <20% of the luminal diameter. Ischemic episodes were accompanied by malignant ventricular arrhythmias and complete heart block. Symptoms were refractory to intensive medical management with nitrates and calcium blocking agents in 1 patient and with nitrates in the other, who was treated before calcium blockers were available. A bypass graft was placed distal to the area of focal spasm and the native artery was ligated proximally in each patient. Both patients are asymptomatic 24 and 66 months after surgery and neither takes antianginal medications regularly. This surgical approach, obviously, should be considered only if therapy to control life-threatening ischemic symptoms with nitrates and calcium blocking agents fails.

Coronary spasm in the denervated transplanted human heart

Although the underlying mechanism of coronary spasm has remained poorly understood, the autonomic nervous system has been implicated. Buda and associates[110] from Stanford, California, demonstrated for the first time that coronary arterial spasm can occur in the transplanted denervated human heart. They reported coronary spasm in a 43-year-old man 2 years after he had received a cardiac transplant. Provocative pharmacologic testing suggested functional denervation of the patient's heart. Thus, autonomic innervation of the heart is not essential for coronary spasm, and circulating catecholamines and/or metabolic or hormonal products may play an important role.

PERCUTANEOUS TRANSLUMINAL CORONARY ANGIOPLASTY

Medical College of Virginia experience

Percutaneous transluminal coronary angioplasty (PTCA) was developed by Gruntzig, who initiated the clinical application of this technique in 1977. Although several medical centers now utilize the procedure, few reports of detailed clinical experience with PTCA have appeared. Thus, important questions need to be answered concerning patient selection, clinical factors that influence early and late results, the frequency of complications, and recurrence of symptomatic CAD.

The experience at the Medical College of Virginia in Richmond, Virginia, in 25 patients and 29 vessels during a 12-month period was reported by Cowley and associates.[111] In 6 additional patients scheduled for PTCA, the procedure was cancelled when repeat angiography identified progression to occlusion, coronary spasm, or other adverse factors not previously apparent. PTCA was successful in 14 (56%) of 25 patients and in 18 (62%) of 29 vessels; success was associated with symptomatic improvement in all patients, and by exercise testing and/or myocardial RNA. Beneficial results were particularly evident with LAD narrowings of <90% in diameter. One peripheral arterial complication occurred and no patients required emergency surgery. Although coronary dissection was detected angiographically in 4 patients and evidence of coronary spasm was present in 3 patients after PTCA, neither was accompanied by untoward clinical events. Multivessel dilation in 3 patients was initially successful, but symptoms returned in 2 during follow-up. Restenosis developed in 3 of 14 patients (21%) after 3 months. These authors concluded that the specific vessel attempted and the severity of the CAD influence the likelihood of PTCA success, the infrequently induced coronary dissection or spasm does not necessarily represent a serious complication, and angiography repeated in preparation for PTCA identified a significant minority of patients who are no longer candidates for the technique.

Mayo Clinic experience

In the first year of the use of PTCA at the Mayo Clinic, it was applied to 34 selected patients whose severe angina pectoris was related to a single, high-grade narrowing. The outcome of the dilations in the 34 patients was summarized by Vlietstra and associates[112] from Rochester, Minnesota. Successful dilation (stenotic diameter widened by 40% or more) was achieved in 22 patients (65%). Early postangioplasty assessment indicated relief of angina in all but 1 patient who had coronary spasm that was responsive to medication. The median hospital stay was 3 days. Failure of PTCA in the remaining 12 patients was usually due to an inability to manipulate the balloon catheter across the stenotic segment; 11 of them had coronary artery bypass grafting (CABG) immediately after the attempted angioplasty. There were no deaths, but 3 patients sustained a transmural AMI. This initial experience indicates that PTCA is a relatively safe and a frequently effective method of relieving coronary stenosis in selected patients with symptomatic CAD.

Providence, Rhode Island, experience in unstable angina pectoris

Williams and associates[113] from Providence, Rhode Island, utilized PTCA in 17 patients with unstable angina pectoris whose chest pain was not satisfactorily relieved by vigorous medical therapy, including 10 patients with refractory in-hospital angina. PTCA was judged successful in 13 patients and resulted in decreased coronary diameter narrowing from 80% to 34% and in a trans-stenotic pressure gradient reduced from 69 mmHg to 23 mmHg. Regional coronary blood flow (CBF) and myocardial metabolism were assessed at rest and during pacing tachycardia in 6 patients with LAD stenosis. Before PTCA, rapid pacing caused neither an increase in regional CBF nor a decline in coronary vascular resistance; myocardial lactate extraction fell, including a shift from aerobic to anaerobic metabolism. Following PTCA, however, rapid pacing resulted in increased regional CBF, a decreased coronary vascular resistance, and a preservation of aerobic metabolism. Following PTCA, successfully dilated patients had marked relief of anginal symptoms, an increase in functional capacity, and objective exercise ECG and thallium scintigraphic evidence of relief of previously ischemic myocardium. This clinical investigation demonstrates that PTCA, when combined with medical therapy, can be performed safely and successfully in selected patients with unstable angina pectoris refractory to medical therapy; it also indicates that PTCA deserves further study as a new therapeutic alternative in this condition.

Morphologic studies

Morphologic studies of coronary arteries in patients who have undergone PTCA are rare. Block and associates[114] from Boston, Massachusetts, and San Francisco, California, described changes in 2 patients who had undergone PTCA and in 1 patient who had undergone percutaneous transluminal angioplasty of the femoral artery. The changes found in these arteries subjected to angioplasty in their 3 patients were similar to those found in coronary arteries of animals that had undergone angioplasty, namely, *superficial plaque disruption* and *intimal splitting*. The disruption and splitting of the atherosclerotic plaque exposes the connective tissue of the plaque to blood elements that favor platelet deposition and thrombus formation. The authors raise the possibility of treating patients who have undergone angioplasty with vasodilators and antiplatelet agents thereafter. Although it seems logical to attribute the splits and/or disruptions of atherosclerotic plaques to the angioplastic procedure in the patients described, the method of studying the arteries in the 3 patients described was not mentioned; artifacts, tears and splits, as illustrated in their 3 photomicrographs, can also be observed in coronary arteries of patients who have not undergone angioplastic procedures. The authors do not include control coronary arteries or femoral arteries in patients who did not have angioplastic procedures.

Baughman and associates[115] from Boston, Massachusetts, performed coronary angiography and coronary arterial balloon angioplasty in 12 human hearts at necropsy. The effect of angioplasty was determined by follow-up coronary angiography, as well as by gross and microscopic inspection of the coronary arteries dilated. Fifty-four dilations were performed in 24 coronary arteries. Angiographically, 50 of the 54 dilations resulted in a mean ($\pm$ standard deviation) increase in luminal diameter ranging from 1.9 ± 0.9–2.7 ± 0.8 mm. Failure to increase luminal size was usually related to a predilation coronary diameter greater than that of the inflated angioplasty balloon. Dilation resulted in mural disruption with intimal or medial tears, or both, in 65% of the arteries dilated. Disruption was more frequent in arteries with atherosclerosis and calcific deposits. The mechanism of luminal enlargement in coronary angioplasty may be focal damage to the arterial wall with intimal or medial splitting, as opposed to the plaque compression initially suggested.

Usefulness in dilating narrowed or totally obstructed aortocoronary conduits

PTCA has been utilized to dilate severely narrowed native coronary arteries in several hundred patients since this procedure was first introduced. Dilation of severely narrowed or totally occluded aortocoronary bypass conduits by percutaneous angioplasty, however, has been infrequently employed. Ford and associates[116] from Pittsburgh, Pennsylvania, utilized PTCA to dilate 6 severely narrowed conduits and to provide lumens in 3 totally occluded conduits. Of the 9 grafts, 8 were successfully dilated. The aortocoronary conduits that were dilated had been in place from 5 months to 7 years (median, 3 years). Thus, this study demonstrates the usefulness of PTCA to relieve severe narrowing or total occlusion in some aortocoronary saphenous vein conduits.

Overview of PTCA

Bourassa[117] from Montreal, Canada, summarized the current status of PTCA. Although far from innocuous and to be practiced only by thoroughly experienced angiographers, it is relatively simple. It requires the use of a guiding coronary catheter located at the ostium of the coronary artery and of a double-lumen dilation catheter with a distensible nonelastic balloon that is passed into the guiding catheter and advanced through the stenotic segment of the artery. The balloon is mechanically inflated and deflated rapidly, usually several times, while it is in the stenotic segment. As a means of reducing the risk of coronary thrombosis and of restenosis, the patient usually receives antiplatelet agents for 2 or 3 days before the dilation, heparin and low molecular weight dextran during the procedure, and oral anticoagulants or antiplatelet drugs for 6 to 9 months after the dilation. In addition, for the prevention of coronary spasm, nitroglycerin and calcium blocking agents are given before and during the procedure.

Candidates for PTCA should fulfill the following criteria to minimize the risk of technical failures and complications: 1) symptoms must justify coronary artery bypass grafting (CABG), 2) the stenosis must be single, proximal, discrete, non-calcific (angiographic), segmental ($\leqslant 1-1.5$ cm), and severe (70%–95% diameter narrowing of the arterial lumen). In such selected patients, dilation is successful about 65% of the time. Most successfully treated patients have complete relief of angina and increased exercise tolerance. Their hospital stay is brief (a few days) and they can resume normal physical activities soon after dismissal from the hospital. Vlietstra and co-workers[112] defined successful dilation as a 40% or more increase in the normal luminal diameter. Other studies defined success as a 10%–20% or greater increase in luminal diameter and an increase of 10–20 mmHg or more in the pressure in the distal coronary artery. Thus, their results are probably slightly better than those reported by others.

The clinical findings are quite similar in the various reports: roughly 80% of the patients are men; the mean age is 51 years; the frequency of prior AMI is approximately 20%; the EF is almost invariably normal; and the distribution of coronary narrowings in patients in whom dilation was attempted is roughly as follows: LAD 65%; right 25%; LC 5%; and LM 5%. The duration of symptoms does not appear to be related to the success of PTCA. In all studies, the percentage of segments successfully dilated among those in whom dilation was attempted was roughly similar for the LAD, right, and LM coronary arteries (60%–70%) and lower for the LC ($<50\%$).

Failure of PTCA occurs in roughly 33% of patients and is usually attributable to the following factors: 1) inability to pass the stenotic area as a result of such anatomic factors as tortuosity or sharp angulation of the artery, tightness of the stenosis, or eccentricity of the lesion (roughly 70% of the failures); 2) inability to dilate the stenotic region once it has been passed, because of rigidity of the lesion (10%), and 3) local complications (20%). The complications include acute coronary occlusions and acute coronary dissections, with about equal frequency, and requiring emergency CABG in approximately 8% of patients. There have been few hospital deaths after PTCA. The NHLBI registry reports a hospital mortality of 1%. The frequency of AMI ranges from 3%–9% and is usually associated with acute coronary occlusions. Vascular complications requiring surgery occur in 1% of the patients. Restenosis during the early follow-up of patients with initially successful PTCA may occur, usually during the first 3 months after the procedure; it happens in approximately 20% of patients. A second PTCA was successful in some patients, but failed in others, and most patients required CABG.

In summary, PTCA is an investigational procedure that must be limited to patients with symptoms justifying CABG and in whom a single coronary artery is suitable for dilation. This combination is realized in <10% of patients who are candidates for CABG. The risk of the procedure is roughly similar to that of CABG for these selected patients. The success rate 3–6 months after the procedure is approximately 50%. The primary indication for this procedure is relief of symptoms, inasmuch as the expected life span with medical therapy in these selected cases is excellent and is not likely to be improved by PTCA or CABG. A definitive advantage of PTCA, as compared with CABG, may be a lower cost in terms of suffering, emotional strain, hospital expenses, and loss of income.

LASER REDUCTION IN SIZE OF CORONARY ATHEROSCLEROTIC PLAQUES

The clinical use of laser energy in medicine has been largely limited to thermocoagulation and excision of pathologic tissue. The potential application of laser phototherapy, however, for the dissolution of atherosclerotic vascular obstruction has not been previously known. Lee and associates[118] from Davis and Sacramento, California, studied the effects of several laser sources on human cadaver coronary arteriosclerotic narrowings. Intact coronary arteries with obstructing atheromatous plaques were extracted at necropsy from patients who had died of CAD. The involved arteries were sectioned transversely and subjected to laser radiation throughout a wide spectrum of specific power intensities and time exposures. The argon-ion vaporization beam strikingly affected patency in fibrous, lipoid, and calcified plaque obstructions. Clinical investigations are now in progress to extend this new therapeutic modality to patients with obstructions in the coronary and other vascular beds.

CORONARY ARTERY BYPASS GRAFTING (CABG)

Magnitude of CABG in the USA

On April 21–23, 1981, the National Center for Health Care Technology (NCHCT), in collaboration with the National Heart, Lung, and Blood Institute (NHLBI), convened a Technology Assessment Forum to examine a wide range of economic, ethical, legal and social considerations regarding coronary artery bypass grafting (CABG) in the USA. A summary of the discussion of that forum was published in the October 9, 1981, issue of JAMA[119] and the document is available from the NCHCT, DHHS, Public Health Service, Rockville, Maryland 20857. The economic impact of CABG in the USA alone is enormous. From 1967–1980, 500,000 CABG operations were performed and, in 1980 alone, 100,000 operations were performed. These operations were performed in at least 600 USA hospitals. The cost per operation, including hospital and professional charges, in 1980 ranged from $11,000–$25,000, including an estimated average surgical fee of $3,000. Thus, the cost in 1980 of CABG operations was about $2 billion. The diagnostic and surgical management of CAD patients in the USA now accounts for nearly 2% of the total health care budget. About 300,000 coronary arteriograms were performed in the USA in 1980 at a total cost of $600–$900 million. About 40% of patients now having coronary arteriography will shortly thereafter undergo CABG. Cardiac radionuclide scanning is estimated to cost in 1981 between $450–$600 million and an estimated 1.5 million procedures will be performed. And, finally, a social note: although the clinical prevalence of CAD in the USA is believed to be similar in blacks and whites, about 97% of patients having CABG in the USA are white.

Predictors of operative and late survival

The risk for CABG surgery performed in 15 major medical centers in the USA and Canada on 6,630 patients during the last half of the 1970's was summarized by Kennedy and associates.[120] The overall operative mortality was 2% (range, 0.3%–6%) in the 15 centers. In the subgroup of 509 patients with additional operative cardiac procedures, the operative mortality was 8% for aneurysmectomy, 8% for plication, and 24% for mitral valve replacement. Twenty clinical and angiographic characteristics were correlated with operative mortality. The operative mortality was 2% for men and 4.5% for women, and significantly higher in every age group for women-vs-men. No increased risk was produced from prior AMI or angina unrelated to exertion, but CHF did increase risk. Mortality with 1-, 2-, or 3-vessel disease was 1.4%, 2%, and 4%, respectively. LM coronary stenosis was the indication for CABG in 1,019 patients and the operative mortality ranged from 1.6% for mild stenosis to 25% for severe stenosis. Operative mortality also varied significantly with the EF (2%, ⩾0.50 and 7% ⩽ 0.19). The operative mortality was 2% for elective surgery, 3.5% for urgent surgery, and 11% for emergency surgery. Of 30 patients with LM coronary stenosis having emergency CABG, 40% died. Although the overall mortality was low, the investigators constructed subsets with enough patients so that the characteristics associated with increased operative mortality did emerge. The age and sex of patients with symptoms of severe unstable angina, CHF, distribution of coronary lesions, ventricular performance, and timing of CABG have a significant bearing on operative mortality.

The National Heart, Lung, and Blood Institute Coronary Artery Surgery Study (CASS) was summarized in the American Heart Association Monograph Number 79, which was Part II of the June 1981 issue.[121] This monograph is too large to summarize here, but this study provides a tremendous amount of information both about the patients undergoing CABG and the procedure itself.

DeRouen and associates[122] of the Seattle, Washington, Heart Watch compared survival of medically and surgically treated CAD patients in subgroups to determine those patients most likely to benefit from CABG after an average 5.5 year follow-up. Of the 2,616 patients analyzed, a statistically beneficial effect of CABG on survival was found in patients with significant 2- and 3-vessel narrowing, EF >30%, age ≥ 48 years, and without a precordial murmur, resting ventricular arrhythmia, significant (>50%) LM coronary narrowing, cardiomegaly, CHF, or diuretic therapy. Patient subgroups defined by the presence or absence of prior AMI or unstable angina and New York Heart Association functional class I-II -vs- III-IV all showed beneficial effects from CABG. The occurrence of significant effects of CABG in patients with both 2- and 3-vessel narrowing is a change from previous reports from the same group that indicated a significant surgical effect only in patients with 2-vessel disease. This excellent analysis of the effects of surgical treatment on CAD is the type of study that provides answers to the questions concerning surgical treatment of various subsets of patients with CHD.

Women undergoing CABG do so at a higher risk and achieve poorer symptomatic results than do men. Douglas and associates[123] from Atlanta, Georgia, compared surgical results in 412 pairs of men and women matched by computer for age, preoperative angina classification, and number of narrowed arteries. The operative mortality was similar in matched patients. Women, however, had smaller distal coronary arteries, a higher frequency of diabetes mellitus, a significantly higher frequency of systemic hypertension, and a higher rate of incomplete revascularization and reduced graft patency than did men. The cumulative survival for men and women at 42 months was 92%. At late follow-up, more men than women were asymptomatic (70% -vs- 62% [p < 0.001]) and men achieved higher activity levels. Saphenous vein graft patency was also higher in men (86% -vs- 74% [p < 0.001]). Thus, the quality of long-term symptomatic results of CABG in women is less favorable than in men because women have smaller arteries, anastomoses are less satisfactory, and flow is lower than in men. Although significantly fewer women than men were asymptomatic after bypass, over 90%, nevertheless, were significantly improved.

Knapp and co-workers[124] from Atlanta, Georgia, analyzed 121 consecutive patients >70 years of age who underwent CABG. Univariant and multivariant analyses showed that patients >70 had a higher frequency of unstable angina, CHF, and cardiomegaly, more severe coronary narrowing, and a higher frequency of severe narrowing of the LM coronary artery (29% -vs- 15%) than did younger patients. The hospital mortality was similar in patients >70 and <70 (1% -vs- 1.6%). Postoperatively, however, the group >70 had a higher frequency of stroke, supraventricular tachycardia, transient psychosis, complete heart block, intraaortic balloon pump usage, and pulmonary embolism. Survival at 36 months, however, was identical in both age groups. The only contraindication to CABG in the older age group, according to these authors, was severe calcification of the ascending aorta.

Berry and associates[125] from Baton Rouge, Louisiana, performed CABG in 65 patients >70 years old, with an operative mortality of 3%. They, too, noted a higher frequency of arrhythmias and mental confusion in the postoperative period, and a longer average hospitalization (14 days) than in younger patients. The long-term survival and symptom-free period postoperatively was excellent. Thus, age per se is not a contraindication for CABG, provided that ventricular function is satisfactory and noncardiac disease is minimal.

Long-term follow-up

Greene and associates[126] from Buffalo, New York, reported survival of various subsets of 1,051 coronary patients having CABG operations from 1973–1977. They compared their results with hypothetical subsets of the USA population, age and sex matched, for 1975. Although not as good as prospective randomized studies, this method provides an independently derived reference point. Of the surgical group, the estimated 5-year survival was 94%. No significant difference from the general population was observed at the 95% confidence interval for 1-, 2-, and 3-vessel or LM coronary disease. Calculation of data of stable and unstable angina against the US population likewise was similar. Although the difference was not statistically significant, survival in females after CABG was considerably lower than that for males, when compared with the hypothetical USA population. The same held true when patients were divided according to the number of coronary arteries narrowed, age, number of arteries grafted, history of AMI, EF, and presence of stable angina.

Phillips and associates[127] from Boston, Massachusetts, analyzed 335 patients without significant LM coronary narrowing or recent AMI who underwent isolated CABG in 1974 or 1975. The hospital mortality was 2% and the 4-year predicted survival was 94%. Neither the preoperative presence or absence of a progressive or unstable anginal pattern, the extent of coronary narrowing, or the LV EF predicted postoperative survival. Of the 25 patients whose EF was ≤30%, none died in the perioperative period or within 36 months of follow-up, giving a predicted 4-year survival rate of 82%. Of these 25 patients, 24 were operated upon because of angina that was unstable in 75%. This study shows that patients with a severely reduced EF should not be refused CABG if symptoms of angina are severe and predominate over symptoms of CHF.

Role of CABG in management of unstable angina pectoris manifested by pain at rest

Although there have been many papers on unstable angina, few have been limited to analysis of patients in whom the instability was characterized entirely by chest pain at rest. Brooks and associates[128] from London, England, analyzed 99 patients admitted to the coronary care unit (CCU) with chest pain at rest without ECG or enzymatic evidence of AMI. They followed the 99 patients from 9–26 months (mean, 14) after their admission to the CCU: 91 underwent cardiac catheterization, most during the period of initial hospitalization, and 78 had fixed coronary arterial narrowing (involving only 1 of the 3 major arteries in 13 patients, 2 arteries in 23, and 3 arteries in 42 patients). Of the 78 patients, 6 (8%) also had severe (>70% diameter reduction) narrowing of the LM coronary artery. Ten (11%) of the 91 patients who had coronary angiography had normal coronary arteries and 3 others had documented coronary spasm without fixed narrowings. In 54 patients, the chest pain disappeared on medical management within 24 hours, and in the other 45 patients, the pain lasted >24 hours. Of the 54 patients in whom the pain subsided in 24 hours, 17 underwent CABG and of the 45 patients in whom the pain lasted >24 hours, 34 underwent CABG. The authors recommended urgent coronary angiography in any patient with rest angina in whom the pain lasts >24 hours and, if the angiogram reveals suitable coronary arterial anatomy, urgent CABG.

Factors influencing patency of aortocoronary conduits

The venous and arterial autografts used for CABG must remain patent to provide long-term benefits, freedom from AMI, and good survival. Mayer and associates[129] from Minneapolis, Minnesota, performed a prospective, randomized trial of platelet aggregation inhibitors in 113 patients undergoing CABG from 1973–1975: 66 control patients had 27 internal mammary artery (IMA) grafts and 93 controls had saphenous vein grafts; 47 treatment patients had 18 IMA grafts and 75 had saphenous vein grafts. The treated patients received 1,300 mg of aspirin and 100 mg dipyridamole daily, and the control patients received neither drug. The patients returned 3–6 months after CABG for repeat angiography: 98/120 grafts (82%) were patent in the control group and 87/93 grafts (94%) were patent in the treatment group (p < 0.02). Of the 45 IMA grafts in both groups, only 1 was occluded (98% patency). In the control group, 72/93 vein grafts (77%) were patent, and in the treatment group, 69/75 (92%) were patent (p < 0.02). Thus, a significant improvement in early patency of saphenous vein grafts was observed in the group treated with aspirin and dipyridamole.

Crosby and associates[130] from Charlottesville, Virginia, in 50 consecutive patients, found the EF, degree of coronary arterial stenosis, and the source of the saphenous vein conduit (from the upper or lower leg) to have no influence on graft patency, but straight grafts had a 96% patency and sequential grafts had only an 80% patency.

Kamath and colleagues[131] from Milwaukee, Wisconsin, analyzed patency of endarterectomized and bypassed coronary arteries in 90 patients who had undergone endarterectomy during a 1-year follow-up period, as revealed by postoperative angiographic and flow studies. Early (<1 month) patency of grafts in endarterectomized arteries was 103/118 (87%) and, in conventional vein grafts in the same patients, 217/233 (93%). Myocardial blood flow, determined by use of zenon-133 with isoproterenol-induced stress, was normal in the endarterectomized arteries. The perioperative AMI rate in patients who received endarterectomy was 3%, similar to that in the non-endarterectomized patient group.

De Rijbel and Schipperheyn[132] from Leiden, The Netherlands, correlated the long-term patency of vein grafts with intraoperative electromagnetic flow measurements. They performed angiography postoperatively in 55 patients with 102 grafts and made flow measurements during operation. By the criteria of acceptable flow pattern analysis, only 6 grafts had abnormally low flow immediately after implantation but, 6 months later, 30/102 grafts (29%) had become occluded. The mean flow levels of the grafts averaged 51 ± 3 ml/min, and no significant difference was observed between grafts that were occluded and those that were patent in the postoperative period. Thus, graft flow measurements by electromagnetic flow meters during operation after implantation of bypass grafts had limited value for predicting long-term graft patency.

CABG of arteries narrowed less than 50%

The predictability of progressive CAD has stimulated a trend toward the grafting of coronary arteries with <50% diameter reduction. To evaluate the patency of these grafts and the effect on the native circulation, Cosgrove and associates[133] from Cleveland, Ohio, reviewed findings in 92 patients with 302 potentially graftable coronary arteries. Of the 226 bypassed arteries, 100 had <50% diameter reduction. All 92 patients were recatheterized postoperatively, 45 routinely and 47 for symptoms of myocardial ischemia. Patency rates were similar for grafts placed to arteries with <50% and >50% stenosis (Table 1-2). No patency rate differences were recorded for vein grafts to the right or LAD coronary arteries. Progression of atherosclerosis (defined as at least a 20% decrease in diameter) occurred in 63% of 100 grafted vessels with <50% stenosis and in 52% of 93 vessels with >50% stenosis. There was a higher frequency of progression in those native arteries in which the conduit was a saphenous vein than in those with an internal mammary artery conduit (67% -vs- 39%). These authors concluded that patency of grafts to arteries with <50% stenosis is similar to that made to arteries with >50% stenosis, the internal mammary artery has a higher patency rate and less progressive atherosclerosis than does the saphenous vein, and for arteries with <50% stenosis, progressive luminal narrowing is greater in grafted than in nongrafted arteries.

P-wave duration as a predictor of atrial fibrillation or flutter after CABG

Atrial fibrillation (AF) and flutter (AFl) occur frequently after CABG. To identify patients at highest risk, Buxton and Josephson[134] from Philadelphia,

TABLE 1-2. *Graft patency rates (%).*

CONDUIT	<50% STENOSIS	>50% STENOSIS
Saphenous vein	77	78
Internal mammary artery	92	96
Overall	79	81
Progression in grafted arteries	63	52

Pennsylvania, measured P-wave duration on a 3-channel ECG in 99 patients undergoing CABG. An intraatrial conduction defect (IACD), defined by conventional criteria as a single standard lead P wave >110 ms, was present in 42 patients. They also identified an IACD by measuring the total P-wave duration (TPWD) from the simultaneous 3-channel recording of the standard leads (IACD-TPWD). Sustained AF-AFl, >1 hour, occurred in 29/99 patients. Of the 29 patients with AF-AFl, 24 had IACD-TPWD. The mean total P-wave duration of patients with and without AF-AFl was 126 ms and 116 ms, respectively (p < 0.001). The mean P-wave duration measured conventionally (ECG lead 2) was 114 ms in the patients with AF-AFl and 110 ms in patients without AF-AFl. An isoelectric interval (IEI), derived by subtracting the ECG lead 2 P-wave duration from the total P-wave duration measured from 3 simultaneous limb leads, was 5.9 ms for patients without AF-AFl -vs- 12.4 ms for patients with AF-AFl (p < 0.001). Of the patients with IACD-TPWD, 24/64 (38%) had AF-AFl; of the patients without IACD-TPWD, 5/35 (14%) had AF-AFl (p < 0.05). The mean ages, number of bypass grafts, preoperative propranolol dose, and prevalence of digoxin use were similar for patients with and without AF-AFl. The presence of IACD-TPWD is a sensitive, but non-specific, predictor of AF-AFl after CABG, and a prolonged IEI enhances the specificity.

Comparison of CABG performed 1969–1973 with that performed 1974–1979

Rahimtoola and associates[135] summarized observations in 2,199 patients who underwent CABG from 1969–1979. The patients were divided into 2 groups: group A, 439 patients undergoing CABG from 1969–1973 and group B, 1,760 patients undergoing CABG from 1974–1979. The operative mortality was 4% for group A and 1% for group B. The 4-year survival was 89% for group A and 93% for group B. The difference between the relative 4-year survival rates of groups A and B was 6%, and the lower operative mortality would account for only 2.6%. The authors concluded that the results of CABG have improved because of 1) lower operative mortality and 2) other factors that cannot be precisely defined at the present time but probably are the long-term result of better and more complete operative and perioperative techniques.

Coronary spasm after CABG

Buxton and colleagues[136] from Philadelphia, Pennsylvania, described 6 patients who had CABG for angina pectoris due to atherosclerotic CAD; each developed sudden circulatory collapse and recurrent ST-segment elevation soon after operation. Clinical, angiographic, and anatomic findings and responses to therapy suggested that the myocardial ischemia was due to coronary spasm in a nonatherosclerotic, nonbypassed artery. All 6 had normal or noncritical luminal irregularities of a dominant right coronary artery and >75% occlusion of a major left coronary artery. Right coronary spasm, demonstrated angiographically in 1 patient, was reversed after intracoronary infusion of nitroglycerin. A patent right coronary artery was found at necropsy in a second patient. Three patients died despite intravenous NTG. Two patients who had been unresponsive to intravenous NTG recovered after direct infusion of NTG into the right coronary artery. Nifedipine was used in 5 of the 6 and intraaortic balloon counterpulsation in 3. All 3 survivors received NTG for 24 hours and nifedipine indefinitely. None in the late postoperative period has had a recurrence of myocardial ischemia or AMI, ST-segment elevation, or chest pain. Thus, coronary spasm may develop soon after CABG and intracoronary infusion of NTG, as well as of calcium blocking agents, and intraaortic balloon counterpulsation may be useful in this setting. Performing coronary angiography in this setting is controversial, because the patients are critically ill, but spasm in both grafted and ungrafted coronary arteries after CABG may account for a small percent of unexplained sudden deaths after CABG.

Although spasm of a native coronary artery has been well documented, spasm of a substitute coronary artery, namely a saphenous vein conduit used between aorta and native coronary artery, had not been documented until Victor and associates[137] from Philadelphia, Pennsylvania, documented by angiography spasm in a saphenous vein between aorta and native coronary artery in a 66-year-old man who began having angina pectoris again about 2 months after CABG. Repeat cardiac catheterization disclosed spontaneous severe narrowing of this sequential saphenous vein venous graft from aorta to posterior descending coronary artery and left obtuse marginal coronary artery. The spasm decreased the luminal diameter by 80%–90% just proximal to its anastomosis to the major marginal branch of the LC. The narrowing was considered to be spasm because it was completely resolved during subsequent injection of contrast material after administration of NTG. The authors speculated that spasm of a venous graft may play a significant role in the early development of AMI, graft closure, or recurrence of angina pectoris after initially successful CABG when venous grafts remain patent.

Cardiac morphologic studies after CABG

Kern and associates[138] from Los Angeles, California, described histologic features observed in 60 operatively excised aortocoronary saphenous vein bypass grafts from 40 patients. In 23 patients, the grafts were occluded by intimal fibrous tissue and in 5 of the 23 it was associated with thrombotic occlusion of the remaining lumen. In 17 patients, graft failure was caused by advanced atherosclerosis and in 13 of them it was associated with thrombotic occlusion, often due to rupture of an atheromatous plaque. The average duration of the failed conduits containing complicated atherosclerotic plaques was 6–7 years and the average period the conduits that contained occlusive fibrous tissue were in place was 3 years. For the conduits containing both fibrous tissue and organized thrombus, the grafts had been in place an average of 7 months.

Moore and Hutchins[139] from Baltimore, Maryland, examined at necropsy 109 hearts in which 1 or more aortocoronary bypass grafts had been inserted including 236 coronary artery grafts. Of the 30 patients who died at operation, 71 (99%) of 72 grafts were patent; of 61 others who died within 1 month, 120 (92%) of 131 were patent. In contrast, in 18 patients who died from 1–70 months after CABG, 20 (61%) of 33 grafts were patent. The coronary anastomotic site was open in 184 (87%) of 211 patent grafts, but in only 13 (52%) of 25 nonpatent grafts. Regional contraction-band necrosis was observed in 83 (45%) of 184 patients with patent grafts and distal anastomoses, and in 11 (21%) of 52 closed grafts. Of the 5 patients with closed distal anastomotic sites, coagulation necrosis was observed in LV myocardium, but it was not observed in any patient with opened conduits. After introduction of cold potassium chloride cardioplegia, significantly less regional contraction-band necrosis (19 [24%] of 79) was found than before (80[51%] of 157). Graft patency is less in the long-term survivors than in short-term survivors, regional contraction-band necrosis is associated with patent grafts and coagulation necrosis with closed grafts, and less myocardial injury occurs with present operative techniques than with those utilized several years ago.

MISCELLANEOUS

Angina pectoris with long-term hemodialysis

Chronic maintenance hemodialysis for chronic renal disease has been considered an accelerator of coronary atherosclerosis. Roig and associates[140] from Barcelona, Spain, studied 9 patients having regular maintenance hemodialysis and associated angina pectoris. Coronary angiograms disclosed that 4 of these patients had entirely normal coronary arteries; all were women significantly younger and with significantly higher BP levels and higher LV wall stress than the other 5 patients with narrowed coronary arteries. The associated anemia and increased myocardial oxygen consumption due to the associated systemic hypertension appears to be the explanation for angina pectoris in the presence of long-term dialysis in patients with coronary arteries that are normal angiographically.

Atherosclerosis in hemophilia

Most patients with hemophilia are believed to have relatively little atherosclerosis, presumably because an intact clotting mechanism is required for atherosclerotic plaques to form; fibrin and platelet deposition on the intimal surfaces are presumably essential to plaque formation. Dalldorf and associates[141] from Chapel Hill, North Carolina, however, described 5 necropsy patients aged 42–75 years, all of whom had severe hemophilia and typical atherosclerotic disease of both aorta and coronary arteries. One had severe CAD with a large healed myocardial infarct. Thus, severe hemophilia may not prevent development of atherosclerosis.

Management of CAD patients for noncardiac surgery

Wells and Kaplan[142] from Atlanta, Georgia, in a lengthy review delineated optimal management of patients with CAD who need noncardiac operations. Their view is based not only on previous reports but on 873 patients with known CAD who underwent noncardiac surgery at Emory University Hospital in 1976. Of those patients, 48 had had an AMI within 3 months of operation and none had another AMI. Significant atrial or ventricular arrhythmias, however, occurred in 15%. In contrast, of the 750 patients without recent AMI but with clinically significant CAD, 1.3% had another AMI perioperatively. These patients were thoroughly evaluated and treated preoperatively by the cardiology staff; early preoperative consultation with anesthesiologists was undertaken; extensive monitoring was used intraoperatively; and many patients were observed postoperatively in the intensive care unit. These improved results in the Emory series reflect increased awareness of the potential problems in CAD and an aggressive approach to perioperative management. These authors also studied 53 patients who had had CABG, then underwent 75 noncardiac operations. Only 1 of them had a perioperative AMI and 2 others had ischemic ECG changes. Thus, patients with successful CABG pose less of an anesthetic risk than do patients with angina pectoris without CABG.

Declining mortality in CAD

Levy[143] from Bethesda, Maryland, reviewed data showing a dramatic unprecedented decline in mortality from cardiovascular disease in the USA, especially CAD and stroke, since 1968. The decline has now been confirmed as real and has been observed in all age, sex, and race groups. Possible causes of the decline in CAD mortality include the development of acute coronary care, new drugs, CABG, noninvasive diagnostic methods for earlier detection, and the identification of specific cardiovascular risk factors. The decline has been temporally related to risk factor awareness and modification (cessation of cigarette smoking, control of systemic hypertension, diet change, and reduction in serum cholesterol). Thus, both primary prevention through lifestyle changes and improved treatment regimes have played a role in the decline in CAD mortality.

References

1. CONNOLLY DC, OXMAN HA, NOBREGA FT, KURLAND LT, KENNEDY MA, ELVEBACK LR: Coronary heart disease in residents of Rochester, Minnesota, 1950–1975. I. Background and study design. Mayo Clin Proc 56:661–664, Nov 1981.

2. ELVEBACK LR, CONNOLLY DC, KURLAND LT: Coronary heart disease in residents of Rochester, Minnesota. II. Mortality, incidence, and survivorship, 1950–1975. Mayo Clin Proc 56: 665–672, Nov 1981.

3. DE FEYTER PJ, MAJID PA, VAN EENIGE MJ, WARDEH R, WEMPE FN, ROOS JP: Clinical significance of exercise-induced ST segment elevation: correlative angiographic study in patients with ischemic heart disease. Br Heart J 46:84–92, July 1981.

4. CORYA BC, PHILLIPS JF, BLACK MJ, WEYMAN AE, RASMUSSEN S: Prevalence of regional left ventricular dysfunction in patients with coronary artery disease. Chest 79:631–637, June 1981.

5. PICHARD AD, WIENER L, MARTINEZ E, HOROWITZ S, PATTERSON R, MELLER J, GOLDSMITH SJ, GORLIN

R, HERMAN MV: Septal myocardial perfusion imaging with thallium-201 in the diagnosis of proximal left anterior descending coronary artery disease. Am Heart J 102:30−36, July 1981.

6. FREEMAN MR, BERMAN DS, STANILOFF H, ELKAYAM U, MADDAHI J, SWAN HJC, FORRESTER J: Comparison of upright and supine bicycle exercise in the detection and evaluation of the extent of coronary artery disease by equilibrium radionuclide ventriculography. Am Heart J 102:182−189, Aug 1981.

7. ELKAYAM U, WEINSTEIN M, BERMAN D, MADDAHI J, STANILOFF H, FREEMAN M, WAXMAN A, SWAN HJC, FORRESTER J: Stress thallium-201 myocardial scintigraphy and exercise technetium ventriculography in the detection and location of chronic coronary artery disease: comparison of sensitivity and specificity of these noninvasive tests alone and in combination. Am Heart J 101:657−666, May 1981.

8. DIAMOND GA, FORRESTER JS: Improved interpretation of a continuous variable in diagnostic testing: probabilistic analysis of scintigraphic rest and exercise left ventricular ejection fractions for coronary disease detection. Am Heart J 102:189−195, Aug 1981.

9. MAURER G, NANDA NC: Two dimensional echocardiographic evaluation of exercise-induced left and right ventricular asynergy: correlation with thallium scanning. Am J Cardiol 48:720−727, Oct 1981.

10. KIRSHENBAUM HD, OKADA RD, BOUCHER CA, KUSHNER FG, STRAUSS HW, POHOST GM: Relationship of thallium-201 myocardial perfusion pattern to regional and global left ventricular function with exercise. Am Heart J 101:734−739, June 1981.

11. PODRID PJ, GRABOYS TB, LOWN B: Prognosis of medically treated patients with coronary artery disease with profound ST-segment depression during exercise testing. N Engl J Med 305:1111−1116, Nov 1981.

12. PROUDFIT WL, WELCH CC, SIQUEIRA C, MORCERF FP, SHELDON WC: Prognosis of 1,000 young women studied by coronary angiography. Circulation 64:1185−1190, Dec 1981.

13. ISNER JM, SALEM DN, BANAS JS Jr, LEVINE HJ: Long-term clinical course of patients with normal coronary arteriography: Follow-up study of 121 patients with normal or nearly normal coronary arteriograms. Am Heart J 102:645−653, Oct 1981.

14. SHUB C, VLIETSTRA RE, SMITH HC, FULTON RE, ELVEBACK LR: The unpredictable progression of symptomatic coronary artery disease: A serial clinical-angiographic analysis. Mayo Clin Proc 56:155−160, March 1981.

15. KIMBIRIS D, SEGAL BL: Coronary disease progression in patients with and without saphenous vein bypass surgery. Am Heart J 102:811−818, Oct 1981.

16. GORDON T, KANNEL WB, CASTELLI WP, DAWBER TR: Lipoproteins cardiovascular disease, and death: The Framingham Study. Arch Intern Med 141:1128−1131, Nov 1981.

17. TATAMI R, MABUCHI H, UEDA K, UEDA R, HABA T, KAMETANI T, ITO S, KOIZUMI J, OHTA M, MIYAMOTO S, NAKAYAMA A, KANAYA H, OIWAKE H, GENDA A, TAKEDA R: Intermediate-density lipoprotein and cholesterol-rich very low density lipoprotein in angiographically determined coronary artery disease. Circulation 64:1174−1184, Dec 1981.

18. WHAYNE TF, ALAUPOVIC P, CURRY MD, LEE ET, ANDERSON PS, SCHECHTER E: Plasma apolipoprotein B and VLDL-, LDL-, and HDL-cholesterol as risk factors in the development of coronary artery disease in male patients examined by angiography. Atherosclerosis 39:411−424, June 1981.

19. MORRISON JA, KHOURY P, MELLIES M, KELLY K, HORVITZ R, BLUECK CJ: Lipid and lipoprotein distributions in black adults: The Cincinnati lipid research clinic's Princeton School Study. JAMA 245:939−942, March 6, 1981.

20. YAARI S, EVEN-ZOHAR S, GOLDBOURT U, NEUFELD HN: Associations of serum high density lipoprotein and total cholesterol with total, cardiovascular, and cancer mortality in a 7-year prospective study of 10,000 men. Lancet 1:1011−1014, May 1981.

21. WILLIAMS RR, SORLIE PD, FEINLEIB M, McNAMARA PM, KANNEL WB, DAWBER TR: Cancer incidence by levels of cholesterol. JAMA 245:247−257, Jan 16, 1981.

22. GILBERT HS, GINSBERG H, FAGERSTROM R, BROWN WV: Characterization of hypocholesterolemia

in myeloproliferative disease: relation to disease manifestations and activity. Am J Med 71:595–602, Oct 1981.

23. HELDENBERG D, RUBINSTEIN A, LEVTOV O, WERBIN B, TAMIR I: Serum lipids and lipoprotein concentrations in young quadriplegic patients. Atherosclerosis 39:163–167, May 1981.

24. SOMER JB, AITKEN JM, ABBOT LK, CHARLESWORTH JA, MACDONALD GJ: Lipoprotein lipids in renal transplant recipients of different pre-transplant etiology of renal disease. Atherosclerosis 39:177–182, May 1981.

25. CARLSON LA, BOTTIGER LE: Serum triglycerides, to be or not to be a risk factor for ischaemic heart disease? Atherosclerosis 39:287–291, June 1981.

26. CABIN HS, ROBERTS WC: Quantification of amounts of coronary arterial narrowing in patients with types II and IV hyperlopoproteinemia and in those with known normal lipoprotein patterns. Am Heart J 101:52–58, Jan 1981.

27. CABIN HS, SCHWARTZ DE, VIRMANI R, BREWER HB, ROBERTS WC: Type III hyperlipoproteinemia: Quantification, distribution, and nature of atherosclerotic coronary arterial narrowing in five necropsy patients. Am Heart J 102:830–835, Nov 1981.

28. SHEKELLE RB, SHRYOCK AM, PAUL O, LEPPER M, STAMLER J, LIU S, RAYNOR WJ: Diet, serum cholesterol, and death from coronary heart disease. The Western Electric Study. N Engl J Med 304:65–70, Jan 1981.

29. KEYS A, ARAVANIS C, VAN BUCHEM FSP, BLACKBURN H, BUZINA R, DJORDJEVIC BS, DONTAS AS, FIDANZA F, KARVONEN MJ, KIMURA N, MENOTTI A, NEDELJKOVIC S, PUDDU V, PUNSAR S, TAYLOR HL: The diet and all-causes death rate in the Seven Countries Study. Lancet 2:58–61, July 1981.

30. SACKS FM, DONNER A, CASTELLI WP, GRONEMEYER J, PLETKA P, MARGOLIUS HS, LANDSBERG L, KASS EH: Effect of ingestion of metal on plasma cholesterol of vegetarians. JAMA 246:640–644, Aug 7, 1981.

31. KANE JP, MALLOY MJ, TUN P, PHILLIPS NR, FREEDMAN DD, WILLIAMS ML, ROWE JS, HAVEL RJ: Normalization of low-density-lipoprotein levels in heterozygous familial hypercholesterolemia with a combined drug regimen. N Engl J Med 304:251–262, Jan 1981.

32. MABUCHI H, HABA T, TATAMI R, MIYAMOTO S, SAKAI Y, WAKASUGI T, WATANABE A, KOIZUMI J, TAKEDA R: Effects of an inhibitor of 3-hydroxy-3-methyl-glutaryl conenzyme a reductase on serum lipoproteins and ubiquinone-10 levels in patients with familial hypercholesterolemia. N Engl J Med 305:478–482, Aug 1981.

33. THOMPSON GR: Plasma exchange for hypercholesterolemia. Lancet 1:1246–1248, June 1981.

34. STOFFEL W, BORBERG H, GREVE V: Application of specific extracorporeal removal of low density lipoprotein in familial hypercholesterolemia. Lancet 2:1005–1007, Nov 1981.

35. SPENGEL FA, DUFFIELD RGM, JADHAW A, WOOD CB, THOMPSON GR: Superiority of partial ileal bypass over cholestyramine in reducing cholesterol in familial hypercholesterolemia. Lancet 2:768–770, Oct 1981.

36. SWANSON JO, PIERPONT G, ADICOFF A: Serum high density lipoprotein cholesterol correlates with presence but not severity of coronary artery disease. Am J Med 71:235–239, Aug 1981.

37. UHL GS, TROXLER RG, HICKMAN JR, CLARK D: Relation between high density lipoprotein cholesterol and coronary artery disease in asymptomatic men. Am J Cardiol 48:903–910, Nov 1981.

38. GUTAI J, LAPORTE R, KULLER L, DAI W, FALVO-GERARD L, CAGGIULA A: Plasma testosterone, high density lipoprotein cholesterol and other lipoprotein fractions. Am J Cardiol 48:897–902, Nov 1981.

39. PETITTI DB, FRIEDMAN GD, KLATSKY AL: Association of a history of gallbladder disease with a reduced concentration of high-density-lipoprotein cholesterol. N Engl J Med 304:1396–1398, June 1981.

40. DEVENYI P, ROBINSON GM, KAPUR BM, RONCARI DAK: High-density lipoprotein cholesterol in male alcoholics with and without severe liver disease. Am J Med 71:589–594, Oct 1981.

41. BROWNELL KD, STUNKARD AJ: Differential changes in plasma high-density lipoprotein-choles-

terol levels in obese men and women during weight reduction. Arch Intern Med 141:1142–1146, Aug 1981.

42. HARTUNG GH, SQUIRES WG, GOTT AM JR: Effect of exercise training on plasma high-density lipoprotein cholesterol in coronary disease patients. Am Heart J 101:181–184, Feb 1981.

43. HOOPER PL, WOO W, VISCONTI L, PATHAK DR: Terbutaline raises high-density lipoprotein-cholesterol levels. N Engl J Med 305:1455–1456, Dec 1981.

44. KANNEL WB: Update on the role of cigarette smoking in coronary artery disease. Am Heart J 101:319–328, March 1981.

45. FRIEDMAN GD, PETITTI DB, BAWOL RD, SIEGELAUB AB: Mortality in cigarette smokers and quitters. Effect of baseline differences. N Engl J Med 304:1407–1410, June 1981.

46. MCNAMARA DG: President's page: confessions of a (reformed) tobacco smoker. Am J Cardiol 48:811–812, Oct 1981.

47. CASTELLI WP, DAWBER TR, FEINLEIB M, GARRISON RJ, MCNAMARA PM, KANNEL WB: The filter cigarette and coronary heart disease: The Framingham Study. Lancet 2:109–113, July 1981.

48. WALD NJ, IDLE M, BOREHAM J, BAILEY A, VAN VUNAKIS H: Serum cotinine levels in pipe smokers: evidence against nicotine as cause of coronary heart disease. Lancet 2:775–777, Oct 1981.

49. DALEN JE, HICKLER RB: Oral contraceptives and cardiovascular disease. Am Heart J 101:626–639, May 1981.

50. STADEL BV: Oral contraceptives and cardiovascular disease. N Engl J Med 305:612–618, 672–677, Sept 1981.

51. HIRVONEN E, MALKONEN M, MANNINEN V: Effects of different progestogens on lipoproteins during postmenopausal replacement therapy. N Engl J Med 304:560–562, March 1981.

52. HOLMES DR JR, KENNEL AJ, SMITH HC, GORDON H, MOORE SB: Coronary artery disease in twins. Br Heart J 45:193–197, Feb 1981.

53. STONE PH, SHERRID MV, COHN KE: Correlation of HLA types in premature coronary artery disease. An attempt to define independent genetic risk factors. Chest 79:381–385, Apr 1981.

54. ROSE G, MARMOT MG: Social class and coronary heart disease. Br Heart J 45:13–19, Jan 1981.

55. SORLIE PD, GARCIA-PALMIERI MR, COSTAS R, HAVLIK RJ: Hematocrit and risk of coronary heart disease: The Puerto Rico Heart Health Program. Am Heart J 101:456–461, Apr 1981.

56. RUBENSTEIN MD, WALL RT, BAIM DS, HARRISON CD: Platelet activation in clinical coronary artery disease. Am Heart J 102:363–367, Sept 1981.

57. ZAHAVI J, BETTERIDGE JD, JONES NAG, GALTON DJ, KAKKAR VV: Enhanced in vivo platelet release reaction and malondialdehyde formation in patients with hyperlipidemia. Am J Med 70:59–64, Jan 1981.

58. STEELE P, RAINWATER J, VOGEL R: Effect of platelet suppressant treatment with dipyridamole and aspirin on exercise performance and platelet survival time in coronary disease. Chest 80:557–561, Nov 1981.

59. HIRSH PD, HILLIS LD, CAMPBELL WB, FIRTH BG, WILLERSON JT: Release of prostaglandins and thromboxane into the coronary circulation in patients with ischemic heart disease. N Engl J Med 304:685–691, March 1981.

60. BERGMAN G, ATKINSON L, RICHARDSON PG, DALY K, ROTHMAN M, JACKSON G, JEWITT DE: Prostacyclin: hemodynamic and metabolic effects in patients with coronary artery disease. Lancet 1:569–572, March 1981.

61. SERNERI GGN, GENSINI GF, ABBATE R, MUGNAINI C, FAVILLA S, BRUNELLI C, CHIERCHIA S, PARODI O: Increased fibrinopeptide a formation and thromboxane A_2 production in patients with ischemic heart disease: relationships to coronary pathoanatomy, risk factors, and clinical manifestations. Am Heart J 101:185–194, Feb 1981.

62. KRAMSCH DM, ASPEN AJ, ABRAMOWITZ BM, KREIMENDAHL T, HOOD WB JR: Reduction of coronary atherosclerosis by moderate conditioning exercise in monkeys on an atherogenic diet. N Engl J Med 305:1483–1489, Dec 17, 1981.

63. ISNER JM, KISHEL J, KENT KM, RONAN JA, ROSS AM, ROBERTS WC: Accuracy of angiographic determination of left main coronary arterial narrowing: angiographic-histologic correlative analysis in 28 patients. Circulation 63:1056–1064, May 1981.

64. MILLER DW, TOBIS FM, IVEY TD, RUBENSTEIN SA: Risks of coronary arteriography and bypass surgery in patients with left main coronary artery stenosis. Chest 79:387–392, Apr 1981.

65. LOOP FD: Risks in diagnosis and therapy of left main coronary atherosclerosis. Chest 79: 386–387, Apr 1981.

66. TYRAS DH, KAISER GC, BARNER HB, PENNINGTON DG, CODD JE, WILLIAM VL: Left main equivalent: results of medical and surgical therapy. Circulation 64(II):7–10, Aug 1981.

67. CABIN HS, ROBERTS WC: Fatal cardiac arrest during cardiac catheterization for angina pectoris: analysis of 10 necropsy patients. Am J Cardiol 48:1–8, July 1981.

68. HECHT HS, CHEW CY, BURNAM M, SCHNUGG SJ, HOPKINS JM, SINGH BN: Radionuclide ejection fraction and regional wall motion during atrial pacing in stable angina pectoris: comparison with metabolic and hemodynamic parameters. Am Heart J 101:726–733, June 1981.

69. KLEIN RC, GREHL TM, STENGERT KB, MASON DT: Evaluation of the effects of systemic nitroglycerin on perfusion of ischemic myocardium in coronary heart disease assessed intraoperatively by antegrade blood flow through intact saphenous vein bypass grafts. Am Heart J 101:292–299, March 1981.

70. SCHWARTZ JB, JACKSON G, KATES RE, HARRISON DC: Long-term benefit of cardioselective beta blockade with once-daily atenolol therapy in angina pectoris. Am Heart J 101:380–385, Apr 1981.

71. SHAPIRO W, PARK J, BIBIANCO R, SINGH SN, KATZ RJ, FLETCHER R: Comparison of nadolol, a new long-acting beta-receptor blocking agent, and placebo in the treatment of stable angina pectoris. Chest 80:425–430, Oct 1981.

72. TELFORD AM, WILSON C: Trial of heparin versus atenolol in prevention of myocardial infarction in intermediate coronary syndrome. Lancet 1:1225–1228, June 1981.

73. LEON MB, ROSING DR, BONOW RO, LIPSON LC, EPSTEIN SE: Clinical efficacy of verapamil alone and combined with propranolol in treating patients with chronic stable angina pectoris. Am J Cardiol 48:131–139, July 1981.

74. JOHNSON SM, MAURITSON DR, CORBETT JR, WOODWARD W, WILLERSON JT, HILLIS LD: Double-blind, randomized, placebo-controlled comparison of propranolol and verapamil in the treatment of patients with stable angina pectoris. Am J Med 71:443–451, Sept 1981.

75. DAWSON JR, WHITAKER NHG, SUTTON GC: Calcium antagonist drugs in chronic stable angina: comparison of verapamil and nifedipine. Br Heart J 46:508–512, Nov 1981.

76. CORBALAN R, GONZALEZ R, CHAMORRO G, MUNOZ M, RODRIGUEZ JA, CASANEGRA P: Effect of a calcium inhibitor, nifedipine, on exercise tolerance in patients with angina pectoris: a double-blind study. Chest 79:302–305, March 1981.

77. SOBEL BE: Introduction to *Symposium on Nifedipine in Angina Pectoris*. Am J Med 71:635–637, Oct 1981.

78. MASERI A, CHIERCHIA S: A new rationale for the clinical approach to the patient with angina pectoris, in *Symposium on Nifedipine in Angina Pectoris*. Am J Med 71:639–644, Oct 1981.

79. MUELLER HS, CHAHINE RA: Interim report of multicenter double-blind, placebo-controlled studies of nifedipine in chronic stable angina, in *Symposium on Nifedipine in Angina Pectoris*. Am J Med 71:645–657, Oct 1981.

80. ENGEL HJ, LICHTLEN PR: Beneficial enhancement of coronary blood flow by nifedipine: comparison with nitroglycerin and beta blocking agents, in *Symposium on Nifedipine in Angina Pectoris*. Am J Med 71:658–666, Oct 1981.

81. LORELL BH, TURI Z, GROSSMAN W: Modification of left ventricular response to pacing tachycardia by nifedipine in patients with coronary artery disease, in *Symposium on Nifedipine in Angina Pectoris*. Am J Med 71:667–675, Oct 1981.

82. DARGIE HJ, LYNCH PG, KRIKLER DM, HARRIS L, KRIKLER S: Nifedipine and propranolol: a beneficial drug interaction, in *Symposium on Nifedipine in Angina Pectoris*. Am J Med 71:676–682, Oct 1981.

83. LUDEBROOK PA, TIEFENBRUNN AJ, SOBEL BE, REED FR: Influence of nifedipine on left ventricular systolic and diastolic function: relationships to manifestations of ischemia and congestive failure, in *Symposium on Nifedipine in Angina Pectoris*. Am J Med 71:683–692, Oct 1981.

84. HOSSACK KF, BRUCE RA: Improved exercise performance in persons with stable angina pectoris receiving diltiazem. Am J Cardiol 47:95–101, Jan 1981.

85. LOW RI, TAKEDA P, LEE G, MASON DT, AWAN NA, DeMARIA AN: Effects of diltiazem-induced calcium blockade upon exercise capacity in effort angina due to chronic coronary artery disease. Am Heart J 101:713–718, June 1981.

86. BROWN CA, HUTTER AM JR, DeSANCTIS RW, GOLD HK, LEINBACH RC, ROBERTS-NILES A, AUSTEN WG, BUCKLEY MJ: Prospective study of medical and urgent surgical therapy in randomizable patients with unstable angina pectoris: results of in-hospital and chronic mortality and morbidity. Am Heart J 102:959–964, Dec 1981.

87. National Cooperative Study Group to Compare Medical and Surgical Therapy: Unstable angina pectoris IV. results in patients with left anterior descending coronary artery disease. Am J Cardiol 48:517–524, Sept 1981.

88. MILLER D, WATERS DD, WARNICA W, SZLACHCIC J, KREEFT J, THEROUX P: Is variant angina the coronary manifestation of a generalized vasospastic disorder? N Engl J Med 304:763–766, March 1981.

89. GERTZ SD, URETSKY G, WAJNBERG RS, NAVOT N, GOTSMAN MS: Endothelial cell damage and thrombus formation after partial arterial constriction: relevance to the role of coronary artery spasm in the pathogenesis of myocardial infarction. Circulation 63:476–486, March 1981.

90. ROBERTSON RM, ROBERTSON D, ROBERTS LJ, MAAS RL, FITZGERALD GA, FRIESINGER GC, OATES JA: Thromboxane A_2 in vasotonic angina pectoris: evidence from direct measurements and inhibitor trials. N Engl J Med 304:998–1003, Apr 1981.

91. BROWN BG: Coronary vasospasm: observations linking the clinical spectrum of ischemic heart disease to the dynamic pathology of coronary atherosclerosis. Arch Intern Med 141:716–721, May 1981.

92. GINSBURG R, LAMB IH, SCHROEDER JS, HARRISON DC: Long-term transtelephonic electrocardiographic monitoring in the detection and evaluation of variant angina. Am Heart J 102:196–201, Aug 1981.

93. FELDMAN RL, PEPINE CJ, WHITTLE JL, CURRY RC, CONTI CR: Coronary hemodynamic findings during spontaneous angina in patients with variant angina. Circulation 64:76–83, July 1981.

94. FREEDMAN B, DUNN RF, RICHMOND DR, KELLY DT: Coronary artery spasm during exercise: treatment with verapamil. Circulation 64:68–75, July 1981.

95. CIPRIANO PR, KOCH FH, ROSENTHAL SJ, SCHROEDER JS: Clinical course of patients following the demonstration of coronary artery spasm by angiography. Am Heart J 101:127–134, Feb 1981.

96. HUCKELL VF, McLAUGHLIN PR, MORCH JE, WIGLE ED, ADELMAN AG: Prinzmetal's angina with documented coronary artery spasm: treatment and follow-up. Br Heart J 45:649–655, June 1981.

97. MAGDER SA, JOHNSTONE DE, HUCKELL VF, ADELMAN AG: Experience with ergonovine provocative testing for coronary arterial spasm. Chest 79:638–646, June 1981.

98. GINSBURG R, LAMB IH, BRISTOW MR, SCHROEDER JS, HARRISON DC: Application and safety of outpatient ergonovine testing in accurately detecting coronary spasm in patients with possible variant angina. Am Heart J 102:698–702, Oct 1981.

99. WATERS DD, THEROUX P, SZLACHCIC J, DAUWE F: Provocative testing with ergonovine to assess

the efficacy of treatment with nifedipine, diltiazem and verapamil in variant angina. Am J Cardiol 48:123−130, July 1981.

100. GINSBURG R, BRISTOW MR, KANTROWITZ N, BAIM DS, HARRISON DC: Histamine provocation of clinical coronary artery spasm: implications concerning pathogenesis of variant angina pectoris. Am Heart J 102:819−822, Nov 1981.

101. GIROTTI AL, RUTITZKY B, SCHMIDBERG J, CROSATTO J, ROSENBAUM MB: Spontaneous remission in variant angina. Br Heart J 45:517−521, May 1981.

102. PEPINE CJ, FELDMAN RL, WHITTLE J, CURRY RC, CONTI CR: Effect of diltiazem in patients with variant angina: a randomized double-blind trial. Am Heart J 101:719−725, June 1981.

103. JOHNSON SM, MAURITSON DR, WILLERSON JT, HILLIS LD: A controlled trial of verapamil for Prinzmetal's variant angina. N Engl J Med 304:862−866, Apr 1981.

104. JOHNSON SM, MAURITSON DR, WILLERSON JT, CARY JR, HILLIS LD: Verapamil administration in variant angina pectoris. JAMA 245:1849−1853. May 8, 1981.

105. FREEMAN WR, PETER T, MANDEL WJ: Verapamil therapy in variant angina pectoris refractory to nitrates. Am Heart J 102:358−362, Sept 1981.

106. MEHTA J, PEPINE CJ, DAY M, GUERRERO JR, CONTI CR: Short-term efficacy of oral verapamil in rest angina: a double-blind placebo controlled trial in CCU patients. Am J Med 71:977−982, Dec 1981.

107. TIEFENBRUNN AJ, SOBEL BE, GOWDA S, McKNIGHT RC, LUDBROOK PA: Nifedipine blockade of er-gonovine-induced coronary arterial spasm: angiographic documentation. Am J Cardiol 48:184−187, July 1981.

108. MOSES JW, WERTHEIMER JH, BODENHEIMER MM, BANKA VS, FELDMAN M, HELFANT RH: Efficacy of nifedipine in rest angina refractory to propranolol and nitrates in patients with obstruc-tive coronary artery disease. Ann Intern Med 94(part 1):425−429, Apr 1981.

109. SUSSMAN EJ, GOLDBERG S, POLL DS, MacVAUGH H, III, SIMSON MB, SILBER SA, KASTOR JA: Surgical therapy of variant angina associated with nonobstructive coronary disease. Ann Intern Med 94:771−774, June 1981.

110. BUDA AJ, FOWLES RE, SCHROEDER JS, HUNT SA, CIPRIANO PR, STINSON EB, HARRISON DC: Coronary artery spasm in the denervated transplanted human heart: a clue to underlying mecha-nisms. Am J Med 70:1144−1149, May 1981.

111. COWLEY MJ, VETROVEC GW, WOLFGANG TC: Efficacy of percutaneous transluminal coronary angioplasty: technique, patient selection, salutary results, limitations and complica-tions. Am Heart J 101:272−280, March 1981.

112. VLIETSTRA RE, HOLMES DR, SMITH HC, HARTZLER GO, ORSZULAK TA: Percutaneous transluminal coronary angioplasty: initial Mayo Clinic experience. Mayo Clin Proc 56:287−293, May 1981.

113. WILLIAMS DO, RILEY RS, SINGH, AK, GEWIRTZ H, MOST AS: Evaluation of the role of coro-nary angioplasty in patients with unstable angina pectoris. Am Heart J 102:1−9, July 1981.

114. BLOCK PC, MYLER RK, STERTZER S, FALLON JT: Morphology after transluminal angioplasty in human beings. N Engl J Med 305:382−385, Aug 1981.

115. BAUGHMAN KL, PASTERNAK RC, FALLON JT, BLOCK PC: Transluminal coronary angioplasty of postmortem human hearts. Am J Cardiol 48:1044−1047, Dec 1981.

116. FORD WB, WHOLEY MH, ZIKRIA EA, SOMADANI SR, SULLIVAN ME: Percutaneous transluminal di-lation of aortocoronary saphenous vein bypass grafts. Chest 79:529−535, May 1981.

117. BOURASSA MG: Percutaneous transluminal coronary angioplasty−still an investigative pro-cedure (editorial). Mayo Clin Proc 56:334−335, May 1981.

118. LEE G, IKEDA RM, KOZINA J, MASON DT: Laser dissolution of coronary atherosclerotic obstruc-tion. Am Heart J 102:1074−1075, Dec 1981.

119. NCHCT Technology Forum: Coronary artery bypass surgery. JAMA 246:1654−1649, Oct 9, 1981.

120. KENNEDY JW, KAISER GC, FISHER LD, FRITZ JK, MYERS W, MUDD JG, RYAN TJ: Clinical and angio-

graphic predictors of operative mortality from the collaborative study in coronary artery surgery (CASS). Circulation 63:793–802, Apr 1981.

121. National Heart, Lung, and Blood Institute Coronary Artery Surgery Study. A multicenter comparison of the effects of randomized medical and surgical treatment of mildly symptomatic patients with coronary artery disease and a registry of consecutive patients undergoing coronary angiography, ed. KILLIP T, Circulation 63 (Part II): I-1–I-81, June 1981 (American Heart Association Monograph 79).

122. DeRouen TA, Hammermeister KE, Dodge HT: Comparisons of the effects on survival after coronary artery surgery in subgroups of patients from the Seattle Heart Watch. Circulation 63:537–545, March 1981.

123. Douglas JS Jr, King SB III, Jones EL, Craver JM, Bradford J, Hatcher CR Jr: Reduced efficacy of coronary bypass surgery in women. Circulation 64:11–16, Aug 1981.

124. Knapp WS, Douglas JS Jr, Craver JM, Jones EL, King SB III, Bone DK, Bradford JM, Hatcher CR Jr: Efficacy of coronary artery bypass grafting in elderly patients with coronary artery disease. Am J Cardiol 47:923–930, Apr 1981.

125. Berry BE, Acree PW, Davis DJ, Sheely CH II, Cavin S: Coronary artery bypass operation in septuagenarians. Ann Thorac Surg 31:310–313, Apr 1981.

126. Greene DG, Bunnell IL, Arani DT, Schimert G, Lajos TZ, Lee AB, Tandon RN, Zimdahl WT, Bozer JM, Kohn RM, Visco JP, Dean DC, Smith GL: Long-term survival after coronary bypass surgery: comparison of various subsets of patients with general population. Br Heart J 45:417–426, Apr 1981.

127. Phillips HR, Johnson RA, Hindman MA, Wagner GS, Harris PH, Dinsmore RE, Gold HK, Leinbach RC, Hutter AM Jr, Erdmann AJ III, Daggett WM Jr, Buckley MJ: Aortocoronary bypass grafting in patients without left main stenosis: relation of risk factors to early and late survival. Br Heart J 45:549–554, May 1981.

128. Brooks N, Warnes C, Cattell M, Balcon R, Honey M, Layton C, Sturridge M, Wright J: Cardiac pain at rest: management and follow-up of 100 consecutive cases. Br Heart J 45:35–41, Jan 1981.

129. Mayer JE Jr, Lindsay WG, Castaneda W, Nicoloff DM: Influence of aspirin and dipyridamole on patency of coronary artery bypass grafts. Ann Thorac Surg 31:204–210, March 1981.

130. Crosby IK, Wellons HA Jr, Taylor GJ, Maffeo CJ, Beller GA, Muller WH Jr: Critical analysis of the preoperative and operative predictors of aortocoronary bypass patency. Ann Surg 193:743–751, June 1981.

131. Kamath ML, Schmidt DH, Pedraza PM, Blau FM, Sampathkumar A, Grzelak LL, Johnson WD: Patency and flow response in endarterectomized coronary arteries. Ann Thorac Surg 31:28–35, Jan 1981.

132. de Rijbel RJ, Schipperheyn JJ: The use of electromagnetic flow measurements for detection of early stenosis in aortocoronary bypass grafts. Ann Thorac Surg 31:402–408, May 1981.

133. Cosgrove DM, Loop FD, Saunders CL, Lytle BW, Kramer JR: Should coronary arteries with less than fifty percent stenosis be bypassed? J Thorac Cardiovasc Surg 82:520–530, Oct 1981.

134. Buxton AE, Josephson ME: The role of P-wave duration as a predictor of postoperative atrial arrhythmias. Chest 80:68–73, July 1981.

135. Rahimtoola SH, Grunkemeier GL, Teply JF, Lambert LE, Thomas DR, Suen YF, Starr A: Changes in coronary bypass surgery leading to improved survival. JAMA 246:1912–1916, Oct 23/30, 1981.

136. Buxton AE, Goldberg S, Harken A, Hirshfeld J, Kastor JA: Coronary artery spasm immediately after myocardial revascularization: recognition and management. N Engl J Med 304:1249–1253, May 1981.

137. Victor MF, Kimbiris D, Iskandrian AS, Mintz GS, Bemis CE, Procacci PM, Segal BL: Spasm of a saphenous vein bypass graft: a possible mechanism for occlusion of the venous graft. Chest 80:413–415, Oct 1981.

138. KERN WH, WELLS WJ, MEYER BW: The pathology of surgically excised aortocoronary saphenous vein bypass grafts. Am J Surg Path 5:491–496, July 1981.

139. MOORE GW, HUTCHINS GM: Coronary artery bypass grafts in 109 autopsied patients: statistical analysis of graft and anastomosis patency and regional myocardial injury. JAMA 246:1785–1789, Oct 16, 1981.

140. ROIG E, BETRIU A, CASTANER A, MAGRINA J, SANZ G, NAVARRO-LOPEZ F: Disabling angina pectoris with normal coronary arteries in patients undergoing long-term hemodialysis. Am J Med 71:431–434, Sept 1981.

141. DALLDORF FG, TAYLOR RE, BLATT PM: Arteriosclerosis in severe hemophilia. Arch Path Lab Med 105:652–654, Dec 1981.

142. WELLS PH, KAPLAN JA: Optimal management of patients with ischemic heart disease for noncardiac surgery by complementary anesthesiologist and cardiologist interaction. Am Heart J 102:1029–1037, Dec 1981.

143. LEVY RI: Declining mortality in coronary heart disease. Arteriosclerosis 1:312–325, Sept/Oct 1981.

Acute Myocardial Infarction and Its Consequences

Acute coronary lesions in AMI

Buja and Willerson[1] from Dallas, Texas, studied 83 necropsy patients with 100 AMIs. Severe atherosclerosis (>75% cross-sectional area narrowing) involved 3 or more major coronary arteries in 65%, 2 arteries in 16%, 1 artery in 15%, and no arteries in 4%. Recent "occlusive" coronary arterial lesions were observed in 61%, including 50 (91%) of 55 grossly apparent transmural AMIs, 9 (35%) of 26 grossly evident subendocardial infarcts, and 2 (11%) of 19 multifocal microinfarcts associated with clinical episodes of acute coronary insufficiency (p < 0.001). The 61 recent occlusive lesions consisted of 2 thromboemboli, 2 isolated plaque hemorrhages, and 57 in situ thrombi. Clinical conditions predisposing to reduced coronary perfusion were identified before the onset of AMI in 26% of infarcts with recent occlusions and in 61% of infarcts without recent occlusions (p < 0.001). The AMI was followed by severe cardiac pump failure or CHF in 64% of infarcts with recent occlusions and in 41% of infarcts without them (p = ns).

Significance of coronary arterial thrombus in transmural AMI

Thrombi in coronary arteries of necropsy patients with transmural AMI obviously have been observed in numerous studies, and for many decades thrombi were believed to have precipitated AMI. They were considered so important in causing AMI that the term "coronary thrombosis" was used for years to describe the event that most physicians now call AMI. In recent years, the primary role of coronary thrombosis in precipitating AMI has been questioned. To evaluate the significance of coronary thrombus in AMI, Brosius and Roberts[2] from Bethesda, Maryland, examined in detail the coronary arteries containing thrombi in 54 necropsy patients with transmural AMI. Among the 54 necropsy patients with transmural AMI and coronary arterial thrombi, histologic sections of the coronary arteries that contained thrombi were examined by video planimetry to determine if the amount of luminal narrowing caused by thrombi was comparable to that produced by underlying atherosclerotic plaques and also the amount of luminal narrowing caused by plaques immediately proximal and distal to the thrombi (Fig. 2-1). The 54 coronary arteries in the 54 patients were narrowed 33%–98% (mean, 81%) by atherosclerotic plaque alone in cross-sectional area at the site of the thrombus (occlusive in 47 and nonocclusive in 7 [Fig. 2-2]), 26%–98%

Fig. 2-1.   Diagram of "average" coronary artery with occlusive thrombus. The four 5 mm segments of coronary artery proximal (P) to thrombus (T) were narrowed an average of 75% in cross-sectional area by atherosclerotic plaque (AP); the 4 segments with occlusive thrombus were narrowed an average of 81% by plaque, and the 4 segments distal (D) to thrombus were narrowed an average of 79% by plaque. Reproduced with permission from Brosius and Roberts.[2]

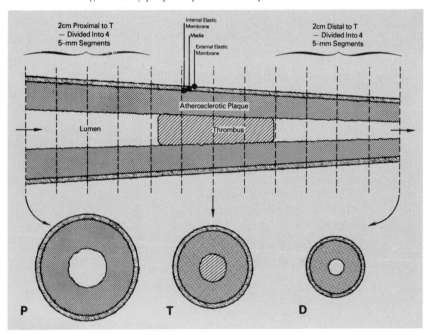

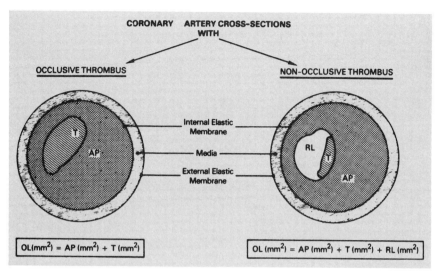

Fig. 2-2. Diagram of cross-sections of coronary arteries with occlusive and nonocclusive thrombi and method of calculating cross-sectional area of atherosclerotic plaque (AP), thrombus (T) and residual lumen (RL). OL = original lumen (area enclosed by internal elastic membrane). Reproduced with permission from Brosius and Roberts.[2]

(mean, 75%) within the 2 cm segment proximal to the thrombus, and 43%—98% (mean, 79%) within the 2 cm segment distal to the thrombus. Of the 54 arteries, 52 (96%) were narrowed 76%–98% in cross-sectional area by atherosclerotic plaque alone at or immediately proximal or distal to the thrombus and 26 (48%) were narrowed 91%–98% by plaque alone. The thrombi were 0.1–6.0 mm² (mean, 1.4) in cross-sectional area and the underlying atherosclerotic plaques were 3.0–21.0 mm² (mean, 8.7). Thus, among necropsy patients with transmural AMI, coronary thrombi occur at sites already severely narrowed by atherosclerotic plaques.

The results of the study raise questions about the importance of coronary thrombi in patients with fatal transmural AMI. The major finding was that, among patients with AMI, thrombi are found in major coronary arteries that already are severely narrowed by old atherosclerotic plaques and are located immediately proximal and/or immediately distal to the site of thrombosis. At the site of most severe narrowing, the lumen of the artery containing thrombus in 96% of their 54 patients was already narrowed 76%–98% in cross-sectional area by atherosclerotic plaque and in 48% of the patients the arterial lumen was narrowed 91%–98%. In contrast, the percent of coronary artery lumen narrowed by thrombus alone averaged 19% (range, 2–67) of the cross-sectional area of the artery in the 47 patients with occlusive thrombi and 7% (range, 2–24) in the 7 patients with nonocclusive thrombi. Thus, if thrombus were the only luminal material, the amount of thrombus within the coronary artery, with few exceptions, probably would not diminish or slow blood flow. Among necropsy patients with fatal AMI and coronary thrombus, the latter is always superimposed on atherosclerotic plaque.

Comparison of degree and extent of coronary narrowing by atherosclerotic plaque in anterior and posterior transmural AMI

Patients with AMI, with rare exception, have severe narrowing by atherosclerotic plaques of at least 1 and usually 2 or more of the 4 major epicardial coronary arteries. Little information also is available on the amount of narrowing by atherosclerotic plaques in the 4 major coronary arteries in patients with either anterior or posterior LV infarcts. AMI of the anterior LV wall is believed by many to indicate a severe "lesion" in the LAD coronary artery or lesser degrees of narrowing of the dominant posterior coronary artery. Similarly, a posterior AMI is generally considered to indicate a severe "lesion" in the right or LC coronary artery and lesser degrees of narrowing of the LAD coronary artery. Brosius and Roberts[3] from Bethesda, Maryland, examined at necropsy, both qualitatively and quantitatively, each of the 4 major epicardial coronary arteries in 50 patients during their first (and fatal) transmural AMI. The percentage of cross-sectional area narrowing by atherosclerotic plaques in each 5 mm segment of the right, LM, LAD, and LC coronary arteries was determined in each patient. The amount and extent of the coronary narrowing in the 22 patients with anterior wall AMI were compared with those in the 28 patients with posterior wall AMI. Although the percentage of coronary arteries narrowed 76%−100% was similar in both groups (74% -vs- 75%; average 3.0 of 4 coronary arteries per patient), the patients with anterior wall AMI had less severe narrowing of each 5 mm segment of the 4 major coronary arteries than did the patients with posterior wall AMI. Of the coronary segments examined in the 22 patients with anterior wall AMI, 23% were narrowed 76%−100% in cross-sectional area by atherosclerotic plaque, whereas 39% of the segments were 76%−100% narrowed in the 28 patients with posterior wall AMI (p < 0.001) (Fig. 2-3). Among the anterior AMI patients, the percentage of 5 mm segments of the LAD coronary artery severely (>75%) narrowed was greater than that for either posterior perfusing coronary artery. The percentage of segments narrowed 76%−100% for each of the major coronary arteries in the posterior AMI patients, however, was similar. Thus, at necropsy, patients with posterior wall AMI appear to have more extensive and severe coronary artery narrowing than do patients with anterior wall AMI. If the coronary arteries had not been examined quantitatively, this difference in severity would not have been apparent.

Nonfatal healed transmural myocardial infarction and fatal noncardiac disease: qualification and quantification of amounts of coronary narrowing and of left ventricular scarring

Much is now known about the amount of LV damage and the extent of coronary narrowing in patients dying either suddenly or with AMI or with chronic CHF after healing of AMI, but information on these 2 points is lacking in patients with healed AMI who subsequently die of noncardiac condi-

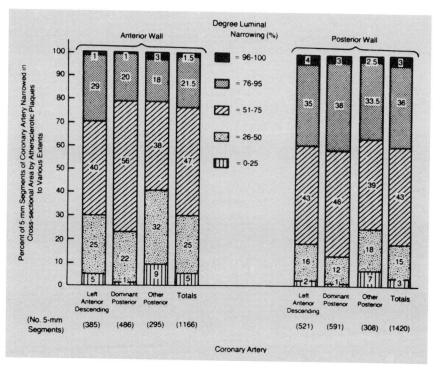

Fig. 2-3.   Percentages of 5 mm segments of each of 3 major epicardial coronary arteries narrowed by atherosclerotic plaques in 22 patients with anterior and 28 patients with posterior transmural AMI. Reproduced with permission from Brosius and Roberts.[3]

tions. To fill this void, Virmani and Roberts[4] from Bethesda, Maryland, performed a quantitative and qualitative analysis of the amount of myocardial scarring and the degree and extent of coronary arterial narrowing by atherosclerotic plaque in the entire lengths of each of the 4 major epicardial coronary arteries in 18 necropsy patients with healed transmural myocardial infarcts and death from a noncardiac condition. An average of 30% of the basal half and 38% of the apical half of the LV wall was scarred. The 9 patients with clinical evidence of previous AMI tended to have larger LV scars than did the 9 patients without such evidence, but the difference was not significant. An average of 26 cm (51 five-mm segments) of coronary artery was examined from each patient and 25 cm (49 five-mm segments) from each of 19 control subjects. Of 924 segments examined in the 18 patients, 292 (32%) were 76%–100% narrowed in cross-sectional area (controls, 5%); 321 (35%) were 51%–75% narrowed (controls, 34%); 210 (23%) were 26%–50% narrowed (controls, 44%), and 101 (11%) were 0–25% narrowed (controls, 17%) (Fig. 2-4). The extent of narrowing > 75% was similar (25%) in the LAD and LC coronary arteries; the right was the most severely narrowed artery and the LM was not severely narrowed in any patient. Excluding the LM artery, the amount of severe narrowing in the proximal and distal halves of

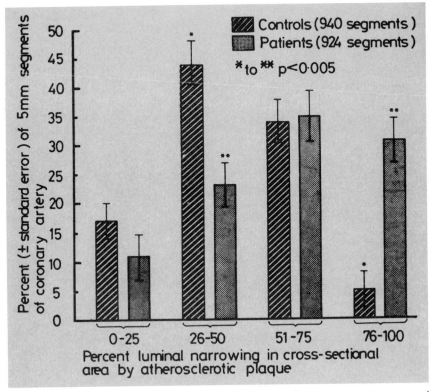

Fig. 2-4. Number and percentage of 5 mm segments of all 4 major coronary arteries narrowed to various degrees in 18 study patients and 19 control subjects. Reproduced with permission from Virmani and Roberts.[4]

the other 3 arteries was similar. The amount of severe narrowing was not related to the age at death or to heart weight, but was greater in patients with systemic hypertension or with a history of AMI.

Comparison of clinical features in autopsied and nonautopsied patients with acute or healed myocardial infarction

Roeske and associates[5] from San Diego, California, examined clinical data from 327 patients with a classic history of AMI who were studied at 1 University center. More than 200 clinical variables were recorded for each patient. More than 90% of these patients were followed for 6 years and, during this time, 140 died and 187 survived. The authors analyzed differences in their large pool of clinical data from the 86 patients autopsied and the 54 who were not. Their purpose was to assert any bias that might be present in use of postmortem data. Of noninvasive aspects examined in the 140 patients, 13 showed significant differences between the autopsied and nonautopsied patients, but the number of noninvasive aspects studied was not given. There had been a greater impairment of vital signs and hemodynamic aspects during early hospitalization in the autopsied than in the nonautopsied patients. Further, the 1-month survival was lower in the autopsied patients than in those not autopsied (31% -vs- 72%). The authors concluded that patients in severe CHF or shock and, presumably, with relatively large or complicated AMI are more likely to die early and, therefore, to be autopsied. Those with better cardiac function live longer and often die after having been released from the initial hospitalization. The latter patients presumably had smaller and uncomplicated infarcts and tended not to be among those autopsied. The authors caution that before investigators correlate pathologic and clinical data from subjects with AMI, it is important to analyze carefully bias inherent in the selection of subjects who have been autopsied. Although not stated by the authors, it is obvious that the patients autopsied had, for the most part, died during the period of AMI, whereas the patients not autopsied had, for the most part, died after healing of the AMI. Thus, the authors are comparing in actuality 2 different sets of patients. In such a comparison there is a bias both ways.

RISK OF AMI FROM SMOKING CIGARETTES, TAKING ORAL CONTRACEPTIVES OR HAVING A VASECTOMY

Hartz and associates[6] from Milwaukee, Wisconsin, studied the association of smoking (not exclusively cigarettes) and a history of AMI in 3,997 men who underwent coronary arteriography. The patients were subdivided into groups based on the amounts of coronary narrowing (minimal, moderate, or severe) and plasma cholesterol level (low, moderate or high). For men >50 years old, smoking was significantly associated with AMI in each occlusion group. For men <50 years, the association was significant for men with moderate or severe arterial occlusion. In the presence of higher cholesterol levels there was a stronger association of smoking with AMI, but a weaker association of smoking with coronary narrowing. These results suggest that the association of smoking with AMI does not depend primarily on the atherogenic effect of smoking. The association seems to be enhanced by greater degrees of coronary narrowing and high levels of serum cholesterol.

It is well established that women have an increased risk of venous thromboembolism, stroke, and AMI while taking oral contraceptives. The risk also is known to diminish soon after the cessation of use, but it is not known whether there is a long-lasting residual effect if oral contraceptives are taken for many years. With regard to AMI, there are particular grounds for concern about a residual effect, since oral contraceptives bring about changes in lipoprotein metabolism, BP, and glucose tolerance that may increase. Slone and associates[7] from Boston, Massachusetts, and Philadelphia, Pennsylvania, evaluated, in a hospital-based case-controlled study, the rate of AMI in relation to both discontinued and current use of oral contraceptives by comparing 556 women (aged 25–49 years) with 2,036 age-matched control subjects. For current users, the rate-ratio estimate was 3.5. For past users 40–49 years of age, the magnitude of the rate-ratio was related to the duration of use: for total durations of past use of <5 years, 5–9 years, and ≥10 years, respectively, the rate-ratio estimates were 1.0, 1.6, and 2.5, and this trend was statistically significant. These findings suggest that an effect on the risk of AMI persists after discontinuation of the long-term use of oral contraceptives.

Vasectomized monkeys have been reported to have accelerated rates of atherogenesis, both when fed high-fat diets and when fed regular monkey chow. No definite evidence of an increase in incidence of atherosclerotic disease, however, has been noted among vasectomized men, but data are limited. Walker and associates[8] determined the incidence of nonfatal AMI among 4,830 vasectomized men and found it to be 0.9/1,000 man-years during 24,420 man-years of observation. This incidence was slightly lower than that in 24,150 nonvasectomized men, each matched with a vasectomized man for calendar year of birth and duration of observation. Thus, no meaningful increase in the incidence of nonfatal AMI was observed in this study of vasectomized men who were compared with a 5-fold larger group of nonvasectomized men. The lack of association between vasectomy and nonfatal AMI does not appear to result from a bias due to confounding risk factors (systemic hypertension, obesity, diabetes mellitus, or smoking).

DIAGNOSIS AND CLINICAL COURSE

Comparison of AMI in hospitalized patients and in nonhospitalized patients

An AMI occurring in a patient already hospitalized for another problem offers an opportunity for early institution of therapy and, possibly, an improved prognosis, at least in the initial phase. However, most hospitalized patients have additional medical or surgical illnesses and occurrence of AMI during hospitalization might portend a less favorable prognosis. Zmyslinski and associates[9] from Columbia, South Carolina, analyzed 510 patients with AMI to investigate differences in clinical characteristics and outcome between those who had AMI while inside the hospital (in-AMI) and those who had an AMI outside the hospital (ex-AMI). Mortality for in-AMI patients was significantly higher than for ex-AMI patients (66% -vs- 22%) and remained higher even after exclusion of high-risk in-AMI patients (surgical patients, those with serious underlying noncardiac illness, and those with underlying cardiac illness as the reason for hospital admission). Medical in-AMI patients experienced fewer typical AMI symptoms and did not reach an intensive care unit significantly sooner than did ex-AMI patients. Time from onset of AMI symptoms to death was not significantly different between in-AMI and ex-AMI groups. Therefore, AMI occurring during hospitalization was associated with poor early prognosis even after exclusion of high-risk patients. These results emphasize the need for improved approaches to prevention, identification, and management of AMI occurring in hospitalized patients.

Leukocyte count, smoking and AMI

Freedman and associates in 1974 were the first to state that the leukocyte count was a predictor of AMI independent of established risk factors, but those workers did not carefully control for cigarette smoking, which is known to increase the leukocyte count. Zalokar and associates[10] from Paris, France, between 1967 and 1972 examined 7,206 Frenchmen aged 43–53 years and free of any clinical manifestation of atherosclerosis at entry, and followed them to the end of 1977; the average follow-up period was 6.5 years. An AMI developed in 104 of the men from 1–118 months (average, 48) after the initial examination. The incidence of AMI rose regularly with increasing leukocyte counts. Men with leukocyte counts of at least 9,000/cu mm (10% of the group) had more than 4 times the incidence of AMI observed among the 50% of men with counts <6,000 (Table 2-1). Other known risk factors for AMI correlated poorly with the leukocyte count, except cigarette smoking. The incidence of AMI in men who had never smoked and in ex-smokers was very low, as compared with that in current smokers of any inhalation category. Noninhalers had twice the incidence and inhalers 6 times the incidence found among nonsmokers, and partial or former inhalers were in an intermediate position. This pattern in relation to smoking was nearly parallel to that of the mean leukocyte count. Within each smoking class, there was no significant trend in the incidence of AMI by leukocyte count category except among inhalers: the inhalers in the high leukocyte category had more than twice the incidence observed in the inhalers of the lower 2 categories. The mean leukocyte count increased regularly with the number of cigarettes smoked. The incidence of AMI was substantially higher in the high count category (≥7,800) than in the lower categories for any number of cigarettes smoked except <10 a day. The increasing incidence of AMI with increasing leukocytes count was seen only among inhalers of cigarette smoke and appeared to start at counts of 7,000/cu mm. Inhalers with counts

TABLE 2-1. *Incidence of MI according to leukocyte count. Reproduced with permission from Zalokar.* [10]

LEUKOCYTE COUNT	PERSON-YEARS OF FOLLOW-UP	CASES OF INFARCTION	INCIDENCE (per 1000 person-years)	95% CONFIDENCE INTERVAL
<6000	22,154	27	1.2	0.8–1.8
6000–6999	10,738	21	2.0	1.2–3.0
7000–7999	6,280	20	3.2	1.9–4.9
8000–8999	3,739	13	3.5	1.8–6.0
≥9000	4,267	23	5.4	3.4–8.1
Total population	47,178	104	2.2	1.9–2.6

⩾9,000/cu mm had nearly 4 times the risk incurred by inhalers with counts <7,000/cu mm.

This study confirms earlier findings that the leukocyte count is an important predictor of AMI, at least in middle-aged men, but this relationship was limited to current smokers who inhaled. Although the degree of inhalation of cigarette smoke was an important risk factor for AMI, among inhalers the leukocyte count provided important additional information on risk. The current number of cigarettes smoked, however, was not a consistent dose-related risk factor.

Further investigation of the inhalers smoking ⩾25 cigarettes daily revealed that the incidence of AMI remained at a plateau between 20 and 34 cigarettes a day, but that the 5% of the inhalers who smoked 35 or more cigarettes had only 1 subsequent case of AMI. The number of cigarettes smoked daily may give an unreliable estimate of the amount of smoke inhaled in any one individual. At least the inhalers who later had AMI smoked in such a manner that their average exposure to cigarette smoke was greater than that of any of the other inhalers, regardless of the number of cigarettes smoked. The mean leukocyte count of subjects with AMI was 8,230/cu mm, as compared with 7,760 among inhalers who smoked 30−34 cigarettes a day. Whether or not the predicted value of the leukocyte count for AMI can be totally explained by smoker's leukocytosis, the leukocyte count does indicate which smokers are at the highest risk. It would, therefore, be reasonable to include this commonly performed measurement among the standard risk factors for AMI, at least in the case of middle-aged male smokers.

Plasma urea after AMI

Moseley and associates[11] from Leeds, England, measured plasma and urine urea and creatinine levels in 50 patients admitted consecutively to a coronary care unit. Of this group, 40 had AMI, and their average plasma urea level increased substantially by the third day after admission, a time when 50% of the patients had abnormally higher plasma urea levels. No change in plasma urea levels occurred in the 10 patients who did not have an AMI. These results indicate that a rise in plasma urea level is common, if not universal, after AMI and is caused by either a decrease in glomerular filtration rate or an increase in urea production, rather than by a mixture of the 2.

Usefulness of the creatine kinase curve area and peak creatine kinase after AMI

Serial determinations of creatine kinase (CK) activity in the serum have been used to assess the extent of myocardial necrosis or infarct size. The integrated area of the CK curve (CK area) also has been employed as an index of the relative size of an AMI and applied in the evaluation of ECG methods of assessing the extent of myocardial damage. To assess the practicality of a number of approaches utilizing serial determinations of CK, Ryan and associates[12] from La Jolla, California, determined CK curve areas in 112 patients with AMI. Two-hour sampling was performed for the first 24 hours or until peak CK was reached, and a gamma density function was used to calculate curve areas from all available samples. Attempts to predict CK curve area by means of the portion of the curve prior to peak CK proved to be inaccurate; not until values 2 hours or more beyond peak CK were utilized did predicted and actual CK areas agree well. A close correlation (r = 0.93) was found between CK area and peak CK. To establish an approach for detecting peak CK in the clinical setting, a range of sampling intervals (4–24 h) was assessed; 4-hour and 6-hour sampling intervals for 48 hours produced maximum CK values at or above 85% of true peak CK in 90% and 89% of patients, respectively, and average maximum CK at both sampling intervals exceeded 94% of that obtained with 2-hour samplings. It was concluded that this simplified approach can provide a basis for estimating infarct size in individual AMI patients.

MB-creatine kinase activity in transmural and nontransmural AMI

The early release patterns of creatine kinase isoenzyme MB (CK-MB) in myocardial ischemia and AMI are largely unknown. Shell and associates[13] from Los Angeles, California, utilized a sensitive column chromatographic assay of CK-MB activity and sequential CK-MB samples during the first 6 hours of AMI to define the early time course of enzyme release. The mean CK-MB in 39 normal subjects was 2.4 ± 0.93 IU/liter. The 22 patients with ischemic chest pain in whom AMI did not develop had normal CK-MBs (2.4 ± 1.0 IU/liter). Of 39 patients in whom transmural AMI developed, 28 (72%) had abnormal CK-MB, either initially or over a 20-minute sampling period. In contrast, 11% of the patients considered to have sustained a nontransmural AMI had abnormal initial CK-MBs and subsequently demonstrated significant increases in CK-MB from 28 ± 19 IU/liter initially to 41 ± 30 IU/liter over the 20-minute sampling period (p < 0.01; n, 16). Thus, CK-MB appears earlier in plasma after nontransmural AMI than after transmural AMI, probably reflecting perfusion to ischemic myocardium.

Long chain free fatty acid and magnesium in AMI

Flink and associates[14] from Morgantown, West Virginia, studied plasma magnesium and long-chain free fatty acid (FFA) levels in 16 patients with AMI. In each, magnesium levels rose and FFA levels fell shortly after onset of pain (Fig. 2-5). Magnesium and FFA values returned to normal within 3 days. An absolute fall in total magnesium level and probable fall in magnesium ion concentration could be important factors in arrhythmias during the first 2 days after AMI. The simultaneous rise in FFA and fall in magnesium levels in a variety of pathologic and physiologic conditions afford an explanation for divergent changes in FFA and magnesium concentrations in AMI. The FFA rise appears to be the primary change and, therefore, provides an explanation for the fall in magnesium levels.

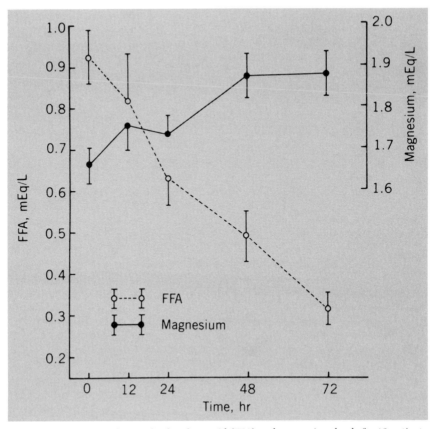

Fig. 2-5.   Mean ± SE of mean for free fatty acid (FFA) and magnesium levels for 16 patients. Values at 0, 12, and 24 h show consistent divergence, with no cross-over of individual values (p < .005). Reproduced with permission from Flink et al.[14]

PROGNOSTIC INDICES

Ventricular arrhythmias

The Lown grading system for ventricular arrhythmias has been used in observational and experimental studies of patients with CAD. The grading system uses 3 levels of ventricular premature depolarization frequency and 4 complex features to assign patients to 1 of 7 grades (Table 2-2). Bigger and Weld[15] from New York City tested several major assumptions of the Lown grading system in 400 patients who had recently had AMI. The Lown grading system assumes that the frequency of VPC exerts a negligible risk force in patients who have complex VPC. Bigger and Weld, however, found that the frequency of VPC contributed significant additional risk for cardiac death,

TABLE 2-2. *The Lown grading system for ventricular arrhythmias. Reproduced with permission from Bigger and Weld.*[15]

LOWN GRADE	DEFINITION
0	No ventricular premature depolarizations
1	Less than 30 ventricular extrasystoles per hour
2	30 or more ventricular extrasystoles per hour
3	Multiform ventricular extrasystoles
4A	2 consecutive ventricular extrasystoles
4B	3 or more consecutive ventricular extrasystoles
5	R on T (RV/QT less than 1·0)

even in the 3 highest Lown grades, 4A, 4B, and 5 (Table 2-3). The Lown grading system assumes that, of the 4 complex features used, R-on-T VPC has the greatest risk for subsequent cardiac death. Bigger and Weld found that paired VPC and VT had more prognostic significance than R-on-T VPC. The authors found it important for prognostic stratification that subgroups merged into a given Lown grade should be relatively homogeneous with respect to outcome. They found a lack of homogeneity in the 3 highest Lown grades. Grade 5 contained 16 subgroups with a mortality risk ranging from 0–75%; statistically significant differences in subsequent mortality were found among these subgroups. Most shortcomings of the Lown grading system in AMI patients resulted from failure to give sufficient weight to VPC frequency and to repetitive VPC.

Campbell and associates[16] from Newcastle-upon-Tyne, England, determined the prevalence of ventricular arrhythmias in the first 12 hours after onset of AMI. They chose 17 patients because of their developing primary ventricular fibrillation (VF) and compared findings in them with those in 21

TABLE 2-3 *Relation between Lown grade and mortality in 400 patients after AMI. Reproduced with permission from Bigger and Weld.*[15]

LOWN GRADE	GROUP TOTAL	DEATHS #	DEATHS %
0	64	9	14
1	85	9	11
2	2	0	0
3	68	10	15
4A	44	9	20
4B	21	7	33
5	116	34	29
All	400	78	20

other patients also with AMI, but without primary VF. None received or had been receiving antiarrhythmic therapy, digitalis, or diuretics. Continuously recorded ECGs were analyzed by a specially developed computer system. The frequency of primary VF and R-on-T ventricular ectopic complexes was highest in the first 3 hours after AMI and was lower thereafter. By contrast, other ventricular arrhythmias, including VT, increased in frequency in hours 4–12. Primary VF in 16 of the 17 patients was initiated by an R-on-T ventricular ectopic complex (QR'/QT ≤ 0.85), whereas only 4 of 265 episodes of VT were so initiated. In the 22 patients (11 with primary VF and 11 without) who had R-on-T ventricular ectopic complexes, the average rate of their occurrence was higher in those with primary VF. In the 10 minutes before primary VF there was a striking increase in the incidence of R-on-T ventricular ectopic complexes. This study shows that different ventricular arrhythmias have a different and changing rate of occurrence in AMI. A close relation was observed between R-on-T ventricular ectopic complexes and primary VF.

Prolonged ventricular repolarization is common during the first 4 days of AMI and, in retrospective studies, it appeared to predispose to early phase inhospital VT and VF. Inhomogeneous recovery or temporal dispersion of the refractory period of the ventricles has been considered to provide the milieu for such tachyarrhythmias in conjunction with acute dysautonomia. A recent retrospective investigation suggested that relative lengthening of the QT interval following AMI at hospital discharge was associated with increased likelihood of sudden death in the subsequent 1 year. Taylor and Associates[17] from Charlottesville, Virginia, prospectively assessed the time course of changes in repolarization during AMI in 32 patients admitted 2 hours after AMI onset. The initial corrected QT interval (QTc) upon hospitalization was longer (0.52 s) in the 14 patients developing VT within the first 48 hours than the QTc (0.47 s) in 8 patients with frequent VPC or the QTc (0.46 s) in 10 patients with infrequent VPC. By the fifth day after AMI onset, the QTc shortened significantly only in the VT group, suggesting a greater initial abnormality of repolarization in these patients. All 32 patients had coronary angiography, RNA, and myocardial perfusion scintigraphy before hospital discharge. Significant discriminating factors relating to early phase VT in AMI included initially longer QT and QTc intervals, faster heart rates, higher peak serum levels of creatine kinase, anterior wall location of the AMI, angiographically documented proximal stenosis of the LAD, and scintigraphic evidence of hypoperfusion of the ventricular septum. Prior AMI, angina pectoris, systemic hypertension, multivessel CAD, and depressed LV EF did not provide discrimination among the 3 different ventricular arrhythmia AMI groups. Thus, the QT interval is frequently prolonged early in AMI, the initial transiently prolonged ventricular repolarization facilitates and predicts a complex ventricular tachyarrhythmia within the first 48 hours of AMI, jeopardized blood supply to the ventricular septum frequently coexists, and therapeutic enhancement of rapid recovery of the ventricular repolarization process merits investigation for prevention of VT in AMI.

Taylor and associates[18] from Baltimore, Maryland, performed coronary and LV angiograms and 24-hour ECG monitoring 10–24 days after AMI in

61 medically treated patients, then did serial 24-hour ECGs for 13 ± 11 months after the AMI. Complex ventricular arrhythmias (2 or more sequential VPC, multiform VPC, bigeminy) during follow-up were associated with a high mortality rate and occurred most commonly in the setting of 3-vessel CAD, proximal LAD CAD, and low LV EF. By contrast, no patient without complex VPC in either the late hospital or posthospital phase of AMI died during the year following AMI; furthermore, these patients had a higher frequency of single-vessel CAD and less LV dysfunction. These results emphasize the adverse prognostic significance of complex ventricular arrhythmias in the year after AMI and their association with extensive CAD and LV damage.

Morrison and associates[19] from Hull, UK, studied cardiac rate and rhythm by 24-hour ambulatory ECG recording in 44 patients before, during, and after their discharge from hospital after an AMI. The first recordings were started 48 hours before discharge, the second on the morning of the day of discharge, and the third 48 hours after discharge (at home). While patients were in hospital and after they had returned home, the heart rate fell during sleep, but there was no diurnal variation in the frequency of VPC. Daytime heart rate and both the frequency and grade (severity) of ventricular arrhythmias were significantly raised 48 hours after discharge. The frequency of VPC during sleep also was increased in the recording made 48 hours after discharge. Rises in heart rate and frequency and severity of VPC were observed on the morning of the day of discharge, increasing up to the time of leaving hospital, but they all diminished during the journey home. No relation was found between ventricular arrhythmias during early convalescence and ventricular arrhythmias during the acute phase of AMI. Thus, at the time of leaving the hospital after AMI, there does not appear to be a serious risk of development of major cardiac arrhythmias.

Usefulness of T-wave changes and recurrent angina pectoris in predicting recurrent AMI

Lofmark[20] from Huddinge, Sweden, studied the predictive value of angina pectoris and T-wave changes in 177 patients with AMI. Of them, 21 had another AMI within 3 months and 11 (52%) of these 21 had at least 1 ECG recorded while in the hospital that showed a steeply ascending limb of negative T wave, as compared with 20 (13%) of the 156 patients who did not have another AMI. Of the 21 patients with recurrent angina pectoris at rest during the hospital stay, 10 (48%) developed another AMI within 3 months. Combining the ECG criteria and recurrent angina at rest led to correct prediction of the 14 (67%) of 21 patients with another AMI and to a false prediction about 30 (19%) of the 156 patients who did not develop another AMI.

Comparison of a new invasive prognostic index with the noninvasive prognostic index of Norris and Peel

Wolffenbuttel and associates[21] from Rotterdam, the Netherlands, studied 132 patients with AMI and followed them over a 2-year period. The noninvasive index of Norris and Peel was compared with a new invasive prognostic index (PI), derived from heart rate (HR), systolic blood pressure (SBP), pulmonary capillary wedge pressure (PCW), and cardiac index (CI). It was shown that $100 \times (SBP \times CI)/(PCW \times HR)$ proved to be the most discriminant formula to predict outcome. In a second series of 123 individuals, studied prospectively, this index showed the same discriminatory power. The data indicate further that patients in Norris classes III–VI should receive hemodynamic monitoring by means of a Swan-Ganz thermodilution catheter and/or arterial line to determine the need for and the response to interventions within the first 24 hours. In addition, patients in Norris classes I and II should receive hemodynamic monitoring when severe conduction disturbances, VT, recurrent VF, or CHF are present. Determination of enzyme levels or the occurrence of VT or VF during the first 24 hours and a variety of noninvasive parameters, such as age, sex, and history of a previous AMI, proved to have little or no value in predicting the immediate or long-term outcome. Only in patients in Norris classes I and II without any complications will monitoring the ECG alone suffice. In these patients, VF or VT will occur sufficiently often to warrant admission to a coronary care unit.

Left ventricular filling pressure

Elevation of LV filling pressure (FP) following AMI is related to both short- and long-term mortality. In previous studies, hemodynamic measurements did not represent a homogeneous sample because LV FP was obtained over a wide range of time after AMI onset, and the invasive procedures were reserved primarily for clinically ill patients. Shell and associates[22] from Los Angeles, California, measured LV FP within 12 hours of onset of AMI in 99 patients, including 21 nonsurvivors. The initial LV FP for survivors was 18 mmHg and, for nonsurvivors, 24 mmHg. Of all patients, 87% had initial LV FP $\geqslant 12$ mmHg and all nonsurvivors were in this group. Life-table analysis was employed to determine LV FP-related mortality rates. If initial LV FP was < 18 mmHg, 72-hour mortality rate was 4% and 30-day mortality rate was 10%. For initial LV FP > 18 mmHg, 72-hour mortality rate was 21% and 30-day mortality rate was 33%. When final LV FP was analyzed, 30-day mortality rate for final LV FP < 18 mmHg was 5%. Mortality rate of 60% was observed for final LV FP > 18 mmHg. This study also compared sequential measurements of LV FP in a subset of survivors and nonsurvivors and found that the long-term average trend was for survivors to increase their LV FP. Thus, AMI mortality rate is related to the LV FP, and LV FP > 18 mmHg is associated with a very high mortality rate, as compared with LV FP < 18 mmHg. Reduction of LV FP either spontaneously or from therapy may lower the AMI mortality rate.

Extent of left ventricular wall thickness infarcted: transmural -vs- nontransmural

Hutter and associates[23] from Boston, Massachusetts, compared the hospital and long-term course of 67 patients with nontransmural AMI with that of 66 patients with transmural anterior AMI and of 63 patients with transmural posterior (inferior) AMI. Patients were matched for age, sex, previous AMI, and previous CHF. During their hospital stay, patients with nontransmural AMI had significantly less CHF and fewer intraventricular conduction defects than did patients with transmural anterior AMI; fewer atrial tachycardias and less sinus bradycardia and AV block than did patients with transmural posterior AMI; and an incidence of hypotension, pericarditis, and ventricular irritability similar to that of patients in the other 2 groups. Patients with nontransmural AMI had a significantly lower coronary care unit mortality rate (9%) than did patients with transmural anterior or posterior AMI (20% and 19%, respectively) (Fig. 2-6). By 3 months, the mortality rate had risen to 14% in the patients with nontransmural AMI, but was significantly higher (29% and 27%, respectively) in patients with transmural anterior or posterior AMI. Angina pectoris was common in all 3 groups, occurring in >50% of patients during a mean follow-up period of 29 months after

Fig. 2-6. Survival curves of 3 patient groups. The arrow identifies curves at 3 months after MI. NTMI = nontransmural MI. TAMI = transmural anterior MI. TIMI = transmural inferior MI.

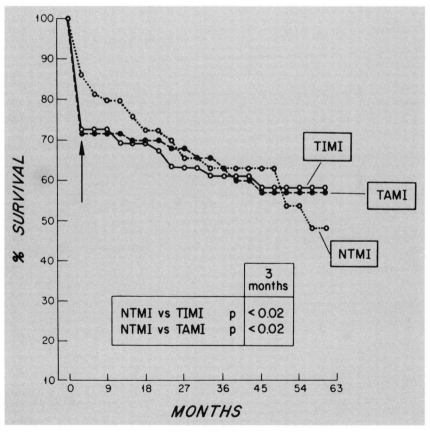

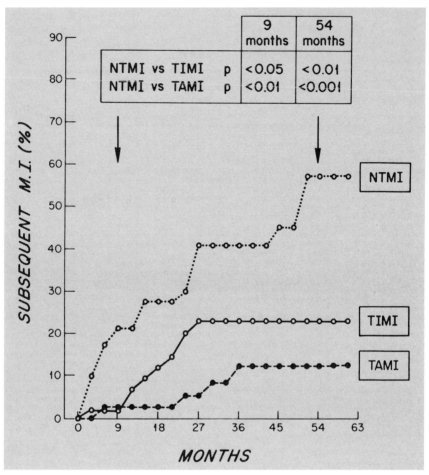

Fig. 2-7. Subsequent MI in 3 patient groups. Arrows identify curves at 9 and 54 months. Abbreviations as in Fig. 2-6.

hospital discharge. In contrast, the incidence of subsequent AMI was significantly greater in patients with nontransmural AMI, occurring in 21% at 9 months, as compared with 3% of patients with transmural anterior and 2% of those with transmural posterior AMI (Fig. 2-7). By 54 months, 57% of patients with nontransmural AMI had sustained a new AMI, in contrast to only 12% of patients with transmural anterior and 22% of patients with transmural posterior AMI. The late mortality increased in patients with nontransmural AMI and, although this group had a significantly better survival rate at 3 months, the overall late mortality of the 3 groups was compatible. Thus, this study suggests that nontransmural AMI is an unstable ischemic event associated with great risk of later AMI and high late mortality rate.

Treadmill exercise testing after AMI

Starling and associates[24] from San Antonio, Texas, evaluated 89 patients with predischarge and 6-week-later post-AMI treadmill exercise tests to determine the importance of repeat tests in identifying abnormalities of prognostic value, and to assess the individual variability of treadmill responses. Nineteen patients (21%) completed only a predischarge exercise test; 9 of them experienced an early cardiac event that precluded repeat testing. All 9 had a prognostically important treadmill abnormality during the predischarge test. ECG ST-segment depression was highly reproducible between the early and 6-week tests. Angina, inadequate BP response, and ventricular arrhythmias showed limited reproducibility and substantial individual variability. Thus, a predischarge treadmill exercise test is important for determining the immediate short-term prognosis after AMI. ST-segment depression is highly reproducible, whereas other treadmill abnormalities show substantial variability between the predischarge and 6-week tests.

Schwartz and associates[25] from Birmingham, Alabama, performed limited treadmill graded exercise testing and both coronary and LV angiography in 48 patients within 3 weeks of AMI. Nineteen (90%) of 21 patients with positive exercise tests (≥1 mm ST depression, angina, or both) had multivessel CAD. In the 27 patients with negative exercise test results, 15 (56%) had multivessel CAD, 11 (41%) had 1-vessel CAD, and 1 (4%) had no CAD. Exercise-induced ST-segment elevation occurred in 24 patients and predicted a significantly lower EF and higher angiographic abnormally contracting segment size. Patients having angina during or after exercise had a significantly shorter 2-year survival (54% ± 21%) than patients without exercise-induced angina (97% ± 3%) (p < 0.03). Thus, limited exercise testing after AMI is useful in evaluating the presence of multivessel CAD and LV dysfunction and in predicting long-term survival.

The study by Schwartz and associates indicates that the prevalence of multivessel CAD in their post-AMI population was 71%. A positive early exercise test identified most patients, although a negative test did not rule out multivessel CAD. Their study also shows that limited exercise testing does not serve to identify all patients with multivessel CAD who might potentially benefit from CABG. The criteria for early post-AMI angiography remain controversial. Certainly angiography should be strongly considered in all patients having a positive limited exercise test and in patients convalescing from AMI complicated by intractable CHF, chest pain, and arrhythmias. Angiography might also be seriously considered in selected patients with negative exercise tests, particularly those under age 65 who are asymptomatic and wish to return to vigorous lifestyles.

Fuller and associates[26] from Houston, Texas, performed (heart rate, ≤120 beats/min) standardized treadmill stress testing before hospital discharge in 40 survivors of uncomplicated AMI. Each patient subsequently underwent coronary arteriography. The AMI was "inferior" in 21, anterior in 10, and nontransmural in 9. In 30 patients, this AMI was their first. A positive ECG response, angina, or both occurred in 15 patients and correctly identified most patients with multivessel disease (sensitivity 67%, predictive value 87%) and patients at risk for coronary events: 35% of positive responders had angina in the first month after discharge, as compared with 4% of patients with a negative test (p < 0.05). During a 7-month follow-up period, 73% of patients with a positive test result developed angina, as compared with 16% of those with negative tests results (p < 0.001). Thus, predischarge post-AMI limited stress testing correctly identifies the high-risk subset of patients with multivessel CAD and thereby allows intelligent selection of patients for early coronary arteriography.

Modified treadmill exercise testing before hospital discharge has been shown to be feasible and safe in uncomplicated post-AMI patients. In addition, ST-segment depression, angina pectoris, and an inadequate BP response have demonstrated predictive value for future untoward cardiac events. It has been suggested that the poor prognosis in patients with these treadmill abnormalities early post-AMI may reflect the high prevalence of coexistent multivessel CAD. The results of prior studies in which post-AMI patients were evaluated with standard stress tests and coronary arteriography several months to years following AMI tend to confirm this contention. Little information exists concerning the predictive value of early post-AMI treadmill exercise testing results or angiographically documented CAD. Also, no study has determined the coronary arteriographic and left ventriculographic correlates of an inadequate BP response during exercise testing early after AMI. Accordingly, Starling and associates[27] from San Antonio, Texas, evaluated 57 patients with modified treadmill exercise testing (MTET) and angiography early post-AMI to determined the predictive value of ST-segment depression, angina, and an inadequate BP response for multivessel CAD. ST-segment depression alone identified multivessel CAD stenoses (>70% diameter narrowing in 2 or more vessels) with a sensitivity of 54%, a specificity of 75%, and an accuracy of 60%. When ST-segment depression and angina were considered a positive treadmill test result, significant improvements in sensitivity (88%) and accuracy (82%) for multivessel CAD were observed. An adequate BP response was associated with multivessel CAD (12/13 patients) and with a significantly reduced average LV EF of 39%, as compared with 58% for patients without this treadmill abnormality. Thus, ST-segment depression and angina on early post-AMI MTET appear to be superior predictors of multivessel CAD, as compared with ST-segment depression alone, and an inadequate BP response during MTET early following AMI is observed in patients with multivessel CAD and reduced LV performance.

PROLONGED (≥20 YEARS) SURVIVAL AFTER TRANSMURAL AMI

Although several reports have described follow-up of patients for up to 5 years after AMI, few have described follow-up for >10 years. Because morphologic and clinical data on patients surviving 20 years or longer without operative intervention after AMI are lacking, McManus and Roberts[28] from Bethesda, Maryland, described clinical and necropsy findings in 8 patients

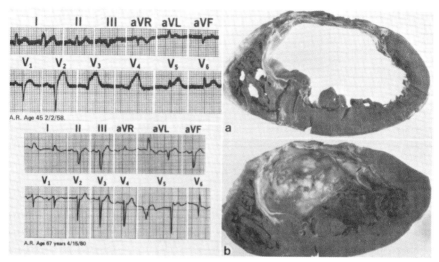

Fig. 2-8. ECGs recorded at time of AMI in 1958 and 4.5 months before death in 1980. Transverse sections of ventricle aneurysm (*a*) with calcific deposits (*b*). Reproduced with permission from McManus and Roberts.[28]

Fig. 2-9. Approximate cumulative survival (%) at selected year periods of published reports of nonoperated patients followed at least 15 years after their first nonfatal AMI. Reproduced with permission from McManus and Roberts.[28]

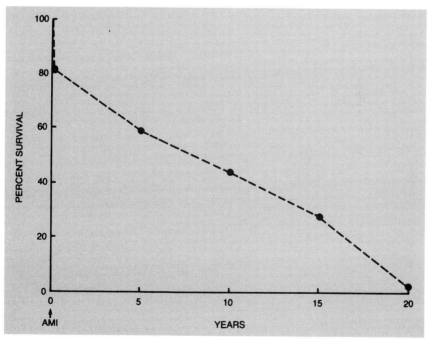

who lived 20–31 years (mean, 24) after healing of a transmural AMI (Fig. 2-8). Two had LV aneurysms and 1 had both RV and LV infarcts. Survival for 2 decades or more after healing of a transmural AMI rarely has been documented, and descriptions of hearts at necropsy in patients with well-documented infarcts 20 years or more earlier are virtually nonexistent prior to this report. A review of reported studies of patients followed for at least 10 years after AMI disclosed that about 40% survived 10 years, but <1% for >20 years (Fig. 2-9). Obviously, for a survivor to live >20 years after AMI, the AMI must occur at a relatively young age and death must occur at a relatively late age. Of the 6 patients studied by McManus and Roberts for whom this information was available, the mean age at the time of AMI was 47 years and the mean age at death was 78 years. The interval from the first AMI to death in 25 reported patients ranged from 20–38 years (mean, 27). Thus, from analyses of the previously reported patients surviving >20 years after AMI, factors that allowed their prolonged survival are not clear. Evidence of myocardial ischemia after healing of the AMI was absent or minimal in most patients.

MANAGEMENT DURING THE ACUTE PHASE

Hospital or home treatment

Of the 600,000 yearly coronary deaths in the USA, about 67% occur suddenly outside the hospital, mostly from VF. Many victims of out-of-hospital sudden coronary death can be saved by prompt application of modern emergency techniques. In the USA, over 300 emergency medical technician (EMT) and paramedic services now operate, and cities with >1 million people have a paramedic service. From the impact of paramedic units, it has been estimated that 220 out-of-hospital cardiac arrests would occur among half a million people each year, and that 30 to 40 individuals would leave the hospital alive, yielding 6–8 lives saved per 100,000 people per year. Another estimate indicated that mobile intensive care can prevent 35,000 cardiac deaths per year in the USA. Nevertheless, doubts about the ability of prehospital coronary care to reduce community death rate persist and Adgey and Crampton[29] from Belfast, Northern Ireland, and Charlottesville, Virginia, reviewed the subject. Some physicians question whether a patient with a suspected AMI should be hospitalized, since mortality of patients cared for at home appeared similar to that in the Coronary Care Units (CCU). In the UK, surveys in 3 regions confirm this view. The Bristol study, confined to men aged <70 years after AMI in the preceding 48 hours, excluded women because care at home would have been difficult for social reasons. Of the 1,203 episodes of AMI, only 343 (29%) were randomized, with 77% treated in-hospital and only 23% at home. The median interval from onset of AMI to arrival of the family doctor was 4 hours. Four weeks later, 10% of the patients in the random home group had died, and 14% of the random in-hospital group had died. This study showed that for some patients seen late after onset of AMI, admission to hospital conferred no benefit.

Significant numbers of patients with AMI, however, always will need hospitalization. Since 20%–40% of patients will not be at home at the time they develop symptoms of a heart attack, they will require hospitalization. Neither the patient nor the family doctor can distinguish whether the illness is AMI, unstable angina pectoris, or an acute ischemic episode. Because of the early high mortality from CAD, some form of prehospital coronary care is mandatory. Emphasis also must be placed upon educating the public about symptoms of heart attack and dealing with sudden death. Training the public to resuscitate is essential. Trained personnel with the necessary drugs and a small portable defibrillator must reach the patient as rapidly as possible after the onset of chest pain, thereby offering the patient the best chance for survival. The physician must aggressively take responsibility for rigorous medical control to improve the quality of prehospital care of patients with a coronary attack and thereby increase survival.

Improved criteria for admission to coronary care units

Fuchs and Scheidt[30] from New York City analyzed 414 patients admitted consecutively to a coronary care unit (CCU) with known or suspected AMI. The patients were divided into a high-risk group that had 1 or more of 3 findings, viz., ongoing chest pain, pulmonary rales, or 1 or more PVC on 12-lead ECG, and a low-risk group that had none of these 3 findings. Of the 306 high-risk patients, 41% received at least 1 intervention while in the CCU and these interventions included administration of lidocaine hydrochloride, atropine sulfate, sodium nitroprusside, or vasopressors; Swan-Ganz or arterial catheterization; insertion of temporary pacemaker; or electroshock. Four percent of the high-risk group died in the CCU. In contrast, of the 108 low-risk patients, only 6% received any intervention in the CCU and none died in the CCU. This study suggests that patients who do not have ongoing chest pain, CHF, or VPC when first evaluated have a low risk of early complications and may not require intensive care.

Exercise therapy and rehabilitation

Approaches to cardiac rehabilitation have changed rapidly in the past 10 years. Prolonged bed rest and convalescence with restriction of activity lead to marked cardiovascular deconditioning, which has adverse physical, psychological, and economic consequences. To reduce these effects, patients are now being allowed to walk and are discharged from the hospital earlier than previously. This approach is safe in patients without complications and in those in whom complications have subsided. There also has been a trend toward early initiation of exercise therapy to facilitate rehabilitation after AMI. The benefits and hazards of such early exercises have not been studied. Sivarajan and associates[31] from Seattle, Washington, studied the effects of early, supervised exercises in preventing deconditioning after AMI. Enrollment in the exercise program occurred an average of 4.5 days after admission (range, 1–9). Discharge from the hospital occurred an average of 10 days after admission in both the control and exercise groups. Most patients had a low-level treadmill test on the day before hospital discharge. There were no differences between the 2 groups in the clinical, hemodynamic, or ECG responses to the treadmill test. Frequencies of complications and deaths (1 death in each group) during hospitalization were similar in the 2 groups, although 6 patients (3%, all in the exercise group) required cardiac surgery —4 because of recurrent chest pain and 2 because of ventricular rupture. Thus, neither beneficial or deleterious effects of an early, in-hospital exercise program were demonstrable.

Treatment with molsidomine

Nitroglycerin (NTG) and the other organic nitrates are frequently used for the treatment of angina pectoris, CHF, and AMI. Because the duration of action of nonparenteral nitrates is relatively short, frequent administration is necessary to maintain a sustained response. Molsidomine (M), a new antianginal vasodilator drug, has been shown to produce hemodynamic responses similar in nature to NTG in patients with chronic stable angina, and the duration of M action appears to be considerably longer. The hemodynamic effects of M, however, require evaluation in AMI patients to assess the drug's potential role in treatment of postinfarction angina and CHF. Aptecar and associates[32] from Buenos Aires, Argentina, evaluated the hemodynamic effects and duration of action of 4 mg intravenous M as compared with those of 10 mg sublingual isosorbide dinitrate (ISDN) in 12 patients with uncomplicated AMI. Both M and ISDN produced marked decreases in the mean right atrial (RA) pressure, mean pulmonary capillary wedge (PCW) pressure, and mean PA pressure. The maximal decreases in RA (-56%) and PCW (-35%) pressure with intravenous M were more pronounced than with sublingual ISDN (RA, 35%; PCW, 29%). Modest physiologic declines in systemic vascular resistance, cardiac output, and arterial BP were similar with both drugs; the duration of action of M was longer (average 5 h) than that of ISDN (2 h). No patient experienced hypotension, tachycardia, or other adverse responses following M, suggesting that M is well tolerated by normotensive patients with AMI.

Treatment with both nitroglycerin and propranolol

Come and associates[33] from Baltimore, Maryland, investigated the hemodynamic effects of combined nitroglycerin (NTG) and propranolol in 15 patients with AMI. After NTG infusion had decreased the mean arterial pressure by 20 mmHg for 1 hour, NTG was continued and patients were given 0.033 mg/kg propranolol every 5 minutes for a total dose of 0.1 mg/kg, or until heart rate decreased to <60 beats/min, LV filling pressure (FP) increased to >15 mmHg, or systolic arterial BP decreased to <85 mmHg. Seven of 8 patients with initial LV FP ≤ 15 mmHg and 3 of 7 with initial LV FP >15 mmHg received 0.1 mg/kg propranolol. Propranolol significantly decreased heart rate. Although pressure $\times$ heart rate decreased significantly, the magnitude of its decrease was small, suggesting only a minimal effect on myocardial oxygen demands. The LV FP increased after propranolol, but remained below control value. Simultaneous administration of NTG likely prevented further increases in LV FP, since LV FP increased after cessation of NTG infusion, and 3 patients subsequently developed pulmonary edema. Propranolol administration resulted in a significant increase in peripheral vascular resistance and a decrease in cardiac output.

Effect of alprenolol on infarct size

A broad spectrum of measures diminishes the amount of myocardial damage after AMI. Several beta adrenergic blocking agents, particularly propranolol, have been studied extensively. Jurgensen and associates[34] from Copenhagen, Denmark, investigated the effects of the beta adrenergic blocking agent alprenolol on myocardial infarct size, as estimated from serial determinations of serum creatine kinase (CK) in 282 patients <66 years of age. Treatment was started immediately on admission with 5–10 mg alprenolol or placebo intravenously, followed by 200 mg alprenolol or placebo orally twice a day for 1 year. In 178 patients, a definite AMI was diagnosed. The infarct size could be estimated from CK in 42 patients treated with alprenolol and in 43 patients receiving placebo. The median infarct size was 21 CK g Eq/m² body surface in the alprenolol group and 34 CK g Eq/m² body surface in the placebo group. The median rate of release of CK from the ischemic myocardium was 28 U/liter/h in the alprenolol group and 48 U/liter/h in the placebo group. Thus, alprenolol limited infarct size significantly when treatment was started within 12 hours of the onset of AMI.

Effect of metoprolol on mortality

Hjalmarson and associates[35] from Goteborg, Sweden, compared the effect of metoprolol on mortality with that of placebo in a double-blind, randomized trial in 2,619 patients with definite or suspected AMI. Treatment with metoprolol or placebo started as soon as possible after the patient's arrival in hospital and was continued for 90 days. Metoprolol was given as a 15 mg intravenous dose, followed by oral administration of 100 mg twice daily. One thousand three hundred ninety five patients (697 on placebo and 698 on metoprolol) were included in the trial. Definite AMI developed in 809 and probable AMI in 162. Patients were allocated to various risk groups and within each group the patients were randomly assigned to treatment with metoprolol or placebo. There were 62 deaths in the placebo group (9%) and 40 deaths in the metroprolol group (6%), a reduction of 36% (p < 0.03) (Fig. 2-10). Mortality rates were given according to the treatment group to which the patients were initially allocated at random.

Effect of nitroprusside-induced fall in systemic arterial pressure on left ventricular hemiaxial shortening

The effect of nitroprusside-induced progressive systemic pressure reduction on segmental function in patients with AMI is unclear. Bodenheimer and associates[36] from Philadelphia, Pennsylvania, obtained control RNA in 15 patients within 24 hours of the onset of chest pain and during the admin-

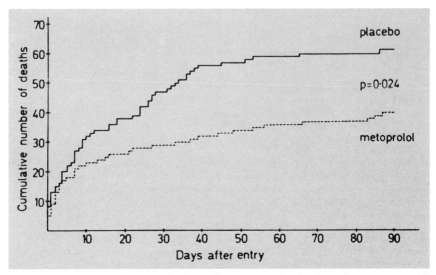

Fig. 2-10. Cumulative number of deaths in all patients randomly allocated to treatment with metoprolol and placebo. Reproduced with permission from Hjalmarson et al.[35]

istration of nitroprusside intravenously. The initial study showed a significant reduction in hemiaxial shortening in the zone of AMI. With nitroprusside, systolic pressure decreased from a mean of 133 mmHg to an intermediate pressure of 116 mmHg. At this pressure, central chord hemiaxial shortening increased in 8 of 15 zones (average increase, 10%−28%). After further reduction in pressure to 87 mmHg, an additional 5 of the 7 remaining zones of AMI improved. Of the 8 zones that improved initially, however, 4 deteriorated at the lowest pressure. Similar changes were seen in the lateral chords. Thus, afterload reduction can improve hemiaxial shortening of the AMI zone. However, the degree of reduction in systemic pressure must be individualized to avoid adverse effects of an excessive decrease in perfusion pressure.

Effect of methylprednisolone on hemodynamics and blood lactate

Henning and associates[37] from Los Angeles, California, investigated hemodynamic and metabolic effects of methylprednisolone in a double-blind study of 28 patients with AMI. Measurements were performed before and at 1.5, 3, 4, 4.5, 12, and 24 hours after infusion of methylprednisolone (13 patients) or placebo (15 patients). Although systemic vascular resistance decreased from 1,750 to 1,420 dynes/sec/cm^{-5} (p < 0.001) and cardiac index increased from 2.8 to 3.1 liters/min/M^2 (p < 0.02) between 0 and 4.5 hours, an abnormal increase in blood lactate was observed in 10 of the 13 patients after administration of methylprednisolone (3.0 -vs- 1.2 mM/L, p < 0.001). Lactate elevation appeared 1 hour after infusion of methylprednisolone, was maximal at 12 hours, and persisted for >24 hours. No significant change in

blood lactate occurred in placebo-treated patients. A transient but significant decrease in plasma volume also was observed after infusion of methylprednisolone. The elevation of blood lactate was not explained by reduction
in plasma volume, since the most striking increases in lactate were observed
12 hours after the initial infusion of methylprednisolone, when the plasma
volume was returning to the control value. No significant differences in other
hemodynamic or metabolic parameters, infarct size, or patient survival were
observed between the 2 groups. Thus, the hemodynamic benefits of gluco-
corticoids (increased cardiac output and lowered systemic vascular resistance) are counterbalanced by the potentially unfavorable conditions (lactate
elevation and volume depletion). Caution is warranted in use of methylprednisolone during AMI.

Effect of glucose-insulin-potassium on plasma free fatty acids and on left ventricular function

Plasma free fatty acids (FFA) are important in CAD because they supply a
major part of the energy requirements to the heart. Their utilization, unlike
that of glucose or glycogen, is oxygen-dependent for energy generation. The
build-up in fatty acids contributed to by elevated circulating levels of plasma
FFA and breakdown of endogenous lipids is thought to have toxic effects that
exacerbate the injury occurring during AMI. The release of membrane lipids
is thought to contribute to generation of arrhythmias associated with AMI.
Fatty acids are also necessary for formation of new membranes or repair of
reversibly damaged membranes, with individual fatty acids having different
roles. Linoleic acid is a major component of cardiolipin, which is a prominent part of the lipid structure of mitochondria. Arachidonic acid is the precursor for prostaglandins and, therefore, has a role relevant to vascular tone,
platelet aggregation, and thromboxane formation in CAD. McDaniel and associates[38] from Birmingham, Alabama, determined if glucose-insulin-potassium (GIK) infusion in patients with AMI altered individual FFA in addition
to providing for overall suppression of total plasma FFA levels. Total and individual plasma FFA were measured on admission and over the next 4 days
in 24 patients with AMI. In a prospective randomized fashion, these patients
were given an infusion of 300 g glucose, 50 units of insulin, and 80 mEq of
KCl/liter at a rate of 1.5 ml/kg/h over the initial 48 hours of hospitalization,
or they served as controls receiving conventional therapy. Eleven patients
were in the control group and 13 were in the GIK group. Of the 24 patients
with suspected AMI, 21 had an AMI by CK-MB rise and ECG changes (in the
GIK group, 3 did not evolve an AMI). The total plasma FFA was 840 μM/liter
in the controls and 933 μM/liter in the GIK group initially (pre-study). Total
FFA rapidly fell in the GIK group and then rebounded when GIK was discontinued. In contrast, total FFA fell gradually in the control group over the 4-
day period. Individual FFAs had similar percentages initially in 2 groups. In
the control group, the percent of individual plasma FFA was unchanged over
the period studied, although there was some mild random day-to-day fluc-
tuation. In contrast, in the GIK group, linoleic acid fell both during and after
the infusion was stopped (27% to 19%). Arachidonic acid doubled in percentage of the total FFA value during GIK infusion (3.1% to 6.4%) and returned to

the control value when administration of GIK was discontinued. Thus, GIK infusion during AMI reduces the total level of plasma FFA while increasing the percent of arachidonic and decreasing the percent of linoleic acid, presumably reflecting improved membrane stability of the ischemic myocardium in AMI.

The in-hospital mortality from AMI in the past 15 years has fallen from 35% to 15%, especially in patients with a smaller AMI. In addition to the treatment of arrhythmias and CHF, a major clinical goal that is the subject of active investigation is reduction or limitation of the extent of AMI by use of hyaluronidase, beta adrenergic blockade, afterload reduction, glucose-insulin-potassium (GIK), intraaortic counterpulsation, intracoronary thrombolytic enzymes, and emergency CABG. Previously, it has been shown that the infusion of GIK solution in AMI patients significantly reduces circulating free fatty acids,[38] diminishes ventricular arrhythmias, and lowers hospital mortality. Mantle and associates[39] from Birmingham, Alabama, examined the effects of GIK on hemodynamics and LV function in a prospective randomized clinical trial in AMI patients. Following completion of baseline hemodynamic measurements, patients were randomly allocated to 48-hour infusions of 300 g glucose, 50 units of insulin, and 80 mEq of KCl/liter at a rate of 125 ml/kg/h or to conventional therapy. In addition to serial hemodynamic measurements, LV function curves were constructed during the second and third days to assess the extent of LV injury. Of the 118 patients who were initially randomized, 85 had AMI documented by diagnostic rise and fall of CK-MB isoenzyme. Baseline characteristics and hemodynamics were similar for GIK and control patients with AMI. The GIK patients who presented with their initial AMI had a significant reduction in PA-end-diastolic pressure from prerandomization value of 16 mmHg to 10 mmHg by day 3, as compared with 16–18 mmHg for control patients, and an increase in cardiac index (CI) from 2.8 liters/min/M^2 to 3.4 liters/min/M^2, as compared with an increase from 2.8 liters/min/M^2 to 3.0 liters/min/M^2 for control patients. In response to dextran infusion, GIK patients had a significant further increase in CI to 3.9 liters/min/M^2 and an ascending slope to their LV function curve, as compared with no significant change in CI and a flat LV function curve for control patients. These data demonstrate that acute intervention with GIK improves hemodynamics and LV function in AMI patients beyond the infusion period by preserving ischemic myocardium.

INTRACORONARY STREPTOKINASE THROMBOLYSIS

Extensive myocardial damage is now the most common cause of death and morbidity among patients hospitalized with AMI. Since massive myocardial ischemia and necrosis produce cardiac pump failure and serious ventricular arrhythmias, new methods have been sought for reducing the degree of myocardial damage associated with AMI. In the past, such techniques have focused on decreasing myocardial oxygen demand, augmenting collateral blood flow, and ameliorating ischemic cellular defects.

Because such interventions have not been generally satisfactory in the clinical setting, there has developed a growing conviction that reduction in AMI size can best be provided by improving reduced coronary blood flow with early restoration of antegrade flow through the infarct-related occluded coronary artery.

After experimental studies in dogs confirmed the feasibility and safety of rapid intracoronary thrombolysis by local infusion of thrombolysin (streptokinase and plasmin), Ganz and associates[40] from Los Angeles, California, attempted intracoronary thrombolysis in 20 patients with evolving AMI who were hospitalized within 3 hours from the onset of symptoms during the day and within 2 hours at night. Thrombolysin was infused in the immediate vicinity of the site of coronary occlusion through a special 0.85 mm diameter catheter advanced through the lumen of the Judkins catheter. Reperfusion was achieved in 4 patients after an average of 53 minutes of thrombolysin infusion at a rate of 2,000 IU per minute, and in 15 patients after an average of 21 minutes of thrombolysin infusion at a rate of 4,000 IU per minute. Rethrombosis occurred in 1 patient 8 days after reperfusion and 2 days after discontinuation of anticoagulants because of a history of chronic alcoholism. LV wall motion and myocardial perfusion radionuclide studies showed improvement following thrombolysin-induced reperfusion. Patency of the involved coronary artery was achieved an average of 4 hours after the onset of AMI symptoms. Early reperfusion is essential to achieve this new therapeutic modality for evolving AMI.

Following this paper by Ganz and associates,[40] many others[41-44] followed and the subject was reviewed in a symposium published in the December 1981 issue of The American Heart Journal.[45-56] The information comprising this monograph establishes some broad preliminary knowledge for proceeding cautiously and judiciously with further clinical application of this clearly salutary and novel therapeutic approach to treatment of AMI (Fig. 2-11). As summarized by Mason,[45] data have now been analyzed from 337 patients with AMI who underwent angiography for consideration of intracoronary thrombolytic therapy. Despite the seeming disparity of methodology constituting the percutaneous transluminal coronary recanalization (PTCR) procedure and the apparent differences in the temporal features, clinical status, and cardiocirculatory characteristics of the AMI patients studied in the 8 medical centers involved, a number of commonalities emerged that allow the formulation of important principles relative to the performance and effectiveness of streptokinase (STK)-PTCR treatment in AMI at the present time. These principles pertaining to the modality of intracoronary thrombolysis in evolving AMI concern the indications, technique, safety, initial recanalization success, early reperfusion benefits, myocardial salvage, ventricular function, complications, adjunctive medical management, hospital course, reinfarction and reocclusion, complementary surgical intervention, and effects on symptoms and survival.

The prevalence of occluding thrombus in the infarct-related artery is strikingly consistent at 81% overall (80% of the 105 American patients and 81% of the 232 West German patients). Similarly, the thrombotic occlusion was successfully recanalized by STK-PTCR therapy in 81% of all such patients

PRE-STK

POST-STK

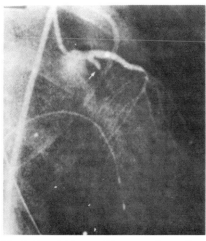 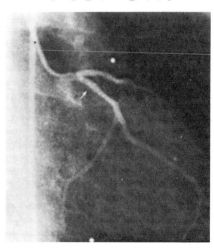

Fig. 2-11. A 38-year-old woman in cardiogenic shock with acute lateral wall MI caused by complete LC occlusion (*arrow*) before STK administration (PRE-STK, *left panel*). Following STK infusion (POST-STK), the LC is now widely patent beyond previous site of obstruction (*arrow*, *right panel*). Right anterior oblique (RAO) projections. Following PTCR procedure, patient fully recovered without complications and was subsequently discharged from hospital in asymptomatic state. Reproduced with permission from Lee et al.[49]

(80% and 81% of American and West German patients, respectively). In the 19% of all AMI patients without presenting occlusion, the subtotal obstruction was generally not affected by regional STK infusion. Intracoronary nitroglycerin was invariably ineffective in achieving patency of the occluding thrombus, and soft-tipped guide wire passage was of little value and was associated with some risk. The PTCR procedure using STK infusion was absolutely safe in terms of mortality; there were no cardiac deaths due to utilization of the technique in the setting of evolving AMI, and no deaths occurred as a consequence of the small number of complications. The overall incidence of hemorrhage requiring transfusion was 5%; hemorrhage was transient and without untoward sequelae. STK-produced thrombolysis was best achieved by rapid initial intracoronary injection, with patency visualized usually by 30 minutes (with < 100,000 IU STK); the infusion was continued at a lesser rate for 30–60 more minutes to dissolve residual clots (total STK administered usually about 300,000 IU, to avoid hemorrhage). Rapid thrombolysis was closely related to shorter duration from symptom onset to STK therapy, but ultimate STK clot lysis with reperfusion occurred as frequently but at longer intervals (Fig. 2-12).

Reperfusion onset was accompanied by relief of chest pain, normalization of ST segments, and easily managed ventricular ectopic activity. Thallium scintigraphy evidenced approximately 50% myocardial salvage of the infarcting segment, associated later with substantially enhanced LV EF (Fig. 2-13). Post-STK reperfusion was best maintained by full-dose (>20,000 IU daily) heparin anticoagulation throughout hospitalization, replaced by warfarin at hospital discharge. Nonlethal reinfarction occurred in the CCU in approximately 10% of all recanalized patients, and late-hospital reocclusion (unaccompanied by infarction) rate was about 5%. Since high-grade residual stenosis remained following STK-recanalization, early CABG was performed safely in suitable patients and afforded the best protection against reinfarc-

Fig. 2-12. Occurrence of reperfusion patency within 1 h (*hatched area*) or after 1 h (*open area*) following initiation of STK infusion to complete thrombus-occluded coronary artery supplying related AMI area. Numerals indicate % of patients successfully reperfused, relative to interval from AMI symptom onset to time of STK-PTCR therapy, within less than 5 h, within 5–7 h, and after more than 7 h. Total height of bars represents all patients successfully reperfused by STK. *n* = Number of instances of AMI thrombotic occlusion in which STK-PTCR was carried out. For *left*, *middle*, and *right bars*, *hatched areas* include 6 cases, 4 cases, and 1 case, respectively; *open areas* include 1, 2, and 4 cases, respectively; and instances without angiographic documentation of STK-PTCR patency are 1 case, 2 cases, and 1 case, respectively. Total number of cases reperfused within less than 5 h = 8; within 5–7 h = 8; and after more than 7 h = 6. Reproduced with permission from Lee et al.[49]

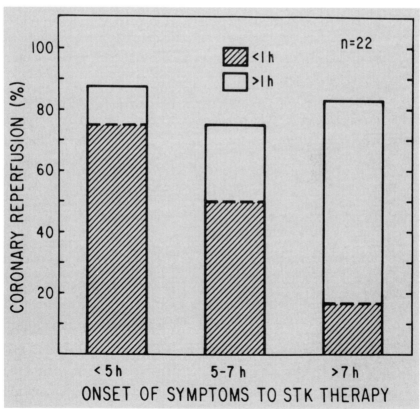

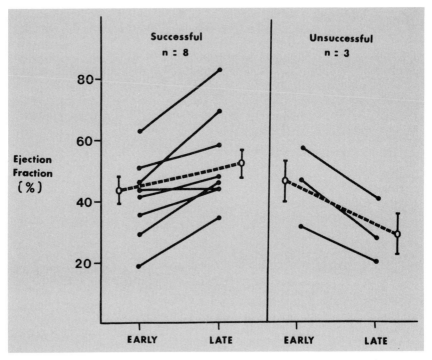

Fig. 2-13.   LV ejection fraction (LV EF) early (prior to SK infusion) and late (8–60 days, mean, 23 days) in patients with successful (*left panel*) and unsuccessful (*right panel*) recanalization. In patients with successful recanalization, LV EF increased from 42% ± 5% to 52% ± 5%. In contrast, LV EF decreased from 45% ± 8% to 30% ± 6% in patients with unsuccessful recanalization. The change in LV EF in successful-vs-unsuccessful groups was significant (p < 0.001). Reproduced with permission from Cowley et al.[50]

tion and chronic angina. Overall in-hospital mortality in patients recanalized with STK averaged only 3%, in contrast to 20% in nonrecanalized patients. In addition, anginal frequency after discharge was less than before AMI in STK-reperfused patients, whereas the reverse was true in nonrecanalized patients with AMI. The possibility of spontaneous clot lysis in AMI taking place at the time of STK reperfusion or during subsequent hospitalization was essentially excluded by the finding that control AMI patients receiving conventional management without STK had a high incidence of infarct-vessel total occlusion 1 month post AMI, similar to that in patients with evolving AMI who presented for STK-PTCR therapy.

It is recognized that considerably more experience with the STK-PTCR procedure is necessary to ascertain its true impact on short- and long-term mortality and morbidity from AMI, and to determine the appropriate place and range of application for this exciting new therapeutic modality in the management of AMI in the future. In addition, clarification is required concerning a number of important aspects of the thrombolytic effectiveness of

STK and its optimal utilization in patients with AMI and related CAD states. The observation that the systemic infusion of STK effects lysis of coronary occluding thrombus in AMI patients requires thorough assessment because of the enormous advantages of this route of administration. In view of the successful clinical introduction of intracoronary thrombolysis for AMI treatment and other therapeutic advances necessitating implementation of invasive techniques, the cardiac catheterization laboratory has become a stimulating therapeutic arena, in addition to its traditional function as an arena for definitive diagnosis, for patients with heart disease. To define the benefits and role of STK-PTCR therapy in AMI, an international registry is recommended, like that currently maintained for the PTCA procedure in coronary artery stenosis, instead of the confusing and expensive undertaking of a large-scale, randomized, controlled trial of the PTCR procedure that possesses inherent multiple variables, such as those that led to misleading assessments of CABG during the past decade.

BETA BLOCKERS CHRONICALLY AFTER AMI

When a survivor of AMI leaves the hospital, all concerned tend to relax, knowing that the greatest risk is past. Unfortunately, the coronary circulation and myocardium remain in an unstable state, and about 1 in 10 of those who survive AMI die in the next year.

Over the past 8 years, hopes have been raised by a series of trials of beta adrenergic blockers, but for various reasons none has been generally accepted by clinicians. The *alprenolol* trial was encouraging. Then for a time it seemed that *practolol* was the answer, with an impressive 35% reduction in deaths, but its unpleasant complications made it unacceptable. In the international *propranolol* trial, the investigators were disappointed at early negative results and gave up (prematurely) when the true benefit (based on a 90% confidence interval) might have been as much as 40%. Preliminary results of the UK *oxprenolol* trial were reported last year, but a final assessment must await the full report, including follow-up of withdrawals. Thus, the position has been unsatisfactory, and the report of the Norwegian *timolol* trial will be studied with keen interest.[57]

The timolol trial was initiated, directed, and reported by physicians advised by an international review committee. The financing came from the manufacturers, who also provided administrative, data-processing, and statistical services.

Twenty clinical center, among them covering one-third of Norway's population, admitted 11,125 patients with suspected AMI over 21 months. Of these, 4,155 were confirmed and 1,884 (52%) of the survivors entered the trial, between 7 and 28 days from the start of their illness. Half received timolol (10 mg, b.i.d.) and the other half a placebo; the trial was randomized and, insofar as this is possible with a beta blocker, double-blind. The groups were well balanced at entry and statistical adjustment for minor differences did not alter the conclusions materially. Withdrawals from randomized treatment occurred in 23% of control patients and 29% of the timolol group, the difference due mainly to the usual side effects of a nonselective beta blocker. Withdrawn patients were followed-up for survival, but not for rein-farction.

The trial was terminated when the last patients to enter had been fol-lowed for 12 months. At that time, 98 patients (10%) randomized to timolol had died, as compared with 152 (16%) of the control group, a reduction in total mortality of 36% (p < 0.001) (Fig. 2-14). The gap between the 2 groups widened through the first 2 years of treatment, with irregular trends beyond that point. Three-quarters of the deaths were sudden (<24 hours), and these accounted for most of the timolol advantage, but the trend was similar for other cardiac deaths. The absolute reduction in mortality was not related to severity of the entry AMI nor to a history of previous AMI, so that the propor-tionate benefit was actually largest in the group with the lowest risk. This finding suggests that the deaths that timolol prevented were not related to the amount of previous myocardial injury. The reduction in deaths was sub-stantially larger in those aged >65 years than in those <65 years. No sepa-rate results were given for women, who formed 20% of the subjects; for the time being, therefore, the results can only be taken as applying to men.

Fig. 2-14. Life-table cumulated rates of sudden cardiac death during administration of medi-cation or within 28 days of last dose. Reproduced with permission from the Norwegian Study.[57]

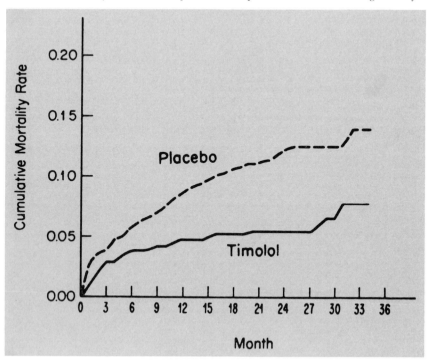

Reinfarction was reported in 88 patients randomized to timolol, as compared with reinfarction in 141 controls, an apparent reduction of 38% in the rate (Fig. 2-15). This result, however, is more open to question than the similar benefit seen for deaths—first, because diagnostic bias cannot be wholly excluded and, second, because nothing is reported of episodes in patients withdrawn from randomized treatment. The commonest causes for withdrawal of timolol were bradycardia, CHF, and hypotension, which could well identify a group with special risk of reinfarction. The claim that a beta blocker is as effective against reinfarction as against fatal arrhythmias is challenging and important. It will be a pity if these suggestive results cannot be put on a firmer basis.

Those who conducted this trial are to be congratulated on an excellent study with a splendid result. They have shown beyond reasonable doubt that, in these patients, timolol achieved a major reduction in deaths and, possibly, in the rate of reinfarction. The full implications are far-reaching. Experience with earlier large trials, however, has taught the danger of hasty judgments. The timolol trial now begins the important process of questioning and debate, aided, it is hoped, by a further, more detailed report. Until this process has taken place, conclusions must still be tentative.

Fig. 2-15. Life-table cumulated rates of first reinfarction during administration of medication or within 28 days of last dose. Reproduced with permission from the Norwegian Study.[57]

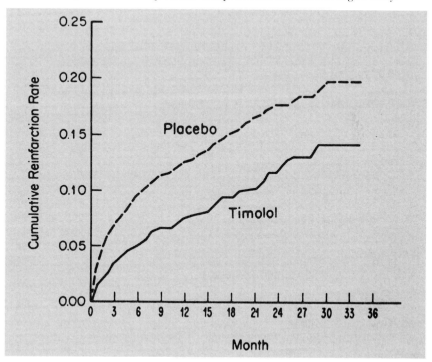

The findings are based on a broad cross-section of Norwegian hospital cases of confirmed AMI that are likely to be similar to those in other countries. The trial cases, however, amounted to no more than 17% of all patients admitted with suspected AMI. The beneficial findings of this trial do not necessarily apply to unconfirmed cases of AMI, including those treated at home without full investigation.

Has timolol now been shown to be superior to other beta blockers for survivors of AMI? Certainly the results show that intrinsic sympathomimetic activity (which timolol lacks) is not essential to the benefit, but we cannot yet answer questions on the importance in this situation of other differences between beta blockers, in pharmacokinetics, pharmacodynamics, and dosage. The various trials are not comparable in terms of the age and severity of cases, the interval between onset (or hospital admission) and start of treatment, dosages, or duration, nor is there a statistically significant difference between their outcomes. One can, however, say that so far only timolol and alprenolol are of demonstrated value for AMI survivors. Questions of dosage and duration of treatment remain unresolved. The results of this post-AMI trial should not be extrapolated to the very different situation of hypertension treatment. Timolol is a useful antihypertensive, but there is no evidence that this or any other beta blocker reduces the coronary risk in systemic hypertension.

If the conclusions of the timolol trial survive the process of intensive scrutiny that they will now face, a beta blocker (timolol or alternative) will become a part of the normal care given to many AMI survivors, in the absence of a reason to the contrary. That being so, then in trials of other forms of treatment—such as platelet-acting drugs—timolol or some other appropriate beta blocker would either have to replace placebos or would have to be available to all trial participants.

The National Heart, Lung, and Blood Institute (NHLBI), Bethesda, Maryland, has taken the unusual step of curtailing one of its major clinical trials (the β-Blocker Heart Attack Trial [BHAT]) on the advice of its Policy and Data Monitoring Board.[58] The step was taken after data indicated that the group of patients receiving *propranolol* hydrochloride experienced a 26% lower mortality from all causes than did a control group.

The BHAT was a randomized, double-blind, multicenter clinical trial of propranolol -vs- placebo in patients enrolled 5–21 days after the onset of AMI. The primary objective was to determine if long-term administration of propranolol would result in a significant reduction in total mortality over the follow-up period. Thirty-one clinical centers, a coordinating center, a resting ECG reading center, a 24-hour ambulatory ECG reading center, a central laboratory, a drug distribution center, and an NHLBI program office were involved in the study.

From June 1978–October 1980, 3,837 men and women, aged 20–69 years, with AMI were enrolled and randomized to 1 of the 2 study groups (1,916 to propranolol and 1,921 to placebo). Baseline comparability between the groups was excellent. There was close agreement with regard to demographic factors, known cardiovascular risk factors, medical history, use of medications, physical findings, and laboratory data. The average time from AMI to randomization was 14 days.

All patients were initially assigned to receive 40 mg propranolol hydrochloride or placebo 3 times a day before hospital discharge. Depending on serum propranolol levels, as measured several days after enrollment, a maintenance dose of 60 mg, t.i.d., or 80 mg, t.i.d., was prescribed at the 1-month follow-up visit. To maintain the blinding, control patients were assigned matching placebo tablets. Patients were seen in the clinical centers every 3 months for evaluation and distribution of additional study medication. Intervention was originally scheduled to end in June 1982.

An independent Policy and Data Monitoring Board met semiannually to review the status of the trial and the accumulating data. One of the charges to the Board was to recommend an early end to the study in cases of greater-than-expected benefit or toxic effects. Since the chance of falsely declaring a difference to be statistically significant increases with frequent reviews of the data, the Board was guided by data monitoring methods. To declare a treatment beneficial, this method requires very large effects early in a trial, and differences between groups closer to those necessary for standard statistical tests toward the end of a trial. At the regularly scheduled meeting of the Board on Oct 1–2, 1981, the BHAT mortality results had substantially crossed the monitoring boundary associated with overall p level <0.05. In fact, the boundary for $p < 0.02$ significance level was crossed. In addition, conditional probability calculations showed that there would be a very high likelihood of declaring the results significant at the scheduled end of the trial even if there were no real treatment benefit during the remainder of the study. Because of these findings, because the effect of propranolol appeared to be consistent across clinics and patient subgroups, and because it was judged important to make these results known, the Board recommended that the BHAT be ended early.

Data reported as of Oct 2, 1981, show a mortality of 9.5% in the placebo group (183 deaths), and 7.0% in the propranolol group (135 deaths), a reduction of 26% (Fig. 2-16). Using life-table analysis, this difference has a Z value of 2.82 (associated with a nominal $p = 0.005$). The results are only minimally changed by adjusting for baseline covariates using the Cox model. The survival experience of these patients is included up to the time they were last known to be alive. All patients were analyzed according to treatment assignment, regardless of subsequent compliance. Site of infarct, age, and sex had no impact on the efficacy of propranolol.

Patients in the propranolol group did not have an increased frequency of CHF. Hypotension, tiredness, faintness, depression, and gastrointestinal problems were more common in the propranolol group. Mean heart rate at the 1-year visit was 65 beats/min in the propranolol group and 73 beats/min in the placebo group. Approximately two-thirds of the patients in each group complied with the treatment regimen. Another 15% were receiving less than protocol dose, and the remainder took no study medication.

The results of the BHAT strengthen and extend the conclusions of previous studies of beta blockers in survivors of AMI. This large study of a noncar-

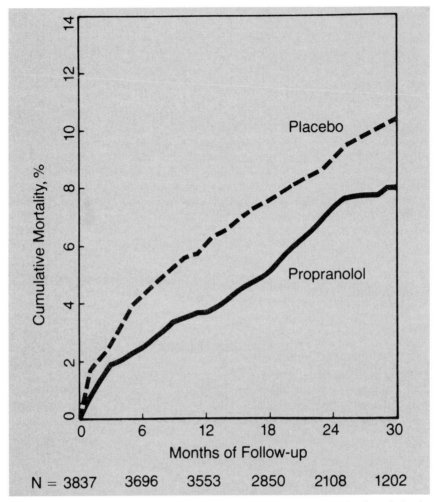

Fig. 2-16. Life-table cumulative mortality curves for propranolol hydrochloride and placebo groups. N denotes total number of patients followed-up through each time point. Reproduced with permission from the Beta Blocker Study.[58]

dioselective agent is in accord with the results of the recent trial of timolol maleate.[57] Contrary to an earlier study of practolol (*Br Med J* 3:735, 1975), the site of AMI appears to be immaterial. Also, as in the timolol study, but contrary to an alprenolol study (Lancet 2:865, *1979*), patients > 65 years) benefited from the treatment as much as younger ones.

The BHAT results indicate that the beneficial effects of propranolol appear to occur primarily in the first year after an AMI. None of the completed beta blocker trials addresses the issues of possible benefit from institution of therapy at a time remote from the AMI or at what point treatment can be discontinued.

CORONARY ARTERY BYPASS GRAFTING (CABG) DURING AMI

Berg and associates[59] from Spokane, Washington, who pioneered the early surgical treatment of AMI, described findings in 227 consecutive patients who presented at their hospital with chest pain and with ECG, coronary angiographic, ventriculographic, and retrospective enzyme findings consistent with AMI. These investigators differentiated AMI, an established entity with myocardial necrosis, from *evolving* AMI, which suggests reversibly damaged myocardium. This study was conducted from March 1971 through April 1979. The LAD coronary artery was the primary occluded artery in 46%, the right in 37%, the LC artery in 11%, combinations in 4%; the site of occlusion was uncertain in 2%. The SGOT and CPK were elevated preoperatively in 76 patients and rose further in the postoperative period. Coronary angiography averaged 34 minutes, and the time for CABG operation averaged 194 minutes, with an average of 2.2 grafts/patient. The average time from onset of chest pain to beginning of operation was 5 hours, 23 minutes, the shortest time being 80 minutes and the longest, nearly 14 hours. The operative mortality was 2% (4/227). Postoperatively, 86 non-fatal complications occurred, including hypotension in 22 and requiring intraaortic ballooning in 9. Of the 227 patients, 102 were restudied angiographically an average of 13 months postoperatively: 94% of the grafts to ischemic areas were patent and 88% of the grafts to nonischemic areas were patent; 88 patients had a normal, unchanged or improved EF. Three patients died within 1 year. Mild angina was present in 30.

This study has 2 major drawbacks. First, there are no controls and second, some of the patients believed to have AMI may have had only unstable angina. Nevertheless, this approach is unique and it needs to continue.

Jones and associates[60] from Atlanta, Georgia, reported 116 patients who underwent urgent CABG for clinical instability within 30 days of AMI: 8 patients within 1 day; 20, 2–7 days after AMI; and 88, 8–30 days after AMI. Indications for bypass included persistent or recurrent angina (81%), pain plus ventricular arrhythmias (12%), and pain plus "compelling anatomy" (7%). The AMI was subendocardial in 32 and transmural in 84. Propranolol was given to 89% of the 116 patients before CABG, intravenous nitroglycerin to 33%, and the intraaortic balloon was used preoperatively in 4 patients. The mean EF was 55%. Only 1 artery was significantly narrowed in 28% of the patients. Heart rate, systemic BP, PA wedge pressure, cardiac output, and some precordial leads were recorded during operation. Anesthetics employed were morphine sulfate, nitrous oxide, and oxygen. Hyperkalemic cardioplegia was employed. A single aortic cross clamp was used for all distal anastomoses. Single CABG was used in 18% of the patients and 3 or more conduits were used in 54 patients. The average number of grafts per patient was 2.6. There were no hospital deaths. The requirement for inotropic drugs was higher in the patients operated on within 1 week after onset of AMI than in those operated on later. Only 1% of the patients required balloon support for elective operations. Actuarial late survival was projected to be 97% at 18 months, freedom from chest pain to be 71%, and graft patency to be 84%.

One reason for these good results described is good myocardial protection during CABG. Data from 939 patients in the CASS multicenter study[61] showed that the addition of potassium cardioplegia during CABG lowered both operative mortality and perioperative AMI ($p < 0.01$ and $p < 0.001$, respectively).

COMPLICATIONS OF AMI

Left ventricular thrombus

DETECTION BY 2-D ECHO

William Bean in the 1930s pointed out the frequency of LV thrombus in patients with AMI. Although LV thrombus is commonly observed at necropsy in patients with fatal transmural AMI, its frequency in survivors of transmural AMI has not been determined. Asinger and associates[62] from Minneapolis, Minnesota, performed serial 2-D echo in 70 consecutive patients with transmural AMI: 35 had posterior (inferior) AMI without LV thrombus; the other 35 had anterior-wall AMI, with LV thrombi in 12. The thrombi were diagnosed from 1–11 days (mean, 5) after onset of the AMI. All patients with LV thrombi had severe apical wall motion abnormalities (akinesis or dyskinesis). Of the 35 patients with anterior AMI, 26 had apical akinesis or dyskinesis on echo and LV thrombi developed in 11 of the 26. Thus, patients with severe apical wall abnormalities during transmural AMI are at high risk for LV thrombosis. This high-risk group can be identified before the development of LV thrombi. Conversely, patients with posterior AMI or anterior AMI without a severe apical wall motion abnormality are at low risk. The presence or absence of LV thrombi could not be explained solely on the basis of the severity of the CHF or the extent of the AMI as determined clinically by peak cardiac enzyme rise or Q-wave evolution on ECG. The study of Asinger and associates certainly suggests that anteriorly located infarcts are more serious than posteriorly located ones. Other studies have shown that, during the early period among patients with AMI of comparable size as determined by creatinine kinase release, anterior infarcts are fatal twice as often as are posterior infarcts.

DETECTION BY COMPUTED TOMOGRAPHY

To investigate the potential of computed tomography (CT) in the detection of LV mural thrombi, Nair and associates[63] from Omaha, Nebraska, studied 16 patients suspected of having LV mural thrombi. All patients had had transmural AMI, and 15 had a LV aneurysm. One had had systemic emboli. The interval between AMI and study ranged from 1–79 months (mean, 15). All patients underwent CT of the heart, M-mode echo, and 2-D echo. Eight patients underwent LV cineangiography. Five patients had surgical confirmation of thrombus. Computerized tomography, 2-D and M-mode echo predicted LV mural thrombi in 10, 8, and 1 of the 16 patients, respectively. LV cineangiography predicted LV mural thrombi in 4 of 8 patients. Both CT and LV cineangiography correctly predicted the presence or absence of LV thrombi in all 5 patients who underwent operation. In the same group, however, 2-D-and M-mode echo failed to predict the presence of thrombi in 1 and 3 patients, respectively. Among the 11 patients without surgical confirmation, 1, in whom no LV thrombi were shown by M-mode and 2-D echo, was shown to have thrombi on CT. In another, 2-D echo was positive, but this finding was not confirmed either by CT or by LV angiography.

Tomoda and associates[64] from Kanagawa, Japan, using a third-generation CT system, detected LV thrombus in 3 patients and confirmed its presence by angiographic methods. In 1 patient the thrombus was not detected by 2-D echo. This experience further indicates that CT may be very useful in detecting LV thrombus.

DETECTION BY RNA

Stratton and associates[65] from Seattle, Washington, assessed the usefulness of RNA in detecting proved LV thrombi and compared results with 2-D echo findings. For 39 patients studied by RNA, 13 RNAs were interpreted as positive or equivocally positive for thrombus and 26 were judged negative. The sensitivity of a positive or equivocally positive RNA for detection of thrombus was 77%, the specificity 88%, the positive predictive value 77%, the negative predictive value 88%. All thrombi were visualized in the anterior view in an area of akinetic or dyskinetic wall motion. For 13 patients undergoing 2-D echo (8 with thrombus, 5 without), this procedure was 100% sensitive and specific. Thus, the finding of a discrete filling defect or squared or cut-off ventricular apex in an area of abnormal wall motion in the anterior view of the RNA suggests the presence of LV thrombus.

Left ventricular aneurysm

LATE FOLLOW-UP AFTER ANEURYSMECTOMY WITHOUT CORONARY ARTERY BYPASS GRAFTING (CABG)

Otterstad and associates[66] from Oslo, Norway, reinvestigated 26 patients (mean age, 55 years) 9–62 months (mean, 30) after LV aneurysmectomy for anterior wall healed LV aneurysm secondary to CAD. LV angiography disclosed the aneurysm to be large in 15 patients and small to medium in 11 others. At follow-up, a large residual LV aneurysm was found in 5 patients, a small to medium one in 13, and akinesia without aneurysm in 8. Following aneurysmectomy, the sum of ST elevation in the precordial leads in the ECG dropped from a mean of 11.2 mm to 7.7 mm. In no patient did the ST segments return to normal after operation. Preoperatively, the mean ST-segment elevation was identical in the patients with large and small-to-medium-sized aneurysms. LV end-diastolic pressure before angiography preoperatively was reduced from a mean value of 21 mmHg to 15 mmHg and, after angiography, from 27 mmHg to 21 mmHg. Of the 6 patients who also had CABG at the time of LV aneurysmectomy, the LV end-diastolic pressure was unaltered at follow-up. In the patients in whom the LV end-diastolic pressure did not return to normal, the amount of coronary narrowing revealed angiographically had progressed postoperatively. These authors suggested that progressive coronary narrowing may be responsible for an eventual further deterioration in LV function after aneurysmectomy.

COMPARISON OF PATIENTS HAVING CABG WITH ANEURYSMECTOMY TO PATIENTS HAVING CABG WITHOUT ANEURYSMECTOMY

Jones and associates[67] from Atlanta, Georgia, compared patients having CABG and LV aneurysm resection (n, 40) or plication (n, 32) with patients having CABG without aneurysmectomy. (n, 2,782). The primary indication for surgery in the aneurysm patients was angina pectoris; CHF was a lesser factor. The aneurysms were anteroapical in 55 and posterior in 7. There was total occlusion of the LAD coronary artery in 75% of the patients having aneurysmectomy and in 38% in those having plication. More grafts were utilized in the plication group (2.6 -vs- 2.0). Hospital mortality was 3% in the aneurysm patients and 1.4% in the patients without aneurysms. Postoperative requirements for "inotropes" or balloon assist were much higher in the aneurysm group. The actuarial survival rate at 42 months for the aneurysm patients was 90%; the frequency of disappearance or lessening of angina was higher in the patients without aneurysmectomy.

Right ventricular infarction

CLINICAL FEATURES

Rackley and associates[68] from Birmingham, Alabama, reviewed clinical features of RV AMI (Table 2-4). RV infarction should be suspected in any patient with inferior (posterior) wall AMI. If the Swan-Ganz catheter is introduced, pullback pressures from the PA should be recorded to compare the PA, RV, and RA pressures, with particular attention to elevation of RA pressure as compared with PA end-diastolic or capillary pressure. RV AMI also should be suspected in severe LV dysfunction and cardiogenic shock, since volume overloading may enhance the hemodynamic evidence of RV dysfunction and improve LV performance. Finally, RV function may be crucial to survival after ventricular septal rupture.

To evaluate the frequency, clinical characteristics, and course of patients with RV AMI, Cintron and associates[69] from San Juan, Puerto Rico, studied 96 patients with AMI: 44 had acute posterior (or inferior) wall LV AMI and 16 of them had evidence of RV dysfunction; all had a positive Kussmaul's sign, and 12 had either a RV third or fourth heart sound. Inspiratory elevation of RA and RV end-diastolic pressures was documented in 9 patients. Three had advanced AV block. All 16 patients survived and were alive 3 months after the onset of the AMI.

TABLE 2-4. *Features of right ventricular infarction. Reproduced with permission from Rackley et al.*[68]

INFERIOR-POSTERIOR MI
CLINICAL FINDINGS MAY INCLUDE:
   Normal or depressed RV function
   Shock
   Tricuspid regurgitation
   Ruptured ventricular septum
HEMODYNAMIC MEASUREMENTS
   Abnormally elevated right atrial pressure
   Normal RV and pulmonary artery systolic pressures
   Increased ratio of RV to LV filling pressure
   Depressed RV function curve
SCINTIGRAPHY
   Uptake in RV free wall
   Increased RV dimensions and decreased wall motion
ECHOCARDIOGRAPHY
   Increased RV dimension
   Absence of pericardial effusion
CARDIAC ENZYMES
   Increased magnitude of enzyme values to LV dysfunction
CARDIAC CATHETERIZATION
   Involvement of right or LC coronary arteries
   RV akinesis
DIFFERENTIAL DIAGNOSIS
   Hypotension with AMI
   Pericardial tamponade
   Constrictive pericarditis
   Pulmonary embolus

ECG FEATURES

The specific ECG findings in patients with RV AMI have not been delineated, other than the occurrence of inferior wall LV AMI. Chou and associates[70] from Cincinnati, Ohio, reviewed ECG findings in 11 patients with RV AMI associated with LV posterior AMI. In 5 of their 11 patients, the presence of RV AMI was confirmed at necropsy. In the other 6, the RV AMI was suspected because of hemodynamic observations. Nevertheless, in 8 of the 11 patients, transient ST-segment elevation occurred in lead V_1. The authors suggested that, in the absence of other explanations for ST-segment elevation in the right precordial leads, RV AMI was the most likely cause.

Candell-Riera and associates[71] from Barcelona, Spain, investigated the relationship between ST-segment elevation in the right precordial lead V_{4R} and the hemodynamic, echo and myocardial scintigraphic signs suggesting RV AMI in 42 patients with documented posterior wall LV AMI. Of the 42 patients, 22 had ST-segment elevation in V_{4R} and, among them, a significant correlation was demonstrated between V_{4R} ST-segment elevation and the hemodynamic, scintigraphic, and echo criteria of RV AMI. These results support the validity of this new ECG sign as a practical means for aiding in the clinical detection of RV AMI associated with posterior wall LV AMI.

HEMODYNAMIC FEATURES

It is well recognized that a significant percentage (about 25%) of patients with transmural AMI involving the posterior (inferior) wall of the LV also have associated AMI of the RV free wall, and that associated RV infarction with anterior transmural LV AMI is virtually nonexistent. Lloyd and associates[72] from Cape Town, South Africa, diagnosed RV AMI in 19 patients with posterior wall LV AMI on the basis of clinical evidence of elevation of systemic venous pressure and an absence of pulmonary congestion. Catheterization documented elevated RV end-diastolic (mean, 15.5 mmHg) and right atrial (RA) pressures (mean, 15 mmHg). In all patients, the PA capillary wedge pressure (CWP) (mean, 13 mmHg) was exceeded or equalled by the RV end-diastolic pressure, suggesting a disproportionate reduction in RV compliance, contractile function, or both. Thirteen patients were hypotensive (systolic systemic arterial pressure <100 mmHg on admission), including 6 patients with clinical evidence of cardiogenic shock. In the 6 patients with hypotension, the RV end-diastolic pressure was significantly higher than in the 13 patients with systemic arterial systolic pressures >100 mmHg (17 mmHg -vs- 13 mmHg). A PA CWP of 15 mmHg or more was present only among the 13 hypotensive patients, and their PA CWP (mean, 15 mmHg) was significantly greater than that in the 6 normotensive patients (mean, 10 mmHg). RV peak systolic pressure was significantly higher in the 13 hypotensive than in the 6 normotensive patients (30 mmHg -vs- 24 mmHg), and there was a linear correlation between this pressure and the PA CWP. Only 1 of the 19 patients died in the hospital. Clinical management generally consisted of administration of fluids and digitalis and implantation of a temporary pacemaker. This study emphasizes the relatively favorable prognosis of RV AMI associated with posterior wall LV AMI.

RNA OBSERVATIONS

It has been shown previously that the extent of myocardial necrosis is virtually identical in patients with anterior and posterior (inferior) AMI, despite a more favorable prognosis associated with the latter. Marmor and associates[73] from St. Louis, Missouri, postulated that the damage associated with posterior AMI is shared by both ventricles, thereby causing less hemodynamic impairment than anterior AMI, which involves only the left ventricle. To further explore this hypothesis, global and regional function of both right and left ventricles were assessed by gated RNA in 50 patients with AMI within 48 hours after admission and again on the tenth day. RNA also was performed in 10 normal subjects. In 22 patients who had anterior AMI, the mean global LV EF was decreased (27 ± 15% [±SD] -vs- 64 ± 10% in normal subjects), reflecting regional abnormalities, and increased only slightly by the tenth day (33 ± 11%). The global RV EF was decreased (28 ± 11% -vs-

43 ± 9% in normal subjects), reflecting a uniform depression of function without localized abnormalities, and returned to normal by the tenth day (43 ± 12%). In 20 patients who had posterior AMI, global LV EF was only slightly decreased (51 ± 11%), reflecting inferoapical dysfunction, and did not change (55 ± 10%) by the tenth day. In contrast, global RV EF was severely and persistently decreased (23 ± 9% -vs- 28 ± 9%), reflecting abnormalities primarily of the posterior region. The decreased RV EF after posterior AMI correlated inversely with enzymatic estimates of infarct size, although there was no correlation between LV EF and infarct size. Thus, the functional responses of the ventricles to AMI are markedly influenced by the site of damage. In patients with anterior AMI, there was persistent regional and global impairment of LV function, but only transient impairment of the right ventricle, whereas posterior AMI was associated with severe persistent regional and global impairment of the right ventricle. These results indicate that the site of AMI is a major determinant of ventricular function and recovery, and that RV AMI is much more common with posterior AMI than is generally appreciated.

VENTRICULAR FIBRILLATION COMPLICATING TEMPORARY PACING

Ventricular fibrillation (VF) is a well-recognized complication of temporary ventricular pacing in the setting of AMI. This complication of temporary pacing has been sporadic and not associated with specific clinical features of the AMI. In a 4-year period, Sclarovsky and associates[74] from Petah-Tikva, Israel, and Chicago, Illinois, noted VF complicating temporary pacing during AMI in 5 of 30 patients with AMI requiring pacing. In all 5 patients, there was clinical evidence, postmortem evidence, or both of associated RV AMI, suggesting that the RV AMI may have been physiologically involved in the occurrence of VF.

TREATMENT BY ATRIAL PACING

If RV hemodynamic decompensation is severe, LV underfilling may result in inadequate systemic perfusion. Therapy in such cases consists chiefly of volume administration aimed at increasing RV filling pressure and thereby augmenting RV cardiac output (CO). The importance of preserving active and synchronous right atrial (RA) pump in RV AMI, however, has not been previously delineated. Isner and associates[75] from Bethesda, Maryland, and Washington, DC, described a patient with "massive" RV and LV AMI in whom appropriately timed atrial contraction was demonstrated both spontaneously and by transvenous atrial pacing to be the critical factor that preserved right-sided contribution to LV filling pressure and thereby maintained adequate systemic perfusion following combined RV and LV AMI. The critical importance of preserving an active and synchronous RA contraction in patients with RV AMI has potential therapeutic implications. First, patients in whom atrial fibrillation accompanies RV AMI with hemodynamic decompensation should be considered candidates for emergency electrical cardioversion. In at least some of these patients, death was preceded for several days by prolonged hemodynamic decompensation associated with protracted AF. Second, in patients like those in the clinical example described, in whom accelerated junctional or ventricular pacemaker overtook the sinus pacemaker but in whom AV conduction remains intact, attempts to restore physiologic atrial function should be quickly and aggressively pursued. Administration of intravenous atropine may be effective in restoring normal sinus rhythm, although in some patients this has been successful on only some occasions, and in these situations, only transiently. Under such circumstances, transvenous physiologic atrial pacing, either from the RA appendage or coronary sinus, may produce substantial CO increment. Finally, patients with RV AMI appear to be at increased risk for the development of complete heart block (CHB). In those patients with RV AMI in whom hemodynamic decompensation is associated with CHB refractory to atropine therapy, ventricular pacing is likely to have deleterious hemodynamic consequences. In contrast, use of a sequential AV pacemaker may provide significant hemodynamic improvement.

Pericarditis

Symptomatic pericarditis may occur days to weeks after AMI. Its discomfort frequently awakens memories and anxieties associated with the recent AMI. Many physicians distinguish 2 separate syndromes of post-AMI pericarditis: an *early* form, said to occur with mild or no discomfort, and a *delayed* form (so-called Dressler's syndrome), associated with severe discomfort, pericardial effusion, and pulmonary infiltrates. Recent reports have pointed out that these 2 entities are not distinct and that the "delayed" form of post-AMI pericarditis can develop within a few days of AMI. In addition, the clinical presentation of these conditions can be indistinguishable. Regardless of when pericarditis develops after AMI, this entity rarely affects the clinical course or prognosis. Since patients are usually distressed by the discomfort of post-AMI pericarditis, analgesic or anti-inflammatory therapy is often initiated with aspirin or indomethacin. Berman and associates[76] from Worcester and Boston, Massachusetts, studied the efficacy of aspirin and indomethacin therapy in relieving the discomfort of post-AMI pericarditis in 2 studies: 1) a retrospective evaluation of patients with symptomatic post-AMI pericarditis during a 5-year period and 2) a prospective, randomized, single-blind comparison of aspirin and indomethacin in similar patients. In the retrospective study, 36 episodes of symptomatic pericarditis in 34 patients were identified; in the prospective study, 25 episodes occurred in 24 patients. Relief from the discomfort of pericarditis was noted within 48 hours in almost all patients given either indomethacin or aspirin therapy. Minor gastrointestinal bleeding developed in 2 patients in the retrospective study and in 2 patients in the prospective study. In the retrospective study, mild discomfort of pericarditis abated within 48 hours in 5 of 8 patients who received either no treatment or minor analgesic therapy. Thus, aspirin and indomethacin are equally efficacious in relieving the discomfort of post-AMI pericarditis.

Ventricular septal rupture

DETECTION BY 2-D ECHO

Bishop and associates[77] from Charlottesville, Virginia, examined by 2-D echo 18 consecutive patients in whom a new precordial murmur appeared during AMI: in 10 patients 2-D echo permitted direct visualization of a ruptured ventricular septum and in 8 others it correctly excluded septal rupture. In 3 patients with rupture, 2-D echo was the first technique to establish the diagnosis. In all patients with rupture, the 2-D echo diagnosis was confirmed by catheterization, operation, and/or necropsy. In 6 patients with rupture, 2-D echo contrast studies were performed and were positive. 2-D echo permitted localization of the rupture in all patients (5 inferior, 5 anterior). To evaluate LV function, a 2-D echo wall motion index (WMI) was calculated, using an 11-segment LV model. Although there was no difference ($p > 0.2$) in AMI-rupture survivors -vs- nonsurvivors in age, Norris Coronary Prognostic Index, rupture location, initial Killip classification, Qp/Qs, peak creatine kinase, and AVO_2 difference, there was no overlap in WMI ($p = 0.004$) of survivors (0.8 ± 0.36) -vs- nonsurvivors (1.7 ± 0.19). Thus, 2-D echo allows accurate detection and localization of post-AMI septal rupture and helps to determine the prognosis of such patients.

OPERATIVE TREATMENT

The proper timing of surgical treatment of post-AMI ventricular septal defect (VSD) is debated. Gaudiani and associates[78] from Stanford, California, analyzed 43 consecutive patients who had closure of post-AMI VSD to determine the optimal time for operative intervention and to identify factors responsible for failure of operative treatment. The AMI in 24 patients (56%) was "anterior" and in 19 patients (44%) it was "posterior" in location. The overall operative mortality was 42%: 90% for those operated on within 24 hours and 11% for those operated on after 4 weeks. Five variables predicted hospital death: 1) emergency operation; 2) the interval from septal rupture to operation; 3) the presence of shock; 4) altered mental status, and 5) posterior location of the AMI. A shunt via the VSD persisted after operation in 7, with recurrence in 4 within 1 week and in 3 others later. The 25 late survivors were followed a mean of 54 months; at 5 years, 90% of discharged patients were alive. The authors recommended immediate operation for all patients with post-AMI VSD unless there was no deterioration after admission and, because of the high risk of the posterior AMI group, they recommend immediate surgery in them, regardless of the symptomatic status.

Killen and associates[79] from Kansas City, Kansas, analyzed 36 patients undergoing operation for post-AMI VSD. Of 8 who stabilized after medical treatment, all survived operation. Of 22 patients in cardiogenic shock treated by surgery, 13 died (17 early). All 8 in shock treated medically died early. These authors concluded that any patient in cardiogenic shock should undergo prompt diagnostic studies and emergency surgery and that repair should be delayed only in those patients in stable condition after initial medical therapy.

Matsui and associates[80] from Los Angeles, California, described results of cardiac operations in 24 patients with septal rupture during AMI. Of the 24 patients, 14 survived hospitalization for the AMI. Of the 13 patients with cardiogenic shock on admission, 8 died in the hospital, but of 11 patients not in shock at the time of referral, only 2 died. Of 12 current survivors, 11 are in NY Heart Association class I or II. Of 11 patients who had bedside cardiac catheterization with a balloon catheter and were operated on immediately thereafter, 8 survived and none died during the next 5 years. Of 13 patients who had formal cardiac catheterization followed by operation, only 6 survived. This group advocates not moving a patient with suspected ventricular septal rupture from the coronary care unit to the catheterization laboratory. Instead, they recommend a limited bedside catheterization with a Swan-Ganz balloon catheter to confirm the septal rupture, then immediate operation.

Radford and associates[81] from Boston, Massachusetts, analyzed 41 patients with post-AMI ventricular septal rupture treated from 1971–75. Cardiogenic shock developed after rupture in 55%, and was unrelated to the site of the AMI, extent of coronary narrowing, LV EF or pulmonary:systemic flow ratio. The mean PA pressure was lower in shock than in non-shock patients, suggesting that the shock was produced primarily by RV impairment. The mean age of the 41 patients was 63 years; 25 were men and 16 were women. In 13 patients, operative repair of the VSD was not attempted; all died within 3 months. Operative repair was done in 28 patients: 8 of 22 with cardiogenic shock preoperatively died in the perioperative period and 3 of 17 without shock died during this period ($p < 0.05$). The overall perioperative survival was 61%. After a minimum 4-year follow-up, 76% of the 17 operative survivors were alive and not disabled. Thus, the presence of shock, regardless of the use of the intraaortic balloon and other factors, is an extremely grave prognostic factor in patients with rupture of the ventricular septum during AMI.

Recurrent ischemic pain

INDICATION FOR READMISSION TO CORONARY CARE UNIT

As many as 30% of all in-hospital deaths due to AMI occur after initial transfer from the coronary care unit (CCU). Singer and associates[82] from Boston, Massachusetts, analyzed the incidence, type, and time of occurrence of complications serious enough to prompt readmission to the CCU during the same hospitalization to answer the following questions: Do such complications result from premature transfer from the CCU? Could they be avoided through longer stays in the CCU? What is the clinical course of patients who have complications after transfer? To what extent can patients at greatest risk of complications after transfer be identified beforehand? Over a 2-year period, 485 of 536 consecutive patients admitted with AMI survived their first stay in the CCU. Complications severe enough to warrant readmission developed in 61 (13%). Readmissions occurred early: half were within 2.7 days of initial transfer from the unit. The subsequent course was severely complicated: 16 readmitted patients (26%) died in the hospital. These high-risk patients could not be identified during their first stay in the CCU. Several previously cited indicators of poor prognosis did not help to identify those later readmitted, but *recurrent ischemic pain* that occurred for the first time after 24 hours in the CCU did. The absence of rales on admission, coupled with absence of recurrent chest pain, was indicative of a subgroup with a favorable short-term prognosis.

FACTORS PRESAGING RECURRENCE

In a prospective study of 200 consecutive patients with AMI, Marmor and associates[83] from St. Louis, Missouri, characterized the frequency and severity of early recurrent AMI (extension), manifested by secondary plasma creatine kinase-MB isoenzyme (CK-MB) and myoglobin peaks, and identified patients at particular high risk. Serial CK-MB and myoglobin determinations and continuous ECG recordings were obtained in all patients for 14 days, and serial radioventriculograms were obtained in selected patients. Chest pain and ST-segment changes occurred often, in 57% and 43%, respectively. A secondary rise in plasma CK-MB levels indicative of recurrent AMI occurred an average of 10 ± 4 days after the initial AMI in 17% of patients. Of 58 patients with initial subendocardial AMI, 25 (43%) had recurrent AMI compared with only 8% of those with initial transmural AMI (Fig. 2-17). The mortality rate was 7% in patients with subendocardial AMI without early recurrence, as compared with 16% in patients with recurrence. Obese women with initial subendocardial AMI and repeated episodes of prolonged chest pain had a high probability (60%) of recurrence, in contrast to the low probability (2%) for patients without these features. Thus, early recurrent AMI is frequent after subendocardial AMI and is associated with a marked increase in mortality.

EARLY POST-AMI ANGINA PECTORIS

Angina pectoris, of course, may precede or follow AMI. Schuster and Bulkley[84] from Baltimore, Maryland, studied over a 40-month period 70 patients with AMI documented by ECG and enzymatic changes and the appearance of chest pain within 10 days from onset of the AMI accompanied by transient ST-segment or T-wave changes. The authors identified the post-AMI chest pain as angina pectoris and described it as being of 2 types: "ischemia at a distance" and "ischemia in the infarct zone." Ischemia at a distance was defined as angina with new ECG changes distant from the AMI, and ischemia in the infarct zone as angina with new ECG changes in the leads originally involved by the AMI. Of their 70 patients followed an average of 6 months, 43 had ischemia at a distance, and 27 had ischemia in the infarct zone. Mortality in the entire group was 56%, but was 72% (31 of 43 patients) among the patients with ischemia at a distance and 33% (9 of 27) among the patients with ischemia in the infarct zone. Thus, post-AMI angina is asso-

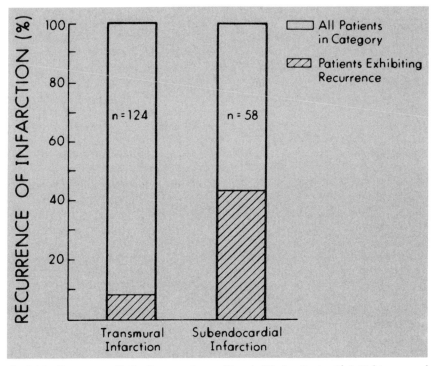

Fig. 2-17. Recurrence of infarction was observed in only 8% of patients with initial transmural infarction in contrast to 43% of patients with initial subendocardial infarction.

ciated with a high mortality, particularly in patients with "ischemia at a distance" who have large areas of viable but jeopardized myocardium.

Mitral regurgitation

MECHANISM AFTER HEALING OF AMI

Burch and colleagues in 1963 introduced the concept of papillary muscle dysfunction as a cause of mitral regurgitation (MR). They suggested 2 mechanisms by which the MR might occur: 1) ischemia or fibrosis of 1 or both papillary muscles preventing normal contraction, which would weaken systolic support for the leaflets and result in leaflet eversion or prolapse into the left atrium, and 2) ischemia or necrosis of the LV myocardium at the base of a papillary muscle, producing dyskinesis in this region, which would pull the papillary muscle away from the valvular orifice, thus increasing tension on the leaflets and preventing complete closure. Angiographic studies have shown the occurrence of MVP in association with ischemia involving a papillary muscle, supporting the occurrence of the first of these 2 phenomena. Angiography, however, is poorly suited to demonstrate displacement of a leaflet

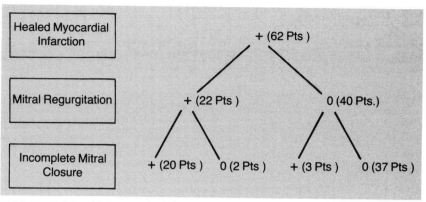

Fig. 2-18. Relationship between healed MI, MR and incomplete mitral valve closure (from God-ley[85]).

downward into the LV cavity and, as a consequence, leaflet arrest with resultant malapposition and valvular regurgitation has not been proven. Cross-sectional echo, however, can assess mitral leaflet motion throughout the cardiac cycle and, therefore, could determine whether abnormal leaflet motion or closure patterns were observable in patients with clinical evidence of papillary muscle dysfunction. If abnormal motion did occur, the technique could determine how this motion related to the mechanisms proposed for leaflet malapposition. To evaluate this possible association, Godley and associates[85] from Indianapolis, Indiana, performed echoes in 22 patients with healed AMI and clinical evidence of papillary muscle dysfunction, in 40 patients with healed AMI and no clinical evidence of papillary muscle dysfunction, and in 20 normal subjects. A unique pattern of incomplete mitral leaflet closure occurred in 91% of the infarct patients with MR, and in these patients, 1 or both leaflets were effectively arrested within the LV cavity during ventricular systole (Fig. 2-18). Dyskinetic wall motion in the region immediately surrounding 1 of the papillary muscles was present in 23 (96%) of 24 patients with demonstrated incomplete closure. Thus, this study provides the first objective evidence that *de novo* MR in patients with healed AMI is due to dyskinesis involving the LV myocardium beneath 1 papillary muscle, producing increased tension on the mitral leaflets and preventing normal closure.

References

1. BUJA LM, WILLERSON JT: Clinicopathologic correlates of acute ischemic heart disease syndromes. Am J Cardiol 47:343–356, Feb 1981.
2. BROSIUS FC, ROBERTS WC: Significance of coronary arterial thrombus in transmural acute myocardial infarction: a study of 54 necropsy patients. Circulation 63:810–816, Apr 1981.
3. BROSIUS FC III, ROBERTS WC: Comparison of degree and extent of coronary narrowing by ath-

erosclerotic plaque in anterior and posterior transmural acute myocardial infarction. Circulation 64:715–722, Oct 1981.

4. VIRMANI R, ROBERTS WC: Non-fatal healed transmural myocardial infarction and fatal noncardiac disease: qualification and quantification of coronary arterial narrowing and of left ventricular scarring in 18 necropsy patients. Br Heart J 45:434–441, Apr 1981.

5. ROESKE WH, SAVAGE RM, O'ROURKE R, BLOOR CM: Myocardial infarction: how representative are autopsied subjects with this clinical entity? Arch Path Lab Med 105:642–646, Dec 1981.

6. HARTZ AJ, BARBORIAK PN, ANDERSON AJ, HOFFMANN RG, BARBORIAK JJ: Smoking, coronary artery occlusion, and nonfatal myocardial infarction. JAMA 246:851–853, Aug 21, 1981.

7. SLONE D, SHAPIRO S, KAUFMAN DW, ROSENBERG L, MIETTINEN OS, STOLLEY PD: Risk of myocardial infarction in relation to current and discontinued use of oral contraceptives. N Engl J Med 305:420–424, Aug 1981.

8. WALKER AM, HUNTER JR, WATKINS RN, JICK H, DANFORD A, ALHADEFF L, ROTHMAN KJ: Vasectomy and non-fatal myocardial infarction. Lancet 1:13–15, Jan 1981.

9. ZMYSLINSKI RW, LACKLAND DT, KEIL JE, HIGGINS JE: Increased fatality and difficult diagnosis of in-hospital acute myocardial infarction: comparison to lower mortality and more easily recognized pre-hospital infarction. Am Heart J 101:586–592, May 1981.

10. ZALOKAR JB, RICHARD JL, CLAUDE JR: Leukocyte count, smoking, and myocardial infarction. N Engl J Med 304:465–468, Feb 1981.

11. MOSELEY MJ, SAWMINATHAN R, MORGAN B: Raised plasma urea levels after myocardial infarction. Arch Intern Med 141:438–440, March 1981.

12. RYAN W, KARLINER JS, GILPIN EA, COVELL JW, DELUCA M, ROSS J Jr: The creatine kinase curve area and peak creatine kinase after acute myocardial infarction: usefulness and limitations. Am Heart J 101:162–168, Feb 1981.

13. SHELL WE, DEWOOD MA, KLIGERMAN M, GANZ W, SWAN HJC: Early appearance of MB-creatine kinase activity in nontransmural myocardial infarction detected by sensitive assay for the isoenzyme. Am J Med 71:254–262, Aug 1981.

14. FLINK EB, BRICK JE, SHANE SR: Alterations of long-chain free fatty acid and magnesium concentrations in acute myocardial infarction. Arch Intern Med 141:441–443, March 1981.

15. BIGGER JT, WELD FM: Analysis of prognostic significance of ventricular arrhythmias after myocardial infarction: Shortcomings of Lown grading system. Br Heart J 45:717–724, June 1981.

16. CAMPBELL RWF, MURRAY A, JULIAN DG: Ventricular arrhythmias in first 12 hours of acute myocardial infarction: natural history study. Br Heart J 46:351–357, Oct 1981.

17. TAYLOR GJ, CRAMPTON RS, GIBSON RS, STEBBINS PT, WALDMAN MTG, BELLER GA: Prolonged QT interval at onset of acute myocardial infarction in predicting early phase ventricular tachycardia. Am Heart J 102:16–24, July 1981.

18. TAYLOR GJ Jr, HUMPHRIES JO, PITT B, GRIFFITH LSC, ACHUFF SC: Complex ventricular arrhythmias after myocardial infarction during convalescence and followup: a harbinger of multi-vessel coronary disease, left ventricular dysfunction and sudden death. Johns Hopkins Med J 149:1–5, July 1981.

19. MORRISON GW, KUMAR EB, PORTAL RW, ABER CP: Cardiac arrhythmias 48 hours before, during and 48 hours after discharge from hospital following acute myocardial infarction. Br Heart J 45:500–511, May 1981.

20. LOFMARK R: T-wave changes and postinfarction angina pectoris predictive of recurrent myocardial infarction. Br Heart J 45:512–516, May 1981.

21. WOLFFENBUTTEL BHR, VERDOUW PD, HUGENHOLTZ PG: Immediate and two year prognosis after acute myocardial infarction: prediction from non-invasive as well as invasive parameters in the same individuals. Eur Heart J 2:375–387, Oct 1981.

22. SHELL W, PETER T, MICKLE D, FORRESTER JS, SWAN HJO: Prognostic implications of reduction of left ventricular filling pressure in early transmural acute myocardial infarction. Am Heart J 102:335–340, Sept 1981.

23. HUTTER AM, DESANCTIS RW, FLYNN T, YEATMAN LA: Nontransmural myocardial infarction: a comparison of hospital and late clinical course of patients with that of matched patients with transmural anterior and transmural inferior myocardial infarction. Am J Cardiol 48:595–602, Oct 1981.

24. STARLING MR, CRAWFORD MH, KENNEDY GT, O'ROURKE RA: Treadmill exercise tests predischarge and six weeks post-myocardial infarction to detect abnormalities of known prognostic value. Ann Intern Med 94:721–727, June 1981.

25. SCHWARTZ KM, TURNER JD, SHEFFIELD LT, ROITMAN DI, KANSAL S, PAPAPIETRO SE, MANTLE JA, RACKLEY CE, RUSSELL RO JR, ROGERS WJ: Limited exercise testing soon after myocardial infarction: correlation with early coronary and left ventricular angiography. Ann Intern Med 94: 727–734, June 1981.

26. FULLER CM, RAIZNER AE, VERANI MS, NAHORMEK PA, CHAHINE RA, EMENTEE CW, MILLER RR: Early post-myocardial infarction treadmill stress testing: an accurate predictor of multivessel coronary disease and subsequent cardiac events. Ann Intern Med 94:734–739, June 1981.

27. STARLING MR, CRAWFORD MH, RICHARDS KL, O'ROURKE RA: Predictive value of early postmyocardial infarction modified treadmill exercise testing in multivessel coronary artery disease detection. Am Heart J 102:169–175, Aug 1981.

28. MCMANUS BM, ROBERTS WC: Survival for 20 years or longer after transmural acute myocardial infarction: analysis of eight well-documented necropsy patients. Am Heart J 102:176–182, Aug 1981.

29. ADGEY AAJ, CRAMPTON RS: Hospital or home for acute myocardial infarction: another look at whether or not we should bother to care. Am Heart J 102:473–477, Sept 1981.

30. FUCHS R, SCHEIDT S: Improved criteria for admission to cardiac care units. JAMA 246:2037–2042, Nov 6, 1981.

31. SIVARAJAN ES, BRUCE RA, ALMES MJ, GREEN B, BELANGER L, LINDSKOG BD, NEWTON KM, MANSFIELD LW: In-hospital exercise after myocardial infarction does not improve treadmill performance. N Engl J Med 305:357–362, Aug 1981.

32. APTECAR M, GARZON CAO, VASQUES A, VARINI S, COLLIA L, ESTEGUY A, CARUSO S: Hemodynamic effects of molsidomine vasodilator therapy in acute myocardial infarction. Am Heart J 101:369–373, Apr 1981.

33. COME PC, FLAHERTY JT, BECKER LC, WEISFELDT ML, GREENE HL, WEISS JL, PITT B: Combined administration of nitroglycerin and propranolol to patients with acute myocardia infarction. Chest 80:416–424, Oct 1981.

34. JURGENSEN HJ, FREDERIKSEN J, HANSEN DA, PEDERSEN-BJERGAARD O: Limitation of myocardial infarct size in patients less than 66 years treated with alprenolol. Br Heart J 45:583–588, May 1981.

35. HJALMARSON A, HERLITZ J, MALEK I, RYDEN L, VEDIN A, WALDENSTROM A, WEDEL H, ELMFELDT D, HOLMBERG S, NYBERG G, SWEDBERG K, WAAGSTEIN F, WALDENSTROM J, WILHELMSEN L, WILHELMSSON C: Effect on mortality of metoprolol in acute myocardial infarction: a double-blind randomized trial. Lancet 2:823–826, Oct 1981.

36. BODENHEIMER MM, RAMANATHAN K, BANKA VS, HELFANT RH: Effect of progressive pressure reduction with nitroprusside on acute myocardial infarction in humans. Ann Intern Med 94(part 1):435–439, Apr 1981.

37. HENNING RJ, BECKER H, VINCENT JO, THIJS L, KALTER E, WEIL MH: Use of methylprednisolone in patients following acute myocardial infarction: hemodynamic and metabolic effects. Chest 79:186–194, Feb 1981.

38. MCDANIEL HG, PAPAPIETRO SE, ROGERS WJ, MANTLE JA, SMITH LR, RUSSELL RO JR, RACKLEY CE: Glucose-insulin-potassium induced alterations in individual plasma free fatty acids in patients with acute myocardial infarction. Am Heart J 102:10–15, July 1981.

39. MANTLE JA, ROGERS WJ, SMITH LR, MCDANIEL HG, PAPAPIETRO SE, RUSSELL RO JR, RACKLEY CE: Clinical effects of glucose-insulin-potassium on left ventricular function in acute myocardial infarction: results from a randomized clinical trial. Am Heart J 102:313–324, Sept 1981.

40. GANZ W, BUCHBINDER N, MARCUS H, MONDKAR A, MADDAHI J, CHARUZI Y, O'CONNER L, SHELL W, FISHBEIN WC, KASS R, MIYAMOTO A, SWAN HJC: Intracoronary thrombolysis in evolving myocardial infarction. Am Heart J 101:4–13, Jan 1981.

41. HECHT HS, TAYLOR R, WONG M, SHAH PM: Comparative evaluation of segmental asynergy in remote myocardial infarction by radionuclide angiography, two-dimensional echocardiography, and contrast ventriculography. Am Heart J 101:740–749, June 1981.

42. MADDAHI J, GANZ W, NINOMIYA K, HASHIDA J, FISHBEIN MC, MONDKAR A, BUCHBINDER N, MARCUS H, GEFT I, SHAH PK, ROZANSKI A, SWAN HJC, BERMAN DS: Myocardial salvage by intracoronary thrombolysis in evolving acute myocardial infarction: evaluation using intracoronary injection of thallium-201. Am Heart J 102:664–674, Oct 1981.

43. LEE G, AMSTERDAM EA, LOW RI, DEMARIA AN, MASON DT: Coronary thrombolysis by intravenous streptokinase in clinical acute myocardial infarction. Am Heart J 102:783–786, Oct 1981.

44. MARKIS JE, MALAGOLD M, PARKER A, SILVERMAN KJ, BARRY WH, ALS AV, PAULIN S, GROSSMAN W, BRAUNWALD E: Myocardial salvage after intracoronary thrombolysis with streptokinase in acute myocardial infarction. N Engl J Med 305:777–782, Oct 1981

45. MASON DT: International experience with percutaneous transluminal coronary recanalization by streptokinase-thrombolysis reperfusion in acute myocardial infarction: new, safe, landmark therapeutic approach salvaging ischemic muscle and improving ventricular function. Am Heart J 102:1126–1133, Dec 1981.

46. SHERRY S: Personal reflections on the development of thrombolytic therapy and its application to acute coronary thrombosis. Am Heart J 102:1134–1139, Dec 1981.

47. LEE G, GIDDENS J, KRIEG P, DAJEE A, SUZUKI M, KOZINA JA, IKEDA RM, DEMARIA AN, MASON DT: Experimental reversal of acute coronary thrombotic occlusion and myocardial injury in animals utilizing streptokinase. Am Heart J 102:1139–1144, Dec 1981.

48. GANZ W, NINOMIYA K, HASHIDA J, FISBEIN MC, BUCHBINDER N, MARCUS H, MONDKAR A, MADDAHI J, SHAH PK, BERMAN D, CHARUZI Y, GEFT I, SHELL W, SWAN HJC: Intracoronary thrombolysis in acute myocardial infarction: experimental background and clinical experience. Am Heart J 102:1145–1149, Dec 1981.

49. LEE G, AMSTERDAM EA, LOW R, JOYE JA, KIMCHI A, DEMARIA AN, MASON DT: Efficacy of percutaneous transluminal coronary recanalization utilizing streptokinase thrombolysis in patients with acute myocardial infarction. Am Heart J 102:1159–1167, Dec 1981.

50. COWLEY MJ, HASTILLO A, VETROVEC GW, HESS ML: Effects of intracoronary streptokinase in acute myocardial infarction. Am Heart J 102:1149–1158, Dec 1981.

51. REDUTO LA, FREUND GC, GAETA JM, SMALLING RW, LEWIS B, GOULD KL: Coronary artery reperfusion in acute myocardial infarction: beneficial effects of intracoronary streptokinase on left ventricular salvage and performance. Am Heart J 102:1168–1177, Dec 1981.

52. RUTSCH W, SCHARTL M, MATHEY D, KUCK K, MERX W, DORR R, RENTROP P, BLANKE H: Percutaneous transluminal coronary recanalization: procedure, results and acute complications. Am Heart J 102:1178–1181, Dec 1981.

53. MERX W, DORR R, RENTROP P, BLANKE H, KARSCH KR, MATHEY DG, KREMER P, RUTSCH W, SCHMUTZLER H: Evaluation of the effectiveness of intracoronary streptokinase infusion in acute myocardial infarction: postprocedure management and hospital course in 204 patients. Am Heart J 102:1181–1187, Dec 1981.

54. RENTROP P, BLANKE H, KARSCH KR, RUTSCH W, SCHARTL M, MERX W, DORR R, MATHEY D, KUCH K: Changes in left ventricular function after intracoronary streptokinase infusion in clinically evolving myocardial infarction. Am Heart J 102:1188–1193, Dec 1981.

55. MATHEY DG, RODWALD G, RENTROP P, LEITZ K, MERX W, MESSMER BJ, RUTSCH W, BUCHERL ES: Intracoronary streptokinase thrombolytic recanalization and subsequent surgical bypass of remaining atherosclerotic stenosis in acute myocardial infarction: complementary combined approach effecting reduced infarct size, preventing reinfarction, and improving left ventricular function. Am Heart J 102:1194–1201, Dec 1981.

56. VETROVEC GW, COWLEY MJ, OVERTON H, RICHARDSON DW: Intracoronary thrombus in syndromes of unstable myocardial ischemia. Am Heart J 102:1202–1208, Dec 1981.

57. THE NORWEGIAN MULTICENTER STUDY GROUP: Timolol-induced reduction in mortality and reinfarction in patients surviving acute myocardial infarction. N Engl J Med 304:801–807, Apr 1981.

58. BETA BLOCKER HEART ATTACK STUDY GROUP: The beta blocker heart attack trial. JAMA 246(18):2073–2074, Nov 6, 1981.

59. BERG R JR, SELINGER SL, LEONARD JL, GRUNWALD RP, O'GRADY WP: Immediate coronary artery bypass for acute evolving myocardial infarction. J Thorac Cardiovasc Surg 81:493–497, Apr 1981.

60. JONES EL, WAITES TF, CRAVER JM, BRADFORD JM, DOUGLAS JS, KING SB, BONE DK, DORNEY ER, CLEMENTS SD, THOMPKINS T, HATCHER CR JR: Coronary bypass for relief of persistent pain following acute myocardial infarction. Ann Thorac Surg 32:33–43, July 1981.

61. BERGER RL, DAVIS KB, KAISER GC, FOSTER ED, HAMMOND GL, TONG TGL, KENNEDY JW, SHEFFIELD T, RINGQVIST I, WIENS RD, CHAITMAN BR, MOCK M: Preservation of the myocardium during coronary artery bypass grafting. Circulation 64:61–66, Aug 1981.

62. ASINGER RW, MIKELL FL, ELSPERGER J, HODGES M: Incidence of left ventricular thrombosis after acute transmural myocardial infarction. Serial evaluation by two-dimensional echocardiography. N Engl J Med 305:297–302, Aug 1981.

63. NAIR CK, SKETCH MH, MAHONEY PD, LYNCH JD, MOOSS AN, KENNEY NP: Detection of left ventricular thrombi by computerised tomography: a preliminary report. Br Heart J 45:535–541, May 1981.

64. TOMODA H, HOSHIAI M, FURUYA H, SHOTSU A, OOTAKI M, MATSUYAMA S: Evaluation of left ventricular thrombus with computed tomography. Am J Cardiol 48:573–577, Sept 1981.

65. STRATTON JR, RITCHIE JL, HAMMERMEISTER KE, KENNEDY JW, HAMILTON GW: Detection of left ventricular thrombi with radionuclide angiography. Am J Cardiol 48:565–572, Sept 1981.

66. OTTERSTAD JE, CHRISTENSEN O, LEVORSTAD K, NITTER-HAUGE S: Long-term results after left ventricular aneurysmectomy. Br Heart J 45:426–433, Apr 1981.

67. JONES EL, CRAVER JM, HURST JW, BRADFORD JA, BONE DK, ROBINSON PH, COBBS BW, THOMPKINS TR, HATCHER CR JR: Influence of left ventricular aneurysm on survival following the coronary bypass operation. Ann Surg 193:733–742, June 1981.

68. RACKLEY CE, RUSSELL RO, MANTLE JA, ROGERS WJ, PAPAPIETRO SE, SCHWARTZ KM: Right ventricular infarction and function. Am Heart J 101:215–218, Feb 1981.

69. CINTRON GB, HERNANDEZ E, LINARES E, ARANDA JM: Bedside recognition, incidence and clinical course of right ventricular infarction. Am J Cardiol 47:224–227, Feb 1981.

70. CHOU T, VAN DER BEL-KAHN J, ALLEN J, BROCKMEIER L, FOWLER NO: Electrocardiographic diagnosis of right ventricular infarction. Am J Med 70:1175–1180, June 1981.

71. CANDELL-RIERA J, FIGUERAS J, VALLE V, ALVAREZ A, GUTIERREZ L, CORTADELLAS J, CINCA J, SALAS A, RIUS J: Right ventricular infarction: relationships between ST segment elevation in V_{4R} and hemodynamic, scintigraphic, and echocardiographic findings in patients with acute inferior myocardial infarction. Am Heart J 101:281–287, March 1981.

72. LLOYD EA, GERSH BJ, KENNELLY BM: Hemodynamic spectrum of "dominant" right ventricular infarction in 19 patients. Am J Cardiol 48:1016–1022, Dec 1981.

73. MARMOR A, GELTMAN EM, BIELLO DR, SOBEL BE, SIEGEL BA, ROBERTS R: Functional response of the right ventricle to myocardial infarction: dependence on the site of left ventricular infarction. Circulation 64:1005–1011, Nov 1981.

74. SCLAROVSKY S, ZAFRIR N, STRASBERG B, KRACODD O, LEWIN RF, ARDITI A, ROSEN KM, AGMON J: Ventricular fibrillation complicating temporary ventricular pacing in acute myocardial infarction: significance of right ventricular infarction. Am J Cardiol 48:1160–1166, Dec 1981.

75. ISNER JM, FISHER GP, DEL NEGRO AA, BORER JS: Right ventricular infarction with hemodynamic

decompensation due to transient loss of active atrial augmentation: successful treatment with atrial pacing. Am Heart J 102:792–794, Oct 1981.

76. BERMAN J, HAFFAJEE CI, ALPERT JS: Therapy of symptomatic pericarditis after myocardial infarction: retrospective and prospective studies of aspirin, indomethacin, prednisone, and spontaneous resolution. Am Heart J 101:750–753, June 1981.

77. BISHOP HL, GIBSON RS, STAMM RB, BELLER GA, MARTIN RP: Role of two-dimensional echocardiography in the evaluation of patients with ventricular septal rupture postmyocardial infarction. Am Heart J 102:965–971, Dec 1981.

78. GAUDIANI VA, MILLER DC, STINSON EB, OYER PE, REITZ BA, MORENO-CABRAL RJ, SHUMWAY NE: Postinfarction ventricular septal defect: an argument for early operation. Surgery 89:48–55, Jan 1981.

79. KILLEN DA, REED WA, WATHANACHAROEN S, McCALLISTER BD, BELL HH: Postinfarctional rupture of the interventricular septum. J Cardiovasc Surg 22:113–125, Mar–Apr 1981.

80. MATSUI K, KAY JH, MENDEZ M, ZUBIATE P, VANSTROM N, YOKOYAMA T: Ventricular septal rupture secondary to myocardial infarction. JAMA 245:1537–1539, April 17, 1981.

81. RADFORD MJ, JOHNSON RA, DAGGETT WM JR, FALLON JT, BUCKLEY MJ, GOLD HK, LEINBACH RC: Ventricular septal rupture: a review of clinical and physiologic features and an analysis of survival. Circulation 64:545–553, Sept 1981.

82. SINGER DE, MULLEY AG, THIBAULT GE, BARNETT GO: Unexpected readmissions to the coronary-care unit during recovery from acute myocardial infarction. N Engl J Med 304:626–629, March 1981.

83. MARMOR A, SOBEL BE, ROBERTS R: Factors presaging early recurrent myocardial infarction ("extension"). Am J Cardiol 48:603–610, Oct 1981.

84. SCHUSTER EH, BULKLEY BH: Early post-infarction angina. Ischemia at a distance and ischemia in the infarct zone. N Engl J Med 305:1101–1105, Nov 1981.

85. GODLEY RW, WANN LS, ROGERS EW, FEIGENBAUM H, WEYMAN AE: Incomplete mitral leaflet closure in patients with papillary muscle dysfunction. Circulation 63:565–571, March 1981.

3

Arrhythmias and Conduction Disturbances

ARRHYTHMIAS IN APPARENTLY HEALTHY PERSONS

Current knowledge concerning the prognostic importance of VPC has come from studies of patients with heart disease. In the clinical situation of overt heart disease, this arrhythmia has been consistently shown to be associated with an unfavorable prognosis, and in post-AMI patients it is an important precursor for sudden death. In persons without heart disease in whom rhythm disturbances are detected on routine examination, it is not yet known whether VPC portend a similar unfavorable outcome. Rabkin and associates[1] from Winnipeg, Canada, determined whether VPC on routine ECGs in men without apparent heart disease predict the later occurrence of clinical manifestations of CAD. The present Manitoba Heart Study cohort consisted of 3,983 men predominantly 25–34 years of age and free of overt CAD at study entry. During the 29-year collection period, 401 persons without clinical evidence of heart disease had VPC on standard ECG at routine examination. They were followed for an average of 11 years and 13% (54 men) later developed manifestations of CAD. Age-specific total CAD incidence was significantly greater for men 40–59 years of age who had VPC than in men of the same age without VPC.

The clinical manifestation most strongly associated with VPC was sudden death. VPC characteristics of frequency, configuration, coupling interval, and postextrasystolic T-wave change did not distinguish those who developed CAD. The prematurity index (R-R'/QT) showed a trend toward an association of late coupled ectopic beats (R-R'/QT ≥ 1.6) and CAD risk. Faster basic ventricular rate plus VPC on routine ECG in men >40 years of age without apparent heart disease identified those at high risk for subsequent clinical CAD events, especially sudden death.

To define the prevalence, frequency, and characteristics of VPC in adults free of recognizable heart disease, Kostis and associates[2] performed 24-hour ambulatory ECGs on 101 subjects (51 men and 50 women; mean age, 49 years) in whom physical examination, chest radiograph, ECG, echo maximal exercise stress test, right- and left-sided heart catheterization, and coronary arteriography were normal. Of the 101 subjects, 39 had at least 1 VPC/24 h, but only 4 had >100 VPC/24 h, and fewer than 5 had >5 VPC/h. The probability of having at least 1 VPC/24 h increased with age (p < 0.02). The number of VPC/24 h also was positively associated with age (p = 0.001). There was no consistent relation between the presence or number of VPC/24 h and sex, BP, weight, height, body mass index, serum potassium or calcium, cholesterol and triglyceride, hemoglobin, the ingestion of coffee, tea or alcohol, and cigarette smoking. Four subjects had multiform VPC and 2 of the 4 had early VPC.

Horan and Kennedy[3] from Baltimore, Maryland, and Long Beach, California, followed 72 asymptomatic individuals with frequent and/or complex ventricular ectopic activity for various periods (mean, 7 years) and studied 27 (38%) of them by invasive techniques. Of the 27, 22% had angiographically significant CAD and 18% noncritical CAD, but 59% had normal coronary arteries. Catheterization in the 16 patients with normal coronary arteries disclosed that most had subtle abnormalities of myocardial function or cardiomyopathies. Whether these subclinical abnormalities were related to VPC is unclear. None of the 72 patients with frequent and complex ventricular ectopic activity experienced a fatal event, 2 developed angina, and 1 developed CHF during the average 7-year follow-up. Thus, frequent and complex ventricular ectopic activity in apparently healthy patients can be associated with latent CAD, but in most it represents an idiopathic benign syndrome, on the basis of this 7-year follow-up.

Ambulatory ECG recordings have been used to detect and quantify cardiac arrhythmias in individual patients. This technique has been used to estimate the prevalence of transient arrhythmias in patients with specific cardiac conditions, but much less information is available on results of 24-hour ambulatory ECG findings in healthy young people. In 1977 Brodsky and associates from Chicago, Illinois (Am J Cardiol 39:390, 1977) described the results of 24-hour ambulatory ECG monitoring in 50 young healthy men. Sobotka and associates[4] from the same laboratory in Chicago, Illinois, in 1981 described the results of 24-hour ambulatory ECG monitoring in 50 young healthy women. During waking periods, maximum sinus rates ranged from 122–189 beats/min (mean ± SD, 153 ± 14) and minimum rates from 40–

73 beats/min (56 ± 7). During sleeping periods, maximum and minimum rates ranged from 71–128 beats/min (105 ± 13) and from 37–59 beats/min (48 ± 6), respectively. Of 50 women, 32 (64%) had atrial premature beats, with only 1 subject (2%) having > 100 beats/24 h. A total of 27 subjects (54%) had VPC, with only 3 subjects (6%) having > 50 beats/24 h. One subject (2%) had one 3-beat episode of VT, and 2 subjects (4%) had transient type 1 second-degree AV block.

ATRIAL ARRHYTHMIAS

Supraventricular tachycardia in 217 children

Garson and associates[5] from Houston, Texas, analyzed 217 children, half of them males, whose first documented episode of supraventricular tachycardia (SVT) began before the age of 18 years. The SVT began in the first year of life in 43%. In those under 4 months of age, HR was more rapid and CHF more frequent than in those patients with SVT beginning at an older age. Of the 217 patients, 60% had a normal heart and 23% had congenital heart disease. In half the latter, SVT began before a cardiovascular operation. The 2 malformations with unusually high frequencies of SVT were Ebstein's anomaly and L-transposition. In 47 (22%) patients, WPW was present. Among 127 patients for whom information was adequate, 23% had other family members with SVT.

Treatment for the 72% of patients who did not spontaneously revert to normal rhythm was most frequently digoxin; in 68% of patients, it was successful in a median time of 6 hours. Synchronized DC conversion was successful in 12 of the 20 patients in whom it was used. Vagal maneuvers were ineffective in infants and young children, but were successful in 12 of 19 older children. Phenylephrine was effective in only 3 of 9 patients, all older children. Overdrive pacing converted the arrhythmia in 4 of 5 patients. Because of the tendency for SVT to recur, long-term treatment with digoxin was used in 72%. Those not so treated had a higher recurrence rate.

Long-term follow-up averaged 4.6 years. The oldest patient was 25 years old. Three children had died, 2 at < 1 month of age, because of the arrhythmia, and the third after a cardiac operation. The prognosis for no recurrence was best for those in whom SVT first appeared before they were 6 months old and who had a normal heart. Although SVT was present in 56% of the patients on long-term follow-up, some had such infrequent episodes that they were not on medication.

Atrial fibrillation: effect on mortality

Although clinical and prognostic differences between paroxysmal atrial fibrillation (AF) and chronic AF are recognized, the true impact of these conditions on mortality has never been established. Gajewski and Singer[6], in a pioneering effort to use a new system of case identification in life insurance medical records, identified from 680 companies 3,099 life insurance appli-

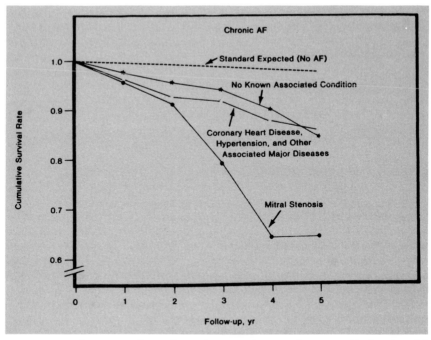

Fig. 3-1. Cumulative survival rate observed in insured men and women with chronic atrial fibrillation (AF) associated with MS, other major conditions, or none. Expected survival was derived from the 1965–1979 Select Basic Tables. Reproduced with permission from Gajewski and Singer.[6]

cants who had AF. Of this number, 71 died over a mean period of 3.3 years; their deaths were compared with deaths expected and derived from standard insurance mortality tables. (Fig. 3-1). Patients with paroxysmal AF but no other identified cardiovascular impairment showed normal mortality. Patients with paroxysmal AF associated with MS or CAD had a significantly increased mortality. Chronic AF, with or without other impairments, entailed a much higher risk than did paroxysmal AF, and patients with associated MS in particular had a very high excess mortality.

Effect of quinidine on digoxin concentration in skeletal muscle and serum in atrial fibrillation

Quinidine causes a rise in serum steady-state concentrations of digoxin and reduces both renal and nonrenal clearances of digoxin. A redistribution of digoxin from tissue stores was suggested as a second underlying mechanism when it was shown that quinidine also increased serum digoxin levels whenever digoxin maintenance therapy had been discontinued before quinidine treatment was begun. In further studies, a quinidine-induced 30%–40% reduction in the apparent volume of distribution of digoxin was found. About 50% of the body's load of digoxin is located in skeletal muscle. Schenck-Gustafsson and associates[7] from Huddinge, Sweden, investigated

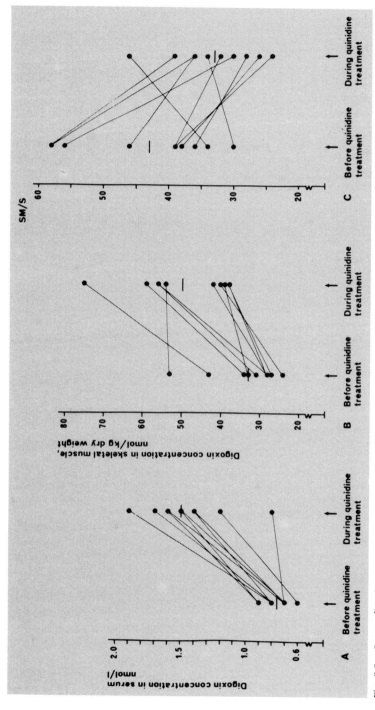

Fig. 3-2. Serum digoxin concentrations (panel A), skeletal muscle digoxin concentrations (panel B), and ratio (SM/S) between skeletal muscle and serum digoxin concentrations (panel C) in 10 patients before and during quinidine treatment. Arithmetic means are indicated by horizontal lines. Reproduced with permission from Schenck-Gustafsson.[7]

whether a redistribution of digoxin from skeletal muscle to serum could be involved in the quinidine-induced reduction in the volume of distribution of digoxin in 10 patients with AF. Their data show that administration of quinidine reduces the ratio of skeletal muscle digoxin to serum digoxin, suggesting reduced binding of digoxin in muscle (Fig. 3-2). In their study, the steady-state digoxin concentration in skeletal muscle increased by approximately 50% during quinidine treatment. It is not known whether an increase in the steady-state digoxin concentration also occurs in heart muscle, but it is likely.

Dual atrioventricular nodal transmission

The electrophysiologic properties of dual AV nodal pathways have been the subject of considerable interest in the past 2 decades. Demonstration of discontinuous AV conduction curves and their relation to AV nodal reentrant tachycardia in particular have been investigated. The ECG manifestations of 2 ranges of PR intervals during sinus rhythm and electrophysiologic demonstration of 2 ranges of A-H intervals during atrial pacing are manifestations of dual AV nodal pathways. The latter electrophysiologic phenomenon, however, has been studied relatively infrequently. Wu and associates[8] from Taipei, Taiwan, performed multiple incremental atrial pacing studies in 24 patients with dual AV nodal pathways to obtain atrial (A) to His (H) basic driven (A_1 and H_1) and extrastimulus (A_2 and H_2) intervals. Discontinuous A_1-A_2 and H_1-H_2 intervals were analyzed for relations between initial coupling times and subsequent A-H responses, and they examined curves of sequential paced cycle lengths (A-A intervals) -vs- A-H intervals. Seventeen patients showed sustained slow pathway (SP) conduction while demonstrating discontinuous A-A and A-H curves. Sustained SP conduction occurred at critical atrial paced rates when the first paced beat was blocked in the fast pathway (FP) with conduction via the SP. Of these 17 patients, 11 had inducible sustained SVT. The A-H interval during SVT in these 11 patients was closely related to SP A-H interval during atrial pacing at the paced rate comparable to SVT rate. The 7 remaining patients showed continuous A-A and A-H curves. In 3 of these 7 patients, sustained SVT was inducible, suggesting an ability to sustain SP conduction. All 3 patients had continuous A_1-A_2 and H_1-H_2 curves during sinus rhythm, so that the first atrial paced beat could not be blocked in the FP for subsequent SP conduction. In the other 4 of the remaining 7 patients, despite block of the first atrial paced beat in the FP with SP conduction, the second paced beat was blocked in the SP, so that all subsequent beats resumed FP conduction. Thus, sustained SP conduction in patients with dual AV nodal pathways requires: 1) an initial beat being blocked in the FP; 2) a critical rate cycle length, and 3) the ability of SP for repetitive conduction at critical rates.

Treatment of supraventricular arrhythmias with verapamil

The WPW syndrome is a well recognized ECG entity that is due to ventricular pre-excitation in sinus rhythm by an accessory AV pathway (bypass). Clinically, it may be complicated by paroxysmal SVT, and it also has been recognized that patients with a normal resting ECG can have a concealed ventriculoatrial (VA) bypass that may play an important role in the genesis of an identical form of tachycardia. The mechanism common to both situations is a reentry circuit consisting of anterograde conduction via the AV node and His-Purkinje system, transventricular conduction to the site of a bypass bridging the AV ring, and return to the atria via the bypass to reach the AV node again. Drugs that act on any part of the reentry circuit to slow conduction or prolong refractoriness may potentially prevent the occurrence of SVT. Verapamil has been shown to be effective in SVT complicating the WPW syndrome, and its action is believed to be predominantly on the AV node, without significant effect on infranodal or atrial tissues. Its effects on accessory bypasses conducting in either direction, or in retrograde direction only, have been studied in a small number of patients; the results indicate that verapamil has little, if any, effect in this regard. Hamer and associates[9] from Los Angeles, California, delineated the efficacy of verapamil in patients with overt or concealed WPW syndrome complicated by recurrent SVT. Verapamil, 0.15 mg/kg, intravenously, was administered to 19 such patients with recurrent SVT who were undergoing electrophysiologic evaluation. Twelve patients had overt WPW syndrome and 7 had concealed accessory pathways conducting in the retrograde direction only. Verapamil had a significant effect in delaying conduction and prolonging refractoriness in the AV node, but no significant action on any of the other cardiac tissues that formed the tachycardia circuit in these patients. In particular, it had no significant effects on antegrade or retrograde bypass conduction or refractoriness. Sustained SVT was initiated in 15 patients and was terminated in 13 patients in 60–105 seconds by a 30-second injection of verapamil. Cycle length alteration during SVT was seen in 6 patients before reversion, and spontaneous VPC were observed following verapamil administration in 5 patients. Two patients with apparently normal sinus node function had prolonged sinus node recovery times immediately after reversion of the SVT by verapamil. Echo zones were assessed before and after verapamil, and sustained or self-terminating SVT could still be induced after administration of the drug in 13 of the 15 patients who had sustained SVT beforehand. Thus, intravenous verapamil was effective in terminating sustained SVT in most patients with overt or concealed WPW and, despite a potential for sinus node depression and the initiation of VPC, the drug had no clinically significant side effects. The ability to reinitiate SVT following verapamil administration suggests a need for immediate follow-up with maintenance drug therapy.

Gonzales and Scheinman[10] from San Francisco, California, administered verapamil or placebo as a bolus infusion in a double-blind fashion to 24 patients with either AF or atrial flutter and to 10 patients with paroxysmal SVT. Patients whose heart rate did not decrease below 100 beats/min were given a second dose. Of the 24 patients with AF or atrial flutter, 11 received placebo first. Control heart rate and BP were not modified by placebo; however, verapamil significantly reduced heart rate and systolic BP in the 24 patients. Of the 10 patients with paroxysmal SVT, 1 reverted to sinus rhythm after the administration of placebo. For the remaining 9, the heart rate was not modified by placebo, but was significantly reduced by verapamil. BP was not modified by verapamil or placebo in these 10 patients. Long-term oral verapamil treatment was maintained without interruption in 18 patients for a mean of 16 ± 7.5 months, and 15 patients required concomitant therapy with other antiarrhythmic drugs to achieve control of arrhythmia. All patients reported symptomatic improvement, and the number of hospitalizations required for control of arrhythmia decreased significantly. Verapamil is safe and effective for acute control of SVT. Long-term oral administration of verapamil, alone or with other antiarrhythmic drugs, is an important contribution to the management of recurrent SVT.

Treatment of supraventricular arrhythmias by surgery

Sealy and Gallagher[11] from Durham, North Carolina, reported experiences in 79 patients with supraventricular tachyarrhythmias who had a total of 82 left free wall accessory pathways of AV conduction of the Kent type. The operation consisted of localization of the pathway by mapping the epicardial excitation sequence of the atria and ventricles, followed by a group of maneuvers needed to divide the pathway, which is not visible or palpable. An endocardial incision was made just above the anulus fibrosus extending 1.5—2.0 cm on each side of the pathway's crossing point; the coronary sulcus fat was widely separated from the anulus fibrosus. Complications included postpericardiotomy syndrome (31 patients), constrictive pericarditis (1 patient), hepatitis (1 patient), pancreatitis (1 patient), and bleeding (3 patients). Three patients died. Eight pathways in 8 patients were missed. Four patients underwent second attempts at division of pathways. The overall success rate for interruption of left free wall pathways was 90%, with no failures in the last 34 patients. In another article by Sealy and Gallagher[12], 32 of 36 pathways were successfully divided in 17 patients.

If atrial arrhythmia is refractory to medical management or if the ventricle has other major abnormalities that make even a mild rhythm disturbance intolerable, a serious clinical problem may result from inappropriate ventricular response to intermittent atrial arrhythmias. Sealy and associates[13] also operated on 42 patients with life-threatening or disabling atrial arrhythmias: 15 had Kent bundles as accessory pathways of AV conduction and 27 had arrhythmias that originated in or above the AV node. Of the latter group, 19 had enhanced AV conduction plus an atrial arrhythmia, and 8 others had atrial arrhythmias without enhanced AV node conduction. In the group with enhanced AV node conduction, the mean heart rate was 187 beats/min (range, 123–260) and 17 of the 19 patients had AF or atrial flutter.

The techniques employed for His bundle interruption were blind suture, electrocauterization, and incision of the septal portion of the right atrium in 11 patients and cryothermia in 31 patients. In the 27 patients without Kent bundles, the His bundle was interrupted by cryothermic ablation in 25 and divided with a knife in 2 others. The latter 2 were successful, but only after a second operation. There were 3 failures with cryothermia. Of the 15 patients with Kent bundles, the His bundle was interrupted by suture cautery in 3 and by incision alone in 6 patients. In 6, the His bundle was interrupted by cryothermia, with 1 failure. Thus, of the 42 patients, there were 6 failures, 4 in patients with hypertrophied atria. Interruption of the AV node-His bundle led to junctional rhythm, necessitating installation of a demand pacemaker. These studies indicate that interruption of atrial-to-ventricular conduction is a satisfactory operation for atrial arrhythmias that are disabling or life-threatening and are refractory to vigorous medical therapy. Cryothermic ablation is the preferable technique.

VENTRICULAR ARRHYTHMIAS

Acceleration of ventricular tachycardia induced by a chest thump

A direct blow to the precordium, i.e., a chest thump, is known to be an effective maneuver for terminating a paroxysm of VT. Several authors, however, have indicated that chest thumping can lead to VF and recommended its performance only when equipment for external defibrillation was available. Recent studies have indicated that the electrophysiologic mechanism of digitalis-induced ventricular arrhythmias may be different from those not due to digitalis use. Sclarovsky and associates[14] from Petah-Tikva, Israel, described 3 patients who were receiving digitalis and had VT and in whom chest thump caused an acceleration of the rate of VT. Following discontinuation of the digitalis therapy, however, chest thump converted to sinus rhythm recurrence of VT in 2 patients and did not cause acceleration of the ventricular rate in the third. Thus, these authors suggest that chest thump be used with caution in patients with VT who are taking digitalis.

Occurrence during Swan-Ganz catheterization in the critically ill

Since its first description in 1970, the flow-directed, balloon-tipped catheter has been used routinely for hemodynamic monitoring of critically ill patients. Introduction of the flow-directed catheter into the right ventricle in the cardiac catheterization laboratory rarely has been associated with ventricular arrhythmias, and previous reports of the use of this catheter in intensive care units also have shown only infrequent production of ventricular arrhythmias. Sprung and associates[15] from Miami, Florida, however, found ventricular arrhythmias to be produced in 29 of 60 critically ill patients in whom right-sided cardiac catheterization with a flow-directed, balloon-tipped catheter was performed: 29 patients developed VPC and 20 VT; 2 patients required antiarrhythmic therapy or a precordial thump to convert VT, and in 1 patient the VT was fatal. Thus, serious catheter-induced arrhythmias, including sustained VT, may develop during Swan-Ganz catheterization in critically ill patients. The 60 right-sided cardiac catheterizations described in this report were in 44 patients, (average age, 61 years) and the procedure was difficult in most because of shock, large right ventricles, dilated PAs, or marked pulmonary hypertension. Thus, the duration of catheterization was longer than in previous studies. Ventricular arrhythmias may not occur during the catheterization procedure, and in 9 of their catheterizations, the arrhythmia was not appreciated until the procedure had ended.

Arrhythmogenic right ventricular dysplasia in children

Arrhythmogenic RV dysplasia (ARVD) was proposed by Fontaine in 1976 as a specific cardiomyopathy limited to the right ventricle. Localized hypokinesis in the dilated RV is demonstrated angiographically and the RV subepicardium is stated to have excess adipose tissue. Additionally, the interstitium between the myocardial fibers in the right ventricle contains excessive amounts of fibrous tissue. ARVD is accompanied by episodes of VT having left BBB patterns. The fact that it usually can be induced by electrical stimulation suggests a reentry mechanism. Delayed potentials may be recorded from anatomically abnormal areas of the right ventricle during catheterization or during epicardial mapping for surgical treatment of the arrhythmia. Dungan and associates[16] from Houston, Texas, described 3 children with recurrent VT from ARVD. These 3 children were found in a review of 26 patients with recurring VT. Ten of the 26 had no clinically recognizable cardiac abnormality aside from the arrhythmia, and 3 of these 10 had ARVD. The 3 patients were seen initially at 1, 2, and 14 years of age with VPC and/or VT. Sustained VT occurred spontaneously or during stress testing. Both VPC and VT were of the left BBB contour, suggesting a RV site of origin. The diagnosis of ARVD was based on RV wall motion abnormalities demonstrated angiographically. The authors suggested that ARVD could be a significantly common cause of VT in children with apparently normal hearts.

Exercise-triggered paroxysmal ventricular tachycardia

Wu and associates[17] from Taipei, Taiwan, performed electrophysiologic studies, isoproterenol infusion, and serial treadmill exercise tests before and after administration of propranolol, verapamil, lidocaine, and procainamide in 3 patients with exercise-triggered VT. In all 3 patients, organic heart disease was absent. VT was reproducibly provoked with exercise and with isoproterenol infusion. Propranolol and lidocaine (tested in 2 patients) effectively prevented exercise provocation of VT. Verapamil terminated the tachycardia in all 3 patients but VPC, couplets, and short salvos remained provokable with exercise. Electrical stimulations with incremental ventricular pacing and ventricular extrastimulus testing failed to induce tachycardia in all 3 patients. These findings strongly suggest that repetitive rhythmic activities related to the catecholamine-sensitive after depolarizations are probably responsible for exercise-triggered VT.

Diuretic-induced ventricular ectopic activity

Diuretics are used commonly to treat patients with systemic hypertension, CHF, and other edematous conditions, and in 10%−50% of patients so treated hypokalemia develops. The guidelines for potassium repletion in hypokalemic patients who do not take digitalis remain controversial, largely because few data are available. Some clinicians believe that patients tolerate hypokalemia quite well and recommend potassium repletion only when the potassium depletion is extreme ($K^+ < 2.5$ mEq/liter) or when the patient becomes symptomatic. Other clinicians, however, have been concerned about cardiovascular complications of hypokalemia. The frequency of ventricular ectopic activity in nondigitalized, hypokalemic patients remains unknown. The routine ECG has a low sensitivity in identifying ventricular ectopic activity, in comparison to 24-hour ambulatory ECG monitoring and exercise testing. Holland and associates[18] from Dallas, Texas, assessed the frequency and types of ventricular ectopic activity during diuretic-induced hypokalemia in 21 patients with mild essential hypertension, plasma potassium levels < 3.5 mEq/liter during previous diuretic treatment, and normal findings (i.e., < 6 unifocal VPC/h) on 24-hour ambulatory ECG monitoring and exercise testing. The patients received hydrochlorothiazide (50 mg, b.i.d.) for 4 weeks, then ambulatory ECG monitoring and exercise testing were repeated. Ambulatory ECG monitoring revealed that ectopic activity developed in 7 patients and complex ventricular ectopic activity (multifocal VPC, ventricular couplets and/or VT) developed in 4. Only 2 of the 7 patients had ventricular ectopic activity during exercise testing while they were hypokalemic. Potassium repletion in these 7 patients with spironolactone abolished complex ventricular ectopic activity and reduced unifocal VPC significantly (p < 0.01) from an average of 71 VPC/h/patient during hydrochlorothiazide treatment to 5.4 VPC/h/patient after potassium repletion. Although complex ventricular ectopic activity more likely occurred with plasma potassium < 3.0 mEq/liter, restoration of normokalemia was required in several patients before residual ventricular ectopic activity was abolished. Persistent ventricular ectopic activity in 1 patient suggested that myocardial injury sustained during hypokalemia may initiate chronic ventricular ectopic activity. Even in nondigitalized patients, the hazard of diuretic-induced ventricular ectopic activity warrants correction of hypokalemia.

Treatment with amiodarone

Amiodarone, a benzofurane derivative, was developed as an antianginal agent and has been widely used as such in Europe. Beneficial myocardial hemodynamic effects result from decreased coronary vascular resistance and increased coronary blood flow. Amiodarone also exerts noncompetitive beta adrenoreceptor blocking effects. In addition, experimental animal studies have demonstrated significant antiarrhythmic properties of the agent. Preliminary clinical experience indicates the utility of amiodarone in a variety of atrial and ventricular tachyarrhythmias. Amiodarone is especially useful in controlling the supraventricular mechanisms associated with the WPW syndrome. The drug's unusually long half-life and infrequent side effects make it unique among antiarrhythmic agents. A major limitation in clinical application is the absence of guidelines for therapeutic adequacy, which derives from the drug's delayed onset of action and the absence of blood level data for determining appropriate dosing. Such deficiencies are particularly perplexing when the tachyarrhythmia being treated is potentially life-threatening. Podrid and Lown[19] from Boston, Massachusetts, evaluated amiodarone in 70 patients with symptomatic, sustained refractory tachyarrhythmias. Of these, 29 had atrial arrhythmias; 20 had recurrent AF, and 9 sustained SVT. Control was achieved in 8 patients with SVT and in 16 with AF without recurrence during a mean follow-up period of 13 months. An additional 41 patients had recurrent VT. In 19 whose symptoms consisted of dizziness or light-headedness without syncope or clinically apparent hemodynamic compromise, treatment was limited to amiodarone. Of these, 14 responded (74%) and have been free of arrhythmia during an average follow-up of 13 months. In 22 patients who had either syncope or life-threatening hemodynamic impairment, amiodarone was added to those agents that had only partially suppressed advanced grades of VPC. Fourteen (64%) of these 22 patients have remained free of recurrent ventricular arrhythmia during an average follow-up of 12 months. After drug loading, maintenance therapy consisted of a daily dose of 200–600 mg. Only mild side effects were encountered in the 17 patients (24%) showing any untoward responses. This experience confirms that oral amiodarone is an effective and safely applied agent against recurrent refractory atrial tachyarrhythmias and sustained intractable VT with moderate symptoms. Although amiodarone is also efficacious in refractory sustained life-threatening ventricular tachyarrhythmia, its use in this condition is made difficult by an insufficiency of information about the pharmacokinetics of the drug.

Nademanee and associates[20] from Los Angeles, California, evaluated the efficacy of amiodarone and determined its dose-response relationships in suppressing VPC, VT, and VF in patients with life-threatening ventricular tachyarrhythmias unresponsive to conventional antiarrhythmic therapy. The antiarrhythmic effects and the dose-response relations of amiodarone, 600–1,200 mg daily, were studied in 22 patients with recurrent life-threatening symptomatic ventricular tachyarrhythmias refractory to 2 or more conventional antiarrhythmic agents. In all patients, the presence of the arrhythmia was confirmed on ECG and/or 24-hour Holter readings. In 10, one or more episodes of cardiac arrest had been documented by ECG. Two patients died before initiation or stabilization of therapy; the goal of therapy was achieved in all but one patient. Amiodarone abolished all VPC and paroxysmal or sustained episodes of VT in all 19 remaining patients. In the 15 for whom predrug and serial 24-hour Holter recordings could be obtained and analyzed, the total VPC were reduced 90%–98% by amiodarone. After a mean follow-up of 12 months on chronic amiodarone therapy, there were no recurrences of VT or VF and sustained antiarrhythmic response was confirmed by Holter recordings. One patient died suddenly at home despite complete suppression of VPC. Amiodarone prolonged the PR interval by +17% and the QT_c interval by +23% without affecting QRS duration. Side effects attributable to amiodarone were gastrointestinal discomfort, halo vision, proximal muscle weakness, transient elevations of hepatic enzymes, and skin photosensitivity, all reversible by reduction of dosage to a level that did not compromise antiarrhythmic efficacy. Amiodarone did not aggravate CHF, even in patients with low LV EF. Thus, amiodarone is an extremely potent and safe agent for the prophylactic control of life-threatening VT.

Heger and associates[21] from Indianapolis, Indiana, evaluated the effects of amiodarone in 45 patients with recurrent VT or VF. At a mean follow-up time of 13 ± 9 months (range, 3–36), amiodarone was successful in 9 of 16 patients with recurrent VF and in 21 of 29 with recurrent VT. During amiodarone therapy, VT could be induced in 18 of 19 patients in whom it had been induced before therapy, but only 6 of these 19 had spontaneous recurrence of VT during follow-up. Side effects included corneal microdeposits, hyperthyroidism, nausea, and symptomatic bradycardia. Pulmonary fibrosis occurred in 3 patients. Doses up to 2000 mg a day did not produce cardiac toxicity, but neurologic side effects precluded long-term therapy at this dose. The authors concluded that amiodarone is effective for long-term therapy of recurrent VT, that induction of arrhythmia during therapy does not always predict efficacy, and that side effects are frequent but do not usually limit therapy. Indeed, cardiovascular toxicity from long-term oral amiodarone therapy appears to be minimal. Hemodynamic studies indicate that amiodarone has mild negative inotropic effects, if any, but acts as a coronary and peripheral vasodilator. In none of the patients studied by Heger and associates did amiodarone appear to exacerbate CHF. The drug also increased the rate of spontaneous sinus node discharge in 2 patients with marked sinus bradycardia and, except for 1 patient in whom a tachycardia-dependent right BBB developed, no patient had disturbances in AV conduction.

Hamer and associates[22] from Los Angeles, California, gave oral amiodarone over several months to 9 patients with life-threatening ventricular arrhythmias. Sustained VT was induced during programmed stimulation in 7 of the 9 patients before amiodarone therapy. Despite an excellent clinical response to the drug over a period of 10–24 months (mean, 15 months), sustained VT could still be initiated in 7 patients after 7–20 weeks of therapy, with multiform VT induced in several patients both before and after amiodarone. After amiodarone therapy, the induced VT was often slower, with an increased QRS width and prolonged RV refractory periods. Repeated ambulatory ECG monitoring in 6 patients showed a reduction in the frequency and complexity of spontaneous ventricular arrhythmias, but there was no consistent effect on the prematurity of the ventricular complexes. The reason for the disparity in some patients between the effects of amiodarone on the electrical initiation of VT and its clinical recurrence requires clarification, but the findings suggest that the clinical efficacy of amiodarone in patients with ventricular tachyarrhythmia may not be reliably predicted by electrophysiologic studies. This clinical investigation was based on only 9 patients, the Holter recordings were not standardized, amiodarone blood levels could not be measured, the timing of the electrophysiologic studies was random, and the doses of amiodarone were nonstandardized and generally low. Nademanee et al[20] took these factors into account. Nevertheless, the disparity between the effects of amiodarone on electrical stimulation and on clinical and Holter recordings is of paramount importance.

Treatment with flecainide

Flecainide acetate is a new antiarrhythmic compound that has had favorable pharmacologic effects in animals. Results of electrophysiologic testing place flecainide in antiarrhythmic class I (agents that have electrophysiologic effects similar to those of quinidine or procainamide). Flecainide shows a wide spectrum of antiarrhythmic action, a high degree of effectiveness, and greater potency than do standard antiarrhythmics. Anderson and associates[23] from Ann Arbor, Michigan, assessed the antiarrhythmic efficacy and safety of oral flecainide acetate in 11 patients with chronic frequent VPC (>600/12 h), and the effects were compared with those in 13 similar patients given a placebo. Of 10 patients completing a trial of different doses, 9 responded completely with a mean VPC suppression of 98% (Fig. 3-3). Repetitive VPC were eliminated. The mean effective dose was 189 mg/day and the effective plasma concentration before administration of the next dose averaged 635 ng/ml. Flecainide continued to be effective and well tolerated at the end of a 2-week outpatient trial, and the 9 complete responders maintained an average VPC suppression of 95%. P-R and QRS intervals were mildly prolonged. The echo EF was unchanged during treatment. The elimination half-life was long—19 ± 4 hours. Thus, flecainide appears to be a

Fig. 3-3. Response to flecainide. Frequency of VPC in 10 treated patients is plotted against study periods. Note change on ordinate scale occurring at 3,000 VPC. PL denotes average of frequencies on both days of placebo-control period; FLEC-DR, frequency at end of inpatient-treatment (flecainide dose-ranging) period (part I); PW, frequency on last day of placebo washout period; FLEC-7d and FLEC-14d, frequencies on 7th and 14th days of outpatient-treatment period (part II), respectively. Reproduced with permission from Anderson et al.[23]

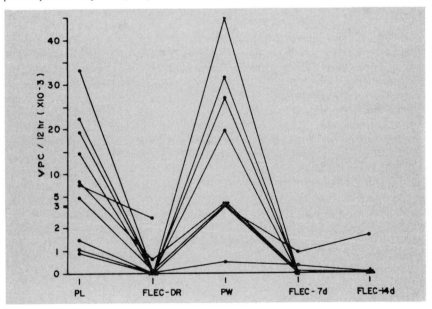

highly effective and well-tolerated antiarrhythmic agent with favorable pharmacokinetics.

Flecainide acetate is one of the few antiarrhythmic drugs that substantially delays myocardial repolarization in tissue preparations. The potential clinical benefit of this mechanism stimulated Olsson and Edvardsson[24] from Göteborg, Sweden, to examine the acute effects of flecainide on intraventricular conduction and repolarization in humans. Three normals and 6 patients were studied before and after an intravenous dose of 2 mg/kg. The study determined ventricular effective refractory period (VERP) and recorded monophasic action potentials (MAP) from the right ventricle during induction of VPC with coupling intervals of VERP $+1$, $+30$, $+40$, and $+50$ ms. Flecainide induced significant prolongations of MAP ($+9.6\%$) and VERP ($+9.8\%$) during regular pacing and delayed intraventricular conduction time ($+17\%$). The MAP of the earliest inducible VPC was even more markedly prolonged ($+19\%$) and, at coupling intervals 30–50 ms longer than VERP, considerable prolongation remained ($+14\%$). In addition, this clinical investigation illustrates the utility of the MAP ventricular recording method, combined with programmed ventricular stimulation, in demonstrating clinical electrophysiologic properties directly comparable with those of microelectrode investigations.

Treatment with encainide

Encainide is a new antiarrhythmic drug used primarily for treatment of ventricular tachyarrhythmias. The agent is unusually effective for suppression of chronic ventricular ectopic activity and is useful for treating patients who have recurrent sustained VT. Although encainide has a short half-life (approximately 3 hours), it can often be administered every 6–8 hours because of a high therapeutic index and the presence of active metabolites with a longer elimination half-life. In microelectrode studies of canine Purkinje cells, encainide markedly depressed the rate of rise of phase 0 of the action potential, similar to other type I antiarrhythmic agents. However, unlike quinidine and procainamide, it does not alter the effective refractory period, and minimally shortens action potential duration. In anesthetized dogs and in humans, intravenous encainide prolongs HV conduction time and QRS duration, but does not significantly alter ventricular refractory periods or Q-T interval. During chronic oral therapy, the P-R and QRS durations and the ventricular refractory period are significantly prolonged and the Q-T interval is unchanged or is slightly prolonged. Winkle and associates[25] from Stanford, California, treated 11 patients with encainide and the agent appeared to cause or exacerbate malignant ventricular arrhythmias. The most common type of arrhythmia associated with encainide toxicity was polymorphic VT resulting in cardiac arrest. In contrast to drug-induced arrhythmias commonly encountered with quinidine and other type I antiarrhythmic drugs, encainide-induced rhythm was not associated with marked Q-T prolongation, was not necessarily initiated by R-on-T VPC, and usually did not end spontaneously. Two patients could not be resuscitated from the rhythm, and several others required prolonged or multiple resuscitations. The risk of encainide-induced ventricular tachyarrhythmias was 11% in 90 patients receiving the drug for recurrent sustained VT and/or VF and 2% in 47 patients receiving the drug for chronic complex ventricular ectopic activity. Encainide-induced arrhythmias occurred 17–48 h (mean, 30) after the start of chronic oral maintenance doses or after dose increases, or 1–2 h after single large doses. Patients experiencing this adverse effect could not be distinguished from those who did not on the basis of encainide dose, degree of QRS widening, or clinical status. The authors recommend that patients with a history of sustained VT or VF have encainide therapy started only in a hospital setting with continuous ECG monitoring and capabilities for cardiopulmonary resuscitation. Dosage should not be changed more often than every 48 hours, and patients should not be discharged from the hospital until they have been on a stable dose of encainide for a minimum of 48 hours.

Treatment with lidocaine

In common with many antiarrhythmic drugs, lidocaine has a low therapeutic index and variable pharmacokinetics. Knowledge of pharmacokinetics can be of great value in designing regimens to achieve an effect rapidly, yet safely, and to maintain that effect throughout the period of treatment. Early clinical experience has shown that major lidocaine toxicity was due to the rapid intravenous administration of large doses, thus precluding the use of a single loading dose. This realization led to the development of regimens, based on sound kinetic principles, that allowed loading over a period of 20–30 minutes. Two alternative methods have been advocated: 1) a series of injections, or 2) a rapid infusion. Although both of these approaches have been used, there has been no formal comparison of their relative merits. It is clear, however, that with the rapid infusion method, it takes a finite time to reach therapeutic concentrations. It has, therefore, been suggested that the optimal regimen for lidocaine administration should involve a priming injection followed by a rapid loading infusion and then a maintenance infusion. Stargel and associates[26] from Durham, North Carolina compared the theoretically optimal regimen (priming dose-rapid infusion loading-maintenance infusion) with a priming dose-triple injection loading-maintenance infusion regimen.

A rapid infusion regimen for lidocaine loading (150 mg infused over 18 minutes following a 75 mg priming injection) was evaluated in 12 patients, in comparison with a multiple injection loading method evaluated in 6 patients that involved three 50 mg injections over 18 minutes following a 75 mg priming dose. Both loading regimens were followed by a maintenance infusion of 2 mg/min. The multiple injection method produced wide variations in lidocaine concentrations, as compared with the rapid infusion method. Some evidence of lidocaine toxicity (drowsiness, tinnitus) was seen in 13 of the 18 patients after the priming injection. During multiple injection loading, all 6 patients experienced side effects (drowsiness, tinnitus, dysarthria, or paresthesias). Only 1 of 12 patients experienced a side effect (drowsiness) during rapid infusion loading. The difference in incidence of adverse reactions was significantly greater with the multiple injection regimen, but was not associated with measurably greater drug levels.

Bretylium -vs- lidocaine in out-of-hospital ventricular fibrillation

Haynes and associates[27] from Seattle, Washington, compared bretylium tosylate and lidocaine hydrochloride as initial drug therapy in 146 victims of out-of-hospital VF in a randomized blinded trial. An organized rhythm was achieved in 89% and 93% and a stable perfusing rhythm in 58% and 60% of patients receiving bretylium and lidocaine, respectively. After initiation of advanced life support, an organized rhythm was first established after mean periods of 10.4 minutes and 10.6 minutes in the 2 respective groups, requiring an average of 2.8 defibrillatory shocks in those who received bretylium and of 2.4 in the lidocaine-treated patients. Comparable numbers of patients were discharged from the hospital: 34% of those given bretylium and 26% of the patients whose initial therapy was lidocaine. No instance of chemical defibrillation was observed with either drug. Thus, bretylium afforded neither significant advantage nor disadvantage, as compared with lidocaine, in the initial management of VF.

Treatment with automatic ventricular defibrillator

Successful clinical application of an automatic ventricular defibrillator was first reported in 1980. This fully implantable device possesses the capability of continuously monitoring cardiac rhythm, recognizing VF and VT characterized by a sinusoidal waveform, and delivering corrective defibrillatory discharges when indicated. The principal goal of the automatic implanted defibrillator is to protect high-risk patients from sudden cardiac death by providing them with a self-contained diagnostic-therapeutic system able to correct malignant ventricular tachyarrhythmias without medical personnel or additional equipment. The total clinical experience to date of 16 patients treated with the implanted automatic defibrillator was reviewed by Mirowski and associates[28] from Baltimore, Maryland. The patients considered potential hosts for the implant had to have survived at least 2 episodes of cardiac arrest (not associated with AMI), with VF or sinusoidal VT documented at least once. One such arrest must have occurred despite prophylactic medical treatment, that was presumably otherwise effective, as judged by the suppression of oral complex ventricular tachyarrhythmias present and/or by simultaneous chronic administration of 2 antiarrhythmic agents resulting in satisfactory, usually salutary, blood levels of these drugs.

During a 1-year period (1980–1981), 12 men and 4 women underwent implantation of the automatic defibrillator; their ages at the time of surgery ranged from 16–74 years (mean, 51). The underlying heart abnormality was CAD in 11 patients and nonischemic cardiomyopathy in 5 (dilated in 2, hypertrophic in 2, and sarcoidosis in 1). Three patients had previous CABG, 1 had ventricular aneurysmectomy, 1 had MVR, 1 had septal myectomy, and 3 had had conventional pacemakers implanted. The average follow-up was 6 months, with the longest being 14 months. Twenty-five episodes of malignant arrhythmias were documented in the hospital following implantation; 8 episodes occurred spontaneously, whereas 17 were induced during electrophysiologic studies. All spontaneous arrhythmias and 14 of 17 induced arrhythmias were correctly identified and converted to sinus rhythm by a single 25-Joule pulse. After nearly 100 defibrillator pulse generator implant-months accumulated to date, no evidence exists of random component failure, premature battery depletion, malfunctioning capacitors, loss of hermeticity, or case fracture. There have been 3 late deaths. Two patients died because of pulmonary edema and 1 patient had cardiac asystole. When removed, the defibrillator devices were found to be operating properly and necropsy did not disclose myocardial damage that could be attributed to the defibrillator.

The clinical efficacy and relative safety of the automatic defibrillator demonstrated to date requires further validation by additional patient studies, with careful attention paid to any potential untoward events related to the device itself. Judging from the limited clinical experience presented, however, the current results are quite promising. Although the overall impact of this innovative approach to the prevention of sudden cardiac death is difficult to estimate at present, the range of available options for effective treatment of refractory malignant ventricular arrhythmias has been markedly extended by the development of this new modality.

Watkins and associates[29] from Baltimore, Maryland, reported the operative features of inserting the automatic implantable defibrillator in 19 patients. Apical ventricular and superior vena caval defibrillating electrodes were implanted via a left lateral thoracotomy if the patient had had previous cardiac surgery or via a median sternotomy if the patient had not. There were no operative deaths or significant surgical morbidity.

Noncoronary bypass operations for ventricular tachycardia

Guiraudon and associates[30] from Paris and Ivry, France, operated on 23 patients with resistant VT not related to CAD. Surgical treatment was guided by intraoperative ventricular mapping. The patients were grouped according to anatomic findings: I, 13 patients with abnormalities of the right ventricle; II, 3 patients with LV aneurysm and normal coronary arteries; III, 2 patients with non-obstructive cardiomyopathy and IV, 5 patients with normal hearts. Surgical indication was the failure of medical treatment or the presence of troublesome side effects of antiarrhythmic therapy. VT had to be inducible by an appropriate triggering technique; when it was not, only patients with a semi-constant VT were operated on.

The surgical procedure consisted of median sternotomy, epicardial mapping in sinus rhythm, and during VT, with cardiopulmonary bypass. Epicardial mapping was done with a hand-held exploring electrode according to an 85-point grid. Operative therapy consisted of ventriculotomy or cryosurgery at the site of origin of VT or exclusion, resection, or undermining of arrhythmogenic areas where delayed potentials were observed. Four patients died during the perioperative period, 2 from low cardiac output, 1 from intractable SVT, and 1 from hemorrhage. Three died later: 1 from gastrointestinal bleeding and 2 from CHF. VT recurred immediately after operation in 4 patients, 3 of whom died during the perioperative period. VT recurred late in 4 patients, 2 of whom were well controlled by drugs. Those patients in whom the site of VT was either right or left ventricle were all successfully treated.

Of the 5 patients in whom the arrhythmic focus was ventricular septum, only 2 were successfully treated. The authors concluded that free wall tachycardias can be successfully managed by this technique, but that arrhythmias arising from the septum need another type of operative treatment.

Coronary artery bypass grafting (CABG) for exercise-induced ventricular tachycardia

The effects of CABG in treadmill stress test-induced VT (≥ 3 consecutive VPC) were analyzed in 9 men operated on by Codini and associates[31] from Chicago, Illinois. Two had had a previous AMI that healed, all 9 had normal (>0.40) LV EF, 3 had 2-vessel disease, and 7 had 3-vessel disease. The preoperative ventricular arrhythmias were brief (3–6 consecutive VPC), and were self-terminating in 6. Two patients had multiple episodes of VT and 1 had ventricular flutter with cardiopulmonary resuscitation. Three patients received 2 grafts, and 6 received three grafts. None had perioperative AMI. All patients were alive and 8 were asymptomatic a mean of 24 months after CABG. Exercise testing postoperatively disclosed isolated VPC in 2 patients and couplets in 1. The double product (*systemic blood pressure* × *heart rate*/100) was significantly higher postoperatively during exercise testing. Thus, among patients with CAD having exercise-induced VT, CABG may improve exercise capacity and suppress the arrhythmia.

Horowitz and associates[32] from Philadelphia, Pennsylvania, provide an excellent review of surgical management of patients with ventricular arrhythmias from CAD.

Ventricular tachyarrhythmias on ambulatory ECG recording after AMI

During the past decade a number of studies have examined the role of ventricular ectopic activity in identifying CAD patients at high risk of subsequent cardiac events. In general, these investigations have shown a correlation between these asymptomatic arrhythmias and subsequent untoward events. Direct comparison of studies from different centers is complicated by differences in duration of ECG monitoring and in definitions of complex ventricular ectopic activity (VEA). Although some studies have commented on the general relationship between the frequency of ectopic beats and the occurrence of complex forms, there have been few systematic studies of this relationship and there is little or no information about the occurrence of complex forms in patients with infrequent VEA. No studies performed in the late hospital or early discharge phase following AMI have used ambulatory ECG recordings beyond 24-hour duration. Given the marked variability of VPC frequency and complexity in patients with chronic frequent VPC taking part in clinical antiarrhythmic drug trials, it is important to consider the day-to-day variability of VPC in the late post-AMI period. Winkle and associates[33] from Stanford, California examined VEA occurring in 57 ambulatory patients during 3 consecutive 24-hour ambulatory ECG recordings performed in the pre-discharge phase of acute AMI (approximately 8–11 days post-AMI). There was considerable additional detection of each type of complex VPC with recordings beyond 24 hours. Multiform, R-on-T, pairs, and bigeminy were often first detected from 24–48 hours, and 5 of 12 patients with VT had this rhythm detected only after 48 hours of monitoring. Complex forms were detected during short recording periods primarily in patients who had complex forms present during a large number of hours of the 72-hour recording session. The occurrence of each type of complex ectopic beat was strongly related to VPC frequency, and some type of complex form was seen in virtually all 24-hour recordings with more than 100 VPC. Of the 24-hour recordings with infrequent VPC (2–10/24 h), 65% also showed complex forms. The day-to-day reproducibility of VPC frequency and complexity was reasonable, but was largely accounted for by the fact that most recordings were free of frequent VPC and a given type of complex VPC. These data suggest that for longer ECG recording periods, the frequency of occurrence of complex forms, rather than their simple presence or absence, may be important for identifying high-risk CAD subgroups post-AMI.

DEFIBRILLATION AND CARDIOVERSION

Influence of paddle size and contact pressure, body weight, chest size, and paddle-electrode location on success rates

Successful defibrillation depends on the delivery of adequate electrical current to the heart; 1 of the major determinants of current flow is transthoracic resistance (TTR). To study the factors influencing TTR, Kerber and associates[34] from Iowa City, Iowa, collected data prospectively from 44 patients undergoing emergency defibrillation. Shocks of 94–450 J delivered energy were administered from specially calibrated Datascope defibrillators that displayed peak current flow, thereby permitting determination of TTR. Shocks were applied from standard (8.5 cm diameter) or large (13 cm) paddles placed anteriorly and laterally. First-shock TTR ranged from 15–143 Ω. There was a weak correlation between TTR and body weight ($r = 0.45$, $p < 0.05$) and a stronger correlation between TTR and chest width ($r = 0.80$, $p < 0.01$). Of 23 patients who were shocked with standard 8.5-cm paddles, the mean TTR was 67 ± 36 Ω, whereas of 21 patients shocked with paddle pairs of which at least 1 was large (13 cm), the TTR was 21% lower (53 ± 24 Ω) ($p = 0.05$). Ten patients received first and second shocks at the same energy level; TTR declined only 8% (from 52 ± 19 Ω to 48 ± 16 Ω) ($p < 0.01$). In closed-chest dogs, shocks were administered by use of a spring apparatus that regulated paddle contact pressure against the thorax. Firmer contact pressure caused TTR to decrease 25%, (from 48 ± 22 Ω to 36 ± 17 Ω) ($p < 0.01$). Thus, human TTR varies widely and is related most closely to chest size. TTR declines only slightly with a second shock at the same energy level. More substantial reductions in TTR and increases in current flow can be achieved by using large paddles and by increasing paddle contact pressure.

Kerber and associates[35] also compared the success rates and energy requirements of 2 electrode-paddle positions (anteroposterior -vs- anterolateral) and different paddle sizes in the elective cardioversion of atrial arrhythmias in 173 patients: 111 with AF and 62 with atrial flutter. The anterolateral paddles used were either both standard size (8.5 cm diameter) or one large (13 cm diameter) anterior paddle with 1 standard size lateral paddle. The anteroposterior paddles used were either a standard size or a 13 cm anterior paddle and a 12 cm posterior paddle. Overall cardioversion success rates for either paddle position were similar (>90%). Use of the larger paddles did not significantly reduce energy requirements for cardioversion of either arrhythmia. Thus, the anterolateral paddles are as effective as anteroposterior paddles for the elective cardioversion of atrial arrhythmias, and there is no demonstrable advantage to using paddles that are larger than the standard size in either position.

CARDIOPULMONARY RESUSCITATION

Cardiac valve motion: its implications regarding the mechanism of blood flow

Questions still exist regarding the actual mechanism of forward blood flow during cardiopulmonary resuscitation (CPR) as conventionally applied. The central issue in this controversy is whether forward blood flow occurs primarily as a result of direct mechanical compression of the heart between the sternum and vertebral bodies or whether the left side of the heart, in particular, is acting passively as a conduit for blood forced out of the lungs along a pressure gradient primarily generated by increasing intrathoracic pressure. The latter theory of blood flow in CPR (the "chest-pump" theory) has recently received considerable physiologic support. Fundamental to this thesis is the demonstration of cardiac valve motion during conventional external chest compression. To demonstrate these changes directly, Werner and associates[36] from Seattle, Washington, performed 2-D echo during CPR by manual external chest compression in 5 patients to assess valve motion. The mitral valve remained open throughout the entire compression-release cycle of CPR. The aortic valve opened during the compression phase of CPR and closed during the release phase. The pulmonic valve moved toward the closed position during the compression phase and the valve leaflets opened during release. Tricuspid valve leaflets were never completely apposed, even during maximum chest compression, and were widely open during release. LV dimensions did not change appreciably during CPR. These findings support the theory that forward blood flow during CPR depends on a generalized increase in intrathoracic pressure and not on direct compression of the heart itself. The left side of the heart appears to act as a conduit for passage of blood, and mitral valve closure is not necessary for forward blood flow during CPR.

CONDUCTION DISTURBANCES

Sinoatrial entrance block

Normally, antegrade cardiac impulse conduction at the AV level in humans proceeds through the AV node and then spreads through the His-Purkinje system; retrograde impulse conduction may or may not be present. The absence of ventriculoatrial (VA) conduction does not indicate abnormal AV nodal function, and is not necessarily associated with prolongation of the A-H interval. Normal impulse conduction at the sinoatrial (SA) level in humans proceeds antegrade from the SA node to the atrium via the perinodal fibers of the SA junction; little is known, however, about retrograde atrio-sinus conduction in humans. In the past decade, the premature atrial stimulus (PAS) method for determining sinoatrial conduction time (SACT) has been developed. Although the PAS technique provides a means to estimate total SACT and to determine the presence of sinoatrial entrance block (SAEB) (the absence of retrograde atrio-sinus conduction), SACT cannot be estimated by the PAS technique when SA entrance block is present. Therefore, nothing has been known about antegrade SA conduction in patients with SAEB.

When AV conduction is normal, the absence of VA conduction is not abnormal; analogous information about retrograde sinoatrial conduction is not available. Although the PAS technique can demonstrate the presence of SAEB, both its prevalence and its relationship to antegrade SA conduction are unknown. Reiffel and associates[37] from New York City determined the incidence of SAEB by using PAS in 59 patients with known or suspected arrhythmias or conduction defects to be 7%. Using catheter-recorded sinus node electrograms (SNE), they measured SACT directly in 3 patients with SAEB. Antegrade SACT was normal in 2 and prolonged in 1. Only the latter had sinus node dysfunction recognized by ECG, conventional sinus node testing, or both. This study concluded that SAEB occurs infrequently, may occur when antegrade SACT is normal, is probably analogous to behavior at the AV node, and should not be used as an indicator of sick sinus syndrome.

Sinoatrial disease in persons under age 25 years

The etiology of sinus node dysfunction occurring without other forms of cardiac disease (sinoatrial disease) is often obscure. Sinoatrial disease is more common in the elderly than in the young, but little is known of its etiology at any age. Few young patients with sinoatrial disease have been studied. Mackintosh[38] from Cambridge, England, surveyed 3 cardiac centers and found 9 patients 25 years of age with sinus node dysfunction in the absence of other forms of heart disease. All were males and 7 were above the 90th percentile for height. Ambulatory monitoring was performed on all the first-degree relatives of 6 of the 9 patients, and 3 families showed conduction system disturbances in the form of sinoatrial disorders or delayed AV conduction. Thus, a genetic factor may be involved in the etiology of sinoatrial disease in persons under age 25 years.

Acquired left or right bundle-branch block (Framingham and Royal Canadian Air Force studies)

It has long been held that complete right BBB is more likely to occur in persons free from other clinically apparent cardiovascular disease and is less likely to be associated with advanced cardiovascular abnormalities than is complete left BBB. This teaching is derived largely from studies of BBB in hospitalized patients and, to a lesser extent, from studies of community-based and young military populations. The available studies of this subject in community-based populations concern relatively small numbers of cases in short duration of follow-up. Accordingly, Schneider and associates[39] from Boston and Framingham, Massachusetts, analyzed cardiovascular abnormalities in 55 persons who acquired left BBB and in 70 persons who acquired right BBB during an 18-year follow-up of the Framingham Study cohort. Those with left and right BBB did not differ from each other in the overall prevalence of systemic hypertension, clinical CAD, or diabetes mellitus (Fig. 3-4). In men,

Fig. 3-4. Prevalence of cardiovascular abnormalities during entire period of follow-up. LBBB = left bundle-branch block. RBBB = right bundle-branch block.

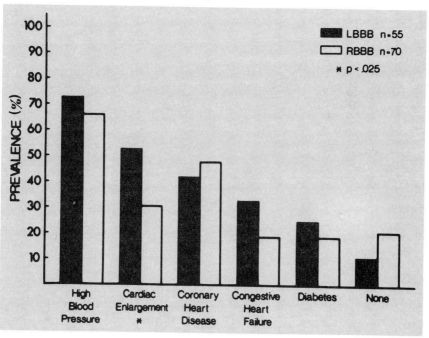

but not in women, left BBB was associated with a significantly greater prevalence of cardiac enlargement and CHF than was right BBB. The trends suggesting a higher mortality rate from cardiovascular disease in those with left BBB than in those with right BBB were more apparent in men than in women (Fig. 3-5). Thus, in the general adult population, men who acquire left BBB are more likely to have or to subsequently acquire advanced cardiovascular abnormalities than are men who acquire right BBB. In women, however, the clinical correlates of the 2 conduction abnormalities are similar.

Rabkin and associates[40] from Manitoba, Canada, examined the characteristics, long-term follow-up, and prognosis of right BBB detected on a routine ECG in men without apparent heart disease. The cohort of this study consisted of 3,983 men who, during World War II, were pilots, pilots in training at the Royal Canadian Air Force, or pilots licensed by the Department of Transport and all had had a routine ECG in addition to the regular medical examination. After release from the service, some continued to fly, but the majority found different occupations in all strata of society. The examination closest to June 30, 1948, was selected as the entry examination. The mean age of the cohort at that examination was 31 years. Medical history, physical examination, and ECG provided evidence that all were without clinical manifestations of CAD at entry. Since then, all were followed by annual mail contact, with physical examination and an ECG at intervals of, at first, 5 years and, later, 3 years. The observation period for the present report was July 1, 1948–June 30, 1977, an average follow-up of 29 years. Annual contact was lost in only 1 living patient. During the 29-year period, right BBB was observed in 59 men with a mean age of 44 ± 2 years. Because marked right or left axis deviation may identify cases with concomitant involvement of the left bundle-branch system, subsets of frontal plane QRS (A QRS) were exam-

Fig. 3-5. Cumulative cardiovascular disease mortality rates after onset of BBB in men-vs-women.

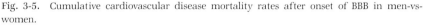

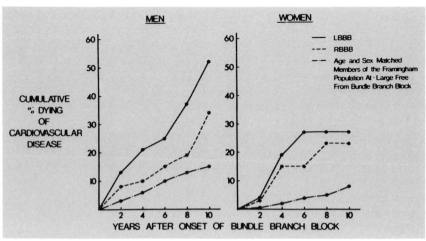

ined. Comparisons were made with groups of similar aged persons free of right BBB. The patients with right BBB were observed for 936 person-years (mean, 16 ± 1.6 years/patient); they showed no excess CAD incidence, no progression to advanced AV block (second- or third-degree), and no sudden deaths. Right BBB was associated with a greater proportion of both right axis and marked left axis deviation, as compared with those of the same age without this conduction disturbance. Thus, in apparently healthy men, right BBB has no adverse long-term prognosis regardless of frontal plane QRS axis.

Additional conduction disorders in left BBB

Barrett and associates[41] from Los Angeles, California, studied 30 patients with left BBB by intracardiac stimulation techniques and found additional conduction disorders in 29 of them: of sinus node function (prolonged maximum sinus node recovery time [corrected] in 23%, prolonged sinoatrial conduction time in 3 of 8 patients), of AV node function (prolonged A-H interval in 33%, and prolonged effective and functional refractory periods in 37% and 74%, respectively), of "His bundle to right bundle branch" conduction (prolonged HV interval in 53%), and of ventriculoatrial conduction (absent in 62%). It was postulated that at least half of the cases with left BBB were incomplete, even though the duration of the QRS complex exceeded 120 ms, because of (further) leftward deviation of the mean frontal QRS axis with sufficiently premature atrial extrastimuli. Block may be complete or incomplete in left BBB with left axis deviation $\geq -30°$ on the standard ECG.

Hemodynamic and angiographic observations in left BBB

Dabizzi and associates[42] from Florence and Legnano, Italy, carried out coronary and LV angiography and hemodynamic studies in 34 patients with CAD and left BBB, and the results were compared with findings in 98 patients with CAD without conduction disturbances. Left axis deviation, common in patients with CAD and left BBB, had no prognostic hemodynamic significance. Left BBB associated with CAD did not imply more severe or more extensive coronary narrowing, although it disclosed a higher frequency of severe narrowing of the LM coronary artery and more severe myocardial dysfunction, with asynergy especially involving the LV anterior wall (Fig. 3-6).

RNA observations in left BBB

Swiryn and associates[43] from Chicago, Illinois, carried out phase analyses of biventricular RNA gated studies in 7 patients with normal conduction and in 8 patients with left BBB, all without significant abnormalities of hemodynamics or LV wall motion. The first Fourier harmonic of time-activity variation in each pixel was computed and displayed as an amplitude image, a phase image, and a phase-distribution histogram. In addition, automatically determined areas of earliest and latest phase for each ventricle were examined and compared. Qualitative analysis revealed relatively uniform

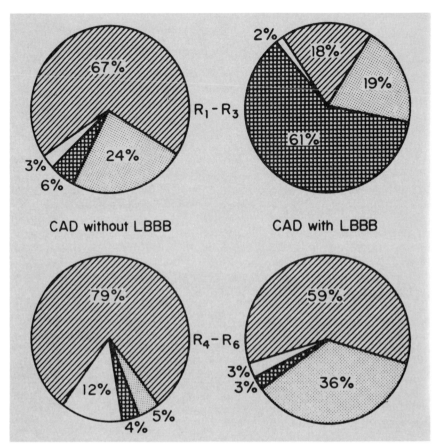

Fig. 3-6. LV wall motion. Relationship between patients with CAD and LBBB and patients with CAD without conduction defects ($p < 0.01$). R_1–R_3 = anterior areas. R_4–R_6 = inferior areas ■ = Normals; ▤ = hypokinesis; ⊞ = akinesis; □ = dyskinesis. Reproduced with permission from Dabizzi et al.[42]

distribution of phase across both ventricles in patients with normal conduction, but markedly delayed phase in the LV of patients with left BBB. In addition, the location within the ventricles of areas of earliest and latest phase was somewhat different for the 2 groups, the most prominent finding being an area of earliest LV phase along the ventricular septum in 7 of 8 patients with left BBB, but in none with normal conduction. Quantitatively, relative measures of mean, early, and late phase calculated by subtracting respective RV from LV values of phase to give ΔMean, ΔEarly, and ΔLate showed marked LV phase delay in left BBB patients. Values of these parameters (normal conduction -vs- left BBB) were ΔMean ($-5°$ -vs- $+36°$), ΔEarly ($-2°$ -vs- $+37°$), and ΔLate ($-7°$ -vs- $+35°$). Thus, phase analysis of ventricular RNA gated studies demonstrated marked differences in both location and timing of LV events in left BBB patients, as compared with normal conduction patients. This noninvasive radionuclide method yields both qualitative and quantitative data reflecting the mechanical correlates of abnormal ventricular activation.

Chronic second degree AV nodal block: natural history

Second-degree AV nodal block is most often recognized in the acute clinical setting, complicating AMI (posterior wall), digitalis intoxication, acute myocarditis, or recovery after open heart operations. In these circumstances, second-degree AV nodal block is usually reversible with time, and usually plays no major role in determining clinical outcome. *Chronic* second-degree AV nodal block also is seen in a variety of circumstances and it, too, is generally considered a benign conduction defect. Few systematic studies on the chronic form of second-degree AV block have been reported. To fill this void, Strasberg and associates[44] from Chicago, Illinois, described their experience with 56 patients with documented chronic second-degree AV block proximal to the His [H] in 46 (82%) men and 10 (18%) women aged 18−87 years. Nineteen patients (34%) had no organic heart disease (including 7 trained athletes) and 37 (66%) did. ECG in all patients demonstrated episodes of type I second-degree block; 5 patients also had periods of 2:1 block. Prospective follow-up of patients with no organic heart disease (157−2,280 days, mean, 1,395 ± 636 days) revealed 1 patient with clear indication for permanent pacing because of bradyarrhythmic symptoms (permanently placed on day 220 of follow-up). Two patients died nonsuddenly. In patients with organic heart disease (prospective follow-up of 60−2,950 days, mean, 1,347 ± 825 days), pacemakers were implanted in 10 patients, primarily for treatment of CHF in 8 and of syncope in 2. Sixteen patients died: 3 suddenly, 7 with CHF, 2 of AMI, and 4 of causes unrelated to cardiac disease. Thus, chronic second-degree AV nodal block has a relatively benign course in patients without organic heart disease. In patients with organic heart disease, the prognosis is related to the severity of the underlying heart condition.

Congenital complete heart block: natural history

Esscher[45] from Uppsala, Sweden, studied 70 patients aged 16−57 years (mean, 31) with isolated congenital complete heart block (CHB). Of the patients < age 30, 70% were free of symptoms and of those > age 30, 29% were free of symptoms. The CHB was diagnosed before age 1 year in 26 patients. Of the 48 patients followed for 12 years, 44 were without symptoms when the study began in 1965 and 28 were without symptoms in 1977. No reliable indicators of bad prognosis were found.

Predictors of need for pacemakers

Karpawich and associates[46] from Houston, Texas, presented data on 24 children with congenital CHB from intracardiac electrophysiologic studies in 1970−80. These 24 were among 70 children with congenital CHB of 19,785 children evaluated at Texas Children's Hospital for possible heart disease. The 24 children were observed from 1–19 years (mean, 5). Stokes-Adams attacks occurred in 8 (33%), in 2 of them before age 2 years. One died at 4 months after an episode of bradycardia. Congenital cardiac defects co-existed in 6 patients (25%): TGA in 2, atrial septal defect (ASD) in 2, ventricular septal defect (VSD) in 1, and both ASD and VSD in 1. Electrophysiologic studies identified the site of block as the AV node in 19 (79%), the His bundle in 3, and distal conduction system in 1. In 1 with fatal syncope, the site of block could not be identified. Of the other 7 with syncope, block was in the AV node in 6 and the distal conduction system in 1. The QRS duration was normal on surface ECG in the 22 children with block in or above the His bundle. Among the 19 with AV nodal block, the resting ventricular heart rate ranged from 40–80 beats/min (median, 50). In the 3 with intra-His block and QRS duration of 0.08 seconds, the ventricular rate was 40–60 beats/min. Thus, the median heart rate was the same, irrespective of site of block, so it was not a predictor of block site, but it was a predictor of the chance of syncope. In those with syncope, the median rate was 45 beats/min (range, 40–50).

On exercise testing (11 patients), the ventricular rate increased to a median of 183% of resting rate, and there was no difference between those with and without syncope. Three children (1 with syncope) had VPC. Of the other 8 tested, 2 also had syncope, but neither had exercise-induced arrhythmia. A pacemaker was implanted in 6 children because of syncope and in 4 because of CHF. After a 1–10-year follow-up, none of the 10 had recurrence of symptoms after pacemaker insertion, and none had complications attributed to the pacemaker. Thus, the resting heart rate was the best predictor of bradycardia-induced syncope. Localization of the site of block did not affect prognosis. The authors recommend pacemakers for symptoms of Stokes-Adams attacks or for CHF.

Chronic acquired complete heart block: histologic studies

The number of studies correlating electrophysiologic and histologic changes in patients with chronic complete heart block (CHB) is limited. Ohkawa and associates[47] correlated ECG findings and the histology of the AV conduction system in 14 patients with chronic CHB and in 13 patients without chronic complete AV block. Patients with chronic complete AV block were divided into 2 groups, based on the width of the QRS complex. The QRS complexes were narrow (<0.12 second) in 4 patients (group 1) and wide (≥ 0.12 second) in 10 (group 2). In group 1, the main lesion was located in the penetrating portion of the His bundle (His_p) in 1 heart, in the branching portion of the His bundle (His_b) in another, and in the combined regions of His_b and the left bundle branch in 2. Three of 4 patients in group 1 had idiopathic fibrosis of the conduction system and 1 had calcific nodules in the central fibrous body. In group 2, the main lesion was located in His_b in 2 cases, in the combined regions of His_b and the right bundle branch in 1, in the His_b and in the bilateral bundle branches in 2, and in the bilateral bundle branches in 5. All patients in group 2 were of the idiopathic type, except 1 who had calcific AS. In 13 patients without chronic CHB the AV conduction system was histologically normal, except for slight-to-moderate aging changes in the His bundle or the bundle branches. Thus, lesions of the His_b, which is believed to be the "distal His" electrophysiologically, may induce CHB with narrow or wide QRS complexes, depending upon the severity of the lesions in His_b or adjacent bundle branches.

PACEMAKERS

Impact of peer review on implantation of permanent pacemakers

Because of a sharp increase in the number of permanent pacemakers inserted at The Brooklyn Hospital from 1972–1976, a peer review committee was established to monitor subsequent pacemaker implantation. Chokshi and associates[48] of New York City reviewed subsequent pacemaker implantations at their hospital. Total number of initial implants declined from 48 to 22 per year in the 2 years that followed (Fig. 3-7). The number of implantations for sinoatrial bradycardias declined from 50 to 27 and the number of implantations for intraventricular conduction defects declined from 32 to 5 in the 2 years after peer review, as compared with the 2 years before. There was no change in the number of pacemakers implanted for complete or ad-

Fig. 3-7. Trend of permanent pacemaker implantations at The Brooklyn Hospital, 1972–1978, shows progressive increase in number of pacemakers implanted from 1972–1976 and dramatic decline after peer review in 1977. Reproduced with permission from Chokshi.[48]

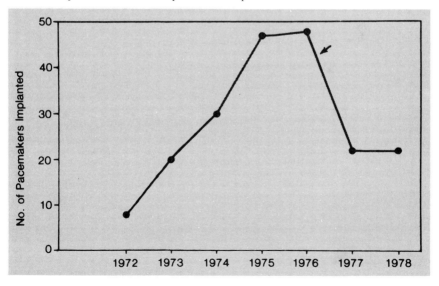

vanced heart block. Almost 10% of patients who received a pacemaker between 1972 and 1976 had other conditions that might have accounted for the events that precipitated the decision to implant a pacemaker. The symptoms for which the pacemaker was implanted persisted in 19% of patients, despite a normally functioning pacemaker system. Patients receiving a permanent pacemaker before peer review had a 17% 1-year and a 43% 3-year mortality. When a more critical patient selection process was instituted, a smaller percentage remained symptomatic (9% -vs- 19%) and 3-year survival rate was improved (86% -vs- 57%). From 1977 through 1978, when permanent pacemaker implantations declined, the number of hospital, medical service, and coronary care unit admissions increased. Thus, peer review can have a substantial impact on permanent pacemaker implantations.

Infections

Choo and associates[49] from Rochester, Minnesota, summarized their experiences in treating 46 patients with infections involving permanent pacing systems. They found that optimal treatment for most patients required removal of the entire infected pacing system.

Prophylactic antibiotics for implantation

Muers and associates[50] from Oxford, England, conducted a prospective trial to assess the value of prophylactic antibiotic treatment in preventing postoperative infection of permanent transvenous pacemaker systems. Of 431 patients, 234 were randomly allocated to treatment and 197 to no treatment. The treated patients received systemic benzylpenicillin and flucloxacillin just before operation and 1 and 6 hours afterwards. Nine primary generator pocket infections occurred without evidence of wound dehiscence or skin erosion: 7 were in the untreated patients and 2 in treated patients. Thus, antibiotic prophylaxis appears to diminish the risk of infection after pacemaker implantation.

Echo features of pacemaker perforation

Gondi and Nanda[51] from Rochester, New York, studied 5 patients with clinically suspected perforation of the RV wall by temporary transvenous pacemakers. Real-time, 2-D echo allowed visualization of the catheter passing through the RV apical wall with the tip located outside the cardiac border in 3 of the 5 patients. In 1 patient, the catheter perforated the AV septum and entered the LV with the tip lodged against the posterior wall. In another patient, the catheter partially penetrated the ventricular septum near the apex. Pericardial effusion was observed in 2 patients, in 1 localized to the site of perforation. No patient had evidence of cardiac tamponade. In 4 patients, the catheters were withdrawn under echo visualization and the catheter tips could be seen moving from the abnormal locations back into the right-heart chambers. Perforation was verified at necropsy in 2 patients, including 1 in whom the catheter was not withdrawn. Thus, real-time, 2-D echo appears to be valuable in diagnosing pacemaker perforation.

Treatment of recurrent tachycardia by programmed stimulation

The initiation and termination of reentry tachycardias by accurately timed electrical stimuli delivered to the heart is a widely used technique for investigation. Kappenberger and Sowton[52] from London, England, applied this technique for long-term clinical control of tachycardias. Eleven patients with recurrent tachycardia refractory to drugs were treated by a pacemaker system that consisted of an implanted QRS-triggered stimulator activated by the application of stimuli to the patient's skin. These skin stimuli were delivered by a small control box carried about in the pocket or handbag and which the patient held in his hands to make contact with the electrode plates during a tachycardia attack. If the heart rate was higher than the preset value on the control box, timed stimuli were delivered to the skin. The tachycardia was stopped by VPC induced during the "termination window," a period that occurred very soon after the refractory period. The skin impulses continued to be delivered until the tachycardia stopped. During >30 months follow-up, about 2,000 episodes were stopped by this pacemaker system. The patients did not feel the skin stimuli and there were few complications.

RELATED TOPICS

Ambulatory ECG: current status

Ambulatory ECG recordings have become an important clinical tool for the diagnosis and management of patients with symptoms suggesting cardiac arrhythmias or with known cardiac rhythm disturbances. One or more forms of long-term ambulatory ECG monitoring are currently available to almost all practicing physicians. Because of the expense of the equipment and considerable technician and physician time required for data reduction and interpretation, these tests are relatively expensive ($150–$250). When used appropriately, however, they can be a cost-effective tool and may prevent hospitalization for continuous ECG recording. To optimize their benefit, the clinician must be familiar with the types of recordings available and the specific clinical situations in which they are likely to yield important information. Their largest proven use is documenting suspected rhythm disturbances in symptomatic patients. Currently, they play a more limited role in the long-term management of patients with arrhythmias, in large part due to our lack of knowledge regarding the benefits of prophylactic therapy for asymptomatic arrhythmias detected on these recordings.

When most clinicians use the term long-term ambulatory ECG recording, what they usually mean is the *continuous* or "Holter" type of ambulatory ECG recorder. The continuous or "Holter" recorders are battery operated and record a continuous ECG signal on magnetic tape for subsequent analysis. Most current recorders permit continuous recording of 2 separate ECG leads for at least 24 hours. These recorders are available in either AM or FM recording modes. They often have timing information recorded on tape and have patient-activated event markers that permit the patient to indicate on the tape those times when specific symptoms occur. The most important positive attribute of continuous recording devices is that all ECG data are retained and are available for subsequent analysis. In contrast, *intermittent* recorders may be activated by the patient when symptoms occur. Since they do not run continuously, they may be worn by the patient for several days before battery depletion occurs. To be of optimal value, patient-activated recording devices should have only a brief delay loop to record the onset of any arrhythmia. These intermittent devices have the shortcoming of not receiving all ECG data and thus there is no way to determine which arrhythmias might have occurred but were not sensed by the patient and recorded by the device. The *transtelephonic monitoring system* has been widely utilized for follow-up of patients with permanently implanted pacemakers, but also has found considerable utility in the diagnosis of arrhythmias. These transtelephonic devices can be kept by the patients for periods of weeks to months.

In recent years, many studies have described the types of arrhythmias that occur on long-term ambulatory ECG recordings in cross-sections of the healthy population and in normal subjects clinically documented to be free of cardiac disease. Sinus tachycardia and sinus arrhythmia are normal occurrences in young children. Detailed studies of young adults indicate that 25%–50% will have occasional atrial or VPC. In middle-aged, apparently healthy subjects, up to 70% may have premature beats; frequent and complex VPC, including short bursts of SVT, VT, or both, may occur in as many as 10%. Although there are few data regarding the long-term prognostic significance of these arrhythmias, most clinicians consider these types of arrhythmias to be relatively benign when they occur in otherwise normal subjects. Such subjects should be told that these rhythm disturbances are probably normal and, in general, therapy should not be initiated.

Monitoring of patients with symptoms that could be due to a cardiac rhythm disturbance represents the most justifiable use of ambulatory ECG recordings. The type of symptom and its frequency of occurrence and duration should indicate the type of ambulatory ECG recording to be utilized. The specific role of ambulatory ECG recordings has been defined for patients with palpitations and with symptoms of presyncope and syncope. In addition, the clinical use of ambulatory ECG recordings has been defined for specific disease states, including the cardiomyopathies, conduction system disease, CAD, denervated states including cardiac transplantation, MVP, evaluation of patients with permanent pacemakers, the pre-excitation syndromes, sinus node dysfunction, and the sleep apnea syndrome.

In the proper application and interpretation of ambulatory ECG monitoring, spontaneous variability in the use of ambulatory recordings to document the suppression of asymptomatic ventricular arrhythmias must be kept in mind. In addition, the use of ambulatory ECG recordings in patients with recurrent sustained tachyarrhythmias remains controversial. The same is true for the use of Holter monitoring for ST-segment changes relative to their implications concerning CAD and the quantification of ST-segment shifts as a prognostic tool for identifying high-risk patients with CAD or for measuring ongoing ischemia in patients with CAD.[53]

Intracardiac electrophysiologic techniques in recurrent syncope of unknown cause

DiMarco and associates[54] from Boston, Massachusetts, evaluated 25 patients with recurrent episodes of syncope, unexplained despite thorough medical and neurologic evaluation, by intracardiac electrophysiologic study with programmed stimulation. Electrophysiologic study yielded a presumptive diagnosis in 17 patients: 9 with rapid VT induced by programmed stimulation, 3 with intra-His conduction delays, 1 with symptomatic atrial flutter, 1 with sick sinus syndrome, and 3 with persistent hypervagotonia manifested as atropine-reversible prolongation of AV nodal refractoriness. Therapy based on these findings provided complete symptomatic relief in 14 and improvement in 1 of these 17 patients during a mean follow-up of 18 ± 10 months. Therapy based on electrophysiologic testing was ineffective in 2 of the 17 patients. Syncope persisted in 4 of the 8 patients in whom electrophysiologic study did not define a probable arrhythmic mechanism. These observations indicate that full electrophysiologic evaluation with programmed stimulation is useful in the diagnosis and therapy of recurrent unexplained syncope.

Relation between Q-T interval and heart rate

The decrease in Q-T interval that occurs with exercise-induced changes in heart rate has long been recognized and has led to the use of formulas that correct the measured Q-T to a basic heart rate. The nonlinear relation first described by Bazett in 1920 has been widely applied to derive this rate-corrected Q-T interval (QT_c). To reevaluate the relationship between the Q-T interval and exercise, Rickards and Norman[55] from London, England, studied 25 patients undergoing a treadmill exercise test, 15 patients undergoing an atrial pacing stress test during cardiac catheterization for evaluation of chest pain without exercise, and 9 patients with complete heart block having ventricular inhibited pacemakers set at 90 beats/min and exercised according to the Bruce protocol. The data for the exercise group indicated that the heart rate–Q-T interval relation could be approximated by a linear regression equation, such that Q-T interval was predicted by Q-T = 522 − (1.87 × heart rate). Thus, a rate change of 100 beats/min would be accompanied by a change in Q-T intervals of approximately 187 milliseconds (ms). With atrial pacing without exercise, the Q-T interval decreased with increasing rates, the slope of the rate–Q-T relation was much flatter [Q-T = 899 − (0.66 × heart rate)]. Thus, an increase of 100 beats/min caused by atrial pacing produced a Q-T decrease of approximately 66 ms. The patients in complete heart block exercised at a fixed ventricular rate controlled by implanted cardiac pacemakers. The ventricular rate remained unchanged throughout exercise and there was a pronounced decrease in stimulus–T interval with increasing atrial rates [Q-T = 530 − (0.95 × heart rate)], so that for a 100 beats/min atrial rate increase, a decrease in Q-T interval of 95 ms would be predicted. Thus, the expected shortening of Q-T interval during physiological exercise was only in part the result of the intrinsic effect of increased rate, since patients undergoing atrial pacing to comparable rates showed only a small decrease in Q-T interval and patients exercising at fixed rates in complete heart block exhibited a decreasing Q-T interval related to an independent atrial rate. Q-T interval changes, therefore, appear to be governed mainly by factors extrinsic to heart rate.

Cardiac arrhythmias in acute cerebrovascular accidents

Mikolich and associates[56] from Atlanta, Georga, assessed the incidence and severity of cardiac arrhythmias during the acute phase of cerebrovascular accident (CVA) in 30 patients in a stroke intensive care unit by 24-hour dynamic ECG recordings. Twenty patients consecutively admitted for elective cataract surgery served as a control group and also had recordings. Of the 30 CVA patients, 15 (50%) had serious ventricular ectopic arrhythmias, as compared with only 3 (15%) of the 20 control subjects. Among the patients with CVA, 2 had VT, 2 had complete AV block, and 2 had asystole, all occurring in CVAs involving the anterior circulation. No control subject had these arrhythmias. Cardiac arrhythmias are common in patients with acute CVA, especially those involving the anterior circulation. Dynamic ECG recordings may detect such arrhythmias and provide data for therapeutic consideration.

Frequency of cardiac arrhythmias during fiberoptic bronchoscopy

To evaluate the occurrence of ECG abnormalities during fiberoptic bronchoscopy in relation to specific states of the procedure and to hypoxemia, Katz and associates[57] from Philadelphia, Pennsylvania, prospectively studied 50 hospitalized patients aged 53 ± 18 years who were undergoing bronchoscopy; they monitored cardiac rhythm with a continuous 2-channel ECG recorder and oxygen saturation by ear oximetry. Major disturbances of cardiac rhythm developed in 20 (40%) patients: ventricular arrhythmias in 10 patients (20%), occurring most often during passage of the bronchoscope through the vocal cords (5 patients); and atrial arrhythmias in 16 patients (32%), but their occurrence was not correlated closely with any specific stage of the procedure. Arrhythmias were most frequent in association with periods of maximum oxygen desaturation in 12 patients. Oxygen desaturation persisted for >1 hour after bronchoscopy in 34 (68%) patients. No correlation was observed between the frequency of arrhythmias during bronchoscopy and patients' age, sex, prior medications, or preexisting cardiac or pulmonary disorders. In no case was an ECG abnormality associated with adverse clinical sequelae.

Treatment of fetal congestive heart failure secondary to tachycardia

Fetal cardiac arrhythmias are being detected with increasing frequency as a result of continuous electronic monitoring of the fetal heart rate. Usually, the arrhythmia has been recognized during labor, and few have been identified during the early antepartum period. Harrigan and associates[58] from Piscataway, New Jersey, reported tachycardia (to 260 beats/min) and scalp edema and ascites as determined by ultrasonography at 26 weeks gestation. After administration of digoxin to the mother, however, the fetal heart rate returned to normal and, after 19 days, the fetal ascites and scalp edema had disappeared. The fetus was delivered vaginally at 38 weeks gestation without complication. After birth, the heart rate, BP, ECG, and M-mode echo were normal. This case shows the importance of recognizing tachycardia in the fetus and of searching for sonographic evidence of CHF in the fetus. Early pharmacologic intervention when the fetal heart rate is persistently >200 beats/min can reduce the threat of fetal death and make the delivery of an immature infant unnecessary.

Sudden death: bibliography of 434 references

Myerburg[59,60] from Miami, Florida, compiled a list of 434 references on sudden death. In Part I[59], the references are related to risk factors and epidemiology, pathology, and pathophysiology. In Part II[60], they are related to clinical, interventional, survival, neurophysiologic and psychophysiologic factors and miscellaneous items. They are a tremendous source of information on fatal cardiac arrest.

References

1. RABKIN SW, MATHEWSON FAL, TATE RB: Relationship of ventricular ectopy in men without apparent heart disease to occurrence of ischemic heart disease and sudden death. Am Heart J 101:135–142, Feb 1981.

2. KOSTIS JB, McCRONE K, MOREYRA AE, GOTZOYANNIS S, AGLITZ NM, NATARAJAN N, KUO PT: Premature ventricular complexes in the absence of identifiable heart disease. Circulation 63:1351–1356, June 1981.

3. HORAN MJ, KENNEDY HL: Characteristics and prognosis of apparently healthy patients with frequent and complex ventricular ectopy: evidence for a relatively benign new syndrome with occult myocardial and/or coronary disease. Am Heart J 102:809–810, Oct 1981.

4. SOBOTKA PA, MAYER JH, BAUERNFEIND RA, KANAKIS C, ROSEN KM: Arrhythmias documented by 24-hour continuous ambulatory electrocardiographic monitoring in young women without apparent heart disease. Am Heart J 101:753–759, June 1981.

5. GARSON A JR, GILLETTE PC, McNAMARA DG: Supraventricular tachycardia in children: clinical features, response to treatment, and long-term follow-up in 217 patients. Pediatrics 6: 875–882, June 1981.

6. GAJEWSKI J, SINGER RB: Mortality in an insured population with atrial fibrillation. JAMA 245:1540–1544. Apr 17, 1981.

7. SCHENCK-GUSTAFSSON K, JOGESTRAND T, NORDLANDER R, DAHLQVIST R: Effect of quinidine on digoxin concentration in skeletal muscle and serum in patients with atrial fibrillation. N Engl J Med 305:209–211, July 1981.

8. WU D, HUNG JS, KUO CT: Determinants of sustained slow pathway conduction and relation to reentrant tachycardia in patients with dual atrioventricular nodal transmission. Am Heart J 101:521–528, May 1981.

9. HAMER A, PETER T, PLATT M, MANDEL WJ: Effects of verapamil on supraventricular tachycardia in patients with overt and concealed Wolff-Parkinson-White syndrome. Am Heart J 101:600–612, May 1981.

10. GONZALES R, SCHEINMAN MM: Treatment of supraventricular arrhythmias with intravenous and oral verapamil. Chest 80:465–470, Oct 1981.

11. SEALY WC, GALLAGHER JJ: Surgical treatment of left free wall accessory pathways of atrioventricular conduction of the Kent type. J Thorac Cardiovasc Surg 81:698–706, May 1981.

12. SEALY WC, GALLAGHER JJ: Surgical problems with multiple accessory pathways of atrioventricular conduction. J Thorac Cardiovasc Surg 81:707–712, May 1981.

13. SEALY WC, GALLAGHER JJ, KASELL J: His bundle interruption for control of inappropriate ventricular responses to atrial arrhythmias. Ann Thorac Surg 32:429–438, Nov 1981.

14. SCLAROVSKY S, KRACOFF OH, AGMON J: Acceleration of ventricular tachycardia induced by a chest thump. Chest 80:596–599, Nov 1981.

15. SPRUNG CL, JACOBS LJ, CARALIS PV, KARPF M: Ventricular arrhythmias during Swan-Ganz catheterization of the critically ill. Chest 79:413–415, Apr 1981.

16. DUNGAN WT, GARSON A JR, GILLETTE PC: Arrhythmogenic right ventricular dysplasia: a cause of ventricular tachycardia in children with apparently normal hearts. Am Heart J: 102:745–750, Oct 1981.

17. WU D, KOU H, HUNG J: Exercise-triggered paroxysmal ventricular tachycardia. Ann Intern Med 95:410–414, Oct 1981.

18. HOLLAND OB, NIXON JV, KUHNERT L: Diuretic-induced ventricular ectopic activity. Am J Med 70:762–768, Apr 1981.

19. PODRID PJ, LOWN B: Amiodarone therapy in symptomatic, sustained refractory atrial and ventricular tachyarrhythmias. Am Heart J 101:374–379, Apr 1981.

20. NADEMANEE K, HENDRICKSON JA, CANNOM DS, GOLDREYER BN, SINGH BN: Control of refractory life-threatening ventricular tachyarrhythmias by amiodarone. Am Heart J 101:759–768, June 1981.

21. HEGER JJ, PRYSTOWSKY EN, JACKMAN WM, NACCARELLI GV, WARFEL KA, RINKENBERGER RL, ZIPES DP: Amiodarone. Clinical efficacy and electrophysiology during long-term therapy for recurrent ventricular tachycardia or ventricular fibrillation. N Engl J Med 305:539–544, Sept 1981.

22. HAMER AW, FINERMAN WB JR, PETER T, MANDEL WJ: Disparity between the clinical and electrophysiologic effects of amiodarone in the treatment of recurrent ventricular tachyarrhythmias. Am Heart J 102:992–1000, Dec 1981.

23. ANDERSON JL, STEWART JR, PERRY BA, VAN HAMERSVELD DD, JOHNSON TA, CONARD GJ, CHANG SF, KVAM DC, PITT B: Oral flecainide acetate for the treatment of ventricular arrhythmias. N Engl J Med 305:473–477, Aug 1981.

24. OLSSON SB, EDVARDSSON N: Clinical electrophysiologic study of antiarrhythmic properties of flecainide: Acute intraventricular delayed conduction and prolonged repolarization in regular paced and premature beats using intracardiac monophasic action potentials with programmed stimulation. Am Heart J 102:864–871, Nov 1981. Goteborg, Sweden

25. WINKLE RA, MASON JW, GRIFFIN JC, ROSS D: Malignant ventricular tachyarrhythmias associated with the use of encainide. Am Heart J 102:857–864, Nov 1981.

26. STARGEL WW, SHAND DG, ROUTLEDGE PA, BARCHOWSKY A, WAGNER GS: Clinical comparison of rapid infusion and multiple injection methods for lidocaine loading. Am Heart J 102: 872–876, Nov 1981.

27. HAYNES RE, CHINN TL, COPASS MK, COBB LA: Comparison of bretylium tosylate and lidocaine in management of out of hospital ventricular fibrillation: a randomized clinical trial. Am J Cardiol 48:353–360, Aug 1981.

28. MIROWSKI M, REID PR, WATKINS L, WEISFELDT ML, MOWER MM: Surgical treatment of life-threatening ventricular tachyarrhythmias with the automatic implantable defibrillator. Am Heart J 102:265–270, Aug 1981.

29. WATKINS L JR, MIROWSKI M, MOWER MM, REID PR, GRIFFITH LSC, VLAY SC, WEISFELDT ML, GOTT

VL: Automatic defibrillation in man: the initial surgical experience. J Thorac Cardiovasc Surg 82:492–500, Oct 1981.

30. GUIRAUDON G, FONTAINE G, FRANK R, LEANDRI R, BARRA J, CABROL C: Surgical treatment of ventricular tachycardia guided by ventricular mapping in 23 patients without coronary artery disease. Ann Thorac Surg 32:439–450, Nov 1981.

31. CODINI MA, SOMMERFELDT L, EYBEL CE, DE LARIA GA, MESSER JV: Efficacy of coronary bypass grafting in exercise-induced ventricular tachycardia. J Thorac Cardiovasc Surg 81:502–506, Apr 1981.

32. HOROWITZ LN, HARKEN AH, JOSEPHSON ME, KASTOR JA: Surgical treatment of ventricular arrhythmias in coronary artery disease. Ann Intern Med 95:88–97, July 1981.

33. WINKLE RA, PETERS F, HALL R: Characterization of ventricular tachyarrhythmias on ambulatory ECG recordings in post-myocardial infarction patients: arrhythmias detection and duration of recording, relationship between arrhythmias frequency and complexity, and day-to-day reproducibility. Am Heart J 102:162–169, Aug 1981.

34. KERBER RE, GRAYZEL J, HOYT R, MARCUS M, KENNEDY J: Transthoracic resistance in human defibrillation: influence of body weight, chest size, serial shocks, paddle size and paddle contact pressure. Circulation 63:676–682, March 1981.

35. KERBER RE, JENSEN SR, GRAYZEL J, KENNEDY J, HOYT R: Elective cardioversion: influence of paddle-electrode location and size on success rates and energy requirements. N Engl J Med 305:658–662, Sept 1981.

36. WERNER JA, GREENE HL, JANKO CL, COBB LA: Visualization of cardiac valve motion in man during external chest compression using two-dimensional echocardiography: implications regarding the mechanism of blood flow. Circulation 63:1417–1421, June 1981.

37. REIFFEL JA, GANG E, LIVELLI F JR, GLIKLICH J, BIGGER JT JR: Clinical and electrophysiologic characteristics of sinoatrial entrance block evaluated by direct sinus node electrography: Prevalence, relation to antegrade sinoatrial conduction time, and relevance to sinus node disease. Am Heart J 102:1011–1014, Dec 1981.

38. MACKINTOSH AF: Sinuatrial disease in young people. Br Heart J 45:62–66, Jan 1981.

39. SCHNEIDER JF, THOMAS HE, SORLIE P, KREGER BE, MCNAMARA PM, KANNEL WB: Comparative features of newly acquired left and right bundle branch block in the general population: The Framingham Study. Am J Cardiol 47:931–940, Apr 1981.

40. RABKIN SW, MATHEWSON FAL, TATE RB: The natural history of right bundle branch block and frontal plane QRS axis in apparently healthy men. Chest 80:191–196, Aug 1981.

41. BARRETT PA, YAMAGUCHI I, JORDAN JL, MANDEL WJ: Electrophysiological factors of left bundle-branch block. Br Heart J 45:594–601, May 1981.

42. DABIZZI RP, AIAZZI L, CAPRIOLI G, BARLETTA G, BALDRIGHT V, FANTANI F: Left bundle branch block: a hemodynamic and angiographic study. Eur Heart J 2:467–473, Dec 1981.

43. SWIRYN S, PAVEL D, BYROM E, WITHAM D, MEYERPAVEL C, WYNDHAM CRC, HANDLER B, ROSEN KM: Sequential regional phase mapping of radionuclide gated biventriculograms in patients with left bundle branch block. Am Heart J 102:1000–1010, Dec 1981.

44. STRASBERG B, AMAT-Y-LEON F, DHINGRA RC, PALILEO E, SWIRYN S, BAUERNFEIND R, WYNDHAM C, ROSEN KM: Natural history of chronic second-degree atrioventricular nodal block. Circulation 63:1043–1049, May 1981.

45. ESSCHER EB: Congenital complete heart block in adolescence and adult life: a follow-up study. Eur Heart J 2:281–288, Aug 1981.

46. KARPAWICH PP, GILLETTE PC, GARSON A JR, HESSLEIN PS, PORTER C-B, MCNAMARA DG: Congenital complete atrioventricular block: clinical and electrophysiologic predictors of need for pacemaker insertion. Am J Cardiol 48:1098–1102, Dec 1981.

47. OHKAWA S, HACKEL DB, IDEKER RE: Correlation of the width of the QRS complex with the pathologic anatomy of the cardiac conduction system in patients with chronic complete atrioventricular block. Circulation 63:938–947, Apr 1981.

48. CHOKSHI AB, FRIEDMAN HS, MALACH M, VASAVADA BC, BLEICHER SJ: Impact of peer review in reduction of permanent pacemaker implantations. JAMA 246:754–757, Aug 14, 1981.

49. CHOO MH, HOLMES DR, GERSH BJ, MALONEY JD, MERIDETH J, PLUTH JR, TRUSTY J: Permanent pacemaker infections: characterization and management. Am J Cardiol 48:559–564, Sept 1981.

50. MUERS MF, ARNOLD AG, SLEIGHT P: Prophylactic antibiotics for cardiac pacemaker implantation: a prospective trial. Br Heart J 46:539–544, Nov 1981.

51. GONDI B, NADA NC: Real-time, two-dimensional echocardiographic features of pacemaker perforation. Circulation 64:97–106, July 1981.

52. KAPPENBERGER L, SOWTON E: Programmed stimulation for long-term treatment and non-invasive investigation of recurrent tachycardia. Lancet 1:909–914, Apr 1981.

53. WINKLE RA: Current status of ambulatory electrocardiography. Am Heart J 102:757–770, Oct 1981.

54. DIMARCO JP, GARAN H, HARTHORNE JW, RUSKIN JN: Intracardiac electrophysiologic techniques in recurrent syncope of unknown cause. Ann Intern Med 95:542–548, Nov 1981.

55. RICKARDS AJ, NORMAN J: Relation between QT interval and heart rate. New design of physiologically adaptive cardiac pacemaker. Br Heart J 45:56–61, Jan 1981.

56. MIKOLICH JR, JACOBS WC, FLETCHER GF: Cardiac arrhythmias in patients with acute cerebrovascular accidents. JAMA 246:1314–1317, Sept 18, 1981.

57. KATZ AS, MICHELSON EL, STAWICK J, HOLFORD FD: Cardiac arrhythmias. Frequency during fiberoptic bronchoscopy and correlation with hypoxemia. Arch Intern Med 141:603–606, Apr 1981.

58. HARRIGAN JT, KANGOS JJ, SIKKA A, SPISSO KR, NATARAJAN N, ROSENFELD D, LEIMAN S, KORN D: Successful treatment of fetal congestive heart failure secondary to tachycardia. N Engl J Med 304:1527–1530, June 1981.

59. MYERBURG RJ: Sudden death. Circulation 64:1070–1074, Nov 1981.

60. MYERBURG RJ: Sudden death. Circulation 64:1291–1296, Dec 1981.

Systemic Hypertension

DETECTION AND METHODS

Healthy blood pressures for children

Systemic hypertension is common in adults and it is reasonable to assume that high BP begins in childhood. Pediatricians now can measure BP with cuffs of appropriate sizes (covers two-thirds to three-quarters of the upper arm) and then compare the reading with the normal for that age and sex. But does such a chart for comparison exist? Adams and Landaw[1] from Los Angeles, California, answer "not yet." Although the Task Force of the National Heart, Lung, and Blood Institute in 1977 attempted to provide these data, the graphs represented many 1-time observations on large numbers of children of different ages. They do not represent longitudinal data and, therefore, the impression given that BP rises as the child grows older may be false. The higher readings after age 10 years may be due to the inclusion of children already becoming hypertensive. Studies on an Indian tribe in South America (with 1-time measurements in many) spanning the adult years show that BP does not rise with age. The answer to the question about normal BP in healthy children needs research and time for its answer. So does the equally important question of the cause(s) of the hypertension designated "essential." Until they have been answered, dietary sodium and potassium, genetics, and body weight receive the most attention. Maintaining ideal body weight is desirable. For feeding of infants and children, *fresh fruits* and *vegetables*, which are low in sodium and high in potassium are recommended in preference to frozen and canned fruits, which increase sodium content 10–200-fold while decreasing potassium.

Prevalence of clinically unsuspected pheochromocytoma

Pheochromocytoma occurs in fewer than 1% of patients with systemic hypertension. Detection of these catecholamine-secreting tumors is important because surgical excision is curative in >90% of patients and because lethal complications often ensue when the diagnosis is not made. In patients with pheochromocytoma, physical signs other than hypertension are unusual and although symptoms may be dramatic, they are often subtle. This fact is unfortunate, because properly selected biochemical tests can establish the diagnosis in >95% of the patients. St. John Sutton and associates[2] from Rochester, Minnesota, reviewed 54 autopsy-proven cases of pheochromocytoma seen at the Mayo Clinic over a 50-year period (1928–1977). There were 31 females and 23 males, and the patients' ages ranged from 40 hours–92 years (mean, 53 years). Pheochromocytoma was multiple in 10 patients (19%), extra-adrenal in 5 (9%), and malignant in 6 (11%). In 13 patients (24%), pheochromocytoma had been correctly diagnosed in life—after the investigation of hypertension in 8 patients, incidentally at laparotomy for unrelated conditions in 4 patients, and in association with the multiple endocrine neoplasia syndrome in 1 patient. For 41 patients (76%) in whom pheochromocytoma had not been suspected clinically, hypertension was present in 22 (54%). Symptoms such as headache, sweating, and palpitations were nonspecific, but all occurred more often among the group of patients in whom the diagnosis had been made. For both groups, hypertensive or hypotensive crisis precipitated by surgery for unrelated conditions was a common cause of death. Prevention of such deaths requires a high degree of clinical alertness and biochemical screening tests for pheochromocytoma in patients with labile or accelerated hypertension.

Cuff and ambulatory blood pressure in hypertension

Floras and associates[3] from London, England, obtained the cuff BP in a clinic on at least 3 occasions and compared it with mean arterial pressures in 59 patients with borderline or essential systemic hypertension who underwent direct ambulatory monitoring of BP. In 22 patients (group I) mean cuff and ambulatory pressures were similar (≤10 mmHg), whereas in 32 subjects (group II) cuff pressures were >10 mmHg higher. Groups I and II could not be distinguished on the basis of clinical examination, indices of sympathetic nerve activity, or BP variability, or by the magnitude of BP rise during physical or mental exercise. Group II has less cardiovascular target organ damage and better baroreflex sensitivity, but there was considerable overlap. There was no reliable way of telling which subjects would have lower ambulatory than cuff pressures. Of the 59 subjects classified as hypertensive by cuff measurements, 20 had awake ambulatory pressures <140/90 mmHg.

A self-recording method of measuring blood pressure

One major drawback in achieving successful antihypertensive control is maintaining satisfactory patient compliance. One method to increase patient compliance is frequent knowledge of the level of his (or her) BP. In the past, usually another family member measured the hypertensive's BP. Often, however, another family member is not available, or is disinclined to perform the task. Recording one's own BP by use of the bulb stethoscope and BP cuff is cumbersome. Accordingly, Gelman and Nemati[4] from Boston, Massachusetts, developed a method by which a patient can take his or her own BP conveniently. The method consisted of elevating the BP cuff to greater than peak systolic pressure, then slowly releasing it until the patient began to feel a throbbing rhythmic pulsation in the arm under the inflated BP cuff. The pressure in the BP cuff at the point where the patient first began to feel this pulsation was recorded as the systolic pressure. Pressure in the cuff was then slowly let down to the point where the patient no longer felt this pulsation, and this point was recorded as the diastolic pressure. Thus, the systolic and diastolic BP were recorded by sensing the appearance and disappearance, respectively, of the pulsatile throbbing sensation in the artery under the pressure cuff. They called this method of BP recording the "sensory detection method" (SDM), and they performed this BP measurement in 21 normal subjects, in 14 patients with systemic hypertension, and in 20 patients in whom cardiac catheterization was performed to obtain direct arterial pressures. In all 3 groups, the SDM showed no significant differences from the routine indirect BP or from the direct arterial BP in patients undergoing cardiac catheterization. Some 15% of patients, however, were unable to use this method of recording BP, but these individuals were easily identified during testing and instructing in the technique.

Ambulatory blood pressure monitoring

Concern for the adequacy of BP measurement prompted investigations into the reliability of office BP determinations as early as 1940. Often office BPs do not correlate well with BPs obtained at home. Subsequently, direct (intraarterial) and indirect methods were developed to obtain BPs during activity for 24 or more hours. Indirect, automatic methods are noninvasive and have a high correlation with intraarterial pressures. Horan and associates[5] from Baltimore, Maryland, and Long Beach, California, reviewed current research uses for indirect, ambulatory BP recordings, including characterization of BP profiles in normotensive and hypertensive populations, evaluation of patients with borderline hypertension, and assessment of the effects of therapeutic interventions. The current cost of the automatic unit ranges from $7,000–$20,000. Depending upon duration of the recording and whether a Holter ECG also is obtained, charges for ambulatory BP recordings have ranged from $130–$305. Since the precise significance of ambulatory BP recordings, methods of data analysis, and the differential utilities of the technology are still being evaluated, it is still premature both from clinical and economic standpoints, to adopt this technique on a widespread basis. Nevertheless, it seems probable that in the near future such instrumentation will provide a useful adjunctive aid to the clinician managing patients with systemic hypertension.

PATHOGENESIS AND EFFECTS OF VARIOUS NATURAL STATES AND SUBSTANCES

Blood viscosity, blood hematocrit and fibrinogen

Arterial pressure depends on 2 hemodynamic variables: cardiac output and total peripheral resistance. The latter is determined by the caliber of resistance vessels and the intrinsic viscous resistance of blood to flow. Consequently, blood viscosity is a determinant of total peripheral resistance and, hence, of blood flow. In hypertensive disorders, little is known concerning the hemodynamic role of blood viscosity in the elevated arterial pressure level. Letcher and associates[6] from New York City measured systemic arterial pressure and components of blood viscosity in 49 normal subjects and in 49 untreated patients with essential systemic hypertension. Blood viscosity values measured at 6 different shear rates were significantly correlated with BP. Blood viscosity was higher in hypertensive patients. This was due to both higher plasma viscosity and increased hematocrit values ($44.4 \pm 4\%$ -vs- $41.5 \pm 3\%$, $p < 0.005$). When blood viscosity was evaluated in subgroups of normal and hypertensive subjects with matched hematocrit values, it remained higher in the hypertensive patients, and the relationship between BP and viscosity was still significant.

Regardless of the hematocrit value, fibrinogen levels were elevated in hypertensive patients ($p < 0.006$) and, in association with the increased globulin concentration, fibrinogen was largely responsible for the increased plasma viscosity in hypertensive patients. Since the viscosity of defibrinated blood was similar in normal and hypertensive subjects with matched hematocrit values, the elevated fibrinogen level also affected whole blood viscosity. Defibrinated blood viscosity and arterial pressures were not correlated.

These studies demonstrate a direct correlation between blood pressure and blood viscosity among normotensive and hypertensive subjects. This relationship is, in part, due to the rheologic effects of an elevated fibrinogen level and to an increased hematocrit value. The basis for hyperfibrinogenemia in hypertensive patients in unclear.

Platelet function

Platelet function was evaluated in 10 patients with systemic hypertension and in 11 normal subjects.[7] In the placebo phase, the plasma beta thromboglobulin level (an index of platelet activation in vivo) was significantly higher in the hypertensive than in the normal subjects; other tests of platelet function gave similar results in the 2 groups. After control of BP with iofexidine (a centrally acting imidazoline derivative), plasma beta thromboglobulin levels decreased in 9 of the 10 hypertensive patients, but increased in 1 who showed no change in BP. These studies suggest that enhanced platelet activation in primary hypertension may be associated with increased vascular resistance.

Acute and chronic vasopressin excess

Whether circulating vasopressin can cause or contribute to systemic hypertension in humans has provoked debate primarily because of evidence that vasopressin has an important role in some forms of hypertension in animals. Although increased antidiuretic activity has been found in the urine of hypertensive persons, plasma levels of vasopressin are not high in essential hypertension or in primary aldosteronism. Padfield and associates[8] from Glasgow, Scotland, studied 29 patients with malignant hypertension and 28 patients with the syndrome of inappropriate antidiuretic hormone secretion to assess the relation of plasma vasopressin to BP in states of acute and chronic vasopressin excess. In the patients with malignant hypertension, vasopressin levels were elevated (13 ± 2 pg/ml [±S.E.M.]), but did not correlate with BP; however, in normal volunteers, BP did not rise when vasopressin was increased beyond these levels through infusion of the peptide. In the patients with inappropriate antidiuretic hormone secretion, BP was not elevated, but vasopressin was raised (39 ± 7 pg/ml) and did not correlate with systolic or diastolic BP. These data do not support the concept that an acute or chronic excess of vasopressin makes an important contribution to the regulation of BP.

Weight loss and plasma renin activity

Tuck and associates[9] from Los Angeles, California, investigated the relation between changes in the renin-aldosterone axis and reduction in BP in 25 obese patients placed on a 12-week reducing diet; sodium intake was either medium (120 mmol) or low (40 mmol). Plasma renin activity (PRA) declined with weight loss, so that by 12 weeks there was a significant decrease in PRA (p < 0.01) and in plasma aldosterone (p < 0.05), regardless of sodium intake. Weight loss with low sodium intake was equal to that with medium intake. The reduction in PRA, but not in aldosterone, correlated with weight loss in both sodium-intake groups. Mean arterial pressure fell significantly and equally in both groups, correlating with weight loss throughout the study and with PRA from the fourth through the twelfth weeks. These results demonstrate that weight loss is accompanied by reductions in PRA and aldosterone; PRA reductions, irrespective of sodium intake, may contribute to the decline in blood pressure.

Effect of obesity

Several studies, of course, have suggested the relationship between body weight and BP. It has been suggested that obesity produces systemic hypertension and that hypertensive persons tend to become obese, and also that obese persons having normal arterial BP tend to become hypertensive. Additionally, weight reduction often leads to a fall in arterial BP. Surprisingly, no data have been reported regarding the effect of increased body weight and elevated arterial BP on basic cardiovascular pathophysiologic mechanisms. To correct this deficit, Messerli and associates[10] from New Orleans, Louisianna, determined systemic hemodynamics, intravascular volume, and plasma renin activity in 135 lean (<105% of ideal weight), mildly obese (105%–125% of ideal body weight), and obese (body weight >125% of the ideal) subjects who were normotensive (all diastolic BPs <90 mmHg) and those with established hypertension (all diastolic BPs >90 mmHg). The cardiac output was higher and the peripheral resistance was lower in obese than in lean subjects, except in borderline (1 diastolic BP <90 mmHg and others >90 mmHg) hypertension. Intravascular volume was increased in obese patients and more so when corrected for body height. Correction for body weight led to relative volume contraction. Intravascular volume correlated directly with cardiac output in the entire population and in the subgroups. Intravascular volume correlated inversely with total peripheral resistance in all subjects and in each subgroup. Both correlations remained significant when an approximation was used to correct influences of obesity on total blood volume. Sodium excretion was higher in obese than in lean subjects. Thus, despite the expanded intravascular volume in obesity, the pathophysiologic relationship between systemic hemodynamics and intravascular volumes remains unchanged. Relatively low peripheral resistance in obesity may decrease the risk of systemic vascular disease. Nevertheless, since circulating volume is increased, the greater venous return adds an additional load to a left ventricle that is already burdened by a high afterload caused by arterial hypertension.

Alcohol-induced hypertension

Saunders and associates[11] from Birmingham, England, measured the BP of 132 alcoholic patients whose mean daily alcohol consumption exceeded 70 g. The BP was measured while drinking, during detoxification from alcohol, and after a period of abstinence. At presentation the BP was >140/90 mmHg in 51.5% of patients. A significant correlation was observed between BP and mean daily alcohol intake over the previous 3 months and between the BP and the severity of alcohol-withdrawal symptoms (Fig. 4-1). No relation was found between BP and degree of histological liver damage, but a correlation was found with serum gamma-glutamyl-transferase activity and with mean corpuscular volume. In most patients, BP fell to normal after detoxification, and remained so for at least a year in those who continued to abstain. Blood pressure rose in those who started drinking again. Thus, excessive alcohol consumption is an important and insufficiently recognized cause of hypertension and, although the exact mechanism is unknown, treatment is simple and effective if patients can be persuaded to abstain.

Sickle cell anemia

It is well recognized that systemic hypertension and the associated cardiovascular and renal complications from it are at least twice as common in

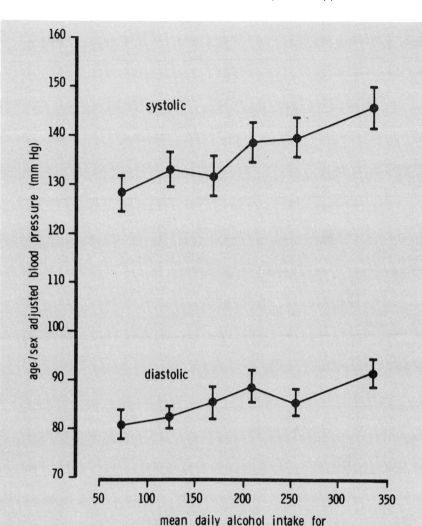

Fig. 4-1. Relationship of systolic and diastolic blood pressure ($\pm$ SEM) to mean daily alcohol intake for 3 months preceding admission. Patients were divided into 6 groups of 22. The coordinate on the x axis represents the mean alcohol intake of each group. Reproduced with permission from Saunders.[11]

North American blacks as in age- and sex-matched whites. Johnson and Giorgio[12] from Los Angeles, California, reviewed the medical records in 187 adults with sickle cell disease (SCD) and found an unexpected small number of patients with systemic hypertension. The BP in the SCD patients was significantly lower than those in the control populations in all ages and did not demonstrate the expected rise with advancing age. In the SCD patients, there was no difference between BP and sex, degree of anemia or hemoglobin genotype. Only 4 patients had diastolic and 2 had systolic hypertension. The prevalence of systemic hypertension was significantly less than that in the black population. These BP findings in SCD may be due to the renal tubular defect responsible for increased sodium and water excretion, which may blunt the plasma volume expansion necessary for sustained hypertension and thus promote lower arterial pressures, similar to the situation observed in patients with salt-losing nephritis.

Low blood pressure in psychiatric inpatients

Arterial BP is known to be lower than normal in patients with schizophrenia, but it is not known if this results from schizophrenia, from its treatment by drugs, or from prolonged residence in a hospital. Masterton and associates[13] from Glasgow, Scotland, recorded BPs in 116 female psychiatric inpatients, 69 with schizophrenia and the other 47 with a variety of non-schizophrenic psychiatric conditions. All had been hospitalized for >1 year, an average of 19 years continuously. An average of 7 recordings of BP per patient were made during that time. On admission to the hospital, the BP of the patients was close to that of 2 normal populations; thereafter, however, it failed to rise at the normal rate and, after an average of 19 years, the systolic arterial pressure was 28 mmHg lower than for controls of the same age, and diastolic pressures were 13 mmHg lower. Lower than control BP was apparent in both schizophrenic and non-schizophrenic women and in women taking no drugs, and in those taking phenothiazines and other drugs. The mean weight of the women was 62 kg, as compared with 64 kg in a local control population of the same age. Prolonged isolation in a hospital appeared to be the most reasonable explanation for the low arterial pressure in the patients described. Psychiatric disease, of course, is a high price to pay for the lower arterial pressure!

Blood pressure after stroke

Wallace and Levy[14] from New Haven, Connecticut, determined BP on the day of admission and during the 10 days thereafter in 334 consecutive patients admitted for acute stroke. On the day of admission, the BP was elevated in 84% of them and decreased spontaneously an average of 20 mmHg systolic and 10 mmHg diastolic in the 10 days following the acute event without specific antihypertensive therapy. It was elevated in only one-third of the patients by the tenth hospital day. The early elevation in BP was believed to be a physiological response to brain ischemia and, as the brain function recovered, BP fell.

Systolic blood pressure before stroke (Framingham study)

Previous epidemiologic investigations have emphasized the importance of systemic hypertension as a contributor to cardiovascular disease in general and to stroke in particular. Indeed, systemic hypertension is the predominant contributor to stroke. Previous studies have established elevated BP in general and systolic BP in particular are predictors of stroke incidence. Kannel and associates[15] from Framingham, Massachusetts, extended these studies by examining the role of isolated systolic hypertension in the role of stroke and attempted to assess its effect, taking arterial rigidity into account. The conclusion is that isolated systolic hypertension predisposed to stroke independent of arterial rigidity. The prevalence of isolated systolic hypertension increased with age and with the degree of blunting of the dicrotic notch of the pulse wave. Subjects with isolated systolic hypertension experienced 2–4 times as many strokes as did normotensive persons. Although diastolic pressure was related to stroke incidence, in the subject with systolic hypertension, the diastolic component added little to risk assessment and, in men in this subgroup, appeared related to stroke incidence.

LEFT VENTRICULAR CONSEQUENCES AS DETERMINED BY ECHO

Cohen and associates[16] from San Diego, California, evaluated by M-mode and 2-D echo 73 patients (35 men, 38 women, aged 28–85 years, mean, 57) with systemic hypertension. All but 2 were receiving antihypertensive therapy at study. LV hypertrophy was found in 37 (51%), concentric in 29 and asymmetric in 8. Factors that did not influence the distribution of patients in the group with LV hypertrophy and normal subjects were 1) duration of hypertension, 2) level of BP, 3) age, 4) body surface area and 5) race. More patients who had a normal LV mass (32 or 89%) than those who had LV hypertrophy (22 or 59%) were receiving 2 or more antihypertensive drugs. Electrocardiography was very insensitive in identifying LV hypertrophy. The presence of increased LV mass was associated with a greater incidence of other target organ disease.

Dreslinski and associates[17] from New Orleans, Louisiana, evaluated echo characteristics of 38 patients with borderline (BP >140/90 mmHg, on occasion interspersed with other readings in the normal range for 6 months) and 38 with mild hypertension (consistent outpatient readings >140/90 mmHg for the preceding 6 months) in the absence of ECG or chest roentgenographic findings consistent with LV hypertrophy. All patients had normal LV function and normal LV wall thickness. Those with borderline hypertension had ventricular septa and LV free walls of similar thickness. The ratio of the LV radius to wall thickness remained normal in both groups, indicating no disproportionate hypertrophy or dilation of chambers during the phase of normal LV function. The patients with mild hypertension had an augmented mean circumferential fiber-shortening rate, as compared with those with borderline hypertension, suggesting an early stage of LV hyperfunction in the development and elaboration of hypertensive heart disease.

Shapiro and associates[18] from Birmingham, England, used computerized apex and echo to study LV dimensions and function in 13 patients with untreated malignant hypertension and in 8 with severe nonmalignant hypertension. All had normal LV cavity dimensions. Five with nonmalignant and 5 with malignant hypertension and a previous history of hypertension had significant thickening of the ventricular septum and LV free wall. In 8 with malignant hypertension without a history of systemic hypertension, wall thicknesses were normal. The absence, of course, of LV hypertrophy in some patients with malignant hypertension suggested that the hypertension was of short duration. Although fractional shortening and peak V_{cf} were normal in all the hypertensives, diastolic LV function was frequently abnormal, with delayed mitral valve opening, reduced peak rate of filling, and outward endocardial motion during isovolumic relaxation. Malignant hypertensives had a cavity shape change during isovolumic contraction and, in those without a previous history, the aortic second heart sound occurred earlier.

To analyze changes in LV diastolic properties in patients with systemic hypertension, Dreslinski and associates[19] from New Orleans, Louisiana, used the atrial emptying index to assess the rapid phase of diastolic LV filling. Ten normal subjects (group 1), 11 hypertensive patients without evidence of cardiac involvement (group 2), and 10 hypertensive patients with echo evidence of LV hypertrophy (group 3) were compared, using M-mode echo and systemic hemodynamic data. Whereas cardiac index (dye-dilution method) and rate of circumferential fiber shortening (echo) were normal in all 3 groups, there was a progressive increase in left atrial index ($p < 0.001$, group 1 -vs- group 2 -vs- group 3) and a progressive decrease in the atrial emptying index ($p < 0.001$, group 1 -vs- group 2 -vs- group 3). No correlation existed between the atrial emptying index and the left atrial index, or between mean arterial pressure or total peripheral resistance in any of the 3 groups. These data suggest that rapid LV filling is reduced early in hypertension, even before ECG or systolic echo abnormalities are detectable. The atrial emptying index, therefore, appears to be an early indicator of abnormalities of LV diastolic compliance in uncomplicated hypertension.

BORDERLINE HYPERTENSION

Relation to labile hypertension

Horan and associates[20] from Baltimore, Maryland, and Long Beach, California, asked the question: "Do patients with borderline systemic hypertension have more labile BP than patients considered to have no hypertension or those with established hypertension?" Labile hypertension is that fluctuating above and below an arbitrarily selected level that is believed to separate normotensive persons from hypertensive persons. It, of course, is purely an operational concept without a true physiologic basis, especially because there are no reliable data showing that these patients' BPs are more labile than others. Horan and associates examined by use of 24-hour ambulatory BP recordings the variability of BPs in patients whose office BPs fluctuated below and above 140/90 mmHg and compared these data with the results from such recordings in normotensive subjects and in patients with fixed hypertension. They recorded BPs every 7.5–15 min, using noninvasive automatic recorders in 21 hypertensive persons, in 21 borderline hypertensive persons, and in 21 fixed hypertensive persons. The mean 24-hour BPs (normotensive, 115 ± 14/74 ± 12 mmHg; borderline hypertensive, 127 ± 16/81 ± 13 mmHg; fixed hypertensive, 143 ± 17/91 ± 12 mmHg) were significantly different from each other, but the standard deviations were not significantly different. The percentages of elevated BPs on the 24-hour recordings of the borderline hypertensive patients were intermediate between those of the normotensive and the fixed hypertensive patients, but within the borderline group there was a broad range in percentage of elevated BPs (8%–81%). Thus, borderline hypertensive patients have BPs no more labile than those in normotensive or fixed hypertensive patients, but because of their broad range of percentage of elevated BPs, their pressures are best evaluated with multiple measurements.

Relation between age, hemodynamics and catecholamines

Messerli and associates[21] from New Orleans, Louisiana, studied the relation between age, systemic and renal hemodynamics, circulating catecholamines (norepinephrine, epinephrine, and dopamine), and intravascular volumes in 38 normotensive subjects and in 77 patients with borderline essential systemic hypertension. Borderline hypertension was defined as diastolic pressures >90 mmHg on several outpatient visits and diastolic pressures <90 mmHg at other times. Borderline hypertensive patients had a higher cardiac index and renal blood flow than normotensive subjects if they were <30 years of age, whereas in older patients no difference was observed. In contrast, total peripheral vascular resistance was normal in young borderline hypertensive patients, but significantly increased in patients >age 40 years. Cardiac output and renal blood flow correlated inversely with age in the entire population and in both subgroups. Cardiac output also increased with age, whereas epinephrine concentration tended to decrease. Plasma and total blood volume correlated directly with cardiac output and inversely with total peripheral vascular resistance. These data indicate that the hyperdynamic circulation (high cardiac output and renal blood flow) of borderline hypertension is found predominantly in patients <age 30 years. Older patients have elevated total peripheral resistances and normal cardiac outputs. The age-dependent increase in circulating norepinephrine and decrease in epinephrine levels may participate in the shift of the hemodynamic profile from high-cardiac-output hypertension in the young to a high-arteriolar-resistance hypertension in the older patient.

SODIUM INTAKE

It is generally believed that salt plays some role in systemic hypertension, but its exact role is unclear. Finn and associates[22] from Liverpool, England, made another attempt to demonstrate an intrapopulation salt/BP relationship using dietary assessment. They studied 537 patients > age 39 years from a random hospital and outpatient population. Patients with systemic hypertension were not specifically excluded or included, but, if they were on treatment, the pretreatment BP was recorded. To assess long-term salt intake, each individual was asked whether he added salt to each of the following types of food: meat, fish, vegetables, salads, potatoes, and eggs. One point was given for each positive answer. Thus, an individual who never added salt at table scored zero and one who added salt to all foods scored 6. This method of scoring proved to be highly repeatable when scoring was carried out by several observers. The BP was then recorded. A clear correlation between salt score and mean systolic BP was observed. Analysis of variance showed a strong dependence of BP on salt score ($p < 0.001$) and age ($p < 0.001$). A separate multiple-regression analysis of BP on salt score, age, sex, and observer collecting the data confirmed the very highly significant dependence on salt score and age, but showed the influence of sex and observer to be nonsignificant. This study confirms the earlier study by Dahl who reported in 1972 an effect due to table-added salt. The analysis also shows an independent age effect that is found only in populations with a high salt intake, and this, therefore, reflects the cumulative effect of the salt already present in the food. The findings of this intrapopulation study are consistent with those of previous interpopulation studies, making a strong case for the dominant role of dietary salt in the etiology of essential systemic hypertension. The National Research Council in 1980 advised that the American population should reduce its average daily salt intake from 10 to 3 g. This would require elimination of salt in cooking and at the table, since non-discretionary salt intake in foods amounts to at least 3 g daily. Finn and associates suggest that the evidence is now sufficiently strong to warrant similar advice in other countries.

Reduction of dietary sodium (Na) has been advocated for the management of hypertension for many years, but its efficacy depended on a regimen that was too restrictive for long-term application. Recently, more modest restrictions of Na intake over periods of 1 month and 2 years were reported to lower BP significantly. Although potassium (K) administration ameliorates salt hypertension occurring in stock and salt-sensitive rats and reduces the BP of Okamoto spontaneously hypertensive rats, few studies of chronic administration to hypertensive people have been done. The possibility that patients with essential hypertension may be specifically sensitive to changes in Na and K intake does not appear to have been investigated. Parfrey and associates[23] from London, England, explored this possibility by studying 16 patients with mild essential hypertension (average diastolic BP 90–110 mmHg) and 8 normotensive subjects (diastolic pressure <85 mmHg) in a randomly allocated, crossover, observer-blind trial in which they received their normal diets supplemented by 100 mmol Na daily for 12 weeks and a no-added-Na diet supplemented by 100 mmol K daily for the same period. During the high-Na diet, the BP rose slowly in both groups. At 12 weeks, systolic BP was significantly (9 ± 13 mmHg) higher than pre-diet levels in the hypertensive group and 5 ± 9 mmHg higher in the normotensive group ($p = $ ns). During the high-K/no-added-Na diet, BP fell sharply in the hypertensive group. At 6 weeks, the mean systolic pressure was 9 ± 11 mmHg lower than pre-diet levels, whereas in the normotensive group it was 4 mmHg higher, the difference in response being significant. There were no significant differences in plasma renin and aldosterone between the 2 groups at the start of the trial, whereas plasma noradrenaline, measured in the supine resting state, was significantly higher in the hypertensive group. During the high-Na phase, the levels of all 3 hormones fell, but only the fall in plasma noradrenaline in the hypertensive group was significant. During the high-K/low-Na phase, there was little change in plasma renin and noradrenaline, whereas plasma aldosterone rose significantly in both groups. Correlations were observed between changes in BP and in the urinary Na/K ratio in the hypertensive group during the trial, but no consistent correlations were found between changes in BP and in hormonal levels. Thus, the BP of patients with mild essential hypertension, but not of normotensive subjects, is lowered by moderately reducing dietary Na and increasing K. It is unlikely that the mechanism of this action is exclusively to involve changes in plasma renin, aldosterone, or noradrenaline.

Parfrey and associates[24] also reported the effects of administering K to young men with a familial predisposition to systemic hypertension; no previous studies on this had been performed. Na intake was lowered and K intake was raised in 2 groups of patients, 1 with and 1 without a family history of systemic hypertension. The BP of the parents of a group of students was determined and 2 subgroups of students were defined: 1 with (PHT group) and 1 without (PNT group) a familial predisposition to systemic hypertension. Observations were made in both groups during 3 periods of modified dietary electrolyte intake: 1) no added Na (low Na), 2) no added Na with K supplementation (low Na/high K), and 3) Na supplementation (high Na). The diets were given in random order. At the start of the trial, while the students continued their customary diet, the PHT group had higher systolic and diastolic pressures and plasma noradrenaline levels than the PNT group. At the end of 4 weeks of the high-Na diet, the BP levels of both groups were significantly higher than those after the low-Na diet. In contrast, when the low-Na diet was supplemented for 2 weeks with potassium, BPs of the PHT group fell significantly, while those of the PNT group rose slightly. BP in the PHT group was significantly lower during the low-Na/high-K diet than during the high-Na diet (systolic 10 ± 2 mmHg; diastolic 11 ± 2 mmHg), the changes being significantly different from those in the PNT group. The changes in plasma renin and aldosterone were similar in both groups during the different diets. Plasma noradrenaline fell in the PHT group, but rose in the PNT group when the low-Na diet was supplemented with potassium. This fall in plasma noradrenaline in the PHT group during the low-Na/high-K diet correlated with the falls in systolic and diastolic BP. It was concluded that, although young adults with a familial predisposition to hypertension behave similar to those without such a predisposition in having a pressor response to a high-sodium intake, they are peculiar in showing a depressor response to a high-potassium intake.

Skrabal and associates[25] from Innsbruck, Austria, investigated 20 normotensive subjects (10 with a family history of systemic hypertension) as to whether moderate salt restriction and/or a high-K intake had a beneficial effect on BP regulation and prevention of hypertension. In all subjects reduction of salt intake from 200−50 mmol/day over 2 weeks reduced the rise in BP induced by various doses of noradrenaline. Furthermore, of 20 subjects 12 (8 with a family history of hypertension) responded to salt restriction with a fall in systolic or diastolic BP of at least 5 mmHg. No significant differences in plasma renin, aldosterone, vasopressin, or catecholamine levels were observed between responders (salt-sensitive subjects) and non-responders, but salt-sensitive subjects had a mean baseline diastolic BP that was higher than that of salt-insensitive subjects by 13 mmHg (77 ± 3 -vs- 65 ± 2). A high-K intake reduced diastolic BP by at least 5 mmHg in 10 of 20 subjects. Of the 10, seven had a family history of hypertension and 9 responded to salt restriction. A high-K intake also improved compliance with a low-salt regimen, promoted Na loss, prevented the rise in plasma catecholamines induced by a low-salt diet, and increased the sensitivity of the baroreceptor reflex. These 4 effects occurred in the group as a whole and were probably the means by which a high-K intake reduced BP. In all subjects, 2 weeks of a combined low-Na/high-K intake reduced BP rises induced by mental stress or noradrenaline infusion by 10 mmHg. Thus, moderate salt restriction combined with a high-K intake helps prevent hypertension, and salt-sensitive subjects would profit most from such a regimen.

TREATMENT

Diuretics plus sodium restriction

Diuretics are used as initial drug therapy for most patients with hypertension and offer both an intrinsic ability to lower the BP and a foundation for additional antihypertensive agents whose effects may be blunted by reactive fluid retention. Various diuretics, differing mainly in their duration of action, are available, but few comparisons of their effectiveness have been performed. The most common and potentially serious side effect of continuous diuretic therapy is hypokalemia. The plasma potassium (K) level usually falls 0.5 to 1.0 mEq/liter, reflecting an increase in urinary K wastage. Before diuretics were used, rigid dietary sodium (Na) restriction to a level <10 mEq/day was shown to lower the BP. When thiazide diuretics became available in 1957, they were substituted for dietary Na restriction in the hope of achieving as much antihypertensive potency with less bother for the patient. Moderate (60−100 mEq/day) dietary Na restriction lowers BP moderately with an average fall in diastolic BP of about 7 mmHg. Another potential advantage of such moderate Na restriction is a decrease in diuretic-induced K wastage, but this effect has not been documented. A decrease in the amount of Na filtered and delivered to the renal distal tubular Na-for-K exchange site should reduce the amount of K swept into the urine. Rigid Na restriction, however, in the presence of diuretic action, by further activation of the renin-aldosterone system, may be counterproductive: even more K wastage has been found in short-term studies on a few patients receiving diuretics given a 1 g low-Na diet.

Ram and associates[26] from Dallas, Texas, determined, in multiple studies on 12 hypertensive subjects ingesting a diet either moderately restricted or higher in Na, changes in total body K level and BP. The 12 patients , 6 men and 6 women, were aged 28–52 years (mean, 41). They had relatively mild primary hypertension, as evidenced by an average BP of 148/100 mmHg without therapy. The data clearly document that the effect of moderate Na restriction is a lessening by almost one-half of diuretic-induced K loss. The decrease in loss with a low-sodium diet accompanied all 3 diuretics tested. *Chlorthalidone* (50 mg/day) induced the greatest reduction in the total body K, whereas the losses with single morning doses of *hydrochlorothiazide*, (50 mg) and two daily doses of *furosemide* (40 mg) were similar. Thus, a greater degree and duration of diuretic action leads to a greater degree of initial K wastage. These results support the use of moderate dietary Na restriction, alone in those with minimally elevated BP and with a diuretic in those in whom Na restriction is not adequate to reduce BP to the desired level. In regard to the choice of a diuretic, for the majority of hypertensive patients who do not have substantial renal damage, a single morning dose of a drug with a 12- to 18-hour duration of action, such as hydrochlorothiazide, may provide the best balance of efficacy and safety.

Beta blockers

ATENOLOL, METOPROLOL, OXPRENOLOL

To insure good patient compliance, individuals with asymptomatic systemic hypertension should take medicine only once daily and that with minimal side effects. Several beta blocking drugs, of course, can be given once daily to control elevated BP. These drugs differ not only in their ancillary pharmacological and physical properties but also in their cost. Wilcox and Hampton[27] from Nottingham, England, performed a single-blind, placebo-controlled crossover study in 25 patients with moderate essential systemic hypertension (standing diastolic BP 100–125 mmHg), comparing 4-week periods of treatment with atenolol (100 mg), metoprolol (100 mg), metoprolol durules (200 mg), slow-release oxprenolol (160 mg) and slow-release oxprenolol (320 mg), respectively. All drugs were significantly better than placebo at reducing resting BP at 24 hours. Atenolol produced the greatest mean reduction of BP and was the most effective drug for most patients, though the differences between atenolol and metoprolol durules were not statistically significant. These 2 drugs, however, were significantly more effective than the remainder. A similar ranking was seen with respect to the reduction of BP and the heart rate response to exercise. None of the treatments had any significant effect on the patients' rating of perceived exertion during the exercise test.

EFFECT ON RIGHT VENTRICULAR PERFORMANCE

Recent studies have shown that RV function and pressures are abnormal in patients with uncomplicated systemic hypertension. To determine if there was a further depression of RV performance in patients with systemic hypertension receiving beta blockade, Ferlinz and associates[28] from Long Beach and Irvine, California, studied 20 patients with essential systemic hypertension by dividing them into 2 groups on a double-blind randomized basis and maintaining 10 on oral *oxprenolol* and 10 on *propranolol* for 5 weeks. Cardiac catheterization and RV angiography were performed at the beginning and again at the end of the 5-week period. RV end-diastolic index did not change significantly in either group. In contrast, RV end-systolic volume index increased and RV EF significantly decreased after chronic beta blockade. Cardiac index decreased in both groups. When the intergroup differences were compared for all measured indices, none of the changes between the 2 groups was significantly different. Thus, RV contractility is clearly diminished after the institution of beta blockade in patients with systemic hypertension, an effect that until this study was believed to be limited to the left side of the heart. A caution, therefore, must be exercised when beta blockade is initiated in patients with severely abnormal RV function, because RV decompensation could result.

COMPARISON TO DIURETICS OR WITH ADDITION OF DIURETICS

Thiazide diuretics and beta adrenergic blocking agents are the most widely used antihypertensive agents today. They have similar hypotensive effects. Thiazide diuretics, however, have been said to induce diabetes mellitus or to impair glucose tolerance, to induce potentially deleterious hypokalemia and decrease body potassium, and to increase serum uric acid and the risk of gout. Berglund and Andersson[29] from Göteborg, Sweden, compared the antihypertensive effects and metabolic side effects of *bendroflumethiazide* with those of *propranolol* in 2 randomly selected groups of 53 previously untreated middle-aged men during 6 years' treatment for systolic hypertension (systolic pressure >170 mmHg or diastolic pressure >105 mmHg). The BP reduction was the same in the 2 groups. None had gout, but serum urate increased in both groups. Glucose tolerance improved significantly in both groups during the first year and this improvement was sustained in the follow-up period. Serum potassium did not differ in the 2 groups during the first 5 years, but during the sixth year it decreased in the diuretic group. Total potassium was unchanged in both groups. These results indicate that the frequency of metabolic side effects during diuretic treatment of mild to moderately severe essential hypertension is low and has been grossly exaggerated. Since the antihypertensive effect and side effects were equal with both drugs, and since the diuretics are cheaper, they should be the drug of first choice in this type of hypertension.

Participants in the Medical Research Council treatment trial for mild hypertension were randomly allocated to 1 of 4 treatment groups:[30] bendrofluazide, propranolol, or a placebo for either of these drugs. The trial was single-blinded; 23,582 patient-years of observation have been completed so far, 10,684 on active drugs and 12,898 on placebos. The results show an association between bendrofluazide treatment and impotence, and impotence also occurred more frequently in patients taking propranolol than in those taking placebo. Other adverse reactions significantly linked with active drugs include impaired glucose tolerance in men and women and gout in men, associated with bendrofluazide treatment, and Raynaud's phenomenon and dyspnea in men and women taking propranolol. No corneal disease was known to have occurred in the propranolol group. Mean serum potassium level fell, and urea and uric acid levels rose, in men and women taking bendrofluazide. In the propranolol group, serum potassium and uric acid levels rose in both sexes, but the urea level rose significantly in women only.

Vander Elst and associates[31] from Brussels, Belgium, and Middlesex, England, completed a double-blind parallel study in 40 patients comparing furosemide (FUR) and hydrochlorothiazide (HCT) when added to a stable dose of beta blocker in the treatment of mild-to-moderate systemic hypertension. This study was carried out by 8 investigators on a multicenter basis. Ambulatory patients of either sex, aged 25–65 years, with supine diastolic BP ⩾100 mmHg but <131 mmHg were studied. Both diuretics caused a significant additional fall in BP when added to propranolol, and there were no differences in the mean BP achieved. However, a higher proportion of patients achieved satisfactory control (BP <160/95 mmHg) on FUR than on HCT and, in addition, there was a more marked dose-response effect with FUR. This study showed that FUR is at least as effective as HCT in the treatment of hypertension when added to propranolol, and it appears to possess certain advantages over the thiazide.

EFFECT ON BLOOD PRESSURE DURING MOTOR CAR DRIVING

The efficacy of antihypertensive drugs is usually assessed by measuring the BP indirectly in the hospital or doctor's office. This method samples only a small amount of data from a subject and at rest, and gives no information on the antihypertensive effects of a drug outside the controlled hospital environment. The development of a method for recording accurately intraarterial BP on magnetic tape in patients who are free to return to their usual activities has made it feasible to undertake more detailed studies. This technique has been used to assess the effect of antihypertensive drugs outside hospital by making paired observations in groups of patients before and during chronic treatment. By means of a diary sheet, detailed correlation of their activities during a recording also may be obtained.

Motor car driving is an activity performed by most adults. Driving is a "stressful" activity, though intraarterial BP changes during driving may be small. There has previously been no attempt, however, to investigate the effects of drug treatment on BP in hypertensive patients while driving a motor vehicle. Millar-Craig and associates[32] from London, England, recorded continuous intraarterial BP during motor car driving in 15 patients with untreated essential systemic hypertension, using the "Oxford" recording technique. Each subject was an experienced driver who used his car every day, and for the study drove from his work place to the hospital during the later afternoon. This drive took place in urban traffic and the average duration was 21 minutes. BP during car driving was remarkably stable, and the average systolic and diastolic pressures were similar to the mean daytime pressures. After 16 weeks of treatment with *oxprenolol*, each patient was restudied. BP during driving had dropped from 176/107 mmHg to 160/93 mmHg, but the BP response to driving and BP variation during driving were unchanged. After treatment, the mean daytime systolic pressure was lower than the mean systolic pressure during driving, but the relative antihypertensive effect during driving was similar to that observed in the same patients during dynamic exercise on a bicycle ergometer. No drug-induced side effects occurred and there were no apparent effects of driving ability. Chronic treatment with oxprenolol reduced BP during car driving without affecting the normal BP response to driving.

Vasodilators

PRAZOSIN WITH LEFT VENTRICULAR DYSFUNCTION

In patients with previously compensated LV dysfunction, a rise in systemic arterial pressure may produce clinical deterioration. Conversely, a reduction in impedance to LV ejection, which may be accomplished by treating systemic hypertension or by lowering peripheral vascular resistence in normotensive persons, may improve performance. Little clinical information, however, is available on the response to antihypertensive therapy in patients with elevated BP and impaired LV function. Accordingly, Massie and Chan[33] from San Francisco, California, evaluated the effect of *prazosin* in 16 patients with moderate (sitting diastolic BP > 95 mmHg while continuing on diuretic therapy) hypertension and reduced EF. Therapy with digoxin and diuretics was continued throughout the study, but other antihypertensive agents were withdrawn at least 1 week before initiation of the study. Measurements of EF, cardiothoracic ratio, and duration of maximal treadmill exercise were made before and after 2 months of prazosin. On prazosin, BP fell from a mean of 169/103 mmHg to 141/84 mmHg. Excellent control was achieved in 13 of 16 patients and significant reductions were noted in the remaining 3. Concomitantly, EF rose ($0.38 \pm 0.02 - 0.43 \pm 0.03$ [$p < 0.02$]), cardiothoracic ratio decreased ($0.55 \pm 0.02 - 53 \pm 0.02$ [$p < 0.05$]), and exercise capacity increased ($9 \pm 0.9 - 12 \pm 1$ minutes [$p < 0.005$]). Prazosin was well tolerated, except in 1 patient whose angina worsened. These findings emphasize the importance of rigorous BP control in hypertensive patients with LV dysfunction and indicate that prazosin is effective in this setting.

COMPARISON OF PRAZOSIN AND HYDRALAZINE

Members of the Veterans Administration Cooperative Study Group on Antihypertensive Agents compared, in a randomized, double-blind trial in 232 adult male hypertensives who could not be controlled with hydrochlorothiazide alone, the antihypertensive efficacy and the incidence of side effects of prazosin and hydralazine.[34] The patients included men aged 21–74 years whose average diastolic pressure on 2 successive clinic visits was 95–114 mmHg. No significant differences were observed between regimens in the percentage of patients who attained goal BP (reduction of diastolic BP to or below 90 mmHg and at least 5 mmHg less than the baseline randomization pressure), effect on pulse rate, or the incidence or reasons for terminations. Absolute reduction of BP was similar for both drugs, except for sitting systolic pressure at 3 and 6 months, when prazosin effected a 3.7 and 3.6 mmHg greater response, respectively. Orthostatic dizziness, sexual dysfunction, and nightmares were more frequent with prazosin than with hydralazine; patient compliance, however, was similar for both drugs. An unexpected finding was the lack of pulse rate increase associated with hydralazine, particularly in older patients.

Converting enzyme inhibitors

Considerable evidence now supports a possible role for the renin-angiotensin system in the pathogenesis and maintenance of essential hypertension. Investigation of the pathogenetic role of angiotensin II was made possible by the availability of the angiotensin II competitive antagonist, *saralasin*, and the converting enzyme inhibitors. Unlike saralasin, the converting enzyme inhibitors have no intrinsic agonistic activity, since they act by blocking the conversion of angiotensin I to angiotensin II, thereby eliminating the cardiovascular effects of circulating angiotensin II. Recently, the new oral active angiotensin I-converting enzyme inhibitor *captopril*, has proved to be a potent pharmacologic blocker of the conversion of angiotensin I to the physiologically active pressor octapeptide, angiotensin II. Fujita and associates[35] from Ibaraki, Japan investigated the role of the renin-angiotensin system in sodium-repleted and sodium-depleted patients with essential hypertension. Captopril was administered to 11 patients with essential hypertension. In the sodium-repleted state (1.50 mEq sodium intake for 6 days) in 11 patients, captopril decreased the average mean BP (113–106 mmHg), plasma renin activity (PRA) increased with sodium depletion (30 mEq sodium intake for 3 days after furosemide treatment (1.26–3.26 ng/ml/h). In the sodium-depleted state, the hypotensive effect of captopril was more pronounced (mean BP, 108–93 mmHg). The decrease in mean BP caused by the inhibitor correlated moderately well with basal PRA. Thus, the renin-angiotensin system participates in the regulation of BP in essential hypertension, even in sodium-repleted patients. This role of the renin-angiotensin system in BP regulation becomes more crucial during sodium depletion.

Huang and associates[36] from Chicago, Illinois, evaluated the antihypertensive effects of *captopril* and *propranolol* in a single-blind trial of 12 weeks in 19 ambulatory men with moderate systemic hypertension (diastolic pressure 100–120 mmHg after they had received placebo for 2 weeks) whose sodium intake was unrestricted. The captopril group included 12 patients and the propranolol group, 7. After the initial dose-finding period of 4 weeks, supine diastolic BP was significantly reduced in 8 patients receiving captopril and in 4 receiving propranolol. Diastolic BP decreased throughout the following 8 weeks. In the remaining patients from each group, diastolic BP was not reduced by either drug given alone at maximum allowable dosages during dose-finding periods, nor by combined administration in the following weeks. No adverse side effects attributable to captopril were noted, except proteinuria in 1 patient. Thus, captopril has value in the treatment of moderate essential hypertension.

Cody and associates[37] from Cleveland, Ohio, assessed the reflex hemodynamic and humoral response to postural change during long-term renin-angiotensin blockade (with captopril) in sodium-depleted hypertensive patients. Orthostatic hypotension was not observed with head-up tilt or repeated pressure recordings. During tilt, a reflex increase of heart rate occurred (76 ± 2 – 98 ± 4 beats/min, [p < 0.001]). Home recordings demonstrated only minor changes in BP with standing. To evaluate these observations, hemodynamic studies were performed during tilt at 3 stages of therapy: control, administration of captopril, and administration of captopril plus diuretic. With tilt, no orthostatic hypotension was noted at all 3 stages of therapy, despite similar peripheral pooling (– 22% cardiac index). Maintenance of BP was due to reflex increase of heart rate (44%, 45%, and 38%) and to systemic resistance (34%, 38%, and 37%). The response to tilt of plasma renin activity was modified by drug therapy, but was not completely blocked. Thus, long-term converting enzyme inhibition and sodium depletion are safe and do not appreciably blunt the cardiovascular reflexes responsible for prevention of orthostatic hypotension.

Case and associates[38] from New York City treated 10 patients with severe and 10 patients with accelerated or *malignant systemic hypertension* with captopril. Captopril acutely reduced BP in all but 2 patients with suppressed plasma renin activity. Four patients with encephalopathy showed immediate improvement after the first dose. Two patients could be withdrawn from nitroprusside infusion upon administration of captopril. Nineteen of 20 patients have remained on captopril for 12 – 32 months and the BP is controlled in 18 and improved in 2. Eleven required the addition of diuretic and 1, the addition of clonidine. The maximal antihypertensive effect of captopril, with or without diuretics, was evident after 3 months of continuous therapy and was associated with elevated plasma renin levels, normal aldosterone excretion, and preservation of renal function. Captopril was well tolerated, but produced occasional rash, loss of taste, and proteinuria. Thus, captopril, alone or in combination with other drugs is effective in both the acute and long-term management of severe malignant systemic hypertension.

Gavras and associates[39] from Boston, Massachusetts, Lausanne, Switzerland, West Point, Pennsylvania, and Rahway, New Jersey, evaluated the effects of the new oral converting enzyme inhibitor "*MK-421*" on BP plasma renin activity, plasma angiotensin II, aldosterone, and angiotensin-converting enzyme in 16 hypertensive patients. Maximum (maintenance) doses ranged from 2.5 – 40.0 mg daily. Average BP decreased from 177 ± 7/111 ± 4 mmHg to 145 ± 6/94 ± 3 mmHg supine and from 174 ± 7/117 ± 4 mmHg to 142 ± 6/101 ± 3 mmHg upright (p < 0.001). Heart rate did not change significantly. Plasma renin activity rose during treatment, whereas plasma angiotensin II, aldosterone, and angiotensin-converting enzyme remained suppressed at 24 hours after the maximum dose. The magnitude of BP reduction after the maximum dose did not correlate with baseline plasma renin activity levels. No side effects occurred during the 2—10-week observation period. Thus, MK-421 is similar to its predecessors in efficacy and clinical and biochemical correlates, the main difference being its higher potency and longer duration of action.

Calcium channel blockers

Nifedipine, the new calcium antagonist drug that can be administered sublingually, can dilate the coronary and peripheral resistance vessels by interfering directly with transmembrane calcium supply. This effect lowers calcium-dependent splitting of adenosine triphosphate, resulting in the uncoupling of the excitation-contraction of vascular smooth muscle. Its effects are to decrease LV systolic and diastolic pressure, mean arterial pressure, total peripheral and coronary vascular resistance, and to increase coronary blood flow, cardiac index, heart rate, and plasma renin activity. Thus, it might be expected that the drug would have a prompt and profound BP-lowering action in systemic hypertension. Accordingly, Beer and associates[40] from New York City assessed the effects of sublingual nifedipine in 43 patients with moderate-to-severe systemic hypertension in an emergency room setting. Following a no-response placebo treatment period, the 17 patients with supine diastolic systemic arterial pressures <110 mmHg (group A) received 10 mg nifedipine sublingually and the 26 patients with supine diastolic BP ≥110 mmHg (group B) received a 20 mg sublingual dose. In group A, systolic BP decreased from 172 ± 19 mmHg to 140 ± 15 mmHg; diastolic pressure, from 109 ± 3 to 88 ± 10 mmHg. In group B, systolic pressure decreased from 204 ± 22 mmHg to 160 ± 24 mmHg; diastolic pressure from 128 ± 11 to 97 ± 14 mmHg. The heart rates increased significantly only in the 20 mg dose group (from 76 ± 2 to 89 ± 6 beats/min). The effects of sublingual nifedipine were seen in 1–5 min, and the maximal effect in 20–30 min, with return to placebo baseline in 4–5 hours. Adverse reactions were minimal in both treatment groups. Thus, nifedipine is an effective and safe hypotensive agent in the rapid management of moderate-to-severe hypertension and seems to be an effective nonparenteral agent for treatment of hypertensive emergencies.

Treatment of mild hypertension: pros and cons

Kaplan[41] from Dallas, Texas, evaluated the results of 3 large clinical trials on the therapy of mild systemic hypertension: 1 from the USA, 1 from Australia, and 1 from Oslo, Norway (The results of these studies were reviewed in *Cardiology 1981.*). Based mainly on the data of the US trial, the Hypertension Detection and Follow-up Program (HDFP), the recent report of the Joint National Committee stated "It is reasonable to reduce BP even in uncomplicated mild hypertension by pharmacologic or nonpharmacologic therapy," and that "the initial goal of antihypertensive therapy is to achieve and maintain diastolic pressure levels at less than 90 mmHg." Careful scrutiny of the results of all 3 trials led Kaplan, however, to a different, more conservative conclusion, namely, that drug therapy for uncomplicated systemic hypertension is indicated only for those whose diastolic BP remained at or above 100 mmHg after 6 months of non-drug therapy. Kaplan emphasized that the difference in these views may look small, but in fact the management of about 20 million Americans is in question. The initial diastolic BP readings on the 158,906 persons aged 30–69 screened by the HDFP found 17% to be between 90 and 100 mmHg. The 20 million figure was derived from interpolating this percentage to the entire USA population—a valid maneuver. Kaplan concluded from analysis of these 3 studies published in 1980 the following: 1) patients with diastolic BP >110 mmHg or >100 mmHg with accompanying target organ damage or other cardiovascular risks should be treated with drugs; 2) patients with diastolic BP <110 mmHg without obvious cardiovascular disease or other risk factors should be encouraged to follow good health habits for 6 months while being closely followed; 3) if the diastolic BP remains <100 mmHg, these patients should be left off drugs and followed at least every 6 months; and 4) if the diastolic BP stays above or goes above 100 mmHg, these patients should be treated with appropriate antihypertensive drugs. These principles seem the best to follow, based on the results of the Australian and Oslo trials. They seem to contradict the results of the HDFP, which showed lesser mortality in those with initial diastolic BP from 90–104 mmHg whose pressures were lowered to an average of 83 mmHg. Moreover, life insurance actuarial data show that the excess mortality associated with hypertension is removed when the diastolic BP is lowered to the same level of 83 mmHg. But before we use antihypertensive drugs in many millions more to achieve a new, lower goal of therapy, we should await the publication of more data from both the HDFP and the Australian Trial studies, as well as the last of the major trials, the Medical Research Council Study, being done in England. For now, a more conservative approach appears best.

Madhaven and Alderman[42] from New York City estimated, by constructing probability tables for extended periods based on the Framingham study data, the risk of cardiovascular disease (CVD) at various levels of systolic BP and the potential benefit of BP reduction. These estimates demonstrate that systolic BP alone delineates subgroups of persons with widely divergent risk of CVD, depending both on their demographic and clinical characteristics. Epidemiologic studies have demonstrated increasing cardiovascular risk with increasing BP, but at any one level of BP the risk for cardiovascular disease differs significantly, depending on the sex and age of the person and the presence of other factors, e.g., a history of smoking or elevated lipid levels. They urge that a method be found to discriminate between so-called low and high risks at any fixed BP, stating that some patients with high levels of systolic BP (>190 mmHg) but no other risk factors may actually be at lower risk than those with lower levels of systolic BP or levels considered normal by most observers, i.e., 135 mmHg if these latter persons have other cardiovascular risk factors.

Madhavan and Alderman urge that physicians not indiscriminately treat patients with lower levels of elevated BP with drugs that may produce side effects; the benefit-risk ratio is low in patients in the low-risk category (i.e., only 1 risk factor, such as mild hypertension) and is especially low in women. They are correct in stating that most of the clinical trials, specifically the Veterans Administration, Public Health, and Hypertension Detection and Follow-up Program studies, base their sole criterion for treatment on BP and their conclusions regarding reduction of mortality on the reduction of BP alone. The fact is that mortality was reduced by reducing BP. The Hypertension Detection and Follow-up Program data demonstrated a decrease of 25% in adjusted mortality and a 50% decrease in strokes in patients with mild hypertension with no evidence of target-organ damage (LV hypertrophy, previous strokes, or AMI) if BP was reduced to goal levels. This reduction in mortality held for patients who initially had diastolic BP of 90–95 mmHg or those of 95–104 mmHg. (Systolic BP was not used as an end point in this study.) It is true that benefit was most notable in patients > 50 years old (where complications are expected to be more common) and in black patients. Treated hypertensive patients have a better prognosis at a set BP than untreated persons at the same BP; insurance companies have greatly reduced life insurance premiums based on the reduction of BP to normal. This improvement in prognosis, as determined by actuarial analysis, has occurred despite the lack of specific measurable changes in other risk factors, although, of course, these also may have changed.

Applying benefit-risk analysis to the treatment of any disease that affects large numbers of people will yield data demonstrating that some persons will not benefit, as compared with the number who will benefit. It is apparent now that a positive method to determine the subset of hypertensive patients in whom cardiovascular disease will develop if untreated is unavailable. We do not, as yet, know how to recognize the 15%–35% of patients whose conditions will progress from mild to more severe hypertension if untreated, but this is not a valid reason to wait for complications to occur before instituting therapy if it can be carried out with minimal side effects (which, in most patients, it can).

Most patients do not fall into a high- or low-risk group, but are found in the intermediate-risk group. Although mild hypertension, by itself, may produce no great immediate risk to a person as compared with the risk of severely elevated BP, the large numbers of so-called mild hypertensive patients (approximately 70% of the hypertensive patients in the USA) make the attributable risk considerable from a public health viewpoint. It is, therefore, important, from a public health point of view, to lower the BP of as many as these patients as possible. Data are clear from numerous studies that the benefit of treatment outweighs the risk, at least in large-scale studies, not just at the higher levels of BP, but at all levels of elevated BP, including mild hypertension.

Certainly physicians should weigh other factors before considering the institution of pharmacologic therapy in a patient with only slight elevation of BP and no other risk factors. These patients are ideal candidates for weight reduction if they are obese, for salt restriction, for institution of exercise programs, for introduction of low-fat diets, and for cessation of smoking. However, based on the data available, an equally strong case can be made for pharmacologic treatment of those patients who do not respond to these measures and whose BP remains elevated. The simplest, least toxic, and least costly medications should be used first.

Step-down therapy

In 1973, of 23 million hypertensive persons, 12 million knew of their condition; 3 million were not treated, nearly 5 million were treated inadequately, and 4 million were treated adequately. In 1977, of 36 million hypertensive persons, 21 million knew of their condition; of these, 7 million were not treated, 7 million were treated inadequately, and 7 million were treated adequately. During the past 6 years, there has been a 25% reduction of strokes in the USA. In 1977, the goal of the National High Blood Pressure Program changed from one of awareness to that of treating patients and continuing their therapy. This change in goal was prompted largely by the high dropout rate in patients being treated. Important in maintaining therapy is the simplification of therapeutic programs, i.e., taking the least number of pills and, particularly, the fewest times of administration. The concept of step care, i.e., starting with a suboptimal dose of medication, then increasing the dosage of that drug and adding another in a stepwise fashion, has obviously emphasized "stepping up." In keeping with the new goals of the National High Blood Pressure Program, it now seems important to emphasize "stepping down" to have patients continue therapy.

To determine the minimum amount of therapy needed to control arterial BP, Finnerty[43] from Washington, D.C., reduced the amount of 1 drug, then discontinued use of 1 or more drugs after the diastolic BP had been <90 mmHg for 6 months in 51 hypertensive patients. By 6 months, 1 drug had been eliminated in 38 patients, and the dosage of another had been decreased in 49 patients. By 12 months, stepping up therapy was necessary in 13 patients; thus, 1 drug therapy had been eliminated in only 27 patients, and the dose had been decreased in another 43 patients. No further therapeutic changes were necessary during the next 6 months. Originally, 161 complaints of side effects were noted. After step-down therapy, 18% of the side effects were reported unchanged, 26% were significantly decreased, and 56% were completely absent.

Withdrawal syndromes after cessation of antihypertensive therapy

Hart and Anderson[44] from Dallas, Texas, reviewed publications concerning sudden withdrawal of antihypertensive drugs, including beta blockers, methyldopa, clonidine hydrochloride, guanabenz, and bethanidine sulfate. Most commonly, the withdrawal syndromes were limited to nervousness, tachycardia, headache, and nausea 36–72 hours after cessation of the drug. Only in rare patients was there serious exacerbation of myocardial ischemia (beta blockers) or hypertension (clonidine, methyldopa) in the posttreatment period. The withdrawal syndromes generally responded promptly to reinstitution of antihypertensive therapy. The infrequent occurrence of withdrawal syndrome should not discourage use of these efficacious agents.

Houston[45] from Nashville, Tennessee, reviewed prospective studies and case reports having to do with complications of abrupt withdrawal of antihypertensive therapy. His conclusion was that abrupt cessation of antihypertensive therapy is usually without immediate consequence but may be associated with signs or symptoms of enhanced sympathetic activity, severe systemic hypertension, or ischemic cardiovascular events. The syndrome is more common following discontinuation of high doses of centrally acting adrenergic and beta adrenergic blocking drugs or combination antihypertensive therapy, but may occur with a variety of antihypertensive agents. Predisposing factors to the adverse reactions include CAD, severe systemic hypertension, renovascular or high-renin hypertension, and large doses of multiple antihypertensive drugs. Gradual tapering of antihypertensive medications over 7–10 days will usually prevent symptoms and dangerous BP elevation. If a post-discontinuation syndrome develops, it should readily respond to the drug previously discontinued.

RENOVASCULAR HYPERTENSION

Duration of hypertension as a predictor of surgical cure

Hughes and associates[46] from New Haven, Connecticut, and Cleveland, Ohio, searched for clinical predictors that might complement the usefulness of renal vein renins (RVR) in selecting patients for successful surgical correction of renovascular hypertension. Among 110 patients who underwent corrective surgery for unilateral renovascular hypertension, they found that the pre-operative duration of hypertension was a highly important predictor of postoperative achievement of normotension. Those with <5-year history of hypertension experienced a 78% incidence of successful outcome, as compared with a 25% incidence of a salutary outcome in patients with a longer duration of hypertension. Although the best RVR ratio (1.4) was less predictive of overall surgical success, the prognostic value of this test improved considerably when analysis of RVR ratio results was confined to patients not receiving renin-suppressing agents during RVR sampling and who had technically satisfactory operations. The highest surgical benefit rate occurred in the patients with both a short duration of hypertension and a high RVR ratio. Conversely, patients with a long duration of hypertension and a low RVR ratio exhibited lower surgical success frequency. Therefore, duration of hypertension is an important factor in the preoperative evaluation of appropriate management in patients with renovascular hypertension.

Percutaneous transluminal dilation

Grim and associates[47] from Indianapolis, Indiana, treated 26 patients with renal vascular hypertension by percutaneous transluminal dilation: 21 were followed for >1 year; 18 underwent repeat angiography. Recurrence of stenosis was shown angiographically in 1 of 6 patients with fibromuscular disease and in all 12 patients with atherosclerotic disease. The procedure was more likely to result in cure of hypertension (6 of 10) in patients with fibromuscular disease than in patients with atherosclerotic disease (1 of 16). Although percutaneous transluminal angioplasty provides the advantages of simplicity, reduced cost, and probably reduced risk, long-term utility of the procedure remains to be established.

ATTITUDES OF PHYSICIANS CONCERNING CONTROVERSIAL ISSUES IN HYPERTENSION

Ten years ago, *Modern Medicine*, under the editorship of Irvine H. Page, distributed questionnaires regarding the definition, work-up, and management of systemic hypertension to 209,000 physicians, 6,747 (3.2%) of whom responded. In light of the report of the Joint National Committee (JNC) on Detection, Evaluation, and Treatment of High BP, the Food and Drug Administration (FDA) and the National Heart, Lung, and Blood Institute (NHLBI) conducted a similar nationwide survey at the end of 1977. Questionnaires were sent to a representative sample of 6,679 physicians, 2,968 (45%) of whom completed them. Traub[48] distributed questionnaires locally concerning comparable issues to 800 physicians and, of the ones returned, 344 (43%) were analyzed. There were differences in the composition of the 3 survey populations. Thus, questionnaires were distributed to all physicians in the *Modern Medicine* poll, to general practitioners, internists, and cardiologists in the FDA survey; faculty members and house staff comprised 50% of the respondents in Traub's poll. Moreover, there were differences in the methods of analyzing the results. In addition, there was a gap of 8–10 years between the first and the last 2 surveys.

These factors may account for some differences in results, but on certain items there were striking similarities. In the initial work-up of hypertensive patients, >90% of the physicians perform a urinalysis (as they did 10 years ago), >90% believe antihypertensive treatment is necessary at diastolic BP levels ⩾105 mmHg and they include a diuretic in the drug therapy for hypertensive patients, while about 45% prescribe drugs for patients with mild hypertension (although it is somewhat differently defined in the 3 studies). Such similarities would suggest that a definite consensus on some items was already established 10 years ago (e.g., the necessity for urinalysis or the benefit from treating moderate and severe hypertension) and that there is a continued lack of consensus on others (e.g., the necessity for drug therapy in mild hypertension at the time of all 3 surveys).

References

1. ADAMS FH, LANDAW EM: What are healthy blood pressures for children? Pediatrics 68:268–270, Aug 1981.
2. ST. JOHN SUTTON MG, SHEPS SG, LIE JT: Prevalence of clinically unsuspected pheochromocytoma: review of a 50-year autopsy series. Mayo Clin Proc. 56:354–360, June 1981.

3. FLORAS JS, HASSAN MO, SEVER PS, JONES JV, OSIKOWSKA B, SLEIGHT P: Cuff and ambulatory blood pressure in subjects with essential hypertension. Lancet 2:107–109, July 1981.

4. GELMAN ML, NEMATI C: A new method of blood pressure recording that may enhance patient compliance. JAMA 246:368–370, July 24/31, 1981.

5. HORAN MJ, PADGETT NE, KENNEDY HL: Ambulatory blood pressure monitoring: recent advances and clinical applications. Am Heart J 101:843–848, June 1981.

6. LETCHER RL, CHIEN S, PICKERING TG, SEALEY JE, LARAGH JH: Direct relationship between blood pressure and blood viscosity in normal and hypertensive subjects: role of fibrinogen and concentration. Am J Med 70:1195–1202, June 1981.

7. MEHTA J, MEHTA P: Platelet function in hypertension and effect of therapy. Am J Cardiol 47:331–334, Feb 1981.

8. PADFIELD PL, BROWN JJ, LEVER AF, MORTON JJ, ROBERTSON JIS: Blood pressure in acute and chronic vasopressin excess: studies of malignant hypertension and the syndrome of inappropriate antidiuretic hormone secretion. N Engl J Med 304:1067–1707, Apr 1981.

9. TUCK ML, SOWERS J, DORNFELD L, KLEDZIK G, MAXWELL M: The effect of weight reduction on blood pressure, plasma renin activity, and plasma aldosterone levels in obese patients. N Engl J Med 304:930–933, Apr 1981.

10. MESSERLI FH, CHRISTIE B, DECARVALHO GR, ARISTIMUNO GG, SUAREZ DH, DRESLINSKI GR, FROHLICH ED: Obesity and essential hypertension: hemodynamics, intravascular volume, sodium excretion, and plasma renin activity. Arch Intern Med 141:81–85, Jan 1981.

11. SAUNDERS JB, BEEVERS DG, PATON A: Alcohol-induced hypertension. Lancet 2:653–656, Sept 1981.

12. JOHNSON CS, GIORGIO AJ: Blood pressure in sickle cell anemia. Arch Intern Med 141:891–893, June 1981.

13. MASTERTON G, MAIN CJ, LEVER AF, LEVER RS: Low blood pressure in psychiatric inpatients. Br Heart J 45:442–446, Apr 1981.

14. WALLACE JD, LEVY LL: Blood pressure after stroke. JAMA 246:2177–2180, Nov 13, 1981.

15. KANNEL WB, WOLF PA, McGEE DL, DAWBER TR, McNAMARA P, CASTELLI WP: Systolic blood pressure, arterial rigidity, and risk of stroke. The Framingham Study. JAMA 245:1225–1229, March 27, 1981.

16. COHEN A, HAGAN AD, WATKINS J, MITAS J, SCHVARTZMAN M, MAZZOLENI A, COHEN AM, WARREN SE, VIEWEG WVR: Clinical correlates in hypertensive patients with left ventricular hypertrophy diagnosed with echocardiography. Am J Cardiol 47:335–341, Feb 1981.

17. DRESLINSKI GR, MESSERLI FH, DUNN FG, SUAREZ DH, PROHLICH ED: Patterns of left ventricular adaptation in borderline and mild essential hypertension. Chest 80:592–595, Nov 1981.

18. SHAPIRO LM, MACKINNON J, BEEVERS DG: Echocardiographic features of malignant hypertension. Br Heart J 46:374–379, Oct 1981.

19. DRESLINSKI GR, FROHLICH ED, DUNN FG, MESSERLI FH, SUAREZ DH, REISIN E: Echocardiographic diastolic ventricular abnormality in hypertensive heart disease: atrial emptying index. Am J Cardiol 47:1087–1090, May 1981.

20. HORAN MJ, KENNEDY HL, PADGETT NE: Do borderline hypertensive patients have labile blood pressure? Ann Intern Med 94:466–468, Apr 1981.

21. MESSERLI FH, FROHLICH ED, SUAREZ DH, REISIN E, DRESLINSKI GR, DUNN FG, COLE FE: Borderline hypertension: relationship between age, hemodynamics and circulating catecholamines. Circulation 64:760–764, Oct 1981.

22. FINN R, McCONNOCHIE K, BOX DEO, FENNERTY AG, GREEN JR: Blood pressure and salt intake: an intra-population study. Lancet 1:1097, May 1981.

23. PARFREY PS, WRIGHT P, GOODWIN JF, VANDENBURG MJ, HOLLY JMP, EVANS SJW: Blood pressure and hormonal changes following alteration in dietary sodium and potassium in mild essential hypertension. Lancet 1:59–63, Jan 1981.

24. PARFREY PS, WRIGHT P, HOLLY JMP, EVANS SJW, CONDON K, VANDENBURG MJ, GOODWIN JF, LEDINGHAM JM: Blood pressure and hormonal changes following alteration in dietary sodium

and potassium in young men with and without a familial predisposition to hypertension. Lancet 1:113–117, Jan 1981.

25. SKRABAL F, AUBOCK J, HORTNAGL H: Low sodium/high potassium diet for prevention of hypertension: probable mechanisms of action. Lancet 2:895–900, Oct 1981.

26. RAM CVS, GARRETT BN, KAPLAN NM: Moderate sodium restriction and various diuretics in the treatment of hypertension. Arch Intern Med 141:1015–1019, July 1981.

27. WILCOX RG, HAMPTON JR: Comparative study of atenolol, metoprolol, metoprolol durules, and slow-release oxprenolol in essential hypertension. Br Heart J 46:498–502, Nov 1981.

28. FERLINZ J, EASTHOPE JL, HUGHES D, SIEGEL J, TOBIS J, ARONOW WS: Right ventricular performance in essential hypertension after beta-blockade. Br Heart J 46:23–29, July 1981.

29. BERGLUND G, ANDERSSON O: Beta-blockers or diuretics in hypertension? A six year follow-up of blood pressure and metabolic side effects. Lancet 1:744–747, Apr 1981.

30. PEART WS, BARNES GR, BROUGHTON P, DOLLERY CT, GREEN KG, GREENBERG G, HUDSON MF, LEVER AF, MEADE TW, ROSE GA, MIALL WE: Adverse reactions to bendrofluazide and propranolol for the treatment of mild hypertension: report of Medical Research Council Working Party on Mild to Moderate Hypertension. Lancet 2:539–542, Sept 1981.

31. VANDER ELST E, DOMBEY SL, LAWRENCE J, VLASSAK W: Controlled comparison of the effects of furosemide and hydrochlorothiazide added to propranolol in the treatment of hypertension. Am Heart J 102:734–740, Oct 1981.

32. MILLAR-CRAIG MW, MANN S, BALASUBRAMANIAN V, CASHMAN P, RAFTERY EB: Effects of chronic beta-blockade on intraarterial blood pressure during motor car driving. Br Heart J 45:643–648, June 1981.

33. MASSIE BM, CHAN S: Antihypertensive therapy with prazosin in patients with left ventricular dysfunction: improvement in cardiac performance and exercise tolerance. Chest 80:692–697, Dec 1981.

34. VETERANS ADMINISTRATION COOPERATIVE STUDY GROUP ON ANTIHYPERTENSIVE AGENTS: Comparison of prazosin with hydralazine in patients receiving hydrochlorothiazide: a randomized, double-blind clinical trial. Circulation 64:772–779, Oct 1981.

35. FUJITA T, YAMASHITA N, YAMASHITA K: Effects of angiotensin-converting enzyme inhibition on blood pressure and plasma renin activity in essential hypertension. Am Heart J 101:259–263, March 1981.

36. HUANG CM, DEL GRECO F, QUINTANILLA A, MOLTENI A: Comparison of antihypertensive effects of captopril and propranolol in essential hypertension. JAMA 245:478–482, Feb 6, 1981.

37. CODY RJ, BRAVO EL, FOUAD FM, TARAZI RC: Cardiovascular reflexes during long-term converting enzyme inhibition and sodium depletion. Am J Med 71:422–426, Sept 1981.

38. CASE DB, ATLAS SA, SULLIVAN PA, LARAGH JH: Acute and chronic treatment of severe and malignant hypertension with the oral angiotensin-converting enzyme inhibitor captopril. Circulation 64:765–771. Oct 1981.

39. GAVRAS H, WAEBER B, GAVRAS I, BIOLLAZ J, BRUNNER HR, DAVIES RO: Antihypertensive effect of the new oral angiotensin converting enzyme inhibitor "MK-421." Lancet 2:543–546, Sept 1981.

40. BEER N, GALLEGOS I, COHEN A, KLEIN N, SONNENBLICK E, FRISHMAN W: Efficacy of sublingual nifedipine in the acute treatment of systemic hypertension. Chest 79:571–574, May 1981.

41. KAPLAN NM: Whom to treat: The dilemma of mild hypertension. Am Heart J 101:867–870, June 1981.

42. MADHAVAN S, ALDERMAN MH: The potential effect of blood pressure reduction on cardiovascular disease: a cautionary note. Arch Intern Med 141:1583–1588, Nov 1981.

43. FINNERTY FA: Step-down therapy in hypertension: Importance in long-term management. JAMA 246:2593–2596, Dec 4, 1981.

44. HART GR, ANDERSON RJ: Withdrawal syndromes and the cessation of antihypertensive therapy. Arch Intern Med 141:1125–1127, Aug 1981.

45. HOUSTON MC: Abrupt cessation of treatment in hypertension: Consideration of clinical fea-

tures, mechanisms, prevention and management of discontinuation syndrome. Am Heart J 102:415–430, Sept 1981.

46. HUGHES JS, DOVE HG, GIFFORD RW JR, FEINSTEIN AR: Duration of blood pressure elevation in accurately predicting surgical cure of renovascular hypertension. Am Heart J 101:408–413, Apr 1981.

47. GRIM CE, LUFT FC, YUNE HY, KLATTE EC, WEINBERGER MH: Percutaneous transluminal dilatation in the treatment of renal vascular hypertension. Ann Intern Med 95:439–442, Oct 1981.

48. TRAUB YM, MCDONALD RH JR, SHAPIRO AP: Attitudes of physicians concerning controversial issues in hypertension. Arch Intern Med 141:571, Apr 1981.

5

Valvular Heart Disease

MITRAL REGURGITATION

---

*Forward stroke volume from aortic valve echoes
in mitral regurgitation secondary to left ventricular
dysfunction*

Corya and associates[1] from Indianapolis, Indiana, developed a clinically
applicable method for calculating aortic valve stroke volume using the echo
recorded initial and late aortic cusp separation, ejection time, and amplitude of posterior aortic root motion during ejection. The formula was tested
prospectively in 55 patients for whom 65 Fick (n, 26) or thermodilution (n,
39) cardiac output determinations were performed simultaneously with
echo. Aortic valve echo (Fig. 5-1) were recorded in all 55 patients and mitral
valve echo (Fig. 5-2) also were recorded in 48. For the 65 studies, linear correlation (r) was excellent between the aortic valve method and Fick or thermodilution method for stroke volume and for cardiac output. Differences between cardiac output values obtained from aortic valve echo and either Fick
or thermodilution techniques ranged from $-1.4-+1.5$ liters/min and were
normally distributed. Of the computed aortic valve data, 90% was within
15% of the Fick or thermodilution data. Aortic valve stroke volume correlated
well (r = 0.93) with stroke volume derived from mitral valve echo in the pa-

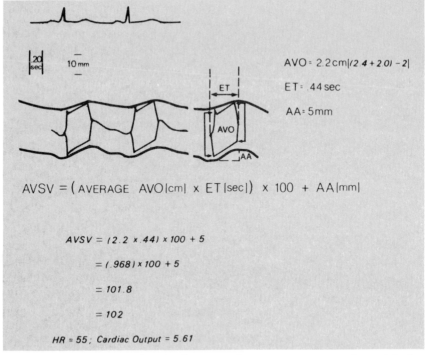

Fig. 5-1. Diagram of aortic valve echo illustrating where measurements are taken and the formula used to calculate aortic valve stroke volume (AVSV). Average aortic valve opening (AVO) is initial plus late aortic cusp separation divided by 2 and measured as internal distance between peripheral-most cusp echoes (cm). ET is ejection time, expressed in seconds and measured as total time aortic valve is open. AA is amplitude (in mm) of echo motion recorded from posterior aortic root during ejection. Heart rate (HR), expressed in beats/min, is calculated by dividing the number 60 by corresponding R-R interval in seconds.

tients without MR, but did not correlate well ($r = 0.78$) in the patients with MR. Mitral valve stroke volume exceeded aortic valve stroke volume by more than 20% in 19 of the 20 patients with MR, as compared with 1 of 28 patients without MR. The presence or absence of ventricular dyssynergy did not alter statistical findings. Data from this study show that 1) aortic valve echo can be used clinically to measure forward stroke volume, and 2) the difference between mitral and aortic valve volume should be a measure of mitral regurgitant flow.

Preoperative left ventricular function in MR: value of end-systolic wall stress systolic ratio

Carabello and associates[2] from Charlottesville, Virginia, evaluated 21 patients with symptomatic, chronic, severe MR without other valvular heart disease or associated CAD to determine which hemodynamic and angiographic factors might be prognostic of surgical outcome. Sixteen patients in

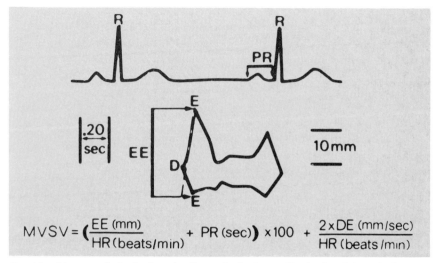

$$MVSV = \left(\frac{EE\ (mm)}{HR\ (beats/min)} + PR\ (sec)\right) \times 100 + \frac{2 \times DE\ (mm/sec)}{HR\ (beats/min)}$$

Fig. 5-2. Diagram of mitral valve echo illustrating both variables (*top*) and formula (*bottom*) used to calculate mitral valve stroke volume (MVSV). EE is measured from outermost echoes of anterior and posterior leaflets. DE is measured as most rapid slope in DE echo. Heart rate (HR) is calculated by dividing the number 60 by R-R interval in seconds.

New York Heart Association functional classes I or II postoperatively formed group A; one patient who remained in class III postoperatively and 4 patients who died perioperatively formed group B. End-diastolic volume index (EDVI) was less for group A than for group B (119 ± 25 ml/m² -vs- 170 ± 28 ml/m²). End-systolic volume index (ESVI) also was lower in group A (39 ± 19 ml/m² -vs- 72 ± 32 ml/m²). The ratio of end-systolic wall stress to end-systolic volume index (ESWS/ESVI) was significantly lower in both groups than in normal persons, indicating relatively greater end-systolic volume at a given wall stress, suggesting LV dysfunction. The ESWS/ESVI ratio in group B (2.2 ± 0.2) was significantly less than in group A (3.3 ± 0.4). The variables of age, PA capillary wedge pressure, EDVI, ESVI, EF, and the ESWS/ESVI ratio were subjected to stepwise discriminant multi-variate analysis to determine if any were independent predictors of outcome, and the only independent predictor determined by this method was the ESWS/ESVI ratio. Thus, the ESWS/ESVI ratio may be helpful in evaluating LV function and operative risk in patients with chronic, symptomatic MR.

MITRAL VALVE PROLAPSE (MVP)

Anthropometric characteristics of women with MVP

Schutte and associates[3] from Dallas, Texas, examined the hypothesis that MVP is often associated with an inherited, anthropometrically distinct habitus. Using standard echo and phonocardiographic techniques, they identified 60 subjects with MVP, 21 first-degree relatives (12 with MVP and 9 normal), and a control group of 57 women. Patients with "silent" (echo only) MVP or the Marfan syndrome were excluded. Analysis of measurements taken of the first 39 patients and 46 control subjects revealed that, in relation to their height, patients with MVP had narrower anteroposterior chest diameters and longer arm spans than did the women in the control group. Linear discriminant analysis produced the equation: $Z = 17.511 + 98.6$ (anteroposterior chest diameter/height) $- 27.3$ (arm span/height). Those with MVP tended to score below zero (mean, 0.39; $p = 0.001$). The equation was tested prospectively on 53 subjects, including the 21 family members, and correctly classified 75% of all unrelated subjects and 86% of the family members as normal or having MVP. Both MVP and discriminant classification followed an autosomally dominant pattern of inheritance. Thus, a significant proportion of the patients with MVP have an autosomal dominant, inherited anthropometrically distinct habitus suggesting that MVP is only 1 component of a generalized developmental syndrome.

Orthostatic hypotension in MVP

To test the hypothesis that orthostatic hypotension could represent an alternative mechanism contributing to symptoms in patients with MVP, Santos and associates[4] from Rochester, New York, measured the systolic and diastolic arterial BP in the supine and standing positions in 86 patients in whom MVP was confirmed by echo. Orthostatic hypotension was demonstrated in 12 patients, 10 of whom presented with recurrent lightheadedness, dizziness, or syncope. Although 9 of these 10 patients reported transient lightheadedness or dizziness during periods of ambulatory ECG recording, in only 1 were the symptoms chronologically related to cardiac arrhythmias; 8 had lightheadedness and 2 near-syncope during the postural test in association with the orthostatic drop in BP. Improvement in symptoms and correction of the orthostatic hypotension occurred in 7 patients after propranolol. Before therapy, the mean systolic BP dropped from 114 ± 3 mmHg in the supine position to 78 ± 1 mmHg upon standing ($p < 0.001$). In repeated postural tests performed after 4 weeks of treatment, the systolic BP changed from 120 ± 3 mmHg supine to 115 ± 1 mmHg upon standing ($p < 0.01$). Thus, orthostatic hypotension is a commonly recognized mechanism in patients with MVP, particularly in those affected by recurrent lightheadedness, dizziness, or syncope.

Diastolic sounds and murmurs in MVP

The usual auscultatory features associated with MVP include a mid-systolic click that may be followed by a late systolic murmur, a late systolic or holosystolic murmur without a click, or the absence of both click and murmur. The presence of a diastolic sound or murmur in MVP is believed to be decidedly uncommon. Wei and Fortuin,[5] however, studied 9 patients with a systolic click or murmur and echo evidence of MVP, and each in addition had a diastolic sound or an early diastolic murmur best heard at the apex or left sternal border. The sound, which was of high frequency and easily audible, followed A$_2$ by 70–110 ms (mean, 94 ± 5 ms), and coincided with the point where the prolapsed posterior leaflet returned from the left atrium and re-coapted with the anterior leaflet. The diastolic sound occurred 40–60 ms (mean, 53 ± 4 ms) before the E point of the echo and 0 point of the apexcar-diogram, and even longer before the rapid-filling wave. The diastolic mur-mur, also of high frequency, was brief and decrescendo, and simulated AR in 2 patients. Thus, MVP may be associated with a sound or murmur in dias-tole. When a diastolic sound or murmur is best heard apically, even if accom-panied by a systolic murmur, MVP should be considered.

Effect of congesting cuffs on the echo-phonocardiographic findings in MVP

Postural changes, tilting, and nitrite administration move the clicks and systolic murmurs earlier in systole in patients with MVP. The explanation proposed for this movement is a decrease in LV volume that allows earlier prolapse of the mitral leaflets toward the left atrium. The application of con-stricting pneumatic cuffs (tourniquets) represents a simple common nonin-vasive procedure whereby venous return is diminished without any drug in-tervention. To evaluate the changes in LV volume and its effect on the systolic click and murmur, Abinader and Oliven[6] from Haifa, Israel, performed simultaneous phonocardiogram and echo in 16 patients with late systolic murmurs, before and after inflation of tourniquets on the upper and lower extremities. The tourniquet administration, known to reduce the venous re-turn, caused a statistically significant movement of the phonocardiographi-cally recorded click toward the first heart sound, associated with reduction of the echo LV and RV and left atrial dimensions. These findings confirm the relation between MVP and LV dimension and suggest that a decrease in LV volume is a tenable explanation for the earlier onset of prolapse.

Systolic anterior motion in the absence of cardiac disease or in the presence of MVP

Systolic anterior motion (SAM) of the mitral valve in the absence of asym-metric septal hypertrophy (ASH) or concentric LV hypertrophy has been re-ported in several conditions other than HC. Gardin and associates[7] from Chi-cago, Illinois, described clinical and echo findings in 15 patients with SAM without associated organic heart disease (10 patients) or in association with MVP (5 patients). Cross-sectional echo disclosed the etiology of SAM in both groups to be early systolic anterior angular motion ("buckling") of mitral chordal structures, rather than movement of the body of the anterior mitral leaflet into the LV outflow tract. In contrast to the patients without asso-ciated organic heart disease, the patients with MVP had auscultatory evi-dence of MVP, a slightly greater mean LV EF, and a greater mean diastolic mitral valve excursion. This spectrum of mitral excursion and LV EF supports the concept that MVP may have as its basis a mitral valve abnormality and/or a hyperdynamic state that predisposes to both chordal buckling and MVP.

Apical cross-sectional echo
in diagnosis of MVP

In light of the nonspecificity of LV angiography and physical examination and the limitations of M-mode echo to define the presence of MVP syndrome, Morganroth and associates[8] from Philadelphia, Pennsylvania, evaluated LV longitudinal and apical 4-chamber tomographic views of cross-sectional echoes in 19 subjects with normal LV cineangiography and in 5 patients with dilated cardiomyopathy. None had auscultatory findings suggestive of MVP syndrome. In all 24 control subjects, the apical view demonstrated the coaptation point and leaflets of the mitral valve to lie inside the LV cavity. A retrospective analysis of 900 consecutive cross-sectional echo studies revealed 105 subjects with no evidence of structural heart disease other than the presence of MVP. Both mitral leaflets were prolapsed in 90% and the apical tomographic cross-sectional echo view was superior to the LV longitudinal view for the detection of anterior leaflet prolapse. These data suggest that the apical cross-sectional view may be the single best technique to define the presence of MVP, and it is much superior to M-mode echo (Table 5-1).

Observer variation in the angiocardiographic
diagnosis of MVP

Kennett and associates[9] from Columbia, Missouri, assessed the reliability of the angiographic diagnosis of MVP by measuring agreement between observers using defined diagnostic criteria. They selected 60 high-quality left ventriculograms, many of which included possible examples of MVP, and these were reviewed by 3 angiographers. Disagreement between observers as to positivity of MVP occurred in 26% and 30% of the cases on 2 reviews, and disagreement as to specific scallop involvement occurred in 68% and 78% of the cases reviewed. A specific intraobserver agreement was positive 80% of

TABLE 5-1. *M-mode echo findings in 99 patients with MVP detected by cross-sectional echo. Reproduced with permission from Morganroth et al.*[8]

	MILD CASES (20)	MODERATE CASES (49)	SEVERE CASES (30)
Age	33.8 ± 16.7	38.9 ± 16.8	42.3 ± 16.5
Sex (% Female)	55	58	70
AO/LA	1.02 ± 0.12	0.96 ± 0.19	0.96 ± 0.22
LV (Dd)	4.80 ± 0.59	4.52 ± 0.45	4.65 ± 0.81
SAM	1/20 (5.0%)	2/48 (4.1%)	5/30 (16.7%)
Holosystolic hammocking	0/20 (0.0%)	17/48 (35.4%)	16/30 (53.3%)
No evidence of MVP	2/20 (10%)	4/49 (8%)	2/30 (6%)

AO = aortic. LA = left atrium. LV (Dd) = left ventricular end-diastolic diameter. SAM = systolic anterior motion of the anterior mitral leaflet.

the time, and in the interpretation of specific scallop involvement, 55%–90% of the time. These results indicate that, in the absence of generally agreed upon quantitative angiographic criteria for the diagnosis of MVP, there is considerable variability among observers in the interpretation of MVP by angiographic studies. In an accompanying editorial by Ginzton and Criley[10] from Torrance, California, the authors utilized the data collected by Kennett and associates to reinforce their view that cineangiography is seldom necessary in the diagnosis of MVP and, indeed, is often misleading and confusing. Ginzton and Criley emphasized that a firm clinical diagnosis of MVP can be established by reproducible findings of a mobile mid-systolic click and a late systolic murmur and they would not be dissuaded by a nondiagnostic echo or cineangiogram. A deficiency of the paper by Kennett and associates is that they did not state how many of their patients had auscultatory or echo evidence of MVP.

Recurrent ectopic junctional tachycardia in MVP

Enhanced AV nodal rhythmicity that is moderately accelerated (70–130 beats/min), lacks sudden onset and abrupt termination, and is accompanied by the presence of AV dissociation has been termed *nonparoxysmal junctional tachycardia*. This arrhythmia typically occurs in digitalis excess, acute rheumatic fever, posterior AMI and after cardiac operations. Goren and associates[11] from Chicago, Illinois, reported the electrophysiologic evaluation of an 11-year-old-girl with MVP in whom the arrhythmia had been documented at age 4 years. The electrophysiologic findings resembled those seen in experimental animal models of triggered automaticity. Triggered automaticity has been described in fibers from the mitral valve of monkeys and in the fibers of the canine coronary sinus. In the patient described by Goren and associates, the rate dependency of tachycardia, its relation to conditions with increased sympathetic activity, and its response to the administration of a beta blocking agent resembled some of the above-described characteristics of the animal models of triggered automaticity.

Conduction system in MVP with sudden death

Despite the frequent occurrence of arrhythmias in MVP, the conduction system in patients with sudden death and MVP has rarely been studied. Bharati and associates[12] from Chicago, Illinois, studied by serial histologic sections a 45-year-old-man who, by Holter monitoring, had frequent VPC and several episodes of rapid nonsustained VT. He died suddenly a year after that study and the posterior mitral leaflet was redundant and the anulus calcified. Histologic studies disclosed marked fatty infiltration of the approaches to the sinus and AV nodes and in the atrial preferential pathways. The AV node was compressed either by the enlarged left atrium, mitral orifice or by calcium in the abnormally formed central fibrous body. The branching bundle lay mostly on the right side of the summit of the ventricular septum. The right part of the bifurcation continued into the right bundle-branch, but some fibers of the left bundle terminated just beneath the summit. The authors believe that some or all of these histologic abnormalities could be related to the episodes of VT.

Platelets, thromboembolism and MVP

Cerebral and retinal ischemic events have been described in MVP. To determine whether platelets play a part in the pathogenesis of thromboembolism, Walsh and associates[13] from Philadelphia, Pennsylvania, studied 29 patients with MVP, including 9 (group I) with thromboembolism (cerebral, retinal, and deep venous), 8 (group II) with transient visual obscurations, and 12 (group III) with neither thromboembolism nor visual complaints. The incidence of platelet coagulant hyperactivity in patients with MVP was 76% (100% in group I, 75% in group II, 58% in group III), as compared with 6% in 18 control patients. These results suggest that platelets play a role in the purported association of thromboembolism and MVP.

MVP in hyperthyroidism

Channick and associates[14] from Philadelphia, Pennsylvania, studied 40 patients with hyperthyroidism; 9 were hyperthyroid at the time of study, and 31 had received treatment and were no longer hyperthyroid. The interval between treatment of hyperthyroidism and the present study ranged from 6 months–18 years (average, 7 years): 16 of the 31 treated patients were taking thyroid hormone at the time of the study. The findings in the patients with hyperthyroidism at some time were compared with those in 40 control subjects without thyroid disease but of similar age and sex. All 40 patients had both M-mode and 2-D echoes. Of the 40 patients with hyperthyroidism, 17 (43%) had MVP, as compared with 7 (18%) of the 40 controls (p < 0.05). No significant differences were observed in the prevalence of MVP between men and women or between white and black subjects in either the study or the control group. The prevalence of MVP did not differ significantly between those patients who were hyperthyroid in the past, those who had become hypothyroid after treatment, and those who remained euthyroid or between those who were taking thyroid hormone and those who were not. The explanation for the increased frequency of MVP in patients with hyperthyroidism is unclear, because palpitations, tachycardia, and other cardiac arrhythmias, with nervousness and anxiety, may be manifestations of either MVP or hyperthyroidism. Mistakenly attributing these symptoms to thyroid disease rather than to MVP may lead to unnecessary testing for hyperthyroidism and, possibly, to inappropriate treatment. Because prophylactic antibiotic treatment is usually recommended for patients with MVP at the time of dental or surgical procedures, physicians should look carefully for this cardiac abnormality in patients with a history of hyperthyroidism.

MVP in type IV Ehlers-Danlos syndrome

To evaluate whether abnormal production of type III collagen, the characteristic biochemical feature of patients with type IV Ehlers-Danlos syndrome, consistently predisposes to MVP, Jaffe and associates[15] from St. Louis, Missouri, evaluated the family of a proband with classic type IV Ehlers-Danlos syndrome. Production of type III collagen was assessed with the use of cultured skin fibroblasts. MVP was detected by M-mode and 2-D echo. Biochemical abnormalities in the production of type III collagen and echo findings of MVP were completely concordant. All patients with abnormal production of type III collagen had MVP and all subjects with normal production of type III collagen had normal echoes. Six of the 8 patients with abnormal production of type III collagen had subtle cutaneous abnormalities. The consistent association of abnormal production of type III collagen and MVP in this family suggests that this abnormality of collagen may give rise to MVP.

MVP and von Willebrand syndromes

Both the MVP and von Willebrand syndromes are forms of mesenchymal dysplasia and the telangiectases, angiodysplasias, and skeletal distortions described in such patients represent genetically determined gross defects that are complementary to the inability of the vascular endothelium to produce factor VIII-related antigen and factor VIII ristocetin-aggregating factor. In heritable disorders of connective tissue, bleeding secondary to multiple events occurs simultaneously with skeletal and vascular anomalies, particularly in the Ehlers-Danlos and Marfan syndromes, and MVP is frequent in both entities. The inherent featues of MVP, with its familial inheritance, associated skeletal deformities, and valvular changes, suggested that it, too, could be grouped with diseases of abnormal mesenchyme. Pickering and associates[16] from Philadelphia, Pennsylvania, searched for MVP by 2-D echo in 15 patients with von Willebrand syndromes to test the hypothesis that this bleeding disorder is actually a mesenchymal dysplasia that resembles other heritable disorders of connective tissue. MVP was found in 9 of the 15 patients, as compared with 4 of 30 sex-matched and age-matched healthy controls ($p < 0.01$). The complex of a von Willebrand syndrome and MVP may be an example of a newly recognized category of related coagulation and cardiovascular disorders.

MVP in mitral stenosis

MVP has been reported to occur in association with MS. Beasley and Kerber[17] from Iowa City, Iowa, determined the frequency with which MS and MVP coexist by studying 20 patients with moderate-to-severe MS. All 20 patients had M-mode and 2-D echo and LV angiograms. M-mode echo criteria for MVP, namely systolic movement posterior to the C-D line, were met in 13 of the 20 patients. In all 13, holosystolic prolapse was suggested by M-mode echo. Two-D echo showed systolic arching of 1 or both leaflets above the AV ring in 4 patients. Subjective evidence of MVP by LV angiogram was present in 5 patients. Using the posterior medial scallop length index, 8 patients were classified as having MVP, but only 4 had angiographic MVP. Two of the 20 patients satisfied all 4 echo and angiographic criteria for MVP. Thus, the coexistence of MVP and MS is relatively uncommon. M-mode echo alone is unreliable in diagnosing MVP when MS is present, since the M-mode criteria for MVP are present in most patients with MS.

Myocardial and urinary taurine in a kindred with MVP and dilated cardiomyopathy

Although MVP and idiopathic dilated cardiomyopathy (IDC) may occur together in any given family, no common biochemical or genetic link has been established between these disorders. Evidence exists that MVP, or at least 1 type of it, is transmitted through autosomal-dominant inheritance. IDC also may be familial, but the pattern of inheritance is less clear. Darsee and Heymsfield[18] from Atlanta, Georgia, and Boston, Massachusetts, found a high incidence of MVP and IDC in a 46-member kindred with consanguineous ancestry (Fig. 5-3). Indeed, 8 progeny in 2 generations had IDC and markedly elevated urinary taurine levels (411–536 mg/g creatinine [normal,

Fig. 5-3. Pedigree of a kindred with a marked incidence of congestive cardiomyopathy and MVP. Fifty-two members are represented (female members are indicated by circles, and males by squares). In the 2nd through 5th generations, 46 consanguineous and 4 nonconsanguineous members are shown; 3 consanguineous members who died before start of investigation are denoted by arrows, and age of each member is given below each symbol. Members with dilated cardiomyopathy are represented by solid symbols, and those with MVP by half-solid symbols. Reproduced with permission from Darsee and Heymsfield.[18]

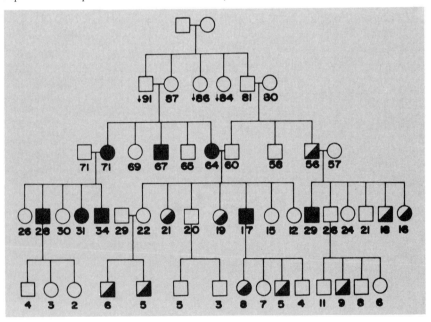

89 ± 32]) and 10 other family members had late or holosystolic MVP and elevated urinary taurine values (215–265 mg/g creatinine). In 2 patients with MVP, IDC eventually developed while the amounts of urinary taurine doubled. One member with MVP died suddenly. The myocardial taurine values in that patient were 17 ± 3 μmol/g protein (normal, 33 ± 4). Four other family members had myocardial fibrosis at autopsy or biopsy and mean myocardial taurine levels of 9 ± 2 μmol/g protein. Thus, hypertaurinuria and depressed levels of taurine in the myocardium may be associated with 1 type of MVP syndrome and a rapidly progressive form of IDC.

Left ventricular function in MVP

The presence of LV contraction abnormalities, chest pain, ventricular arrhythmia, symptoms and ECG abnormalities in patients with MVP has suggested a myocardial component in this condition. To determine systolic LV function in MVP, Gottdiener and associates[19] from Bethesda, Maryland, utilized technetium-99m gated equilibrium radionuclide cineangiography in 47 patients with MVP diagnosed in all 47 by the presence of a mid-systolic click or a late systolic murmur by auscultation and/or the presence of classic findings of MVP on echo. Of the 47 patients, 39 had no MR and the average EF in them was normal at rest (mean, 57 ± 3%; normal, 57 ± 1%) and exceeded the lower limits of normal in all but 1 patient. The EF during maximal exercise, however, was lower in the 39 patients with MVP without MR than in normal subjects (average, 64 ± 2%; normal, 71 ± 2%). Of the 8 patients with MVP and MR, the average EF was normal at rest, but was diminished with exercise, in comparison both with normal subjects and patients with MVP without MR. Chest pain, arrhythmia, and the pattern or extent of MVP on echo were not independently associated with impaired LV functional reserve. Thus, although many patients with MVP have normal LV function, there is a subgroup without MR in whom diminished LV functional reserve is present.

In contrast to the findings by Gottdiener and associates,[19] Newman and colleagues[20] from Durham, North Carolina, evaluated by RNA 34 patients with MVP, 11 of whom (their group III) had associated coronary narrowing by coronary angiography, 12 of whom (their group II) had normal coronary arteries by angiography, and 11 of whom (their group IV) had MVP diagnosed only by echo; there was no clinical evidence of CAD, but no coronary angiography was performed. The findings in these 34 patients were compared with those in 11 patients who had neither MVP nor CAD, as determined by angiography. Their findings are summarized in Table 5-2. In their patients in groups I, II, and IV, the EF and stroke volume increased with exercise. In 6 of the 11 patients with MVP and documented CAD, the EF and stroke volume decreased with exercise, and these patients had wall motion abnormalities detected only during exercise. Thus, this study suggests that MVP alone has no detrimental effect on LV function during rest and exercise and that exercise-induced abnormalities in LV function are related to the presence and severity of CAD and not to MVP.

TABLE 5-2. *Effect of exercise on LV EF and stroke volume in MVP with or without coronary narrowing (from Newman et al[20]).*

				EXERCISE	
GROUP	# Pts	MVP	CAD	EF	SV
I	11	0	0	↑	↑
II	12	+[a]	0	↑	↑
III	11	+[a]	+	↓	↑
IV	11	+[b]	−[c]	↑	↑

[a] Diagnosed by auscultation ± echo; [b] Diagnosed by echo; [c] No clinical evidence of myocardial ischemia. Abbreviations: CAD = coronary narrowing by angiography; SV = stroke volume.

Coronary spasm in MVP and its relation to chest pain

Chest pain is a frequent symptom in patients with MVP. The associated findings of abnormal resting and stress ECGs and ventricular arrhythmias have caused several investigators to postulate an ischemic mechanism for the pain, despite the fact that most patients with MVP have normal coronary arteries by angiogram. A commonly held view contends that traction on the papillary muscles during ventricular systole produces ischemia of these structures and of adjacent subendocardium. Recently, coronary spasm has been suggested as a cause of the chest pain in MVP. Mautner and associates[21] from New Orleans, Louisiana, performed coronary angiograms in 14 patients with MVP, all of whom had recurrent chest pain as their chief complaint. The chest pain had been serious enough in all 14 patients to warrant at least 2 previous emergency visits to medical facilities in the 6 months preceding the coronary angiogram. At catheterization, all had normal LV function and only 1 had a significant fixed obstruction of a major coronary artery. Seven of the 14 patients had evidence of coronary spasm during catheterization; 5 of these 7 had histories highly suggestive of coronary spasm. During the procedure, spasm occurred spontaneously in 3 patients, was ergonovine-induced in 2, and was catheter-tip-induced in 2. Ergonovine was administered to 9 of the 14 patents and induced vasospasm in 2. Of the 7 patients who showed no evidence of spasm, 4 had typical chest pain in association with reversible ST-segment elevation and manifested a variant anginal syndrome. Thus, this study suggests that coronary spasm plays an important role in causing chest pain in some patients with MVP.

Tricuspid valve prolapse with MVP

It is well recognized that tricuspid valve prolapse (TVP) occurs in 20%–50% of patients with MVP, as determined by morphologic or angiographic criteria. Mardelli and associates[22] from Philadelphia, Pennsylvania, evaluated the prevalence of TVP in patients with MVP with 2 cross-sectional echo views, utilizing the apical and longitudinal RV inflow tract views to investi-

TABLE 5-3. *Clinical information in both groups. Reproduced with permission from Mardelli et al.*[22]

	TRICUSPID AND MVP (31) %	MVP (33) %
Age (yrs)	42 ± 22	37 ± 18
Women	21/31 (68)	25/33 (76)
Chest pains	13/22 (59)	11/26 (42)
Palpitations	16/22 (73)	13/26 (50)
Dizziness/syncope	12/20 (60)	10/26 (38)
Fatigue/weakness	15/20 (75)	7/26 (27)*
SOB	10/21 (48)	8/26 (31)
Clicks	12/19 (63)	7/25 (28)*
Murmur	16/26 (62)	15/25 (60)
ST-T changes	10/26 (39)	9/20 (45)
IRBBB	3/26 (12)	2/20 (10)
Ventricular arrhythmias	4/25 (16)	4/20 (20)
Supraventricular arrhythmias	8/25 (32)	4/20 (20)
Severe bony thorax deformity	8/26 (31)	0/26 (0)*
M-mode echo data		
LV end diastolic diameter, cm	4.5 ± 0.5	4.6 ± 0.6
Left atrial end-systolic diameter, cm	3.1 ± 1.0	2.9 ± 1.0
Aortic root end-systolic diameter, cm	3.0 ± 0.3	3.0 ± 0.4
Excursion of mitral valve (DE), cm	2.2 ± 0.4	2.3 ± 0.3

* $p < 0.02$ (Chi square analyses). IRBB indicates incomplete right bundle branch block.

gate the tricuspid valve in 64 patients with MVP and in 16 controls who had neither angiographic nor echo evidence of MVP. The tricuspid valve leaflets and their coaptation point in systole were below (towards the RV apex) the level of the tricuspid valve ring in systole in all controls. TVP, defined as the leaflet(s) of the tricuspid valve lying above the tricuspid valve ring within the right atrium, was seen in 31 (48%) of 64 patients with MVP (Table 5-3). The RV inflow tract view demonstrated TVP most readily, as compared with the apical view, and 29 of the 31 patients with TVP had prolapse of at least 2 leaflets of the tricuspid valve. The 31 patients with both MVP and TVP, when compared with the 33 patients with MVP alone, had more symptoms and abnormal physical findings.

Ebstein's anomaly of the tricuspid valve with MVP

The hearts from 10 patients with Ebstein's anomaly of the tricuspid valve were examined at necropsy by Cabin and Roberts[23] for abnormalities of the mitral valve. Five patients were aged 18–72 years (mean, 36); all had focal fibrous thickening of the mitral leaflets and 3 had prolapse of one or both mitral leaflets. Only one of the 3 patients with MVP had an ASD (secundum type), indicating that the association of MVP with Ebstein's anomaly is not due to the presence of an ASD.

Surgical treatment of mitral regurgitation from MVP

Yacoub and associates[24] from London, England, reported results of operative treatment of 132 patients with MR from MVP. MVR with an antibiotic-sterilized fresh aortic homograft was done in 46 patients, and valve repair in 86 patients. More than 80% of patients in both groups were in functional class III or IV preoperatively and most patients in both groups had ruptured chordae tendineae from the posterior leaflets. Repair, rather than MVR, was done if there was prolapse of the posterior leaflet, with or without chordal rupture, with rectangular resection of the responsible segment of leaflet. Ruptured chordae to the anterior leaflet were treated by excision of the triangular flail segment, retention of normal chordal attachments of the remaining leaflet tissue, and suturing of the defect. No prosthetic rings were used. The repaired valve was tested for residual MR while the heart was actively beating and the LV systolic pressure was 100–120 mmHg. Of the 46 patients having MVR, 5 (11%) died early and 15 (32%) late; of the 86 patients having valve repair, 4 (5%) died early and 5 died (7%) late. Actuarial survival at 5 years was 62% in the MVR group and 90% in the repair group. In the MVR group, 5 patients had bioprosthetic valve failure and 4 required reoperation. Two patients in the repair group developed significant MR and required reoperation. Two patients in the repair group had thromboembolism. Most patients were functionally class I after operation.

Thus, the results from MVR for MR from MVP are poor with use of fresh homograft bioprostheses, but long-term results from mitral repair procedures are good. Whether or not the use of an anuloplasty ring with their repair would have improved results further is unclear.

MITRAL STENOSIS

New formula for calculating area of stenotic cardiac valve from hemodynamic data

Since 1951, the hemodynamic evaluation of the severity of valvular stenosis has relied on the estimation of valve orifice areas, using the equation of Gorlin and Gorlin first published in 1951. The formula states that the valve area (in cm²) is equal to the flow across the valve (in ml/s) divided by the product of 2 constants and the square-root of pressure difference across the valve. One of the constants is the discharge coefficient, which is an empirical constant with an assumed arbitrary value of 1.0 for the aortic valve and 0.7 for the mitral valve. The second constant is 44.5, which is equal to the square-root of twice the gravity acceleration factor (980 cm/s/s). The flow across the valve is equal to the cardiac output (in ml/min) divided by the product of the heart rate (beats/min) and the systolic ejection period or diastolic filling period (s/beat). In 1972, Cohen and Gorlin revised the original formula and suggested the use of 0.85 as the discharge coefficient for the mitral valve (instead of 0.7). Because the original formula is cumbersome and time-consuming, it is rarely used by cardiologists who are not involved with hemodynamic measurements. Hakki and associates[25] from Philadelphia, Pennsylvania, simplified the Gorlin formula and described their results by both the original and simplified formulas as applied to 100 patients with either MS or AS. The valve area was measured by the simplified formula as cardiac output (liters/min) divided by the square-root of pressure differences across the valve. In patients with AS of varying severity, there was an excellent correlation between the original Gorlin formula and the simplified one ($r = 0.96$, $p < 0.001$). The correlation was unchanged when the peak gradient was used instead of the mean gradient in the simplified formula. Excellent correlation also was seen in patients with MS of varying severity ($r = 0.94$, $p < 0.001$). The simplicity of the formula makes it easy to memorize and use.

New formula for calculating area of stenotic mitral valve from echo

Most investigators have had difficulty in quantitating the orifice area by M-mode and 2-D echo in patients with MS. Seitz and Furukawa[26] from Vienna, Austria, and Kyoto, Japan formulated a mitral valve orifice equation from the echo measurable variables of stroke volume (SV) and diastolic filling period (DFP) by the formula, $A = 21 (SV)/(DFP)^2$. The mitral valve area computed from this M-mode echo measurement correlated well ($r = 0.90$) with mitral valve area calculated by the Gorlin formula in the resting state in patients with MS. Thus, in the absence of wall irregularities, the mitral valve area may be quantified on the basis of M-mode echo.

Left atrial thrombus in mitral stenosis: detection by echo or coronary angiography

Although both M-mode and 2-D echo are well-established methods in diagnosing MS, both methods have proved disappointing in diagnosing left atrial thrombi, particularly the M-mode technique. Schweizer and associates[27] from Aachen, West Germany, performed both M-mode and 2-D echo in 111 patients with MS, 92 of whom shortly thereafter underwent open-heart operations on the mitral valve. In 5 of the 111 patients, left atrial thrombi were identified by echo; all 5 were diagnosed by 2-D echo and only 3 of the 5 by M-mode echo.

Arteriographic findings of neovascularity and formation of a fistula from the coronary arteries to the left atrium have occasionally been reported in association with atrial thrombosis in patients with MS. To establish the diagnostic value of these findings, Colman and associates[28] from Santander, Spain, evaluated preoperative coronary angiograms in 507 patients who underwent open mitral valve operations for MS. Atrial thrombi were present in 76 patients (15%) (Table 5-4). In the 30 patients with angiographic neovas-

TABLE 5-4. *Clinical data in 76 patients with mitral valve disease and atrial thrombus.*

Age (yrs)	
Mean ± standard deviation	50 ± 5
Range	41–62
Sex (women/men)	44/32
Functional class	
I	1
II	19
III	42
IV	14
Systemic embolism	31 (41%)
Previous mitral valve surgery	3 (4%)
Rhythm	
Sinus rhythm	1
Atrial fibrillation	75 (99%)
Mitral valve disease	
Mitral stenosis	25 (46%)
Mixed mitral valve disease	41 (54%)
Calcification	
Valve	30 (39%)
Atrial wall	18 (24%)

cularity and fistula formation, the thrombi always arose from the circumflex coronary artery and none of the 30 patients had atherosclerotic CAD. Left atrial thrombosis was present in 25 of these 30 patients. Thus, the coronary angiogram predicted the presence of left atrial thrombus with a predictive accuracy of 83%, a specificity of 99%, and a sensitivity of 33%.

Right ventricular function

Until recently, the dynamic geometry and pump function of the pressure-overloaded RV in patients with MS and pulmonary hypertension had not been well defined. With use of a recently developed method for calculating RV volume in humans, Wroblewski and associates[29] from Philadelphia, Pennsylvania, assessed RV performance by computer-analyzed biplane right ventriculograms in 7 normal subjects and in 8 patients with MS and moderate pulmonary hypertension. The patients with MS and elevated systolic RV pressures (mean, 25 ± 2 mmHg for normal subjects, 57 ± 6 mmHg for patients with MS), but normal values for RV end-diastolic volume index (normal subjects = 95 ± 11 ml/m^2, patients = 81 ± 9 ml/m^2) and EF (normal subjects = 0.49 ± 0.02, patients = 0.58 ± 0.04). Comparison of RV function using group performance curves of stroke work -vs- end-diastolic volume revealed the slope of the MS line to be significantly greater than that of the normal line. A plot of RV stroke volume -vs- end-diastolic volume, which removes pressure from the performance index, revealed that the 2 groups had similar performance indices. LV function measured by EF was reduced in MS. These data suggest that the RV performs normally in patients with MS with moderate pulmonary hypertension and maintains normal size and EF.

Open mitral commissurotomy: results

Gross and associates[30] from New York City reviewed results of open (with cardiopulmonary bypass) mitral commissurotomy in 202 patients operated on from 1967–1978: 144 patients underwent isolated mitral commissurotomy and 58 patients had other cardiac procedures. Closed mitral commissurotomy had been performed previously in 7% and preoperative thromboembolic events occurred in 25% of the patients. The operative mortality was 2% and the late mortality, 3%. Follow-up data from 1–122 months were obtained in 98%. Actuarial survival analysis indicated a cumulative annual mortality of 1%, with a 92% projected survival at 10 years. Anticoagulants were used in 40 of 197 patients postoperatively, with a cumulative annual complication rate of 1%, while the rate of thromboembolic phenomena was 0.3%. The overall frequency of embolic events clinically was small and did not correlate with the cardiac rhythm or anticoagulation therapy, despite a 20% occurrence of left atrial thrombus at operation. Subsequent MVR for MR was performed in 12 patients (6%). Residual MS or MR were the indications for subsequent MVR. Ninety percent of the patients were in functional classes I or II postoperatively.

Vega and colleagues[31] from Santander, Spain, reported results of open mitral commissurotomy in 163 patients. Their operative mortality was 1%, and the late mortality rate was 0.2% per patient-year. Only 2 patients required a later operation, 3 patients had a systemic embolus later, and all survivors were functional class I or II. Thus, excellent results can be obtained with open mitral commissurotomy. The postoperative thromboembolism rate is low and anticoagulation postoperatively is usually not required.

MITRAL ANULAR CALCIUM

Formation of a complete circle or "O" configuration

Mitral anular calcium (MAC) is a common occurrence in hearts of older persons in the Western World. The MAC on radiograph generally is "J-," "C-," or "U"-shaped because it is located nearly always entirely in or below the anulus of the posterior mitral leaflet. Roberts and Waller[32] from Bethesda, Maryland, described 2 patients in whom the MAC not only was located in and beneath the anulus of the posterior mitral leaflet, but extended across the ventricular aspect of the anterior leaflet to form a complete calcific circle or "O". These 2 patients were the only ones encountered by these 2 authors in >200 other patients studied at necropsy with MAC.

Causing mitral stenosis

For years, pathologists suspected from examination of hearts with heavy mitral anular calcium (MAC) that the mitral orifice in some of these patients was stenotic, i.e., produced a pressure gradient between left atrium and left ventricle. In 1978 Hammer and associates (*Am J Med.* 64:371, 1978) confirmed the presence of MS hemodynamically in 4 patients with MAC. All their 4 patients had small LV cavities and associated obstruction to LV outflow. Those investigators believed that the LV outflow tract obstruction and the small size of the LV cavity had something to do with the obstruction produced at the mitral level. Osterberger and associates[33] from Detroit, Michigan, reported 6 patients with massive MAC and they measured mean diastolic gradients across the mitral valve varying from 6–34 mmHg. Additionally, 3 of their 6 patients also had obstruction to LV outflow with pressure gradients across the aortic valve ranging from 57–100 mmHg. For their 3 patients without obstruction to LV outflow, the mean diastolic gradient across the mitral orifice was 12, 19, and 34 mmHg, respectively. Thus, not only can a gradient occur across the mitral valve in the presence of heavy MAC and associated LV outflow obstruction with relatively small LV cavity, but obstruction at the mitral level may occur in association with MAC in the absence of LV outflow obstruction.

Rapid development

Some conditions predispose to mitral anular calcium (MAC); these include elevation of the systolic LV pressure (systemic hypertension, LV outflow tract obstruction), hyperlipidemia, chronic hypercalcemia (renal disease and hyperparathyroidism), and defects of cardiac connective tissue (Hurler and Marfan syndromes). The length of time it takes to develop extensive MAC has received no attention. DePace and associates[34] from Philadelphia, Pennsylvania, described a 52-year-old man with chronic renal disease who had hemodialysis regularly over a 3-year period. At age 49, before hemodialysis was started, M-mode echo demonstrated no MAC and only minimal thickening of the mitral leaflets. Echo about 3-years later demonstrated MAC and additional thickening of both mitral leaflets. Also, the precordial systolic murmur had increased from grade 1/6 to 3/6 during this period. This case shows that extensive MAC can develop in a 3-year period.

AORTIC VALVE STENOSIS

Volume fraction of left ventricular myofibrils in AS

There is virtually no information correlating quantitative ultrastructural findings with hemodynamic data in patients with AS. Schwarz and associates[35] from Bad Nauheim, West Germany, therefore, examined the ultrastructure of transmural myocardial biopsy tissue from 19 patients with AS and quantitated the intracellular volume fractions of myofibrils (contractile material), sarcoplasm, and mitochondria by electron microscopic morphometry, and the interstitial myocardial fibrosis by light microscopic morphometry. Transmural biopsies of the LV free wall perfused by the LAD coronary artery were obtained during AVR. LV function was analyzed from preoperative right- and left-heart catheterization and angiography. Group 1 consisted of 7 patients with EF >55% and mean left atrial (LA) pressure <15 mmHg. Group 2 consisted of 12 patients with EF <55% and mean LA pressure >15 mmHg. Patients in group 1 had lower LV end-diastolic volume (92 -vs- 145 ml/m², p < 0.05) and lower LV muscle mass (148 -vs- 200 g/m², p < 0.05) than patients in group 2. The volume fraction of myofibrils was higher in group 1 than in group 2 (48% -vs- 42%, p < 0.05), while volume fractions of sarcoplasm (32% -vs- 36%) and mitochondria (21% -vs- 22%) were comparable (p < 0.05). Interstitial myocardial fibrosis did not differ between groups (16% -vs- 15%, p < 0.05). Biopsies from the area perfused by the LAD in 10 additional surgical patients with CAD and moderate LAD narrowing and normal wall motion in the area of LV free wall perfused by the LAD were taken as controls for morphometric data. No significant difference of ultrastructural data was found between group 1 and controls. The volume fraction of myofibrils was lower in group 2 than in controls (42% -vs- 53%, p < 0.001), and the volume fraction of sarcoplasm was higher (36% -vs- 21%, p < 0.001). Mitochondria and interstitial fibrosis did not differ in group 2 and controls (p < 0.05). Thus, intracellular reduction in the volume fraction of myofibrils was the major morphologic finding in LV biopsy samples of patients with decompensated pressure overload.

Calcific embolus to retinal artery in AS

Abrupt occlusion of the central retinal artery by embolus, thrombus, or spasm typically causes abrupt loss of all or part of the visual field in 1 eye. If the visual loss if fleeting, the term "amaurosis fugax" is applied to the syndrome. If the visual deficit persists beyond a day, retinal infarction is presumed to have occurred. The usual conditions associated with occlusion of the central retinal artery include systemic hypertension, diabetes mellitus, diffuse arteriosclerosis, arteritis, localized extracranial cerebrovascular atherosclerotic disease, and valvular heart disease. Calcific emboli from the aortic valve have been recognized for years as a potential complication of aortic valve valvuloplasty or replacement, but spontaneous, clinically important calcific emboli from a stenotic aortic valve is rare. Over a 7-month period, however, Brockmeier and associates[36] from Cincinnati, Ohio, observed 4 patients with AS in whom calcific emboli to a central retinal artery or to 1 of its branches had occurred (Fig. 5-4). Their 4 patients ranged in age from 40–60 years and peak systolic pressure gradients between left ventricle and systemic artery (3 patients) were 45, 50, and 130 mmHg. Heavy calcific deposits were present in the aortic valve in all 4 patients and 2 underwent successful AVR. In each of the 4 patients, the central retinal artery embolus was the presenting manifestation of the presence of AS.

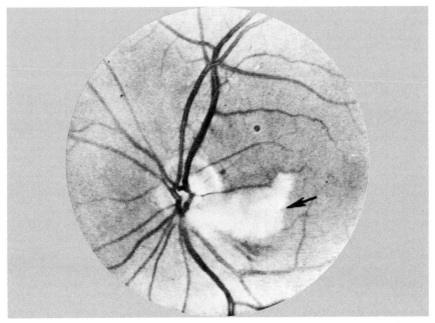

Fig. 5-4. Photograph of left fundus, taken 7 days after onset of visual symptoms, showing wedge-shaped infarction of nerve fiber layer of retina (*arrow*). The arteriolar occlusion is probably at disc margin, obscured by edema. Reproduced with permission from Brockmeier et al.[36]

Assessing its severity by 2-D echo

The severity of AS has been quantitated directly by M-mode echo by measuring aortic cusp separation and by determining the relationship of end-systolic LV wall thickness to LV internal dimension and systolic systemic BP. Although helpful in individual patients, M-mode echo has not been consistently reliable. Two-D echo, however, by providing lateral discrimination and improved spatial orientation, permits examination of the entire aortic valve throughout the cardiac cycle. Godley and associates[37] from Indianapolis, Indiana, studied 81 adults with AS by 2-D echo in the long-axis view. Long-axis systolic aortic cusp separation (MACS) <8 mm was 97% predictive of severe AS and 100% predictive of moderate or severe AS; separation from 8–12 mm had a low predictive value for the severity of AS, and separation >12 mm was 96% predictive of mild AS. Short-axis scans provided a valuable index of severity and were obtainable in 46 patients. When short-axis scans were included in assessment of severity in the subgroup of patients with 8–12 mm MACS, the predictive value improved from 46% to 86%. Direct recording of aortic valve area in the short axis was successful, however, in only 13% of the patients. Thus, the severity of AS can be accurately predicted using the long-axis MACS measurement alone in patients with values <8 mm and

>12 mm. Combining both the long- and short-axis assessment of severity in the 8–12 mm range further enhances the predictive value of the cross-sectional technique.

Rate of left ventricular emptying in AS

The delayed upstroke of the arterial pulse in AS has been attributed, at least in part, to prolonged LV emptying. LV emptying rate, however, has not been measured in AS. Lederman and associates[38] from Philadelphia, Pennsylvania, assessed the rate of LV emptying by computer analysis of biplane cineangiograms in 7 normal subjects, in 6 with mild-to-moderate AS, and in 12 with severe AS. As an indicator of delayed arterial pulse rise, T-time index (time to half-maximum aortic pressure, corrected for heart rate) was measured in each group. T-time index averaged 0.07 ± 0.01 units in normal subjects, 0.14 ± 0.04 in patients with mild-to-moderate AS, and 0.13 ± 0.05 in those with severe AS. Patients with mild-to-moderate and severe AS differed significantly from normal subjects. Relative emptying rates were defined as the percentage of initial systolic volume ejected divided by the percentage of systole elapsed. These relative emptying rates were determined during the first, second, and third thirds of systole in all 3 groups. No significant decrease in the relative rate of LV emptying was noted when each group of patients with AS was compared with the normal subjects. Neither was there slowing in the actual rate of ejection of blood (in ml/s) throughout systole. Thus, the rate of ventricular emptying is normal in AS and the arterial pulse delay cannot be explained by this mechanism.

Effects of nitroprusside in severe AS

The untoward clinical consequences of severe AS are principally due to marked pressure overload imposed on the LV by marked outflow obstruction. In this way, the greatly augmented chronic afterload burden caused by the excessively increased impedance to LV ejection leads to development of CHF as cardiac compensatory mechanisms become overwhelmed, and myocardial ischemia is provoked by the considerably elevated cardiac oxygen requirements resulting from LV hypertrophy as well as increased intramural systolic tension. Therefore, it is logically anticipated that alleviation of LV pressure overloading with its attendant life-threatening complications would prove highly beneficial in this critical setting. Although this goal is successfully achieved by AVR, effective medical therapy has been lacking to reduce the excessive pressure burden on the LV in severe AS. Such a medical approach would be of major clinical importance in improving cardiac deterioration short-term in preparing such patients for safer operative intervention.

Since it has been shown that LV systolic pressure (SP) is ultimately concordant with arterial SP in AS by vasopressors, Awan and associates[39] from Davis and Sacramento, California, evaluated the efficacy of nitroprusside (NP) on LV function, energetics, and myocardial perfusion in 15 severe AS patients. NP infusion (average, 33 μg/min) proved beneficial in each: the average LV SP was reduced from 192 mmHg to 164 mmHg; arterial SP decrement equaled LV SP change; LV end-diastolic pressure declined from 19 mmHg to 10 mmHg; cardiac index (2.7 liters/min/M²) and heart rate were unaltered; total systemic vascular resistance decreased from 1433 dynes · sec · cm⁻⁵ to 1201 dynes · sec · cm⁻⁵; elevated stroke work index diminished from 92 g·m/M² to 74 g·m/M². Simultaneously, LV oxygen consumption decreased, LV diastolic flow was unchanged, and subendocardial perfusion increased. Thus, cautious NP therapy with careful monitoring provides marked reduction of LV afterload and improved LV function, energetics, and coronary flow distribution.

Left ventricular function and 10-year survival after aortic valve replacement for AS in patients ≥age 60 years

Adults with severe AS have an average mortality of about 9%/year. Murphy and associates[40] from Portland, Oregon, analyzed 99 patients aged 60–81 years (mean, 65) with severe AS requiring AVR. Preoperatively, 93% of the 99 patients were in NYHA class III or IV; the average peak systolic pressure gradient across the aortic valve was 76 ± 3 mmHg, the aortic valve index was 0.34 ± 0.01 cm²/m²; average LV systolic pressure was 207 ± 4 mmHg; mean cardiac index was 2.5 ± 0.1 liters/min/M²; LV EF was 0.57 ± 0.02; and LV end-diastolic volume was 408 ± 60 ml/m². The operative mortality was 16%, but that extended back to 1962 when myocardial protection techniques were inferior to those of today. The mean follow-up was 55 ± 4 months. When life-table analysis was used, the 10-year survival (excluding noncardiac deaths) was 57 ± 7%, and 91% of the survivors were in functional class I or II. Thus, the long-term results of AVR in person ≥60 years of age are good.

Gastrointestinal bleeding in AS cured by aortic valve replacement

Sometimes AS is associated with gastrointestinal (GI) bleeding, which may be related to the presence of angiodysplasia of the GI mucosa. Significant bleeding from these lesions appears to occur after chronic underperfusion of the bowel. Danilewitz and associates[41] from Johannesburg, South Africa, and Birmingham, Alabama, described a patient in whom evidence of severe GI bleeding ceased after AVR. Quantitation of blood loss before and after AVR was done by ⁵¹Cr-labeling of the patient's erythrocytes. The patient (a 66-year-old woman) had severe calcific AS. Preoperatively, when the patient was actively bleeding, despite extensive investigation no cause for the GI blood loss was found. It amounted to 176 ml/day (⁵¹Cr-tagged erythrocyte method). Preoperative in-hospital stool blood loss without overt bleeding over a 2-week period was 20 ml/day (normal, <2.0 ml/day). Following AVR, the patient had no evidence of GI bleeding for 14 months. Her average daily blood loss, as measured by stool radioactivity following intravenous injection of ⁵¹Cr-tagged erythrocyes, was <1.5 ml/day. This study indicates the possibility that unexplained GI bleeding of severe magnitude associated with severe AS might be considered an indication for AVR when the blood loss is incapacitating and life-threatening.

AORTIC REGURGITATION

Congenitally bicuspid aortic valve causing severe, pure AR without superimposed infective endocarditis

The congenitally bicuspid aortic valve frequently becomes stenotic, and because most stenotic valves are also regurgitant, the most frequent circumstance in which AR is found with this congenital anomaly is in association with AS. In this situation, the AR is usually of only mild or moderate degree. Also, the congenitally bicuspid aortic valve is often the site of infective endocarditis. Although it may be superimposed on a stenotic congenitally bicuspid aortic valve, infective endocarditis far more commonly involves the previously normally functioning bicuspid valve or the one previously only slightly regurgitant. The usual consequence of the infection in this circumstance is severe pure AR. Mild degrees of pure AR also are commonly observed in patients with a congenitally bicuspid aortic valve and elevated pressure in the ascending aorta from associated aortic isthmic coarctation. However, severe AR due to a nonstenotic and noninfected congenitally bicuspid aortic valve is believed to be decidedly infrequent. Roberts and associates[42] from Bethesda, Maryland, described observations in 13 men who underwent AVR because of severe pure AR unassociated with AS or infective endocarditis and this is the first such report describing this complication of the congenitally bicuspid valve. Among 189 patients having AVR at the National Heart, Lung and Blood Institute because of isolated pure AR, the congenitally bicuspid aortic valve, never the site of infective endocarditis, was responsible for the AR in 13 (7%)

TABLE 5-5. *Etiology of isolated pure AR in 189 patients aged 18–70 years having AVR.*

| | PATIENTS | |
CAUSE	#	%
Rheumatic*	94	49
Infective endocarditis*	41	22
Bicuspid (7)		
Tricuspid (34)		
Marfan and Marfan-type	15	8
Congenital (bicuspid valve)*	13	7
Prolapse from VSD*	10	5
Syphilis	9	5
Aortic dissection	2 ⎫	
Ankylosing spondylitis	2 ⎪	
With subaortic stenosis*	2 ⎬ 7	4
Discrete subaortic stenosis (1)	⎪	
HC (1)	⎪	
Trauma	1 ⎭	
Total	189	100

* Aortic regurgitation resulted from aortic valve abnormality only and not from abnormality of the aorta.

(Table 5-5). This report described certain clinical and morphologic findings in 13 men, aged 26–65 years (mean, 43), who required AVR because of severe AR secondary to noninfected, nonstenotic congenitally bicuspid aortic valve. Although not generally recognized, the noninfected congenitally bicuspid aortic valve is an important cause of pure AR severe enough to warrant AVR.

Significance of a third heart sound in AR

Although acknowledged as an indicator of cardiac decompensation for a century, the ventricular gallop's significance in patients with chronic isolated AR without overt CHF is unclear. Some investigators have associated this sound (S_3) with LV dysfunction and others believe that it reflects only more severe degrees of AR. Abdulla and associates[43] from Augusta, Georgia, examined hemodynamic and clinical data from 42 patients with chronic significant AR and from 31 normal subjects. Of the patients with AR, 28 had a third heart sound gallop and 14 did not. No significant difference in the severity of the AR was noted between the patients with and without an S_3. All patients with an S_3, however, had an abnormally increased LV residual volume and depressed contractile state. Thus, the S_3 gallop in patients with chronic AR reflects LV dysfunction, rather than more severe degrees of AR, and it may, therefore, be useful in selecting patients for cardiac catheterization and consideration for AVR.

Detection of left ventricular dysfunction by exercise echo in AR

Paulsen and associates[44] from London, Ontario, Canada, assessed LV performance in 20 symptom-free patients and in 10 with symptoms, all of whom had isolated AR, by measuring the echo peak velocity of circumferential fiber shortening (echo peak V_{cf}) at rest and during graded bicycle ergometer exercise in the supine position. The normal LV response during exercise was first determined in 20 healthy controls. On the basis of their resting and exercise echo peak V_{cf}, the 30 patients with AR could be separated into 3 groups: group 1 comprised 11 symptom-free patients with a normal resting echo peak V_{cf} that increased normally with exercise; group 2 comprised 9 symptom-free patients with a normal resting echo peak V_{cf}, but with a subnormal response to exercise, and group 3 consisted of 10 patients with symptoms with a depressed resting echo peak V_{cf} that remained subnormal with exercise. Subsequent cardiac catheterization disclosed a normal EF in patients in group 1, borderline EF in those in group 2, and a reduced EF in those in group 3. Thus, echo assessment of LV performance during supine isotonic exercise provides a simple noninvasive method for the early detection of LV dysfunction in symptom-free patients with AR.

Left ventricular function in chronic AR

Debate continues about LV contractile performance in volume overload caused by AR. Depending on the definitions and measures of contractility used, contractility is increased, normal, or decreased. Commonly used isovolumic phase indices may be distorted in severe AR because the isovolumic phase of the cardiac cycle is shortened. The classic Frank-Starling curve, however, which relates performance to end-diastolic length, may be more reliable. Sagawa and associates in 1977 defined a new measure of contractility based on the relation of end-systolic pressure to end-systolic volume. This method is only minimally influenced by preload and afterload and is suitable for evaluation of ventricular performance in volume overload states. Accordingly, Osbakken and associates[45] from Philadelphia, Pennsylvania, studied LV contractile and pump function in patients with chronic AR, using conventional methods such as stroke work index, EF, and the Frank-Starling relation, and also the new method of contractility developed by Sagawa and colleagues. Twelve normal subjects and 21 patients with chronic AR (10 with minimal symptoms and 11 with CHF) were evaluated. A computer-based quantitative analysis of biplane left ventriculograms was used. Both patient groups had significant AR documented by ventriculography. Contractile function, as measured by peak systolic stress/end-diastolic volume and end-systolic pressure/volume curves, was poorer than that in normal subjects in chronic AR patients with CHF, but not in asymptomatic patients. When normalized for muscle mass, stroke work was not depressed in either asymptomatic patients or in AR patients with CHF, by comparison with the value in normal subjects. Angiographically determined cardiac index (CI) increased with increasing volume overload, even though forward CI measured by the Fick method remained essentially unchanged: normal subjects, total CI, 3.7 ± 0.4 liters/min/M^2, Fick CI, 2.4 ± 0.1 liters/min/M^2; asymptomatic patients, total CI, 7.6 ± 0.7 liters/min/M^2; Fick CI, 2.3 ± 0.2 liters/min/M^2; patients with CHF, total CI, 9.1 ± 0.82 liters/min/M^2; Fick CI, 2.1 ± 0.18 liters/min/M^2. LV peak stress increased significantly in patients with CHF (511 ± 55 dynes/cm$^2 \times 10^{-3}$) compared with values in normal subjects (360 ± 33 dynes/cm$^2 \times 10^{-3}$) and in asymptomatic patients (428 ± 50 dynes/cm$^2 \times 10^{-3}$. Thus, the combination of decreased muscle function and increased demands on pump function causes significant increases in end-diastolic pressure only in patients with CHF and this results in symptoms of pulmonary congestion.

Arteriolar dilator (hydralazine) in chronic AR

Arteriolar dilators have beneficial effects on cardiac performance in patients with CHF; reduced impedance enhances LV emptying and increases stroke volume. In MR, the predominant effect of arteriolar dilation is to redistribute total LV stroke volume in a manner favoring forward stroke volume at the expense of regurgitant flow. In patients with chronic severe AR, arteriolar dilation with *hydralazine* improves cardiac performance both at rest and during exercise. The mechanism responsible for the beneficial effects, however, is uncertain. To evaluate the effects of hydralazine on LV performance, volumes, and regurgitant flow in patients with AR, Greenberg and associates[46] from Portland, Oregon, evaluated the acute effects of hydralazine in 10 patients with chronic severe AR. Control measurements of intracardiac and intravascular pressures, cardiac output, and LV volumes were obtained. Hydralazine, 0.3 mg/kg, i.v., (maximal dose, 20 mg) was administered and all measurements were repeated 30 minutes later. A reduction in systemic vascular resistance from 1,264 to 710 dynes-sec-cm^{-5} was associated with significant increases in forward cardiac index (2.9–5.1 liters/min/M^2) and stroke volume index (37 to 55 ml/m^2). LV end-diastolic pressure was reduced from 19 to 12 mmHg. There was a significant reduction in mean arterial pressure (88 to 83 mmHg) and a significant increase in heart rate (81–94 beats/min).

Regurgitant stroke volume was reduced by more than 10 ml/m^2 in 7 patients and, for the group, was significantly reduced (65 to 53 ml/m^2). Regurgitant fraction was reduced in all patients (0.64 to 0.48). EF increased more than 0.10 in 4 patients, by 0.08 in an additional patient and, for the group, increased significantly from 0.50 to 0.57. LV end-diastolic volume decreased by >25 ml/m^2 in 4 patients, by 19 ml/m^2 in an additional patient and decreased significantly, for the group (208 to 190 ml/m^2). Thus, arteriolar dilators improve cardiac performance in AR by reducing the amount of AR and, in some patients, by substantially improving systolic pump function.

Hemodynamic and angiographic evaluation 8 and 27 months after aortic valve replacement for AR

Toussaint and associates[47] from Rouen, France, evaluated 18 patients with chronic AR hemodynamically and angiographically 8 and 27 months after AVR. Both the PA diastolic pressure and the LV end-diastolic volume decreased significantly, but the mean EF and the cardiac output remained identically lowered. The relative reduction in end-diastolic volume was correlated only with the preoperative EF and regurgitant fractions. In the 10 patients whose LV volume remained high or whose EF remained low, a second evaluation was performed 27 months after AVR. The LV end-diastolic volume was significantly lowered, back to normal in 5 patients. The systolic and diastolic LV shape returned to normal. Cardiac index and EF were unchanged. These results show a marked improvement a few months after AVR, with a further improvement several months later, as shown mainly by the decrease of LV end-diastolic volume and the return to normal of LV cavity shape. However, in most cases, the EF remained at its preoperative value, suggesting that AVR should be performed early, before myocardial deterioration appears.

Preoperative criteria predictive of late survival after aortic valve replacement for severe AR

In severe AS following AVR, LV function remains normal when it was normal preoperatively and returns toward or to normal when it was impaired preoperatively, provided no perioperative myocardial damage occurs. In contrast, in severe AR, LV function is impaired in more patients preoperatively than it is in patients with severe AS. Although LV hypertrophy and dilation regress after successful AVR, this regression is not complete in most AR patients. Improvement of impaired LV systolic pump function is unpredictable and occurs in only about 50% of patients operated on for severe AR. Thus, it is possible that late survival after AVR for severe AR and impaired LV function may be worse than in those with normal LV function. To evaluate this question, Greves and associates[48] from Portland, Oregon, studied 45 patients who underwent AVR for severe isolated AR. Patients with other valvular lesions or co-existing congenital cardiovascular anomalies or a mean aortic valve gradient >20 mmHg were excluded. The patients ranged in age from 14–74 years (mean, 45). Six patients with a mechanical prosthesis and not receiving anticoagulants were excluded from further analysis. Of the 39 remaining patients, 2 died perioperatively (4%) (both class IV preoperatively): 35 had mechanical prostheses and received anticoagulants and 2 had a bioprosthesis. Three died late with a 5-year survival of 85%. The 5-year survival with pre-AVR LV EF ≥0.45 was 87% -vs- 54% <0.45, (p < 0.04) (Fig. 5-5); cardiac index ≥2.5 liters/min/M² 92% -vs- 66% <2.5 (p < 0.04) (Fig. 5-6); mean VCF ≥0.75 -vs- <0.75 circ/s (p < 0.09); end-diastolic pressure ≤20 -vs- >20 mmHg (p < 0.08). Late survival was not significantly different between pre-AVR functional class I and II -vs- class III and IV; LV end-diastolic volume index ≥210 -vs- <210 ml/m²; LV end-systolic volume index ≥110 -vs- <110 ml/m²; and LV mass ≥240 -vs- <240 g/m². With EF ≥0.50 there was 1 operative death (functional class IV) and no late deaths. Thus, late survival after AVR for severe isolated AR is better predicted preoperatively by the LV systolic pump function variables of EF and cardiac index than by LV diastolic parameters and clinical status.

Fig. 5-5. Actuarially determined survival curves demonstrating differences in survival for those patients with preoperative EF ≥ 0.45 (*upper curve*) -vs- those patients with preoperative EF < 0.45 (*lower curve*). Reproduced with permission from Greves et al.[48]

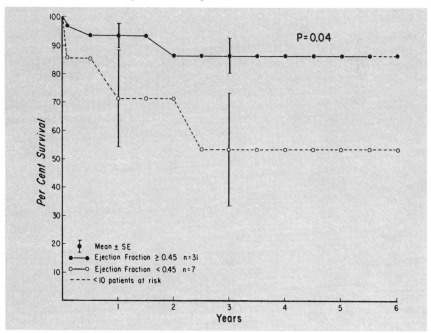

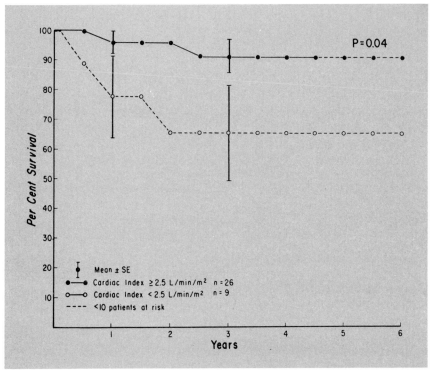

Fig. 5-6. Actuarially determined survival curves demonstrating the differences in survival for those patients with preoperative CI ≥ 2.5 liters/min/M² (*upper curve*) -vs- those patients with preoperative CI < 2.5 liters/min/M² (*lower curve*). Reproduced with permission from Greves et al.[48]

Management of the Marfan syndrome with dilated ascending aorta

Chronic AR, aortic root aneurysm with or without rupture, and aortic dissection are the primary causes of death in patients with the Marfan syndrome. McDonald and associates[49] from Baltimore, Maryland, summarized operative data on 13 patients with the Marfan syndrome who had dilated ascending aortas. By M-mode echo, the aortic diameter at the mid-valve level ranged from 5.3–8.2 cm. The operative techniques included excision of the aortic valve, placement of a composite woven Dacron valve-conduit and separate coronary anastomosis to the graft. Six patients had aortic dissection at operation. On follow-up of 6–96 months (mean, 23) in the 10 operative survivors, 1 died 20 months postoperatively (arrhythmia) and 2 at 4 and 6 months, respectively, (infective endocarditis). These investigators believe that, since the size of the aorta can be monitored by echo, consideration should be given to prophylactic resection when the aortic root diameter is >5.5 cm.

VENTRICULAR WALL MOTION OR MASS OR CAVITY SIZE IN MITRAL OR AORTIC VALVE DISEASE

Reliability of echo and ECG in assessing serial changes in left ventricular mass after cardiac valve replacement

ECG and echo are noninvasive techniques that are, of course, used widely in assessing LV hypertrophy. Previous studies have shown a fair correlation between ECG voltage and LV mass, as determined by echo, angiography and necropsy. Furthermore, echo measurements of LV free wall thickness and internal dimensions and derived estimates of ventricular mass, have closely corresponded to similar measurements determined by LV angiography. The strongest correlation between echo methods of estimating LV mass has been observed when echo dimensions were measured by a nonstandard method (Penn convention) and mass estimates were based on an average of both ventricular septal and LV free wall. To evaluate the reliability of these noninvasive methods in determining serial changes in LV mass in the same patient, Ditchey and associates[50] from La Jolla, California, reviewed concurrent ECG and echoes in 39 patients with aortic or mitral valve disease and in 15 normal subjects. Of the 39 patients, 21 had predominant AS and 18 had MR or predominant AR. Patients with predominant MS were excluded. Pre- and early postoperative echo estimates of LV mass in 17 patients who had valve replacements correlated well (r = 0.96, p < 0.01) and demonstrated little change in mean values despite altered LV dimensions. Echo estimates of LV mass were, therefore, used as a standard for evaluating other noninvasive indices. Precordial ECG voltage showed a weak correlation with LV mass in the study group as a whole (r = 0.59, p < 0.001), and no correlation in patients with volume overload (r = 0.36, p = ns). In 18 patients who had preoperative and 3 postoperative studies at least 8 weeks apart, changes in cross-sectional area (an index of LV mass that corrects for changes in LV volume) closely followed alterations in LV mass. Changes in posterior wall and ventricular septal thickness, however, often resulted from altered ventricular volume and did not accurately reflect directional changes in LV mass. Serial changes in ECG voltage were similarly unreliable. The authors concluded that LV mass and cross-sectional area by echo allow accurate noninvasive assessment of LV mass, whereas wall thickness and ECG changes do not.

Left ventricular regional wall motion and velocity of shortening in chronic MR or AR

Osbakken and associates[51] from Philadelphia, Pennsylvania, studied LV regional wall motion (% systolic shortening) and velocity of shortening in 32 patients with CHF due to chronic volume overloads from AR (21 patients) or MR (11 patients). Ten of the 21 patients with AR and 4 of the 11 patients with MR were asymptomatic, and the other 18 patients had CHF. None of the 32 patients had CAD. The findings were compared with those in 12 normal subjects. Biplane left ventriculograms were analyzed by computer and divided into 4 regions: anterior, inferior, posterolateral and septal. With CHF, EF was decreased in both AR and MR (normal, 62 ± 3%; AR, 48 ± 3; and MR, 51 ± 5). In MR with CHF, the percent segment shortening in anterior and posterolateral regions was significantly decreased, whereas this value in the inferior and septal regions was normal. In AR with CHF, anterior, inferior, and septal segment shortening was significantly decreased, whereas posterolateral segment shortening was normal. In both groups with CHF, mean shortening velocity showed regional variations due to those of percent shortening, whereas peak instantaneous shortening velocity was not reduced in MR, as compared with normal values. In the asymptomatic group, shortening and mean shortening velocity were normal, whereas peak instantaneous shortening velocity was increased in MR. In AR and MR with decreased LV function demonstrated by a reduced EF, regional wall motion abnormalities that are not caused by associated CAD may be present.

Right ventricular function in aortic and mitral valve disease

Although it is well recognized that the right ventricle can be affected in patients with severe left-sided valvular heart disease, RV contrast angiography is seldom performed in these patients because the hyperosmolar contrast injection may be poorly tolerated as an added volume load to patients who already are likely to have elevated left atrial pressures. No widely accepted method for quantitating RV EF is available, and TR during RV angiography may be catheter-induced. RNA methods overcome these difficulties, and, consequently, RNA of the right side of the heart was performed within 2 weeks of cardiac catheterization by Winzelberg and associates[52] from Boston, Massachusetts, in 43 patients with severe aortic or mitral valve disease or both, and in 13 controls. RV EF in the normals was 60 ± 7%; in patients with valvular disease, it was below the normal range in only 2 (14%) of 14 patients with RV peak systolic pressures <50 mmHg, but in 16 (55%) of 29 patients with an RV EF below normal when the RV peak systolic pressure was >50 mmHg. There was no relation of RV EF to right atrial pressure in the patients with valvular heart disease. Of the 35 patients who subsequently underwent valvular operations, no difference in early postoperative course was noted between those with normal or reduced RV EF. Central venous systolic reflux was present in 3 of 12 and in 22 of 25 patients with RV peak systolic pressures below and above 50 mmHg. Thus, radionuclide assessment of RV function in patients with aortic or mitral valvular disease or both provides information that cannot be inferred from right-sided pressure measurements.

Left ventricular size and function 2–4 weeks after valve replacement in AR or MR

Boucher and associates[53] from Boston, Massachusetts, utilized multigated blood pool scanning to examine LV volumes and EF before and 2–4 weeks after valve replacement in 20 patients with isolated AR and in 20 patients with isolated MR. Early postoperatively, EF decreased significantly (p < 0.01) in both patient groups (mean, 0.55 ± 0.12−0.40 ± 0.14 in AR and 0.66 ± 0.09−0.48 ± 0.11 in MR). The decrease in EF was associated with a large decrease in stroke volume with minimal or no change in end-systolic volume; it was unrelated to the preoperative EF. Early postoperative EF correlated best with preoperative end-systolic volume and was normal in 14 (67%) of 21 patients with a preoperative EF >0.60, in 4 (27%) of 15 patients with a preoperative EF of 0.50−0.60, and in 0 of 4 patients with a preoperative EF <0.50 (p < 0.05) (Fig. 5-7). In addition, repeat scan in 16 patients late (1−2 years) after operation showed a further reduction in end-systolic volume in patients with AR with an increase in EF toward preoperative values. There was no significant change in patients with MR. End-diastolic volume decreased significantly (p < 0.001) early postoperatively (162 ± 60 to 102 ± 41 ml/m² in patients with AR and from 131 ± 40 to 78 ± 30 ml/m² in patients with MR). This decrease was closely related to a decrease in stroke volume and was unrelated to preoperative EF. Early postoperative end-diastolic volume correlated best with the preoperative end-systolic volume. The major part of the reduction in end-diastolic volume occurred within 2 weeks of valve replacement. Removal of chronic LV volume overload due to AR or MR produces a decrease in EF and end-diastolic volume. The early reduction is, in part, a result of altered loading conditions and may not necessarily

Fig. 5-7. Mean ventricular volumes (ml/m²) and EF before (PREOP) and early after (POSTOP) valve replacement in patients with AR and MR. There was a comparable decrease in mean EF and mean stroke volume (SV) in both patient groups. Mean end-systolic volume (ESV) decreased slightly in patients with AR (p < 0.05), but did not change significantly in those with MR.

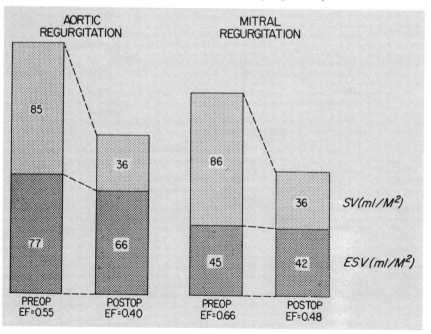

imply alterations in myocardial contractile function. The reduction in EF appears to persist in patients with MR.

CORONARY ARTERIES IN AORTIC VALVE DISEASE

Mechanism of angina pectoris with normal coronary arteries in aortic valve disease

Angina pectoris is common in patients with aortic valve disease and some patients have coronary arterial narrowing and others do not. Bertrand and associates[54] from Lille, France, measured coronary sinus blood flow using a continuous thermodilution method both at rest and during isometric handgrip exercise in 46 patients with aortic valve disease. All 46 had normal coronary angiograms. The patients were separated into 3 groups: 12 with AS; 15 with both AS and AR, and 3 with AR. At rest, the coronary sinus flow was 2 to 3 times normal but, when corrected for LV mass (ml/100 g), flow was normal.The ratio of diastolic pressure-time index/systolic pressure-time index (DPTI/SPTI) was decreased in all 3 groups at rest. During isometric exercise, coronary sinus blood flow increased significantly and there was a reduction in the DPTI/SPTI ratio. Of the 18 patients with angina on effort during the test, 7 were in group I, 6 in group II, and 5 in group III. There were no differences in the coronary sinus blood flow between patients with angina and those who were pain-free, either at rest or during exercise. Angina pectoris does not appear to be caused by a failure of coronary blood flow to increase. There was no discrepancy between myocardial demand, as measured by the pressure-time index and coronary blood flow. However, the DPTI/SPTI ratio was significantly lower during exercise in the patients with angina than in those who were pain-free. Underperfusion of the subendocardial muscle seems to be a causative factor in the patients with angina.

Usefulness of exercise-induced regional wall motion abnormalities on radionuclide angiography in detecting coronary narrowing in valvular heart disease

Exercise-induced regional wall motion abnormalities, as detected by RNA, have been reported only in the presence of coronary arterial narrowing and have been considered specific for CAD. Because coronary and valvular heart disease often co-exist, it would be important to know whether exercise-induced regional wall motion abnormalities are a reliable indicator of CAD in patients with valvular disease. Accordingly, Hecht and Hopkins[55] from Los Angeles, California, evaluated the reliability of exercise-induced wall motion abnormalities in 19 consecutive patients with valvular heart disease and angiographically normal coronary arteries. Of the 19 patients, 14 had AR, 2 had combined AR and AS, and 1 each had AS, MR, and combined AR and MR. Of the 19 patients, 18 were men; their ages ranged from 32–69 years. Exercise-induced regional wall motion abnormalities were found in 42% of the patients with valvular heart disease, in 63% of 35 patients with CAD without valvular heart disease, and in none of 12 normal controls. Thus, exercise-induced regional wall motion abnormalities are not reliable for the detection of CAD in patients with valvular heart disease.

Aortic valve replacement without coronary bypass in combined aortic valvular and coronary heart disease

To test the hypothesis that coronary artery bypass grafting (CABG) is not routinely required in patients undergoing AVR who have co-existent CAD, Bonow and associates[56] from Bethesda, Maryland, compared the results of operation in 55 consecutive symptomatic patients who had CAD and underwent AVR without CABG with results in another 142 patients without CAD who underwent AVR during the same period, and with published results from other centers in which CABG was used in patients with CAD who underwent AVR. The operative mortality was 4% in patients with CAD and 5% in patients without CAD. Late survival was not significantly different between the 2 groups when analyzed for the entire population (80% survival at 3 years in CAD patients, 82% for non-CAD patients), or for the subgroup of patients with AS, AR, or AS plus AR (Figs. 5-8 and 5-9). Eight patients with

Fig. 5-8. Survival after AVR. Long-term survival was not significantly different between patients with associated CAD and patients without CAD. Reproduced with permission from Bonow et al.[56]

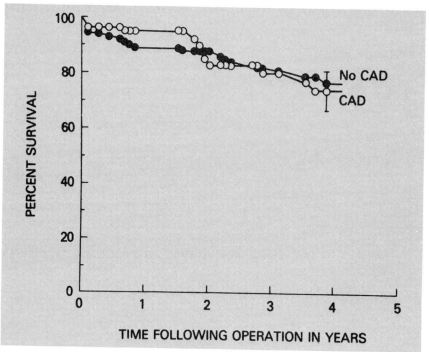

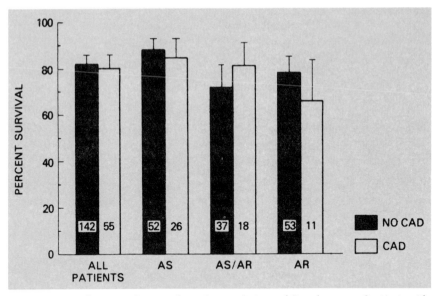

Fig. 5-9. Survival 3 years after AVR for entire population and for subgroups of patients with aortic stenosis (AS), aortic stenosis plus regurgitation (AS/AR), and AR. Number of patients at operation for each group is indicated within each bar. Associated CAD did not significantly affect survival. The SEM is shown at top of each bar. Reproduced with permission from Bonow et al.[56]

CAD (15%) developed recurrent angina after AVR (mean follow-up, 43 months); only 3 patients (6%) required CABG because of medically refractory angina (12–43 months). Operative mortality, operative AMI (9%), recurrent angina and long-term survival in patients with CAD after AVR were similar to those at other centers after AVR plus CABG. These data suggest that preoperative detection of CAD does not necessitate CABG in all patients at the time of AVR.

The article by Bonow and associates[56] was followed by an editorial by Kirklin and Kouchoukos,[57] who disagreed with the view of Bonow and associates that CABG at the time of AVR is not advantageous as a near-routine procedure for patients with combined important aortic valve disease and CAD. Kirklin and Kouchoukos believe that such a conclusion was premature and unwarranted, and their bias was in favor of near-routine choice of the combined procedure. Neither they nor Bonow and associates, however, had demonstrated with certainty that the other was wrong.

Coronary arterial anatomy with bicuspid aortic valve

Several reports beginning in 1975 indicated that patients with congenitally bicuspid aortic valves had a much higher incidence than normal of left coronary dominant systems. This frequency has varied from 25%–60%, whereas the frequency of the left coronary dominant system in patients without congenitally bicuspid aortic valves is about 10%. Additionally, since 1977, several reports also have indicated that the LM coronary artery is shorter than normal in patients with either a congenitally bicuspid aortic valve, a left dominant coronary system, or both. It is not clear whether a short LM coronary artery is actually dependent on the occurrence of left coronary dominance or the bicuspid condition of the aortic valve. Virtually no information is available on the position of the coronary arterial ostia with respect to the sinotubular junction of the ascending aorta in patients with congenitally bicuspid aortic valves. Lerer and Edwards[58] from Rochester, Minnesota, examined 100 hearts at necropsy, 50 of which had what they called congenitally bicuspid aortic valves and the other 50 had acquired bicuspid aortic valves (Fig. 5-10). They sought to determine the frequency of coronary arterial variations in these 100 patients. In the 50 patients with congenitally bicuspid aortic valves, the left coronary ostium arose at or above the sinotubular junction in 44%, whereas this location for the left coronary ostium in the acquired group was only 20%, and that for the right coronary ostium in both congenital and acquired groups was also 20%. In the patients

Fig. 5-10. Schematic diagram of location of raphe in 50 congenitally bicuspid aortic valves (*left*) and of commissural fusion in 50 acquired bicuspid aortic valves (*right*). L = left cusp. P = posterior cusp. R = right cusp. Reproduced with permission from Lerer and Edwards.[58]

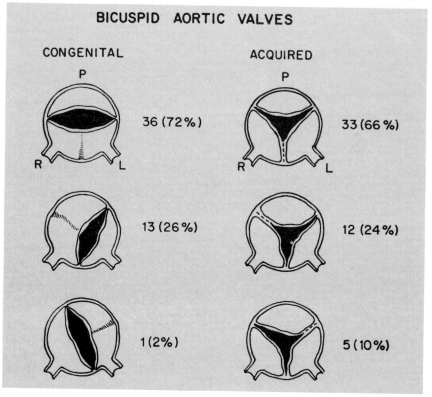

with congenitally bicuspid aortic valves, the frequency of left coronary dominance was 28%, the frequency in the acquired group was 16%, and both figures were significantly higher than the normal of 10%. In both the acquired and congenital patients with bicuspid valves, the length of the LM coronary artery was similar and, in both, was significantly shorter in hearts with left coronary dominance than in those with right or shared dominance.

The functional state of the bicuspid aortic valves in the patients described by Lerer and Edwards was not mentioned. They considered a bicuspid aortic valve congenital if it contained a conjoined cusp and acquired if it showed fusion of a true commissure. The aortic valves in the congenital group all had raphes. Most of their patients with acquired bicuspid aortic valves also had rheumatic mitral valve disease. In both groups, there were 41 men and 9 women. The age range in the congenital group was from 15–86 years (mean, 60) and in the acquired group 39–88 years (mean, 65).

INFECTIVE ENDOCARDITIS

M-mode echo during and after healing of active bacterial endocarditis limited to the mitral valve

Since 1972, many reports have described echo features of vegetations in 1 or more cardiac valves. Most reports described echo features during the period of active infection, and few described long-term follow-up by serial echo in patients with active infective endocarditis (IE). Because of the sparsity of serial echo information in patients with active IE limited to the *mitral valve*, Sheikh and associates[59] from Washington, D.C., and Bethesda, Maryland, analyzed 99 M-mode echoes recorded during and up to 144 months after healing of active *bacterial* endocarditis limited to the mitral valve in 27 patients. Their study produced the following findings: 1) Little or no change occurred in the echo size of the vegetations during the first 6 weeks after diagnosis and institution of appropriate antibiotic therapy unless a major systemic embolus occurred. 2) The echo size of the vegetations did not determine the amount of cardiac damage or dysfunction produced by the valvular infection. 3) The larger the vegetations by echo, the greater was the likelihood of a clinical event compatible with a systemic embolus. 4) The gravest prognostic sign yielded by the echo was evidence of rupture of chordae tendineae. 5) Although echo was a useful adjunct to diagnosis before appropriate antibiotic therapy was instituted, once bacteriologic cure had been achieved it was of limited value in delineating an active from a healed vegetation. 6) The echo appearance of the vegetations was not determined by the type of infecting bacterium.

No change in the echo size of the mitral vegetations occurred in 22 of their 27 patients with active bacterial endocarditis in whom more than 1 echo was recorded during the first 6 weeks after diagnosis. After the first 6 weeks, the echo size of the mitral vegetations decreased in 8 of the 16 patients (Fig. 5-11). Although other investigators have found that the size of the

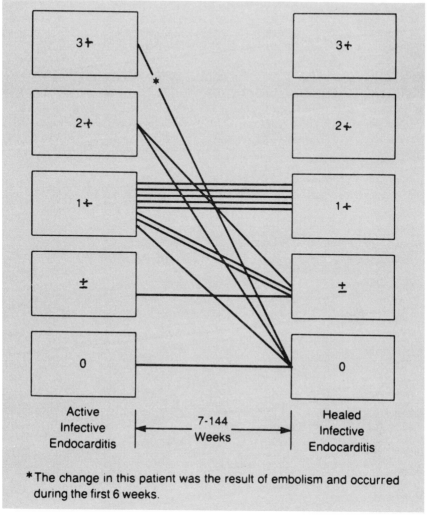

Active Infective Endocarditis ←——— 7-144 Weeks ———→ **Healed Infective Endocarditis**

*The change in this patient was the result of embolism and occurred during the first 6 weeks.

Fig. 5-11.   Size of echo vegetation during and after healing of active bacterial endocarditis in 13 patients with 1 episode of infection. Reproduced with permission from Sheikh et al.[59]

vegetation on a heart valve, as observed by M-mode echo, was 1 of the major determinants of outcome for the patient, the study by Sheikh and associates did not find this to be the case in their patients, in whom the vegetations were limited to the mitral valve. In none of their 3 patients with the largest vegetations by echo did systemic emboli occur, none developed CHF, none required MVR, and none died. In contrast, of their 18 patients with relatively small-sized vegetations by M-mode echo, 7 developed CHF and each patient either died or underwent MVR. Of their 5 patients with large-sized mitral vegetations, each had a systemic embolus. In contrast, of their 19 patients with relatively small-sized vegetations during the period of active infection, only 2 developed systemic emboli that were clinically apparent. Of their 8 patients in whom evidence of rupture of mitral chordae tendineae was observed by M-mode echo, 7 had overt CHF and each died or underwent MVR.

Caution, of course, must be taken when grading the size of a cardiac valvular vegetation by M-mode echo alone. Obviously, this technique views the vegetation from only 1 dimension, and that particular dimension may or may not be the vegetation's largest dimension. Two-D echo, in contrast, is far more accurate in determining the precise size of a cardiac valvular vegetation. Nevertheless, despite this recognized limitation, M-mode echo, as shown by this report, is useful in estimating the relative size of a mitral valvular vegetation, and this information is useful in patient management and in predicting complications and outcome.

M-mode and 2-D echo in active bacterial endocarditis limited to the aortic valve

Sheikh and associates[60] from Washington, D.C., and Bethesda, Maryland, also described M-mode echo findings in 17 patients with active bacterial endocarditis (ABE) involving the aortic valve and compared the observations in this group of patients to those made earlier in patients with infection involving the tricuspid or mitral valve. One or more echo abnormalities involving an aortic valve cusp or their immediate vicinity was present in 15 (88%) of the 17 patients, including "shaggy" echoes indicative of vegetations in 12 (71%). Of the 12 patients with echo evidence of AV vegetations, 11 developed overt CHF and either died or had AVR, and 7 had clinical events compatible with systemic emboli; of the 5 patients without echo-demonstrated vegetations, only 1 had CHF, none had AVR, 2 died, and 1 had a systemic embolus.

The patients with ABE involving the AV, as compared with those with infection on either the mitral valve (MV) or the tricuspid valve (TV), had a higher frequency of CHF (11 of 17 -vs- 12 of 29 [mitral] and 1 of 23 [tricuspid]), a higher frequency of systemic emboli (8 of 17 -vs- 6 of 29 [mitral]), a much higher frequency of valve replacement during the period of active infection (6 of 17 -vs- 4 of 29 [mitral] and 1 of 23 [tricuspid]), and a much higher total mortality (8 of 17 -vs- 9 of 29 [mitral] and 4 of 23 [tricuspid]). Thus, infection involving the aortic valve, as compared with that involving either the mitral or tricuspid valve, is far more liable to produce CHF and systemic emboli, to necessitate valve replacement, and to cause death during the ABE period.

Berger and associates[61] from New York City performed M-mode and 2-D echoes in 14 patients with active infective endocarditis involving the aortic valve. In 12 patients, vegetations were detected by 2-D echo and in 8 patients the vegetations were detected by M-mode echo. In all 8 patients in whom the M-mode echo disclosed a valvular vegetation, the 2-D echo also was positive for a vegetation on the aortic valve. The 2-D echo was superior to the M-mode echo in determining the size, shape, and mobility of the vegetations. Serial 2-D echoes performed after completion of antibiotic therapy in 7 patients disclosed no change in appearance of vegetation in 5 and disappearance of the vegetation in 2. Of the 12 patients with vegetations visualized by 2-D echo, 7 responded to medical therapy alone, 4 had AVR, and 1 died. In the 2 patients in whom the 2-D echo was negative for vegetations, the vegetations were ≤3 mm in diameter at operation or necropsy. Vegetations visualized by 2-D echo were at least 5 mm in diameter at operation. Thus, visualization of a vegetation by 2-D echo was not an absolute indication for operative intervention. In those patients who underwent serial studies, no correlation existed between clinical improvement and change in size of the vegetation. The authors stressed that clinical decisions should not be made solely on the basis of the 2-D echo, but its findings should be interpreted along with other laboratory and clinical factors.

M-mode and 2-D echo assessment of vegetations on any cardiac valve and comparison with radionuclide scanning

Both the M-mode and 2-D echo have proved to be extremely useful in detecting cardiac valvular vegetations in patients with active infective endocarditis (IE). Melvin and associates[62] from New York City not only evaluated the usefulness of M-mode and 2-D echo in detecting valvular vegetations but they also utilized technetium-99m stannous pyrophosphate scanning and gallium-67-citrate scanning to detect vegetations. Of 33 patients with 35 episodes of clinically diagnosed active IE, M-mode echo detected 18 vegetations in 17 of the 35 episodes (49% positive); 2-D echo detected 30 vegetations in 28 of the 35 episodes studied (80% positive). In contrast, no vegetations were detected by radionuclide scanning. The 2-D echo was better than the M-mode in detecting aortic and tricuspid valve vegetations.

In drug addicts

Hubbell and associates[63] from San Francisco, California, reviewed their 11-year experience and follow-up attempts in 79 addicts with 97 separate episodes of active infective endocarditis (IE) from 1965–1976. The patients ranged in age from 19–61 years (mean, 33) and 57 (72%) were men. The site of infection was nearly equally divided among the heart valves in the 97 episodes of active IE (Fig. 5-12): aortic valve (AV) in 37 (38%), mitral valve (MV) in 30 (31%), and tricuspid valve (TV) in 35 (36%). Preexisting cardiac valve lesions were present in 41 episodes. Of these, a previous history of IE was present in 17 episodes (41%). The principal organisms were *Staphylococcus aureus* 36%, group D *Streptococcus* 19%, fungus 12%, and *Serratia marcescens* 8%. Only 1 patient with a typical clinical picture of IE had multiple negative blood cultures. Of the 79 patients, 28% had surgical therapy (with paravalvular leaks occurring in 50% and second infections occurring in 24%) and 60% of them died (16% perioperatively); 73% had medical therapy alone with a mortality rate >70% occurring with *Serratia*, fungus, or aortic valve infection. Of medically managed patients, 17% had second infections. Surgical managment increased survival in hemodynamically severe IE, but long-term postoperative mortality was high.

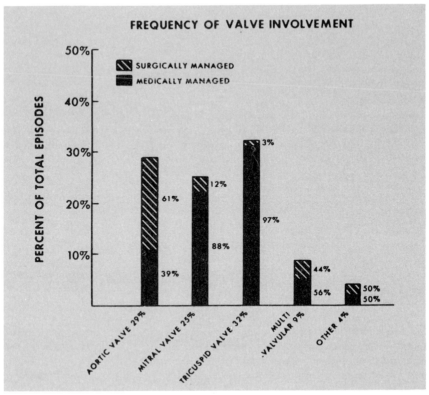

Fig. 5-12. Although site of infection was comparably distributed among aortic, mitral, and tricuspid valves, aortic involvement dominated those managed surgically. Reproduced with permission from Hubbell et al.[63]

Complicating mitral valve prolapse

Infective endocarditis (IE) is well recognized as one of the possible complications of MVP. Nolan and associates[64] from Little Rock, Arkansas, compared clinical features, response to therapy, and outcome of active IE in 10 patients with MVP with those in 23 patients with IE involving nonprolapsed mitral or aortic valves. Of the 23 patients without MVP, 7 had the IE involving the mitral valve and the other 16 of the aortic valve. Signs of active IE were more subtle in the patients with MVP, and antimicrobial therapy was instituted later than in the other 23 patients. Nevertheless, 9 of 10 patients with MVP and active IE responded optimally to antimicrobials. In contrast, only 5 of 23 patients with IE not involving a prolapsed mitral valve responded similarly. Four patients with MVP experienced increasing valvular dysfunction during the year after treatment of the IE and none died. The authors concluded that IE in patients with MVP is more responsive to antimicrobial therapy, even though recognition of the IE often is delayed, compared to patients with IE involving nonprolapsed mitral valves. Progressive valvular dysfunction, however, may be a later complication.

Early aortic valve replacement for active bacterial endocarditis involving the aortic valve

Prager and associates[65] from Nashville, Tennessee, described operative treatment in 14 patients with bacterial endocarditis of the aortic valve. The AVR was done because of severe CHF. Two patients also had arrhythmias, 3 had emboli, and 1 had suspected associated CAD. All were operated on within 2 weeks of the institution of antibiotic therapy. The responsible bacterium was *Streptococcus* (6 patients), *Staphylococcus* (4 patients) and *Escherichia coli* and *Enterococcus* (1 patient each). None died in the perioperative period, 1 died later, and 2 underwent re-operation because of persistent aorto-RV fistula (1 patient) or perivalvular leak (1 patient). Nine patients are now functional class I, and 4 are class II. Thus, AVR is beneficial for active bacterial endocarditis of the aortic valve causing CHF.

NECESSITY OF ROUTINE CARDIAC CATHETERIZATION BEFORE CARDIAC VALVE REPLACEMENT

St. John Sutton and associates[66] described results of an investigation carried out in the Brompton Hospital, London, England, in 1978 to determine the usefulness of *routine* cardiac catheterization before operative replacement of one or both left-sided cardiac valves. The authors concluded that routine cardiac catheterization is unnecessary before valve replacement and this view was supported in an accompanying editorial by Brandenburg[67] from the Mayo Clinic. Before accepting the conclusion of the Brompton Hospital study, another look at the data collected is warranted.[68]

During a single year, 243 patients with valvular heart disease and without previous cardiac catheterization were referred to physicians at the Brompton Hospital. In each patient, a decision to perform cardiac catheterization was delayed until an analysis had been made of the history and physical signs, ECG, and chest roentgenogram and, in those in whom it was obtained, M-mode echo. After these data had been collected, the diagnosis appeared "unequivocal" in 184 patients (76%) and catheterization in them was not performed. In the remaining 59 patients (24%), cardiac catheterization was performed because of "persistent doubt about the severity of the valve lesions, clinical evidence of aortic root disease, evidence of substantial CAD, or discordance between clinical and echocardiographic data." The decision regarding the usefulness of preoperative cardiac catheterization was evaluated postoperatively by comparison of *operative mortality, 2-year mortality, extent of symptom relief*, and *frequency of* "subsequent valve replacement for untreated aortic valve or mitral valve regurgitation" between the groups having and not having this invasive procedure preoperatively. Additionally, 62 other patients with valvular heart disease and previous cardiac catheterization were referred to the Brompton Hospital during the same year and they, too, were included in their analysis.

The operative and 2-year mortality and extent of symptom relief were similar in the groups of patients having and not having preoperative cardiac catheterization and no uncorrected valvular lesions became apparent in the 2-year follow-up period in the uncatheterized patients. Thus, the authors concluded that *routine* cardiac catheterization was unnecessary before valve replacement. But is their conclusion applicable to patients with valvular heart disease being evaluated for valve replacement operations at other medical centers? The Brompton Hospital patients were *younger, less symptomatic,* and had a *much higher frequency of mitral valve disease* than patients having cardiac valve replacement at most Western World medical centers.

Of their 305 patients, 42% were <50 years of age and, of course, significant associated coronary narrowing is relatively infrequent in this younger age group, especially in persons from Third World countries, the source of a significant percentage of their patients. Of their 177 patients (58%) aged 50 years and older, 57 (32%) had coronary angiograms, of which 15 (36%) were abnormal, and 5 patients received aortocoronary bypass conduits. Thus, only 5 (1.6%) of their 305 patients having valve replacement also had aortocoronary bypass, a much lower percent than observed in the USA.

Nearly one half (48%) of their patients were in New York Heart Association functional class I (asymptomatic) or II, a sharp difference from that of most patients having valve replacement in the major medical centers in the USA. Did all those class I and II patients really need a cardiac operation, especially a valve replacement, as compared with a valve commissurotomy (mitral group)?

In comparison to the higher frequency of AVR in the USA, MVR was more frequent than AVR among the Brompton Hospital patients. Of their 305 patients, 209 (69%) had MVR (with or without AVR) and 166 (54%) had AVR (with or without MVR). Of their 235 patients having isolated valve replacement, 59% involved the mitral, and 41%, the aortic valve. Although the specific types of hemodynamic valve lesions present in their patients were not identified, it can be inferred that MS was the most common type of valvular dysfunction because rheumatic heart disease was stated to be the etiology of the valvular heart disease in 164 (67%) of the 305 patients, a much higher percentage than observed in most major medical centers in the USA today, where AS is the most frequent type of valvular dysfunction necessitating valve replacement. The reason that rheumatic heart disease was so frequent in their patients appears to be related to the fact that many were from abroad, particularly from Third World countries, where the frequency of rheumatic heart disease is quite high.

Assuming ideal follow-up (which was not the case with the Brompton study), can comparison of operative and 2-year postoperative mortality, and evaluation of symptoms and new valve lesions between 1 group having and another group not having preoperative catheterization really provide sufficient data to answer the question, "Is *routine* cardiac catheterization necessary before cardiac valve replacement?" The method of follow-up of their patients apparently was primarily by correspondence and not by re-examination by a physician or repeat M-mode echo or hemodynamic study. Meaningful comparisons using 1 type of prosthetic cardiac valve rather than another cannot be obtained simply by analysis of the operative and 2-year postoperative mortality and evaluation of symptoms at 2 years postoperatively, and it is unlikely that these parameters are sensitive enough to provide meaningful information on the usefulness of routine cardiac catheterization as a preliminary to cardiac valve replacement. If the usefulness of a procedure, namely cardiac catheterization, is to be evaluated, it seems unlikely that the necessary information can be obtained simply by avoiding the performance of the procedure being evaluated.

Although the authors stated that only 62 of the 305 patients with valvular heart disease referred to them in 1978 had had cardiac catheterization previously, it is likely that most or all of their 50 patients who underwent reoperation without cardiac catheterization did, indeed, have this invasive procedure performed before the initial cardiac operation. If these 50 patients were added to their 50 (of 243 evaluated) who underwent cardiac catheterization before their first cardiac operation, the patients (excluding those who had catheterization before referral to Brompton) having catheterization before valve replacement would increase from 24% to 45%.

The paper by St. John Sutton and associates[66] does, indeed, indicate that valve replacement can be performed successfully without prior cardiac catheterization, but it does not indicate whether or not valve replacement was necessary in the first place, because the severity of the valve lesion(s) most often was not determined. Nearly half the patients studied by St. John Sutton and colleagues were asymptomatic or had only mild symptoms and it is, of course, difficult to improve on an asymptomatic state when relief or diminution of symptoms and lack of death are the only bases for the judgment of improvement or success. The idea that valve surgery can be performed "successfully" without preoperative catheterization is, of course, not new. In the 1950s many patients having mitral valve commissurotomy had no previous cardiac catheterization or, if they did, it was usually limited to the right side of the heart; the operation was, nevertheless, usually quite beneficial.

In the 1950s, echo was not available. Has the additional information provided by the M-mode and 2-D echo supplanted *routine* cardiac catheterization before cardiac valve replacement today? The answer is "no." Although the echo does record certain aspects of the functional *anatomy* of the cardiac valves and hemodynamic parameters record the functional *effects* of valvular dysfunction, the echo has not proved as useful as originally hoped in diagnosing and in quantitating valvular dysfunction. The M-mode echo, for example, has proved to be highly useful in diagnosing MS, but it has not proved useful in indicating the severity of the obstruction and *it is the severity of the valve lesion, not the presence of it, that is the major determinant of whether or not valve replacement or commissurotomy is indicated.* The 2-D echo has proved to be more useful in predicting the severity of MS, but many pitfalls confront the estimator of mitral valve area by this means alone and, therefore, considerable caution must be exerted in using it quantitatively. Just as the ECG is poor in predicting the severity of AS, both the M-mode and 2-D echo are not only poor in predicting its severity but are frequently not helpful in diagnosis of AS. Likewise, echo has proved highly useful in diagnosing or confirming MVP, but it is not very helpful in indicating the presence or degree of MR, irrespective of the cause. Additionally, the echo has been extremely useful in determining the presence of aortic root dilation (anuloaortic ectasia) but it is not very good in determining the degree of and, at times, even the presence of AR. Of course, the echo has been extremely helpful in evaluating LV size in both phases of the cardiac cycle, but with the exception of pure AR, LV size *per se* does not determine whether valve replacement is indicated or will predictably be successful. And finally, the standard M-mode and 2-D echo is not reliable in delineating associated tricuspid valve disease, especially TR. Contrast echo, however, has been useful in this regard. (It is surprising, incidentally, that associated tricuspid valve stenosis or regurgitation was not mentioned in any of the 305 patients reported by St. John Sutton and associates.) Thus, the echo is helpful in diagnosing some valve lesions, but it is not reliable in predicting the severity of most valvular lesions.

In patients with valvular heart disease, *cardiac catheterization is the only presently available procedure that provides accurate information on the severity of the valvular lesion(s).* Symptoms of cardiac dysfunction are not necessarily proportional to the degree of valvular stenosis or regurgitation. In patients with valvular heart disease, symptoms of cardiac dysfunction cannot be attributed to valvular dysfunction unless the degree of valvular dysfunction is considerable. Some patients with large gradients or severe degrees of regurgitation involving either the mitral valve, the aortic valve, or both have minimal symptoms and some patients with small gradients or mild degrees of regurgitation involving one or both of these valves have severe symptoms. Improvement may occur postoperatively in some patients irrespective of the amount of reduction in valvular gradient or degree of regurgitation. Thus, when nearly one-half of the patients having valve replacement reported by St. John Sutton and associates were functionally class I or II preoperatively, it is impossible to know whether the operation was indicated in the first place or whether it was beneficial in the second place without knowing the degree of valvular obstruction or regurgitation present preoperatively. The only way to obtain that information at the present time is by preoperative cardiac catheterization. Judging degrees of valvular obstruction by visual inspection at operation is fraught with enormous error, as is determining the degree of valvular regurgitation by manual palpation within the downstream chamber.

When a patient enters the operating room for a cardiac valve operation, be it commissurotomy, anuloplasty, or replacement, the surgeon should have as much precise information as possible available to him regarding which valve functions abnormally and the extent of the dysfunction. It is expecting too much for surgeons uniformly to make proper decisions on which valve to excise or incise by visual inspection or palpation alone at operation. The most stenotic orifice of the mitral valve, for example, is at a level corresponding to the distal margins of the leaflets, and this portion of the valve is not necessarily seen well from the left atrium. The gold standard for the degree of obstruction across a valve is that obtained by measurement of pressures on either side of a valve, not by anatomic inspection or palpation. I have seen calcified aortic valves of diminished mobility that, by visual inspection, appeared stenotic, but by catheterization a short time earlier showed no or minimal peak systolic pressure differences across the valve. *The fewest errors are produced when most decisions regarding replacement of cardiac valves have been made on the basis of hemodynamic and angiographic data before the patient and surgeon enter the operating room.* Echo data should be viewed mainly as supplemental and primarily diagnostic, because they provide limited information on the severity of valve lesions.

Information regarding the level of the pulmonary arterial pressure, of course, is useful in following patients with mitral valve disease and this pressure cannot be obtained accurately without cardiac catheterization. Pressures obtained at operation, of course, are not nearly as reliable as those obtained while the patient is awake. The RV systolic pressure is most useful in evaluating the anatomic status of the tricuspid valve in patients with tricuspid regurgitation. Patients having TR associated with high RV systolic pressures usually have anatomically normal tricuspid leaflets and chordae tendineae and dilated tricuspid valve anuli; patients with TR and normal or only mildly elevated RV systolic pressures usually have anatomically abnormal tricuspid-valve leaflets and chordae and these valves, in contrast to the former, are more likely to require replacement.

To determine the status of the epicardial coronary arteries, there is no substitute for coronary angiography. If the patient population is mainly <50 years of age, from Third World countries where the frequency of associated CAD is small, and the majority have mitral rather than aortic valve disease, the likelihood of associated significant coronary narrowing is relatively small. But patients in most Western World medical centers being considered for valve replacement are >50 years of age, have a high frequency of associated coronary narrowing, and more commonly have aortic, rather than mitral-valve disease. The presence of associated significant coronary arterial narrowing in patients with AS and angina pectoris, for example, cannot be determined reliably without cardiac catheterization (coronary angiography). Some patients with valve disease and symptoms of severe myocardial ischemia have insignificant coronary narrowing by coronary angiogram, and vice versa. Knowing the status of the epicardial coronary arteries in patients >50 years of age, or possibly > age 40, being considered for cardiac valve replacement appears to be a fundamental preoperative requirement in 1982. Even when aortocoronary bypass grafting is not planned, if the patient has trouble being weaned from cardiopulmonary bypass after valve replacement, this additional procedure might, nevertheless, be warranted. No one can reliably determine the degree of narrowing of the epicardial coronary arteries by visual inspection or palpation, either in the operating room or in the necropsy room. This information needs to be obtained by selective coronary angiography preoperatively.

When the decision regarding the necessity for cardiac valve replacement arises, no procedure provides the information required as objectively as does preoperative cardiac catheterization. Cardiac catheterization today, including measurements of pressures in all 4 cardiac chambers and in both great arteries, and both selective coronary and LV and aortic root angiography, is a procedure that, in skilled and experienced hands, takes only about 1 hour to perform. It is minimally traumatic to the patient. It not only provides the only conclusive data available regarding the severity of the valvular lesions, but it also provides objective baseline data with which postoperative studies can be compared. Its expense is relatively small, as compared with the expense of the cardiac operation, and it may even prevent the latter from being performed. Cardiac catheterization can be performed many times in a lifetime, but the number of times that thoracotomy and cardiotomy can be performed in a lifetime is limited. Therefore, the indications for the latter must be as precise as possible to achieve the maximal benefit when it is performed, and to prevent its being performed if the valve lesion(s) is not of sufficient severity to expect considerable improvement.

In some *emergency* situations in patients with valvular heart disease, of course, it may be more advantageous to omit preoperative cardiac catheterization and proceed directly to the operating room. These circumstances might include extremely low cardiac output states from a stenosed or detached prosthetic or bioprosthetic cardiac valve, sudden severe valvular regurgitation (mainly aortic valve) from active infective endocarditis, and papillary muscle dysfunction in the setting of acute myocardial infarction. But *for elective valve replacement in a stable patient, preoperative cardiac catheterization will increase the diagnostic accuracy, determine accurately the severity of the valvular dysfunction, provide information on the status of the epicardial coronary arteries, prevent surprises at operation, and provide a baseline of information with which postoperative data can be compared*, and this information cannot be obtained reliably today from any procedure other than cardiac catheterization.

CARDIAC VALVE REPLACEMENT

Caged ball prostheses

The caged ball prosthesis was the first effective prosthetic valve and has been in use for over 20 years (since 1960). Tepley and associates[69] from Portland, Oregon, analyzed their 20-year experience with 2,135 patients with Starr-Edwards caged ball prostheses: AVR in 52%, MVR in 34%, both AVR and MVR in 42%, and triple valve replacement in 2%. The 15-year actuarial survival was $43 \pm 2\%$ (SEM) for AVR; $44 \pm 3\%$ for MVR, $27 \pm 5\%$ for combined MVR and AVR, and $23\% \pm 7$ for triple-valve replacement. Survival curves after AVR and MVR showed significant improvement with time due to a decrease in operative mortality after AVR and a decrease in postoperative and late mortality after MVR. The frequency of emboli and ball variance decreased significantly from the earlier to the current time period ($p < 0.001$), and hemorrhagic episodes increased significantly. Infective endocarditis, prosthetic thrombosis, and repeat valve replacement rates were the same during both periods of time. The percentage of MVR patients emboli-free at 5 years was 95% in the earlier period and 69% in the later period. After isolated AVR, 89% of the patients were embolus-free in the later time frame and 77% in the earlier time frame ($p < 0.001$). Of all late deaths after single-valve replacement, 52% were cardiac related. Valve-related mortality and morbidity have decreased. The embolus-free curves for silicone-rubber ball-valve prostheses showed a significant improvement in the 5-year emboli-free rate after both AVR and MVR.

Tilting disc prostheses

ECHO FEATURES OF THE ST. JUDE BILEAFLET PROSTHESIS

The St. Jude (SJ) prosthesis is a low-profile pyrolytic carbon bileaflet, central flow tilting disc prosthesis, introduced in October 1977. The 2 leaflets have an opening angle of 85° and a closing angle of about 33°, depending on the valve size. Amann and associates[70] from Basel, Switzerland, investigated 10 patients in whom the aortic valve was replaced and 11 patients in whom the mitral valve was replaced by SJ prostheses. In patients with the SJ prostheses in the aortic valve position, M-mode echo allowed visualization during systole of both leaflets and of the anterior and posterior part of the ring. In those with the SJ prosthesis in the mitral position, a part of the anterior leaflet and the entire posterior leaflet, together with the posterior ring, were visualized during diastole. Distinctive opening sounds were missing in the patients with aortic SJ prostheses. An amplitude of the posterior leaflet of 9.8 ± 1.3 mm and a leaflet separation of 4.8 ± 0.9 mm were measured. In the mitral prostheses, the Q-closure interval was 0.07 ± 0.03 s and leaflet separation was 4.4 ± 0.8 mm. In both aortic and mitral positions, high values for opening and closing velocities were measured, and closing velocities exceeded opening rates. These findings established the normal pattern and values by echo for patients with AVR or MVR with SJ prostheses.

DePace and associates[71] from Philadelphia, Pennsylvania, studied by simultaneous phonocardiograms and echoes 43 consecutive patients with a SJ prosthesis in the mitral (28 patients) or aortic (20 patients) position, or in both (5 patients). An opening click was not recorded. A loud aortic or mitral closing click, however, was recorded in all 43 patients. In patients with a SJ mitral prosthesis, an echo-free space separated the 2 leaflets during ventricular diastole; 7 also had a mid-diastolic closing and late diastolic reopening motion, and 2 of the 7 had an associated closing mid-diastolic click. A mid-diastolic rumble was recorded in 6 of the 28 patients with a SJ prosthesis in the mitral position. In the patients with a SJ prosthesis in the aortic valve position, leaflet motion was recorded in 17 of the 20 patients and was indistinguishable in appearance from echoes obtained with various eccentric monocusp valves. Thus, the SJ prosthesis has variable normal phonocardiographic-echo patterns and knowledge of these variable patterns is important in assessing patients with suspected malfunction of a SJ prosthesis.

Tri and associates[72] from San Francisco, California, performed M-mode and 2-D echo on 19 patients with 25 normally functioning SJ prostheses. Satisfactory M-mode echoes were obtained in 17 of the 19 patients and satisfactory 2-D echoes in all. M-mode measurements included the diameter of the orifice ring, leaflet separation, and the opening and closing slopes of the leaflets. The values obtained compared favorably with direct measurements from the prosthesis and were reasonably reproducible. Two-D imaging revealed characteristic systolic and diastolic patterns and provided direct visualization of valvular motion. Echo evaluation of the prosthesis can be facilitated if it is positioned at implantation so that the open leaflets are perpendicular to the echo plane of the long axis of the ventricle.

HEMODYNAMIC OBSERVATIONS AFTER MITRAL OR AORTIC VALVE REPLACEMENT WITH THE ST. JUDE PROSTHESIS AND COMPARISON WITH BJÖRK-SHILEY PROSTHESIS

Chaux and associates[73] from Los Angeles, California, implanted the SJ prosthesis in the mitral position in 57 patients and in the aortic position in 43 patients. The operative mortality was 2% and the late mortality 6%. No death was prosthetic-related. One embolic episode occurred in the 79 of 88 patients who received long-term anticoagulation therapy. The 53 survivors improved at least 2 functional classes (New York Heart Association). Postoperative catheterization at rest, during pacing, and during isoproterenol infusion demonstrated significantly improved hemodynamic performance in both the mitral and aortic positions, as compared with the mitral porcine bioprosthesis in the mitral position ($p < 0.05$). In the mitral area, the prostheses with 25–31 mm anular diameters had calculated valve areas from 2.1–3.1 cm². In the aortic valve area, the prostheses with diameters of 21–25 mm had valve areas from 2.7–3.6 cm².

Wortham and colleagues[74] evaluated the hemodynamics of the SJ prosthesis in 7 patients who had AVR for severe AS or AR. Utilizing 19–21 mm SJ valves, the average peak systolic pressure gradient at rest was 14 mmHg and, with exercise, 32 mmHg.

Horstkotte and associates[75] from Düsseldorf, West Germany, evaluated 22 patients 1 year after implantation of a SJ prosthesis in the mitral position and compared the results with those in 40 patients with Björk-Shiley (B-S) prostheses in the mitral position. In both groups, functional improvement was significant and similar. In the SJ group, no thromboembolic events occurred, whereas 5 patients (12%) in the B-S group had an embolus during the first postoperative year. Hemolysis was significantly lower in the B-S group, but remained subclinical in the SJ group (mean LDH was 241 with the SJ and 199 with the B-S [$p < 0.005$], haptoglobin with the SJ was 26 and with the B-S it was 76 [$p < 0.005$]). With similar-sized prosthetic diameters (29 mm), the calculated effective valve orifice was 3.07 ± 1.36 cm² for the SJ and 1.85 ± 0.53 cm² for the B-S. In both groups, the mean PA pressure was significantly reduced postoperatively at rest, but increased during exercise. Except for the calculated effective valve orifice areas, no significant hemodynamic differences were observed between the 2 prostheses.

Nicoloff and associates[76] from Minneapolis, Minnesota, began utilizing the SJ prosthesis in October 1977 and analyzed their results in 232 patients to December 1980: AVR with another procedure was done in 114 patients; MVR, either alone or in combination with another procedure, in 105, and both AVR and MVR in 13. Postoperatively, all but 7 patients received warfarin chronically. The operative mortality after AVR alone was 5% (6 of 114). Mean follow-up was 13 months and no patient had clinical evidence of valve thrombosis or prosthetic malfunction. The actuarial probability of being embolism-free after AVR was 98%. Of 22 patients recatheterized, 13 had no transvalvular gradient: the mean gradient at rest was 1 ± 1 mmHg and, with exercise, it rose to 4 ± 1.5 mmHg. Of the 105 patients having *MVR*, 8 died in the perioperative period. During follow-up, none had evidence of valve thrombosis or prosthetic malfunction, but 4 patients had thromboembolic events. Actuarial probability of freedom from thromboembolism was 95% at 30 months. Of 7 patients catheterized and exercised 4 months postoperatively, the mean gradient at rest was 1 ± 1 mmHg and, with exercise, it rose to 5 ± 1.5 mmHg (p < 0.005). Of the 13 patients having *double-valve replacement*, 3 died in the perioperative period. At follow-up to 28 months (mean, 14), no episodes of thromboembolism had occurred.

Hemodynamic measurements are usually obtained under resting conditions in the supine position after replacement of 1 or more cardiac valves with various prostheses. The values obtained under resting conditions, however, may not be representative of the patient's usual hemodynamic state. Despite many reports of residual gradients during exercise in patients after MVR, the consistency of the determinants of aortic valve area in their mathematical relationship has not been established for patients under stress after AVR. Thormann and associates[77] from Bad Nauheim, West Germany, therefore, carried out stress evaluations in 26 patients approximately 7 months after AVR with B-S prostheses (13 patients) and SJ prostheses (13 patients). During isoproterenol infusion (0.3 μg/kg/min), cardiac output increased by a factor of 1.5 and aortic valve area decreased by 50% for both valve groups, while transvalvular gradients (rest: 7 ± 2 -vs- 10 ± 5 mmHg, p > 0.05) increased to 42 ± 18 -vs- 51 ± 18 mmHg, (p > 0.05), i.e., to levels of moderate AS. During pacing stress, however, these values progressively decreased with rising heart rates. In other postoperative evaluations that included ergometric stress with isoproterenol and pacing, induced hemodynamic changes after AVR were predictable and consistent with regard to both direction and magnitude, and they differed characteristically according to the type of stress used. The authors found no functional differences between B-S and SJ prostheses. Standardized evaluation with isoproterenol is a sensitive stress test of prosthetic valvular hemodynamics. Because of the apparent magnification of residual obstruction after AVR, it has advantages over pacing.

OPERATIVE RESULTS WITH BJÖRK-SHILEY PROSTHESIS

Karp and associates[78] from Birmingham, Alabama, evaluated 643 patients having replacement of 1 or more cardiac valves with a Björk-Shiley (B-S) prosthesis at their center from 1975–1978. The follow-up ranged from 1–71 months (mean, 38). Survival rates in patients having AVR, MVR, and double valve replacements were similar to that reported in patients having similar valve replacements with other types of mechanical prostheses and bioprostheses. Overall operative mortality was 9%. At 4 years, actuarial survival for patients having AVR was 86%; for MVR, 83%, and for combined AVR and MVR, 72%. Preoperative factors associated with increased late mortality included functional class, previous valve replacement, LV aneurysmectomy, ventricular arrhythmia, or double-valve replacement rather than isolated AVR or MVR. Thromboembolism occurred in 65 (10%) of the 643 patients: in 36 patients after isolated AVR (13 minor and 23 major episodes); in 17 patients after isolated MVR (all major), and in 12 patients with combined AVR and MVR (2 minor and 10 major). The percent free of thromboembolism after isolated AVR was 88%, after isolated MVR 85%, and after combined AVR and MVR, 85%. All patients were treated with anticoagulants long-term. Valve thrombosis occurred in 16 patients and was fatal in 13. After isolated AVR, the risk of thrombosis for 4 years was 3%; after isolated MVR, 13%, and for combined AVR and MVR, 13% (Fig. 5-13). Complications related to anticoagulation occurred in 158 (25%) patients. The major disadvantage of the B-S prosthesis appears to be its relatively high risk of thrombosis and thromboembolism.

Cheung and associates[79] from Milwaukee, Wisconsin, reported a 10-year experience with AVR in 579 patients with a mean follow-up of 49 months, using exclusively the B-S prosthesis. The patients were divided according to associated procedures: group I included 280 patients with isolated AVR; group II, 90 patients with AVR plus coronary bypass; group III, 92 patients with combined AVR and MVR; group IV, 109 patients with other associated cardiac and great vessel procedures, and group V, 8 patients who had had at least 1 previous cardiac operation. The age range was 38–76 years (mean, 55). Anticoagulation with intermittent intravenous heparin was carried out

Fig. 5-13. Actuarial incidence of valve thrombosis for aortic, mitral, and double-valve replacement. Number of valves = 643. Reproduced with permission from Karp et al.[78]

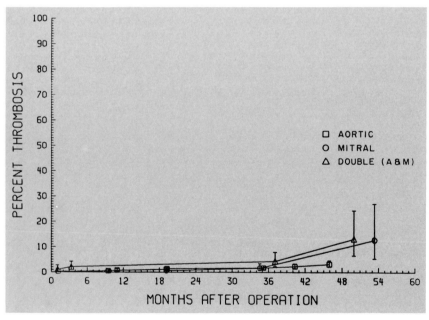

after removal of the chest tubes, and warfarin was begun as soon as the patients could take liquids orally. The operative mortality was 11% (66 of 579) and ranged from 6% in the group with isolated AVR to 21% in those with AVR plus resection of ascending aortic aneurysms. The operative mortality for NYHA functional classes II, III, and IV was 4%, 13% and 22%, respectively (p < 0.001). The overall 5-year survival was 70%: 73% in the patients with isolated AVR and 69% in those with associated procedures (p < 0.02). Five-year survival was similar in patients with either AS or AR, an observation at variance with other reports. Twenty-eight patients had 36 embolic episodes and 15 patients died from thromboembolic complications. Excluding patients who were not on anticoagulants, the embolic rate was 1.2/100 patient-years. Hemorrhage from anticoagulant therapy was fatal in 5 patients (intracerebral) and nonfatal hemorrhages occurred in 18 others. The overall frequency of hemorrhage from anticoagulation was 1.2/100 patient-years. Four patients (0.6%) were known to have had thrombotic obstruction of the prosthesis. Sixteen patients (2.8%) had bacterial endocarditis, 5 early and 11 late. Thus, the earlier the patient with AS or AR was operated on, the lower the operative mortality and the longer the survival. Functional class appears to be the most significant factor in this study determining long-term survival.

Schaff and associates[80] from Baltimore and Bethesda, Maryland, reported results of AVR with size 19 mm B-S prostheses in 43 patients followed a mean of 40 months. Four patients died late. Pre- and post-operative angiograms in 17 patients demonstrated a significant decrease in the mean LV wall thickness and in LV mass. Postoperative cardiac catheterization in an additional 24 patients showed an average peak systolic pressure gradient at rest of 16 mmHg (range, 0–45) and an average effective valve orifice area of 1.06 cm^2 (0.63–2.02) across the prosthesis. Thus, this valve size provides satisfactory hemodynamic alleviation of AS and LV overload, despite a small residual gradient.

Porcine bioprostheses

OPERATIVE RESULTS

Cohn and associates[81] from Boston, Massachusetts, summarized results of cardiac valve replacement with Hancock porcine bioprostheses in 128 patients operated on between January 1972 and January 1975. Pre- and post-operative functional evaluation, frequency of thromboemboli related to valve location and cardiac rhythm, and the frequency of valve dysfunction at these follow-up periods were presented. AVR was performed in 47 patients, MVR in 62, and combined AVR and MVR in 19. Four patients (3%) died within 30 days of operation, and 29 (16%) later. The actuarial probability of survival at 8 years for all patients was 80 ± 4%. Clinical thromboembolic events occurred in 2 of 43 patients after AVR, in 9 of 62 after MVR, and in 4 of 18 after combined AVR and MVR. Actuarial projection of freedom from thromboemboli at 96 months in 56 patients with atrial fibrillation was 70% and in the patients with normal sinus rhythm or heart block, 97% (Fig. 5-14). The probability of freedom from embolus at 96 months after AVR was 97 ± 2%, after

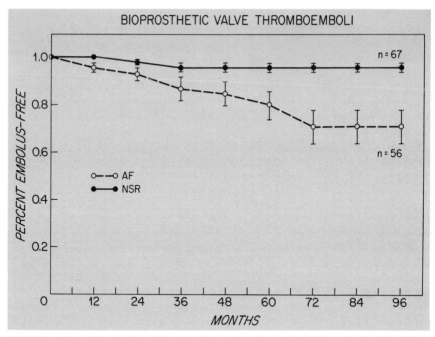

Fig. 5-14. Actuarial projection of freedom from thromboemboli at 96 months for 56 patients with atrial fibrillation (○) and 67 patients with normal sinus rhythm or heart block (●). Bars denote SEM. Reproduced with permission from Cohn et al.[81]

MVR 82 ± 5% and, after combined AVR and MVR, 72 ± 12%. Dysfunction occurred in 10 of 141 bioprostheses at risk: 5 from bacterial endocarditis and 5 from primary valve dysfunction (4 mitral and 1 aortic). The probability of freedom from dysfunction after AVR and MVR at 8 years was 90%. Thus, the probability of dysfunction before 6 years is low, and clinical thromboembolic events are more frequent in patients with atrial fibrillation than in those with sinus rhythm.

Gallo and associates[82] from Santander, Spain, reviewed results of valve replacement with the Hancock bioprosthesis in 491 patients (mitral, 291; aortic, 102; both, 102) operated on between June 1974 and June 1979. The hospital mortality was 10% for MVR, 5% for AVR, and 14% for both MVR and AVR. Actuarial survival for MVR at 6 years was 80%; for AVR, 80%, and for both, 78%. Nineteen patients had nonfatal thromboembolic events, a frequency of 1.5% per patient-year for MVR, 0.1% per patient-year for AVR, and 2.1% for combined MVR and AVR. The probability of being embolus-free at 6 years was 93% for MVR, 99% for AVR, and 94% for combined MVR and AVR. Twelve bioprostheses failed among 577 followed survivors: 6 ruptured; 4 thrombosed; 1 regurgitated, and 1 stenosed. Ten of the 12 failure patients had reoperation, with 1 postoperative death, and 2 other patients died of calcified thrombosis before reoperation. Actuarial curves showed that 95% of the patients with MVR were free of bioprosthetic failure at 6 years, 99% with AVR, and 87% with both MVR and AVR. The quality of life was improved, survival was excellent, and the rate of postoperative embolization was low. Of the embolic incidents in the patients with MVR, 55% occurred within the first 3 months, suggesting that anticoagulants during that period are useful. Among 18 patients with bioprosthetic endocarditis, 7 were treated successfully medically, and of the 7 who underwent reoperation after antibiotic therapy, 4 had normal functioning bioprostheses.

Curcio and associates[83] from Cape Town, South Africa, again documented the high frequency of calcification of glutaraldehyde-preserved porcine bioprostheses implanted in young patients. Seven of 54 patients <16 years of age required reoperation for bioprosthetic calcification and stenosis, and 3 other patients died from calcified and stenotic bioprostheses before reoperation.

Jamieson and associates[84] from Vancouver, British Columbia, Canada, reviewed results from implantation of 509 porcine bioprostheses (1/3 Hancock, 2/3 Carpentier-Edwards). The rate of embolic events was 1.3/100 patient-years for aortic valves, 3.3 for mitral valves, and 4.9 for multiple prostheses. Thirteen of 14 patients with emboli were in atrial fibrillation and only 3 were receiving anticoagulants. These authors believe that anticoagulation is beneficial in those patients with increased risk of thromboemboli with porcine bioprostheses, particularly those with atrial fibrillation and large left atria.

Geha and associates[85] from New Haven, Connecticut, analyzed 253 consecutive adult survivors receiving 294 porcine bioprostheses from 1974—1979. This number was 41% of all valve replacements at their medical center. The mean follow-up was 26 months. Valve dysfunction occurred in 4 of 294 bioprosthetic valves, 3 in the mitral and 1 in the tricuspid, all caused by recurrent infective endocarditis. Thromboembolism occurred in 6 of 294 xenografts, none in the aortic or tricuspid positions, regardless of cardiac rhythm or anticoagulation status. Four of the 6 mitral xenografts associated with thromboembolism were in the 16 patients with atrial fibrillation and they received aspirin and persantin, but not warfarin. Thromboembolism did not occur in any patient with a mitral bioprosthetic valve, sinus rhythm and antiplatelet agents. Thromboembolism did not occur in any patient with atrial fibrillation who received warfarin therapy. Of the 30 late deaths, none resulted from bioprosthetic dysfunction and only 1 resulted from thromboembolism. Xenograft performance was excellent for as long as 75 months; dysfunction occurred from infective endocarditis, whereas thromboembolism occurred after MVR in those who were in atrial fibrillation and not receiving anticoagulants.

Borkon and associates[86] from Bethesda, Maryland, studied 111 patients with a porcine bioprosthesis in the mitral position, with or without 1 or more mechanical prostheses. The hospital mortality was 10%, the mean follow-up was 5.4 years, and 70 patients were followed 5–10 years. The late mortality was 4.3% per patient-year, actuarial survival was 82% at 5 years and 65% at 10 years. The frequency of thromboemboli was 3.3 ± 0.9% per patient-year for all patients and 4.2% in those who had both a mitral bioprosthetic and a mechanical prosthetic aortic valve. Bioprosthetic failure occurred in 10 patients, 5 secondary to perivalvular regurgitation or infective endocarditis. Postoperative cardiac rhythm appeared to be a major determinant of emboli, in that 25% of patients in atrial fibrillation or rhythm other than sinus had thromboembolism. The frequency of structural deterioration was 1% at 5 years, 8% at 7 years, and 30% at 9 years, but the standard error was large and the numbers of patients very small at the late years. The probability of primary bioprosthetic dysfunction before 6 years was <5%.

Lipson and associates[87] from Bethesda, Maryland, studied hemodynamically 18 patients with porcine bioprostheses in the mitral position for >5 years. A significant increase in mitral valve gradient (from 5.9 to 8.6 mmHg [p < 0.01]) and a significant decrease in calculated mitral valve area (from 2.2 to 1.7 cm^2 [p < 0.01]) was observed between early and late catheterization studies postoperatively. Seven patients had a decrease in valve area >1.0 cm^2, 5 with bioprostheses in place for >80 months. Thus, there is hemodynamic deterioration in porcine bioprostheses in the mitral position >5 years, even in patients who are clinically stable.

Zusman and associates[88] from Boston, Massachusetts, analyzed 150 patients with Hancock modified-orifice aortic bioprosthesis in the aortic position, 38% of whom had associated procedures carried out. The operative mortality was 5% and, at a mean follow-up of 26 months, 10 patients had died and the 3-year survival was 80%. The frequency of emboli was 1.5/100 patient-years. No primary bioprosthetic failures had been recognized in 43 patients, transvalvular intraoperative peak systolic pressure gradients averaged 12.5 with the 19 mm valve, 10 with the 21 mm valve, 11 with the 23 mm valve, and 10 with the 25 mm valve.

The Carpentier-Edwards valve has slightly better hemodynamics in both the mitral and aortic positions, with lower transvalvular gradients than the Hancock porcine valves, as reported by Levine and associates[89] from Boston, Massachusetts. The gradient for the 29 mm Hancock bioprosthesis in the mitral position was 3.7 ± 1.2, as compared with 2.8 ± 1.1 for the Carpentier-Edwards bioprosthesis.

The bioprosthetic porcine valve appears to be quite durable up to 6 years postimplantation and it has a low thromboembolic potential, particularly in the aortic position.

ECHO CHANGES IN CUSPAL THICKNESS WITH TIME

To assess the ability of M-mode echo to detect the incidence and frequency of porcine bioprosthetic thickening, Alam and associates[90] from Detroit, Michigan, obtained echoes in 131 patients with 147 porcine bioprostheses in either the mitral or aortic positions. The patients were divided into an early group in whom the echoes were performed within 2 months of valve replacement, an intermediate group studied 2–48 months after operation, and a late group studied ≥48 months after operation. The porcine cusp echoes were visualized with proper gain settings, enlarged, and then recorded on a strip chart. The mean thickness of both the mitral and aortic cusps was measured with the valve in the coapted position. The mean thickness of the porcine mitral valve increased from 1.23 ± 0.12 mm in the early group to 2.3 ± 0.19 mm in the late group ($p < 0.02$). Aortic valve thickness increased from 0.91 ± 0.07 mm in the early group to 2.1 ± 0.37 mm ($p < 0.05$) in the late group. A significant change in valve thickness was not observed in the intermediate group. In the late group, 21/82 (27%) had a thickness >3 mm: 9 (43%) of these bioprostheses have been replaced because of clinical dysfunction. Only 1.6% of the valves in the late group with a thickness <3 mm had or developed severe porcine valve insufficiency ($p < 0.001$). In all 10 instances, echo assessment of valve thickness was validated on gross examination of the valve removed at re-operation. This study indicates that the thickness of both mitral and aortic porcine valves can be measured by M-mode echo. Valve thickness increases after 48 months and those valves with thickening $\geqslant 3$ mm are at a high risk of developing valve dysfunction.

MORPHOLOGIC STUDIES

Ishihara and associates[91] from Bethesda, Maryland, determined the frequency of occurrence of *endothelial cells* by histologic and scanning and transmission electron microscopic studies in 49 porcine valve bioprostheses removed from 43 patients 2 days–113 months (average, 31 months) after implantation. Endothelial cells were found in none of 17 bioprostheses in place <1 year, in 5 (23%) of 22 in place 1–5 years, and in 7 (70%) of 10 in place >5 years. The 12 bioprostheses in which endothelial cells were present were in the AV position (7 of 32 in the mitral position and 5 of 6 in the tricuspid position) for 21–113 months (average, 71). Endothelial cells were not found in any of 11 bioprostheses in the semilunar position (9 in the aortic position and 2 in pulmonary conduits); however, all but 1 of these bioprostheses had been in place for <5 years. Endothelial cells were concentrated along the basal regions of the cusps. These cells did not grow in direct contact with valve collagen, but were attached to fibrin, thrombi, or fibroelastic host tissue (fibrous sheath) on the valve surfaces. The growth of endothelial cells and associated fibrous tissue may serve to increase the structural stability of the bioprosthetic cusps, which may be of functional importance several years after implantation when the porcine connective tissue may have undergone significant deterioration.

Ishihara and associates[92] also studied 16 porcine valve bioprostheses that had been implanted in 14 patients aged 2–65 years because they had *cuspal tears and/or perforations*. Eleven bioprostheses had been in the mitral position 30–123 months, 4 in the aortic position for 15–40 months and 1 in a valved pulmonary conduit for 96 months. The cuspal lesions were classified into 4 types regardless of the location of the bioprosthesis (Fig. 5-15). Cuspal tears and perforations were more frequent in the left and noncoronary cusps than in the right coronary cusps (the latter may be protected by its muscle shelf against this type of damage).

Bovine parietal pericardial bioprostheses: operative results

The Ionescu-Shiley bovine parietal pericardial bioprosthesis was introduced in 1971 as a hemodynamically superior alternative to the porcine bio-

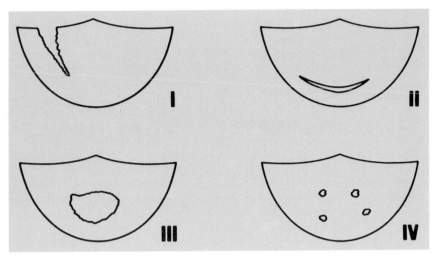

Fig. 5-15. Diagram showing 4 types of tears and perforations in porcine valve bioprostheses according to localization and to presence or absence of involvement of cuspal free edge.

prosthesis. Despite its use for 10 years, little information on its durability and complication rate is available. Becker and associates[93] from New York City reviewed 97 patients who underwent AVR or MVR with the Ionescu-Shiley valve between 1977 and 1980. Of the 45 patients having AVR, the actuarial survival was about 90% at 2 years and the thromboembolism-free rate at 2 years was 95%. Of the 52 patients having MVR, the 2-year survival was 65% and the thromboembolism-free rate at 2 years was 80%. Of the total 97 patients, 42% were in atrial fibrillation, and 80% of the thromboembolic episodes occurred in patients with atrial fibrillation. All but 1 embolic episode was manifested by cerebral ischemia and 1 patient had a residual neurologic impairment. There were no major problems of durability during this short time period.

Comparison of mechanical prostheses with porcine bioprostheses in the mitral position

The long-term outcome after MVR is determined by certain preoperative factors, by the type and size of prosthesis used, and by the skill of the operative team. The preoperative factors were analyzed by Dalby and associates[94] from Johannesburg, South Africa, in 545 patients undergoing isolated MVR with the Starr-Edwards prosthesis in 292 patients and with the porcine bioprosthesis in 253. The operative mortality was 7%. A large ($\geq$75%) cardiothoracic ratio on chest roentgenogram reduced operative survival (81% -vs- 95%, [p < 0.05]), 3-year survival (67% -vs- 84%, [p < 0.005]), and increased the frequency of thromboembolic events (98% -vs- 90%, [p < 0.05]) in the perioperative period. A left atrial diameter $\geq$12 cm reduced operative survival, but did not influence late survival or the frequency of thromboembolism. A cardiac index ≤1.5 liters/min/M² or elevated systolic PA pressure, pulmonary vascular resistance, or LV end-diastolic pressure did not increase mortality or the thromboembolism rate. Patients with poor preoperative hemodynamics had reduced operative survival (91% -vs- 97%, [p < 0.02]), but survival at 3 years and the rate of thromboembolism were unaffected.

Thus, the presence of severe abnormal hemodynamic variables in patients undergoing MVR increases operative mortality, and marked cardiomegaly increases both operative and late mortality and the frequency of thromboembolic events.

Complications of cardiac valve replacement

DIFFERENTIATION OF VALVULAR -VS- MYOCARDIAL CAUSE OF CONGESTIVE HEART FAILURE LATE AFTER VALVE REPLACEMENT

Goldman and associates[95] from Boston, Massachusetts, studied 41 patients who had had AVR (17 patients) or MVR (24 patients) 6 weeks–11 years earlier and who developed chronic CHF thereafter. The patients were studied by gated blood pool scanning (radionuclide ventriculography [RNV]) to analyze the spectrum of EF and its clinical correlates. Of the 17 patients who developed CHF after AVR, 10 had RNV EF >0.5 (all of them had severe valve or prosthetic dysfunction as the primary cause of CHF) and 7 had EF <0.5 (5 with severe myocardial disease and 2 with prosthetic dysfunction) (Fig. 5-16). Of the 24 with CHF after MVR, 13 had RNV EF >0.5 and only 8 of them had mechanical causes of CHF (7 prosthetic dysfunction and 1 constrictive pericarditis); of the 11 patients after MVR with EF <0.5, nine had severe myocardial disease and 2 had prosthetic dysfunction (Fig. 5-17). Thus, reduced EF in patients with CHF after AVR or MVR suggests myocardial disease as the basis for CHF, and normal EF implies a mechanical cause of CHF after AVR, but may be associated with either myocardial or mechanical factors after MVR.

VENTRICULAR ARRHYTHMIAS LATE AFTER AORTIC VALVE REPLACEMENT

Sudden unexplained death is a common mode of death late after AVR. To evaluate the occurrence of ventricular arrhythmias in patients after AVR, Gradman and associates[96] from New Haven, Connecticut, performed two 24-hour ambulatory ECG recordings in 45 such patients (mean age, 55 years) who had undergone AVR an average of 3.3 years previously. In 43 patients, a ventricular arrhythmia was detected; it was rare (mean VPC frequency <1/15 min) in 18 patients (40%), moderately frequent (mean frequency, 1–10/15 min) in 14 patients (31%), and frequent (mean frequency >10/15 min) in 11 patients (24%). Multiformity occurred in 40 (89%), bigeminy in 27 (60%), couplets in 27 (60%), and VT in 16 (36%) of the 45 patients. The occurrence of ventricular arrhythmia was not related to the predominant hemodynamic lesion or to the presence of CAD, as determined at the time of preoperative cardiac catheterization. RNA LV EF, determined at the time of ECG monitoring in 39 patients, demonstrated normal LV function (EF

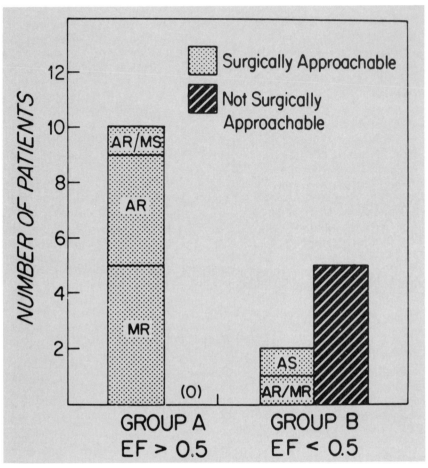

Fig. 5-16. Bar graph illustration of distribution of surgically approachable and surgically unapproachable disease for post-AVR patients in groups A and B. The distribution of surgically approachable-vs-surgically unapproachable patients between groups A and B was significantly different (p < 0.005). Reproduced with permission from Goldman et al.[95]

>50%) in 27 patients (60%), moderately depressed function (EF 36%–50%) in 8 (21%), and severe dysfunction in 4 (10%). When patients with abnormal and normal LV performance were compared, the mean VPC frequency was 21 ± 26/15 min -vs- 5 ± 11/15 min (p < 0.01); couplets occurred in 10 (83%) of 12 -vs- 13 (48%) of 27 patients (p < 0.05), and VT in 8 (75%) of 12 -vs- 6 (22%) of 27 patients (p < 0.01). Patients with VT had a mean LV EF of 47 ± 14%, as compared with 62 ± 13% in patients without this arrhythmia (p < 0.005). This study indicates that significant ventricular arrhythmias, including VT, are common late after AVR. In addition, a relation exists between occurrence of arrhythmia and LV function abnormalities.

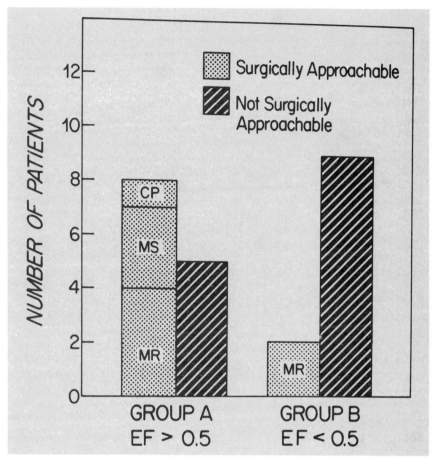

Fig. 5-17. Bar graph illustration of distribution of surgically approachable and surgically un-approachable disease for post-MVR patients in groups A and B. The distribution of surgically approachable-vs-surgically unapproachable patients between groups A and B was significantly different (p < 0.05). CP = constrictive pericarditis. Reproduced with permission from Goldman et al.[95]

PROSTHETIC AORTIC VALVE ENDOCARDITIS: OPERATIVE TREATMENT

Reitz and associates[97] from Stanford, California, described 4 patients with prosthetic valve endocarditis in the aortic valve position treated by removal of the entire prosthesis, curettage of an anular abscess, translocation of a porcine aortic valve above the "anulus" and native coronary artery ostia, and insertion of aortocoronary conduits into all 3 major coronary systems. In each patient, reoperation was done because of CHF from AR: 2 patients had systemic emboli and 2 had uncontrolled infection. The cause of infection was *Enterococcus* species in 3 and unknown in 1. Ischemic times averaged 135 minutes. A 25 mm dacron graft containing a porcine valve was used to replace the ascending aorta and aortic valve. One patient died 40 days postoperatively; another died 12 months postoperatively (of chronic active hepatitis), and 2 are alive within 60 days of the reoperation. Thus, the technique described for prosthetic valve endocarditis is a useful one and can be lifesaving.

REOPERATION TO REPLACE A PROSTHETIC OR BIOPROSTHETIC AORTIC VALVE

Wideman and associates[98] from Birmingham, Alabama, evaluated the incremental risk factors involved with replacement of an aortic valve prosthesis or bioprosthesis in 200 patients. The initial AVR was performed between January 7, 1975, and July 1979. Aortocoronary bypass or aneurysm resection also had been performed in 20 patients (10%). The indications for replacement of the substitute aortic valve were: replacement of a Braunwald-Cutter prosthesis in 65 patients; incompetence of a homograft biologic valve in 63; prosthetic endocarditis in 27; periprosthetic leak in 15; repeated thromboembolism in 10; prosthetic stenosis in 9; prosthetic thrombosis in 4; severe hemolytic anemia in 4; outgrowing the prosthesis in 1; aortic dissection in 1, and poppet escape (from a Braunwald-Cutter prosthesis) in 1. The reoperation was via the previous median sternotomy; ascending aortic and right atrial cannulations usually were performed. Cold ischemic arrest was employed in 76 patients (1975–76), and cold potassium cardioplegia in 123 patients (1977–1979). Hospital mortality for the first aortic re-replacement was similar to that of the initial AVR. Ten patients (5%) died in the hospital, as compared with 24 (3%) among 842 patients undergoing isolated or combined initial AVR. By simple continuous-table analysis, New York Heart Association functional class IV increased the risk of hospital death ($p = 0.002$), as did prosthetic valve endocarditis ($p = 0.005$), and the use of cold ischemic arrest ($p = 0.003$). Excluding those patients having elective re-replacement (Braunwald-Cutter prosthesis), hospital mortality was reduced by operating before severe hemodynamic deterioration occurred, by utilizing a medium sternotomy, by keeping aortic cross-clamp time short, and by employing cold cardioplegia.

TRICUSPID REGURGITATION

Detection by contrast echo

Lieppe and associates in 1978 (*Circulation* 57:128, 1978) suggested that 2-D echo was a sensitive and specific means for diagnosing TR. They used ultrasound contrast from an antecubital vein injection of saline or indocyanine green, and monitored the inferior vena cava (IVC) for appearance of contrast from the subcostal transducer position. Meltzer and associates[99] from Rotterdam, the Netherlands, also utilized this technique and also M-mode and 2-D echo for diagnosing TR in 62 patients. Group 1 consisted of 10 patients with clinical TR; group 2, of 40 patients without definite clinical signs of TR, but with conditions known to be commonly associated with TR (e.g., mitral valve disease, pulmonary hypertension, previous tricuspid valve operations); group 3, 12 normal subjects. The IVC was imaged by 2-D echo followed by M-mode echo. M-mode IVC measurements in the absence of contrast were not sufficient to separate reliably TR patients from non-TR patients. IVC contrast was imaged, frequently during deep inspiration, in all 10 group 1 patients, in 36 of 40 group 2 patients, and in 3 of 12 group 3 normal subjects. Three patterns of contrast appearance in the IVC were observed: "v-wave synchronous" patterns in all but 2 patients with TR, and "a-wave synchronous" or "random" patterns in patients without TR. The presence of TR was independently assessed during angiography or surgery in 26 patients. There were 2 false-negative echo studies, as judged by intraoperative palpation of a thrill over the right atrium. There were no false-positive v-wave synchronous studies. M-mode echo was superior to 2-D echo in detection of the appearance of contrast in the IVC and ease of pattern interpretation. Recognition of false-positive (a-wave synchronous or random) and false-negative patterns (insufficient central contrast, excessively inferior transducer position) improves diagnostic accuracy of contrast IVC echo, which is a sensitive and specific method for diagnosing TR.

Reeves and associates[100] from Hershey, Pennsylvania, utilized 2-D echo to visualize the right superior hepatic vein (RSHV) for detection of TR and for estimation of the central venous pressure (CVP). The patients were divided into 2 groups: 18 in group I on the basis of clinical features of TR (5 patients) or 2-D echo contrast evidence of TR (13 patients); group II included 55 patients without TR. Maximal transverse dimension of RSHV of at least 1.8 cm (range, 1.8–3.8 cm, mean, 2.4) identified all patients in group I (100% sensitivity). One patient in group II had RSHV width of 2.1 cm (96% specificity). Predictive value was 95%. RSHV width ranged from 0.4–2.1 cm (mean, 1.3) in group II. Mean values for groups I and II were significantly different (p < 0.001). Linear regression analysis was utilized to compare CVP and maximal RSHV width in 42 patients (15 group I and 27 group II). The slope of the line was significantly different from zero. In patients with maximal RSHV width >1.5 cm, the predictive value for elevated (>6 mmHg) CVP was 87%, with 69% sensitivity and 78% specificity. In 13 group II patients with technically satisfactory 2-D echoes, the RSHV was indistinct. CVP ranged from 4–12 mmHg with 4 elevated (>6 mmHg) values. Predictive value of normal CVP in the absence of visible RSHV was 69%. This study suggests that determination of maximal RSHV width is useful in detection of TR and may be helpful in estimation of CVP.

Pulsed Doppler echo may allow detection of TR as disturbed or turbulent systolic flow in the right atrium and of pulmonary regurgitation (PR) as turbulent diastolic flow in the RV outflow tract. Of 121 patients (101 with heart disease of various causes and 20 without), Waggoner and associates[101] from Houston, Texas, utilized pulsed Doppler echo to detect TR and PR. Results were compared with right-sided pressure measurements and M-mode echo findings in all, and with RV angiography in 21 patients. Pulsed Doppler study detected TR in 61 of 100 patients, 12 (20%) of whom had clinical evidence of

TR. Angiographic evidence of TR was present in 18%, 17 of whom had positive Doppler findings (sensitivity 94%), and absent in 3, all with negative Doppler findings. PR was found on pulsed Doppler study in 47 of 91 patients, 3 of whom (all after pulmonary valvotomy) had clinical evidence of PR. Increased (>35 mmHg) RV systolic pressure occurred more often in patients with (55 [90%] of 61) than in those without (22 [37%] of 59) TR (p < 0.01). PA mean pressure was elevated (≤22 mmHg) more often in patients with (38 [88%] of 43) than in those without (24 [38%] of 64) PR (p < 0.01). Thus, pulsed Doppler echo appears to be an accurate technique for detection of right-sided valve regurgitation. The absence of diagnostic physical findings in many patients indicates that the hemodynamic severity of the Doppler-detected valve regurgitation was probably insignificant. Because of its high incidence rate (87%) and association with pulmonary hypertension (87%), pulsed Doppler detection of TR, PR, or both (in the absence of pulmonic stenosis) was superior to M-mode echo measurements (RV size, pulmonic valve motion) in the prediction of pulmonary hypertension.

Detection by intracardiac phonocardiography

Cha and associates[102] from Browns Mills, New Jersey, obtained intracardiac phonocardiograms from the right atrium (RA) to study the relationship between clinical signs of TR, intracardiac murmurs, and the degree of TR demonstrated by right ventriculography with the use of a pre-shaped catheter. In 5 patients without heart disease, right ventriculograms showed no evidence of TR and intracardiac phonocardiograms in the RA demonstrated no murmur. Among 35 patients with valvular heart disease, a Carvallo sign (increased intensity of systolic murmur during inspiration) was present in 19 and absent in 16. All 19 patients with the Carvallo sign had variable degrees of TR on right ventriculography, and intracardiac phonocardiograms were positive for TR in 18. Among 16 patients with an absent Carvallo sign, neither right ventriculography nor intracardiac phonocardiography was indicative of TR in 5. Five patients had 1+ TR and the intracardiac phonocardiogram was positive in 3. The other 6 patients showed 3+ to 4+ TR and the intracardiac phonocardiogram was positive for TR in all. Thus, the Carvallo sign is a reliable indicator of TR, but its absence does not rule out TR, and right ventriculography is useful in detecting clinically unrecognized TR.

Tricuspid valvulectomy without prosthetic valve replacement

In 1970, tricuspid valvulectomy was performed without prosthetic replacement because of unremitting sepsis resulting from bacterial endocarditis of the tricuspid valve in a drug addict. Arbulu and Asfaw[103] from Detroit, Michigan, pioneered the nonreplacement therapy of tricuspid valve endocarditis. They now report 61 patients who underwent tricuspid valvulectomy from 1970–1980, 29 operated upon by them and 32 by others. All patients required this operation because of severe right-sided endocarditis: in 56, it was due to a bacterium (Gram-negative in 37 and Gram-positive in 19); in 3 patients, due to a fungus (*Candida albicans*); 1 was due to trauma to the tricuspid valve, and another was due to cancer of the tricuspid valve. Of the 61 patients, 52 were addicted to drugs given intravenously. Twelve of the 61 patients died within 60 days of the operation and 7 later. Eleven patients subsequently underwent insertion of a prosthetic valve in the tricuspid valve position. The results in the long-term follow-up of these 11 patients, as compared with the 50 patients who did not have a tricuspid valve inserted, were not significantly different. Actuarial survival for those who underwent tricuspid valvulectomy and not prosthetic valve replacement was 86% at 10 years. These authors concluded that, in the patients described, tricuspid valvulectomy without prosthetic valve replacement was the operation of choice.

RELATED TOPICS

Mitral anular size and motion in normals and in patients with dilated left ventricles

It is recognized that patients with LV dilation often develop MR. The exact mechanism by which MR occurs in this setting, however, remains uncertain. Initially, it was believed that dilation of the mitral valve ring (anulus) was important, but subsequently that viewpoint has not been popular, and malalignment of the papillary muscles with dysfunction has been viewed in recent years as the most likely mechanism of MR in patients with dilated left ventricles. Chandraratna and Aronow[104] from Long Beach, California, assessed the role of dilation of mitral valve anulus in the genesis of MR in 23 normal subjects (group 1), in 11 patients with dilated cardiomyopathy (DC) who had MR (group 2), and in 11 patients with DC and no MR (group 3). Through cross-sectional echo in the long axis, the maximum anteroposterior diameter of the mitral ring in diastole (Dd), the smallest diameter in systole (Ds), and the LV end-diastolic dimension (LVED) were measured. Percentage of shortening of the ring in systole (ΔD%) and ratio Dd/LVED were calculated. The LVED, Dd, and Ds were significantly higher than normal in group 2 and group 3 patients, whereas ΔD% and Dd/LVED were significantly lower. Dd was within normal limits in 8 patients in groups 2 and 3, 4 of whom had MR. Thus, dilation of the mitral anulus occurs only in some patients with DC and does not occur proportionally to the degree of LV dilation. MR that occurs in association with LV dilation may be due to a mechanism independent of mitral ring dilation, such as loss of sphincteric action of the anulus or malalignment of the papillary muscles.

Using wide-angle, phased-array, 2-D echo, Ormiston and associates[105] from Los Angeles, California, recorded mitral leaflets and their anular attachments from a view close to the standard apical 4-chamber view. The transducer was rotated and recordings were made at 30° rotational intervals around the circumference of the mitral anulus. To reconstruct the anulus, diameters (or chords) from each rotational interval were arranged around a reference point. This was done 12 times during the cardiac cycle. Anular areas were planimetered and circumferences were measured. Correlation was good for areas reconstructed and measured by the same observer on separate occasions (r = 0.96) and by 2 different observers (r = 0.99). In 11 normal subjects, the anular area index (area divided by body surface area) increased during diastole to a maximum of 3.8 ± 0.7 cm²/m² (mean ± SD) in late diastole. Presystolic narrowing was followed by systolic narrowing to a minimum in midsystole. The mean reduction in area was 26 ± 3%. The maximal anular circumference was 9.3 ± 0.9 cm and the mean reduction in circumference was 13 ± 3%. Mitral anular reconstruction may provide new information about normal and abnormal function of the mitral valve apparatus.

Maternal and fetal complications of pregnancy in the Marfan syndrome

Pyeritz[106] from Baltimore, Maryland, found reports of 32 women affected by the Marfan syndrome who had at least 1 pregnancy: 16 died of and 4 survived acute aortic dissection. Most women who had an aortic complication in association with pregnancy had preexisting AR, aortic root dilation, or another severe cardiovascular problem. Because women with the Marfan syndrome usually desire children, clinic records were reviewed and patients were contacted to determine a more representative estimate of maternal risks. The pregnancy histories of women with the Marfan syndrome were compared with those of spouses of men with the Marfan syndrome and those of mothers of a sporadic (new mutation) child with the Marfan syndrome. One of 26 women with the Marfan syndrome died shortly after pregnancy of infective endocarditis; she was the only woman to have a severe, preexisting cardiovascular condition. The prevalences of milder pregnancy-associated cardiovascular and general complications did not differ among the study groups. The rate of early spontaneous abortion was higher in women with the Marfan syndrome than in either control group. These results suggest that the risk of maternal death is low in women with the Marfan syndrome who have minimal cardiovascular disease. Women with the Marfan syndrome should be counseled regarding pregnancy risks only after review of their cardiovascular status, including an echo- determined aortic root diameter.

References

1. CORYA BC, RASMUSSEN S, PHILLIPS JF, BLACK MJ: Forward stroke volume calculated from aortic valve echograms in normal subjects and patients with mitral regurgitation secondary to left ventricular dysfunction. Am J Cardiol 47:1215–1222, June 1981.

2. CARABELLO BA, NOLAN SP, McGUIRE LB: Assessment of preoperative left ventricular function in patients with mitral regurgitation: value of the end-systolic wall stress-end-systolic volume ratio. Circulation 64:1212–1217, Dec 1981.

3. SCHUTTE JE, GAFFNEY FA, BLEND L, BLOMQVIST CG: Distinctive anthropometric characteristics of women with mitral valve prolapse. Am J Med 71:533–538, Oct 1981.

4. SANTOS AD, PUTHENPURAKAL KM, HILAL A, WALLACE WA: Orthostatic hypotension: a commonly unrecognized cause of symptoms in mitral valve prolapse. Am J Med 71:746–750, Nov 1981.

5. WEI JY, FORTUIN NJ: Diastolic sounds and murmurs associated with mitral valve prolapse. Circulation 63:559–564, March 1981.

6. ABINADER EG, OLIVEN A: The effect of congesting cuffs on the echo-phonocardiographic findings in mitral valve prolapse. Chest 80:197–200, Aug 1981.

7. GARDIN JM, TALANO JV, STEPHANIDES L, FIZZANO J, LESCH M: Systolic anterior motion in the absence of asymmetric septal hypertrophy: a buckling phenomenon of the chordae tendineae. Circulation 63:181–187, Jan 1981.

8. MORGANROTH J, MARDELLI TJ, NAITO M, CHEN CC: Apical cross-sectional echocardiography: standard for the diagnosis of idiopathic mitral valve prolapse syndrome. Chest 79:23–28, Jan 1981.

9. KENNETT JD, RUST PF, MARTIN RH, PARKER BM, WATSON LE: Observer variation in the angiocardiographic diagnosis of mitral valve prolapse. Chest 79:146–150, Jan 1981.

10. GINZTON LE, CRILEY JM: Mitral valve prolapse palpating the pachyderm. Chest 79:129–130, Jan 1981.

11. GOREN C, SANTUCCI BA, BUCHELERES HG, DENES P: Chronic recurrent ectopic junctional tachycardia resembling triggered automaticity in mitral valve prolapse syndrome. Am Heart J 101:504–507, Apr 1981.

12. BHARATI S, GRANSTON AS, LIEBSON PR, LOEB HS, ROSEN KM, LEV M: The conduction system in mitral valve prolapse syndrome with sudden death. Am Heart J 101:667–670, May 1981.

13. WALSH PN, KANSU TA, CORBETT JJ, SAVINO PJ, GOLDBURGH WP, SCHATZ NJ: Platelets, thromboembolism and mitral valve prolapse. Circulation 63:552–559, March 1981.

14. CHANNICK BJ, ADLIN EV, MARKS AD, DENENBERG BS, McDONOUGH MT, CHAKKO CS, SPANN JF: Hyperthyroidism and mitral-valve prolapse. N Engl J Med 305:497–500, Aug 1981.

15. JAFFE AS, GELTMAN EM, RODEY GE, UITTO J: Mitral valve prolapse: a consistent manifestation of type IV Ehlers-Danlos syndrome: the pathogenetic role of the abnormal production of type III collagen. Circulation 64:121–125, July 1981.

16. PICKERING NJ, BRODY JI, BARRETT MJ: Von Willebrand syndromes and mitral valve prolapse. N Engl J Med 305:131–134, July 1981.

17. BEASLEY B, KERBER R: Does mitral prolapse occur in mitral stenosis?: echocardiographic-angiographic observations. Chest 80:56–60, July 1, 1981.

18. DARSEE JR, HEYMSFIELD SB: Decreased myocardial taurine levels and hypertaurinuria in a kindred with mitral valve prolapse and congestive cardiomyopathy. N Engl J Med 304:129–135, Jan 1981.

19. GOTTDIENER JS, BORER JS, BACHARACH SL, GREEN MV, EPSTEIN SE: Left ventricular function in mitral valve prolapse: assessment with radionuclide cineangiography. Am J Cardiol 47:7–13, Jan 1981.

20. NEWMAN GE, GIBBONS RJ, JONES RH: Cardiac function during rest and exercise in patients with mitral valve prolapse. Am J Cardiol 47:14–19, Jan 1981.

21. MAUTNER RK, KATZ GE, ITELD BJ, PHILLIPS JH: Coronary artery spasm: a mechanism for chest pain in selected patients with the mitral valve prolapse syndrome. Chest 79:449–453, Apr 1981.

22. MARDELLI TJ, MORGANROTH J, CHEN CC, NAITO M, VERGEL J: Tricuspid valve prolapse diagnosed by cross-sectional echocardiography. Chest 79:201–205, Feb 1981.

23. CABIN HS, ROBERTS WC: Ebstein's anomaly of the tricuspid valve and prolapse of the mitral valve. Am Heart J 101:177–180, Feb 1981.

24. YACOUB M, HALIM M, RADLEY-SMITH R, McKAY R, NIJVELD A, TOWERS M: Surgical treatment of mitral regurgitation caused by floppy valves: repair versus replacement. Circulation 64:210–215, Aug 1981.

25. HAKKI A, ISKANDRIAN AS, BEMIS CE, KIMBIRIS D, MINTZ GS, SEGAL BL, BRICE C: A simplified valve formula for the calculation of stenotic cardiac valve areas. Circulation 63:1050–1055, May 1981.

26. SEITZ WS, FURUKAWA K: Hydraulic orifice formula for echographic measurement of the mitral valve area in stenosis: Application to M-mode echocardiography and correlation with cardiac catheterization. Br Heart J 46:41–46, July 1981.

27. SCHWEIZER P, BARDOS P, ERBEL R, MEYER J, MERX W, MESSMER BJ, EFFERT S: Detection of left atrial thrombi by echocardiography. Br Heart J 45:148–156, Feb 1981.

28. COLMAN T, DE UBAGO JLM, FIGUEROA A, POMAR JL, GALLO I, MORTERA C, PAJARON A, DURAN CMG: Coronary arteriography and atrial thrombosis in mitral valve disease. Am J Cardiol 47:973–977, Apr 1981.

29. WROBLEWSKI E, JAMES F, SPANN JF, BOVE AA: Right ventricular performance in mitral stenosis. Am J Cardiol 47:51–55, Jan 1981.

30. GROSS RI, CUNNINGHAM JN, SNIVELY SL, CATINELLA FP, NATHAN IM, ADAMS PX, SPENCER FC: Long-term results of open radical mitral commissurotomy: ten year follow-up study of 202 patients. Am J Cardiol 47:821–825, Apr 1981.

31. VEGA JL, FLEITAS M, MARTINEZ R, GALLO JI, GUITIERREZ JA, COLMAN T, DURAN CMG: Open mitral commissurotomy. Ann Thorac Surg 31:266–270, March 1981.

32. ROBERTS WC, WALLER BF: Mitral valve "anular" calcium forming a complete circle or "O" configuration: clinical and necropsy observations. Am Heart J 101:619–621, May 1981.

33. OSTERBERGER LE, GOLDSTEIN S, KHAJA F, LAKIER JB: Functional mitral stenosis in patients with massive mitral anular calcification. Circulation 64:472–476, Sept 1981.

34. DEPACE NL, ROHRER AH, KOTLER MN, BREZIN JH, PARRY WR: Rapidly progressing, massive mitral anular calcification. Occurrence in a patient with chronic renal failure. Arch Intern Med 141:1663–1665, Nov 1981.

35. SCHWARZ F, SCHAPER J, KITTSTEIN D, FLAMENG W, WALTER P, SCHAPER W: Reduced volume fraction of myofibrils in myocardium of patients with decompensated pressure overload. Circulation 63:1299–1304, June 1981.

36. BROCKMEIER LB, ADOLPH RJ, GUSTIN BW, HOLMES JC, SACKS JG: Calcium emboli to the retinal artery in calcific aortic stenosis. Am Heart J 101:32–37, Jan 1981.

37. GODLEY RW, GREEN D, DILLON JC, ROGERS EW, FEIGENBAUM H, WEYMAN AE: Reliability of two-dimensional echocardiography in assessing the severity of valvular aortic stenosis. Chest 79:657–662, June 1981.

38. LEDERMAN SM, GASH AK, BOVE AA, SPANN JF: Normal rate of ventricular emptying in valvular aortic stenosis. Br Heart J 46:415–420, Oct 1981.

39. AWAN NA, DEMARIA AN, MILLER RR, AMSTERDAM EA, MASON DT: Beneficial effects of nitroprusside administration on left ventricular dysfunction and myocardial ischemia in severe aortic stenosis. Am Heart J 101:386–394, Apr 1981.

40. MURPHY ES, LAWSON RM, STARR A, RAHIMTOOLA SH: Severe aortic stenosis in patients 60 years of age and older: left ventricular function and 10-year survival after valve replacement. Circulation 64:184–188, Aug 1981.

41. DANILEWITZ D, MCKIBBIN J, DERMAN D: Cessation of gastrointestinal bleeding after valve replacement of aortic stenosis. Am Heart J 101:686, May 1981.

42. ROBERTS WC, MORROW AG, MCINTOSH CL, JONES M, EPSTEIN SE: Congenitally bicuspid aortic valve causing severe, pure aortic regurgitation without superimposed infective endocarditis. Analysis of 13 patients requiring aortic valve replacement. Am J Cardiol 47:206–209, Feb 1981.

43. ABDULLA AM, FRANK MJ, ERDIN RA, CANEDO MI: Clinical significance and hemodynamic correlates of the third heart sound gallop in aortic regurgitation: a guide to optimal timing of cardiac catheterization. Circulation 64:464–471, Sept 1981.

44. PAULSEN W, BOUGHNER DR, PERSAUD J, DEVRIES L: Aortic regurgitation: detection of left ventricular dysfunction by exercise echocardiography. Br Heart J 46:380–388, Oct 1981.

45. OSBAKKEN M, BOVE AA, SPANN JF: Left ventricular function in chronic aortic regurgitation with reference to end-systolic pressure, volume and stress relations. Am J Cardiol 47:193–198, Feb 1981.

46. GREENBERG BH, DeMOTS H, MURPHY E, RAHIMTOOLA SH: Mechanism for improved cardiac performance with arteriolar dilators in aortic insufficiency. Circulation 63:263–268, Feb 1981.

47. TOUSSAINT C, CRIBIER A, CAZOR JL, SOYER R, LETAC B: Hemodynamic and angiographic evaluation of aortic regurgitation 8 and 27 months after aortic valve replacement. Circulation 64:456–463, Sept 1981.

48. GREVES J, RAHIMTOOLA SH, McANULTY JH, DeMOTS H, CLARK DG, GREENBERG B, STARR A: Preoperative criteria predictive of late survival following valve replacement for severe aortic regurgitation. Am Heart J 101:300–308, March 1981.

49. McDONALD GR, SCHAFF HV, PYERITZ RE, McKUSICK VA, GOTT VL: Surgical management of patients with the Marfan syndrome and dilatation of the ascending aorta. J Thorac Cardiovasc Surg 81:180–186, Feb 1981.

50. DITCHEY RV, SCHULER G, PETERSON KL: Reliability of echocardiographic and electrocardiographic parameters in assessing serial changes in left ventricular mass. Am J Med 70:1042–1050, May 1981.

51. OSBAKKEN MD, BOVE AA, SPANN JF: Left ventricular regional wall motion and velocity of shortening in chronic mitral and aortic regurgitation. Am J Cardiol 47:1005–1009, May 1981.

52. WINZELBERG GG, BOUCHER CA, POHOST GM, McKUSICK KA, BINGHAM JB, OKADA RD, STRAUSS HW: Right ventricular function in aortic and mitral valve disease. Relation of gated first-pass radionuclide angiography to clinical and hemodynamic findings. Chest 79:520–528, May 1981.

53. BOUCHER CA, BINGHAM JB, OSBAKKEN MD, OKADA RD, STRAUSS HW, BLOCK PC, LEVINE FH, PHILLIPS HR, POHOST GM: Early changes in left ventricular size and function after correction of left ventricular volume overload. Am J Cardiol 47:991–1004, May 1981.

54. BERTRAND ME, LABLANCHE JM, TILMANT PY, THIEULEUX FP, DELFORGE MR, CARRE AG: Coronary sinus blood flow at rest and during isometric exercise in patients with aortic valve disease: mechanism of angina pectoris in presence of normal coronary arteries. Am J Cardiol 47:199–205, Feb 1981.

55. HECHT HS, HOPKINS JM: Exercise-induced regional wall motion abnormalities on radionuclide angiography: lack of reliability for detection of coronary artery disease in the presence of valvular heart disease. Am J Cardiol 47:861–865, Apr 1981.

56. BONOW RO, KENT KM, ROSING DR, LIPSON LC, BORER JS, McINTOSH CL, MORROW AG, EPSTEIN SE: Aortic valve replacement without myocardial revascularization in patients with combined aortic valvular and coronary artery disease. Circulation 63:243–251, Feb 1981.

57. KIRKLIN JW, KOUCHOUKOS NT: Editorial: Aortic valve replacement without myocardial revascularization. Circulation 63:252–253, Feb 1981.

58. LERER PK, EDWARDS WD: Coronary arterial anatomy in bicuspid aortic valve. Br Heart J 45:142–147, Feb 1981.

59. SHEIKH MU, COVARRUBIAS EA, ALI N, LEE WR, SHEIKH NM, ROBERTS WC: M-mode echocardiographic observations during and after healing of active bacterial endocarditis limited to the mitral valve. Am Heart J 101:37–45, Jan 1981.

60. SHEIKH MU, COVARRUBIAS EA, ALI N, SHEIKH NM, LEE WR, ROBERTS WC: M-mode echocardiographic observations in active bacterial endocarditis limited to the aortic valve. Am Heart J 101:66–75, July 1981.

61. BERGER M, GALLERSTEIN PE, BENHURI P, BALLA R, GOLDBERG E: Evaluation of aortic valve endocarditis by two-dimensional echocardiography. Chest 80:61–67, July 1981.

62. MELVIN ET, BERGER M, LUTZKER LG, GOLDBERG E, MILDVAN D: Noninvasive methods for detection of valve vegetations in infective endocarditis. Am J Cardiol 47:271–278, Feb 1981.

63. HUBBELL G, CHEITLIN MD, RAPAPORT E: Presentation, management, and follow-up evaluation of infective endocarditis in drug addicts. Am Heart J 101:85–94, July 1981.

64. NOLAN CM, KANE JJ, GRUNOW WA: Infective endocarditis and mitral prolapse: a comparison with other types of endocarditis. Arch Intern Med 141:447–450, March 1981.

65. PRAGER RL, MAPLES MD, HAMMON JR JW, FRIESINGER GC, and BENDER JR HW: Early operative intervention in aortic bacterial endocarditis. Ann Thorac Surg 32:347–350, Oct 1981.

66. ST. JOHN SUTTON MG, SUTTON M, OLDERSHAW P, SACCHETTI R, PANETH M, LENNOX SC, GIBSON RV, GIBSON DG: Valve replacement without preoperative cardiac catheterization. N Engl J Med 305:1233–1237, Nov 1981.

67. BRANDENBURG RO: No more routine catheterization for valvular heart disease. N Engl J Med 305:1277–1278, Nov 1981.

68. ROBERTS WC: No cardiac catheterization before cardiac valve replacement—a mistake. Amer Heart J 103:930–933, May 1982.

69. TEPLY JF, GRUNKEMEIER GL, D'ARCY SUTHERLAND H, LAMBERT LE, JOHNSON VA, STARR A: The ultimate prognosis after valve replacement: an assessment at twenty years. Ann Thorac Surg 32:111–119, Aug 1981.

70. AMANN FW, BURCKHARDT D, HASSE J, GRADEL E: Echocardiographic features of the correctly functioning St. Jude medical valve prosthesis. Am Heart J 101:45–51, Jan 1981.

71. DEPACE NL, KOTLER MN, MINTZ GS, LICHTENBERG R, GOEL IP, SEGAL BL: Echocardiographic and phonocardiographic assessment of the St. Jude cardiac valve prosthesis. Chest 80:272–277, Sept 1981.

72. TRI TB, SCHATZ RA, WATSON TD, BOWEN TE, SCHILLER NB: Echocardiographic evaluation of the St. Jude medical prosthetic valve. Chest 80:278–284, Sept 1981.

73. CHAUX A, GRAY RJ, MATLOFF JM, FELDMAN H, SUSTAITA H: An appreciation of the new St. Jude valvular prosthesis. J Thorac Cardiovasc Surg 81:202–210, Feb 1981.

74. WORTHAM DC, TRI TB, BOWEN TE: Hemodynamic evaluation of the St. Jude medical valve prosthesis in the small aortic anulus. J Thorac Cardiovasc Surg 81:615–620, Apr 1981.

75. HORSTKOTTE D, HAERTEN K, HERZER JA, SEIPEL L, BIRCKS W, LOOGEN F: Preliminary results in mitral valve replacement with the St. Jude medical prosthesis: comparison with the Bjork-Shiley valve. Circulation 64:203–209, Aug 1981.

76. NICOLOFF DM, EMERY RW, AROM KV, NORTHRUP WF III, JORGENSON CR, WANG Y, AND LINDSAY WG: Clinical and hemodynamics results with the St. Jude medical cardiac valve prosthesis: a three-year experience. J Thorac Cardiovasc Surg 82:674–683, Nov 1981.

77. THORMANN J, GOTTWIK M, SCHLEPPER M, HEHRLEIN F: Hemodynamic alterations induced by isoproterenol and pacing after aortic valve replacement with the Bjork-Shiley or St. Jude medical prosthesis. Circulation 63:895–904, Apr 1981.

78. KARP RB, CYRUS RJ, BLACKSTONE EH, KIRKLIN JW, KOUCHOUKOS NT, PACIFICO AD: The Bjork-Shiley valve: intermediate-term follow-up. J Thorac Cardiovasc Surg 81:602–614, Apr 1981.

79. CHEUNG D, FLEMMA RJ, MULLEN DC, LEPLEY D JR, ANDERSON AJ, WEIRAUCH E: Ten-year follow-up in aortic valve replacement using the Bjork-Shiley prosthesis. Ann Thorac Surg 32:138–145, Aug 1981.

80. SCHAFF HV, BORKON AM, HUGHES C, ACHUFF S, DONAHOO JS, GARDNER TJ, WATKINS L JR, GOTT VL, MORROW AG, BRAWLEY RK: Clinical and hemodynamic evaluation of the 19 mm Bjork-Shiley aortic valve prosthesis. Ann Thorac Surg 32:50–57, July 1981.

81. COHN LH, MUDGE GH, PRATTER F, COLLINS JJ JR: Five to eight-year follow-up of patients undergoing porcine heart-valve replacement. N Engl J Med 304:258–292, Jan 29, 1981.

82. GALLO JI, RUIZ B, CARRION MF, GUTIERREZ JA, VEGA JL, DURAN CMG: Heart valve replacement

with the Hancock bioprosthesis: a 6-year review. Ann Thorac Surg 31:444–449, May 1981.

83. CURCIO CA, COMMERFORD PJ, ROSE AG, STEVENS JE, BARNARD MS: Calcification of glutaralde-hyde-preserved porcine xenografts in young patients. J Thorac Cardiovasc Surg 81:621–625, Apr 1981.

84. JAMIESON WRE, JANUSZ MT, MIYAGISHIMA RT, MUNRO AI, TUTASSURA H, GEREIN AN, BURR LH, ALLEN P: Embolic complications of porcine heterograft cardiac valves. J Thorac Cardiovasc Surg 81:626–631, Apr 1981.

85. GEHA AS, HOLTER AR, LANGOU RA, LAKS H, HAMMOND GL: Dysfunction and thromboem-bolism associated with cardiac valve xenografts in adults. Circulation 64:172–176, Aug 1981.

86. BORKON AM, McINTOSH CL, VON RUEDEN TJ, MORROW AG: Mitral valve replacement with the Hancock bioprosthesis: five-to-ten-year follow-up. Ann Thorac Surg 32:127–137, Aug 1981.

87. LIPSON LC, KENT KM, ROSING DR, BONOW RO, McINTOSH CL, CONDIT J, EPSTEIN SE, MORROW AG: Long-term hemodynamic assessment of the porcine heterograft in the mitral position: late development of valvular stenosis. Circulation 64:397–402, Aug 1981.

88. ZUSMAN DR, LEVINE FH, CARTER JE, BUCKLEY MJ: Hemodynamic and clinical evaluation of the Hancock modified orifice aortic bioprosthesis. Circulation 64:189–191, Aug 1981.

89. LEVINE FH, CARTER JE, BUCKLEY MJ, DAGGETT WM, AKINS CW, AUSTEN WG: Hemodynamic eval-uation of Hancock and Carpentier-Edwards bioprostheses. Circulation 64:192–194, Aug 1981.

90. ALAM M, GOLDSTEIN S, LAKIER JB: Echocardiographic changes in the thickness of porcine valves with time. Chest 79:663–668, June 1981.

91. ISHIHARA T, FERRANS VJ, JONES M, BOYCE SW, ROBERTS WC: Occurrence and significance of en-dothelial cells in implanted porcine bioprosthetic valves. Am J Cardiol 48:443–454, Sept 1981.

92. ISHIHARA T, FERRANS VJ, BOYCE SW, JONES M, ROBERTS WC: Structure and classification of cuspal tears and perforations in porcine bioprosthetic cardiac valves implanted in pa-tients. Am J Cardiol 48:665–678, Oct 1981.

93. BECKER RM, SANDOR L, TINDEL M, FRATER RWM: Medium-term follow-up of the Ionescu-Shiley heterograft valve. Ann Thorac Surg 32:120–126, Aug 1981.

94. DALBY AJ, FIRTH BG, FORMAN R: Preoperative factors affecting the outcome of isolated mitral valve replacement: a 10 year review. Am J Cardiol 47:826–834, Apr 1981.

95. GOLDMAN MR, BOUCHER CA, BLOCK PC, BUCKLEY MJ, AUSTEN WG, STRAUSS HW, POHOST GM: Spectrum of congestive heart failure late after aortic valve or mitral replacement: dif-ferentiation of valvular versus myocardial cause by radionuclide ventriculogram-ejec-tion fraction. Am Heart J 102:751–756, Oct 1981.

96. GRADMAN AH, HARBISON MA, BERGER HJ, GEHA AS, SHAW RK, CROCCO CJ, STOTERAU S, PYTLIK L, ZARET BL: Ventricular arrhythmias late after aortic valve replacement and their relation to left ventricular performance. Am J Cardiol 48:824–831, Nov 1981.

97. REITZ BA, STINSON EB, WATSON DC, BAUMGARTNER WA, JAMIESON SW: Translocation of the aor-tic valve for prosthetic valve endocarditis. J Thorac Cardiovasc Surg 81:212–218, Feb 1981.

98. WIDEMAN FE, BLACKSTONE EH, KIRKLIN JW, KARP RB, KOUCHOUKOS NT, PACIFICO AD: Hospital mortality of re-replacement of the aortic valve: incremental risk factors. J Thorac Car-diovasc Surg 82:692–698, Nov 1981.

99. MELTZER RS, HOOGENHUYZE DV, SERRUYS PW, HAALEBOS MMP, HUGENHOLTZ PG, ROELANDT J: Diagnosis of tricuspid regurgitation by contrast echocardiography. Circulation 63:1093–1099, May 1981.

100. REEVES WC, LEAMAN DM, BUONOCORE E, BABB JD, DASH H, SCHWITER EJ, CIOTOLA TJ, HALLAHAN

W: Detection of tricuspid regurgitation and estimation of central venous pressure by two-dimensional contrast echocardiography of the right superior hepatic vein. Am Heart J 102:374–377, Sept 1981.

101. WAGGONER AD, QUINONES MA, YOUNG JB, BRANDON TA, SHAH AA, VERANI MS, MILLER RR: Pulsed Doppler echocardiographic detection of right-sided valve regurgitation. Am J Cardiol 47:279–286, Feb 1981.

102. CHA SD, GOOCH AS, MARANHAO V: Intracardiac phonocardiography in tricuspid regurgitation: relation to clinical and angiographic findings. Am J Cardiol 48:578–583, Sept 1981.

103. ARBULU A, ASFAW I: Tricuspid valvulectomy without prosthetic replacement: ten years of clinical experience. J Thorac Cardiovasc Surg 82:684–691, Nov 1981.

104. CHANDRARATNA PAN, ARONOW WS: Mitral valve ring in normal-vs-dilated left ventricle: cross-sectional echocardiography study. Chest 79:151–154, Feb 1981.

105. ORMISTON JA, SHAH PM, TEI C, WONG M: Size and motion of the mitral valve anulus in man: I. a two-dimensional echocardiographic method and findings in normal subjects. Circulation 64:113–120, July 1981.

106. PYERITZ RE: Maternal and fetal complications of pregnancy in the Marfan syndrome. Am J Med 71:784–790, Nov 1981.

6

Myocardial Heart Disease

CLASSIFICATION

Brandenburg and associates[1], in a report of the WHO/ISFC task force, defined *cardiomyopathies* as *heart muscle diseases of unknown cause* or *heart muscle diseases of known cause* or *associated with disorders of other systems*. The idiopathic cardiomyopathies were of 3 types: 1) *dilated cardiomyopathy* (formerly called congestive cardiomyopathy); 2) *hypertrophic cardiomyopathy* (previously called idiopathic hypertrophic subaortic stenosis, muscular subaortic stenosis, obstructive cardiomyopathy, asymmetric hypertrophy, asymmetric septal hypertrophy, etc.), and 3) *restrictive cardiomyopathy*, which includes endomyocardial fibrosis and Loffler's endoplastic parietal endocarditis. The specific heart muscle diseases included infective, metabolic, general system diseases, heredofamilial, and sensitivity and toxic reactions.

IDIOPATHIC DILATED CARDIOMYOPATHIES

Natural history

Although idiopathic dilated cardiomyopathy (IDC) is a relatively common cardiac condition, surprisingly few clinical or necropsy studies comprising large numbers of patients are available. Fuster and associates[2] from Rochester, Minnesota, analyzed 104 patients (64 men and 40 women, median age, 49 years) with IDC who were seen at the Mayo Clinic between January 1960 and December 1973. All 104 patients were followed for a minimum of 6 years or until death if it occurred in <6 years. The median follow-up period was 11 years and the longest was 20 years. At entry into the study, all 104 patients also had selective coronary cineangiography. At catheterization, 85% of the patients were taking digoxin, diuretic drugs, or both. Patients were excluded if they had an obstruction of least 50% in luminal diameter in 1 of the 4 major coronary arteries. The 46 patients who had selective coronary cineangiography were free of significant coronary narrowing and 14 other patients who had postmortem examination were free of significant coronary narrowing. Thus, the lack of significant coronary narrowing was determined either angiographically or morphologically in 60 of the 104 patients. Patients with diseases of cardiac muscle or associated with a general systemic disease also were excluded. Of the 104 patients, 21% had a history of excessive consumption of alcohol, 20% had had a severe influenza-like syndrome within 60 days before the appearance of cardiac manifestations, and 8% had had rheumatic fever in the past without involvement of cardiac valves. Thus, possible etiologic risk factors of infectious-immunologic type may have been important in some patients. Of the 104 patients, 80 (77%) had an accelerated course to death, with two-thirds of the deaths occurring within the first 2 years (Fig. 6-1): 24 patients (23%) survived, and 18 of them had clinical improvement and a normal or reduced heart size. Univariate analysis at the time of diagnosis revealed 3 factors that were highly predictive (p < 0.01) of the clinical course: *age, cardiothoracic ratio on chest roentgenogram,* and *cardiac index.* Systemic emboli occurred in 18% of the patients who did not receive anticoagulant therapy and in none of those who did; thus, anticoagulant agents should probably be prescribed unless their use is contraindicated.

Autonomic function

Impaired parasympathetic function, increased peripheral sympathetic activity, and depletion of cardiac catecholamine stores have been reported in patients with CHF. These changes are believed to occur as a direct result of the poor cardiac output and are, therefore, nonspecific. In patients with CHF due to idiopathic dilated cardiomyopathy (IDC), a beneficial effect of beta adrenergic blockade together with deterioration on withdrawal of therapy was reported in 1980 and this observation suggested that increased sympathetic activity contributed to the underlying disease process. Since the presence of CHF invalidates any study of autonomic mechanisms specific to cardiomyopathy, Amorim and associates[3] from London, England, studied 5 patients with presumed cardiomyopathy before onset of CHF and 5 additional patients who had had an episode of CHF but were completely compensated at the time of study. The observations in these 10 patients with IDC were compared with those in 5 healthy control subjects. Heart rate and BP were recorded during physiological and pharmacological interventions and

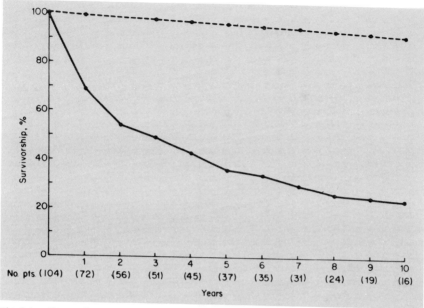

Fig. 6-1. Observed survival plotted against time in years in 104 patients with diagnosis of idiopathic dilated cardiomyopathy (*solid line*). The *dashed line* represents control expected survival, on basis of age and sex distribution, according to death rates of The Minnesota 1970 White Population Life Table. The number of alive patients under observation at each follow-up interval is indicated in parentheses.

plasma noradrenaline concentration was measured at rest and when the physiological interventions produced a peak response. The results indicate that even at an early (pre-CHF) state of IDC parasympathetic function is impaired, but no significant increase in sympathetic activity occurs at this stage. At rest, the heart rate and BP values of controls and patients were similar, whether CHF had occurred in the past or not. Plasma noradrenaline concentrations were similar in controls and in both groups of patients with IDC. During handgrip exercise, the percentage increase in heart rate at 120 seconds was similar in controls and pre-CHF IDC patients, while in the post-CHF group the maximum response was significantly less. Cardiac acceleration, however, during the first 10 seconds of exercise and cardiac deceleration during the first 10 seconds after cessation of exercise was considerably less in the IDC patients than in controls. The increase in heart rate after atropine administration was less in the post-CHF group than in controls. The BP response to cold stimulation was impaired, but surprisingly only the diastolic level seemed to be impaired in the post-CHF group. The mechanism responsible for the impaired autonomic function was unclear. Thus, autonomic function appears to be impaired even at an early pre-CHF stage in patients with IDC. These results, furthermore, do not show any evidence of important primary increase in adrenergic activity. Therefore, benefit from therapeutic intervention aimed at depressing sympathetic nerve function, at least in patients with IDC who are not in CHF, would not be expected.

Chronic beta blockade therapy

Ikram and Fitzpatrick[4] from Christchurch, New Zealand, administered acebutolol, a beta adrenergic blocking drug, or placebo in a double-blind, cross-over trial, to 15 patients with idiopathic dilated cardiomyopathy (IDC). Acebutolol significantly reduced maximum exercise tolerance and also ventricular function, as shown by an increase in cardiothoracic ratio. These results argue against routine administration of beta blocking agents in IDC.

Cardiac transplantation

Cardiac transplantation has become a relatively successful mode of treatment for some patients with end-stage cardiac disease. At Stanford University Medical Center in Stanford, California, the current expected 1-year survival after cardiac transplantation is 70%, with a yearly attrition rate of 5% thereafter. Most patients who have undergone cardiac transplantation have had the operation because of end-stage CAD, but recently an increasingly higher percentage of the patients undergoing this operation have had idiopathic dilated cardiomyopathy (IDC). Hassell and associates[5] from Stanford, California, reviewed results in 46 patients who underwent cardiac transplantation because of IDC and compared the findings in them with those in 59 patients who underwent cardiac transplantation because of CAD (Fig. 6-2). The overall 1-year survival rate was similar in the 2 groups: IDC-transplant = 64% and CAD transplant = 55%. The 3-year survival for IDC-transplant patients since 1974 was nearly 60%. In contrast, of 36 similarly ill patients with IDC not undergoing transplantation, the 1-year survival rate was 23% and the 3-year survival rate, 4%. Survival rates in the IDC-transplant group were unaffected by age, but patients in the age group <40 years of age had a lower frequency of infection, and a significantly longer interval to second rejection episodes (a measure of rejection frequency). IDC-transplant patients <40 years of age had fewer deaths due to rejection (17%), as compared with older patients in this group (36%). Thus, cardiac transplantation appears to be effective treatment for some patients with end-stage IDC.

Comparison of M-mode echo findings in chronic alcoholics with dilated cardiomyopathy and in asymptomatic chronic alcoholics

To assess the type and prevalence of cardiac abnormalities in heavy drinkers with and without overt CHF, Matthews and associates[6] from Bethesda, Maryland, performed M-mode echo in 11 symptomatic chronic alcoholics with dilated cardiomyopathy and in 22 asymptomatic chronic alcoholics. Echo data in both groups were adjusted for age and body surface area, using previously derived regression equations. All 11 symptomatic patients had a significantly decreased LV percent fraction shortening (mean, 14%;

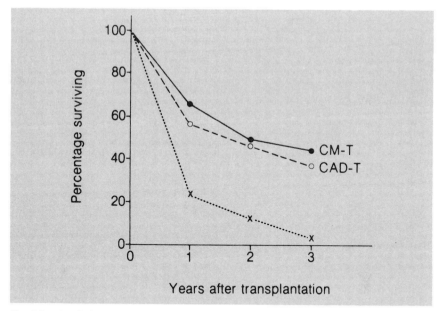

Fig. 6-2. Survival curves for patient groups under comparison. The proportion surviving is plotted against time for patients undergoing transplantation because of end-stage cardiomyopathy (CM-T, *solid circles*) or CAD (CAD-T, *open circles*). The group with cardiomyopathy not undergoing transplantation is represented by *crosses*.

normal range, 28–44) along with significant increases in LV systolic and diastolic dimensions (mean increases of 105% and 48% above normal, respectively), left atrial dimension (mean increase, 21%) and estimated LV mass (mean increase, 105%). Among the 22 asymptomatic patients, 15 (68%) demonstrated significant increases in at least 1 of the following echo variables: LV mass, LV dimensions, septal and LV wall thicknesses, and left atrial dimension.

Asymptomatic patients could be classified into 2 subgroups: 1) those with a LV diastolic dimension <10% above the normal predicted value and an increased LV wall thickness-to-radius ratio (mean increase, 16% above normal) and upper normal percent fractional shortening, and 2) those with a LV diastolic dimension 10%–24% above normal and a slightly subnormal thickness-to-radius ratio and lower normal percent fractional shortening. Echo abnormalities in asymptomatic chronic alcoholics did not correlate with the presence or absence of auscultatory abnormalities on physical examination and appear to reflect an earlier stage in the spectrum of alcoholic disease before the development of dilated cardiomyopathy.

Clinically occult cardiomyopathy in habitual alcoholism

It is well known that some patients with habitual alcoholism develop overt evidence of dilated cardiomyopathy. It is also known experimentally that ethyl alcohol damages myocardium directly and that the damage may lead to low-cardiac output CHF. Relatively few studies at necropsy have been performed on the heart in patients with fatal alcoholic cirrhosis. Steinberg and Hayden[7] from Detroit, Michigan, examined the heart at necropsy in 43 patients with histories of alcohol abuse and necropsy evidence of micronodular hepatic cirrhosis. None of the 43 patients had clinical evidence of heart disease and none at necropsy had significant CAD, congenital, valvular or pericardial heart disease. Patients with histories of systemic hypertension, diabetes mellitus, and high-output CHF or pulmonary heart disease also were eliminated. The mean absolute heart weight and the mean heart weight-to-body weight ratio in their 43 necropsy patients were significantly increased, as compared with a group of 33 similarly selected, age-matched nonalcoholics who died mainly of trauma or neoplasms. The mean value of absolute heart weight in the alcoholic group was 347 g, which was at the upper limit of normal (250–350 g). In 22 of the 43 alcoholics, 1 or more morphologic features observed frequently in dilated cardiomyopathy patients were seen. Additionally, 15 of these 22 patients had heart weights above the mean absolute heart weight in the alcoholic group. Focal interstitial myocardial fibrosis occurred in only 3 of the 33 controls. The presence of morphologic features consistent with dilated cardiomyopathy in the alcoholic with heart weights below the upper limits of normal, namely 7 patients, suggests that there is a subclinical form of alcoholic cardiomyopathy.

Cardiovascular status in asymptomatic alcoholics

King and associates[8] from Osaka, Japan, studied 145 alcoholics without known causes of heart disease to determine the frequency of cardiac abnormalities and dose-related effects of ethanol. All patients were admitted to their alcohol detoxification center. All patients were classified as either heavy drinkers (consumed more than the equivalent of 125 ml ethanol daily for 10 years or more) or moderate drinkers (consumed 75–125 ml ethanol daily). All were ambulatory and free from symptoms of cardiac dysfunction. There was no difference between heavy and moderate drinkers in the frequency of abnormalities detected by the ECG and chest roentgenograms. In the alcoholics, the most frequent finding was a prolonged $Q-T_c$ interval of >0.44 sec on the ECG (62 patients, 43%), unrelated to serum electrolyte imbalance. Cardiomegaly on chest roentgenogram was observed in 25 patients (17%). M-mode echo was recorded in randomly selected patients and compared with age- and sex-matched controls. Both ventricular septum and ventricular muscle mass were significantly increased only in heavy drinkers. LV function at rest was not depressed at an average of 31 days after the last drink of ethanol. CHF was not found even among the group of heavy drinkers, of whom more than 90% had hepatic dysfunction. Cardiac hypertrophy occurs in heavy drinkers, but is clinically well compensated in most.

A symposium on alcohol and cardiovascular diseases was published as Part II of the September 1981 issue of *Circulation*.[9] This monograph contains a large amount of information regarding the effect of alcohol on the cardiovascular system.

HYPERTROPHIC CARDIOMYOPATHY

Prognosis and predictors

McKenna and associates[10] in a retrospective analysis of the clinical course of 254 patients with hypertrophic cardiomyopathy (HC), followed 1–23 years (mean, 6), found that 38 had died, 32 of them suddenly (Fig. 6-3). They compared the 196 survivors with the 38 dead patients (6 from chronic CHF), and found that the combination of young age (≤ 14 years), syncope at diagnosis, severe dyspnea at last follow-up, and a family history of HC and sudden death best predicted sudden death (false negative rate, 30%; false positive rate, 27%). A "malignant" family history was associated with poor prognosis, particularly in the younger patients; a family history of HC without sudden death was more frequent in the survivors (12%) than in the dead (5%). Patients who had a diagnosis in childhood were usually asymptomatic and had an unfavorable family history and a 6% annual mortality rate. In those aged 15–45 years at diagnosis, there was a 2.5% annual mortality rate and syncope was the only prognostic feature. Among those diagnosed between ages 45 and 60 years, dyspnea and exertional chest pain were more

Fig. 6-3. Cumulative survival curve from year of diagnosis for 211 medically treated patients. Probability of death = total number of deaths for year divided by adjusted number at risk, minus number of deaths due to other causes.

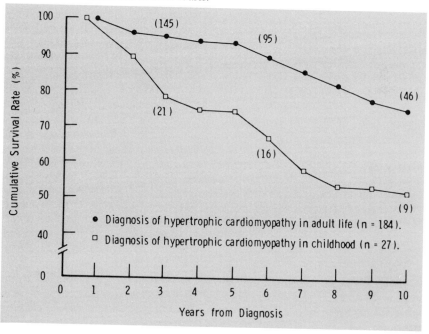

common in the patients who died, and the annual mortality rate was 2.6%. Poor prognosis was better predicted by the history at the time of diagnosis and by changes in symptoms during follow-up than by any ECG or hemodynamic measurement.

Echo observations

The M-mode echo is generally very good in detecting LV hypertrophy and the presence of, or lack of, LV dilation. Because HC is characterized anatomically by hypertrophied nondilated ventricles, the M-mode echo is highly useful in identifying asymmetric septal hypertrophy, which is present in about 90% of these patients. On occasion, however, the conventional M-mode echo may not show LV hypertrophy, yet the patient may present other clinical features highly suggestive of HC, including abnormal ECG and a strong family history. Maron and associates[11] from Bethesda, Maryland, studied 21 patients without evidence of LV hypertrophy by M-mode echo. Each patient was suspected clinically of having HC because of an abnormal ECG and either a family history of HC or symptoms of cardiac dysfunction. The 21 patients were aged 5–49 years (mean, 16) and 16 of the 21 were asymptomatic. The most common ECG abnormalities were deep Q waves, T-wave inversion, and RV hypertrophy. By use of 2-D echo to reconstruct the geometry of the LV wall, 16 of the 21 patients (76%) were found to have prominent, but unusually located, focal LV wall hypertrophy. In each patient, the hypertrophy involved regions of the LV wall through which the M-mode ultrasound beam does not usually pass, i.e., the posterior portion of the ventricular septum (7 patients), anterior or anterolateral LV free wall (7 patients), and the ventricular septum near the apex (2 patients). No patient had echo or hemodynamic evidence of LV outflow obstruction. Thus, some patients with HC have substantial LV hypertrophy in unusual locations. Although ECG abnormalities suggested the presence of myocardial disease, conventional M-mode echo (performed from standard parasternal positions) did not reliably identify such sites of hypertrophy, which were limited to LV regions not accessible to the M-mode beam. Only wide-angled 2-D echo permitted definitive identification of these unusually located regions of LV hypertrophy.

To characterize more completely the distribution of hypertrophy throughout the LV free wall and ventricular septum (VS) and to determine whether different patterns of hypertrophy were of particular clinical significance, Maron and associates[12] from Bethesda, Maryland, studied by wide-angle 2-D echo 125 patients with HC and identified 4 patterns of septal and LV free wall hypertrophy (Figs. 6-4 and 6-5). *Type I hypertrophy* occurred in 12 (10%) of the 125 patients and was confined to the anterior portion of the VS, the region of VS through which the M-mode ultrasonic beam passes. In contrast, the LV free wall and posterior portion of VS appeared normal. *Type II hypertrophy* occurred in 25 patients (20%) and involved both the anterior and posterior segments of VS, and the LV free wall appeared normal. *Type III hypertrophy* occurred in 65 patients (52%) and involved substantial portions of both the VS and LV free wall. Most commonly (41 of 65 patients), the predominant region of LV hypertrophy was the anterior or posterior VS; in 4

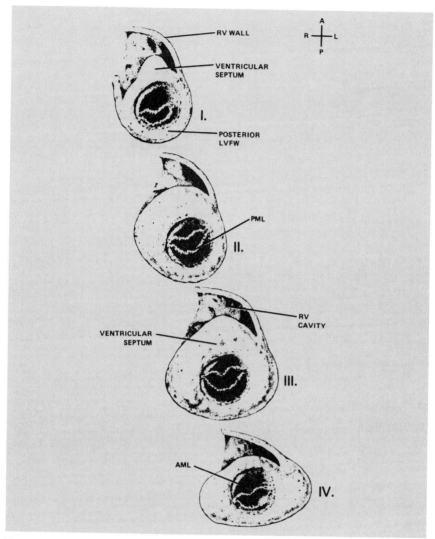

Fig. 6-4.   Artistic representation of the 4 patterns of hypertrophy identified with wide angle 2-D echo in 125 patients with hypertrophic cardiomyopathy. Shown only are cross-sectional planes at level of the mitral valve. AML = anterior mitral leaflet LVFW = left ventricular free wall. PML = posterior mitral leaflet.

other patients the hypertrophy was predominant in the anterolateral free wall and, in the remaining 20 patients, the hypertrophied segments of VS and LV free wall were relatively equal in thickness. *Type IV hypertrophy* occurred in 23 (18%) patients and the anterior VS in the basal portion and the LV free wall were either of normal or of only slightly increased thickness. Two-D

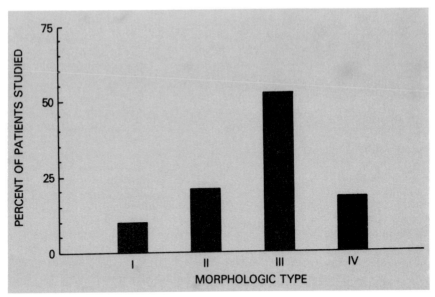

Fig. 6-5.   Prevalence of 4 patterns of hypertrophy identified with wide angle 2-D echo in 125 patients with hypertrophic cardiomyopathy.

echo, however, disclosed substantial hypertrophy in other regions of the LV wall, i.e., those inaccessible to the M-mode echo beam. Patients with the most widespread hypertrophy involving most of the VS and portions of the free wall (type III) differed from patients having the other patterns of hypertrophy: 1) they more commonly had moderate-to-severe functional limitation (38 of 65 [58%] -vs- 16 of 60 [27%]), and 2) they more often demonstrated obstruction of LV outflow under basal conditions (36 of 65 [55%] -vs- 11 of 60 [18%]) (Fig. 6-6). Hence, in patients with HC, wide-angle 2-D echo is capable of detecting myocardial hypertrophy that involves a variety of patterns and is more extensive than may be appreciated with M-mode echo. Although LV hypertrophy is "asymmetric" in most patients with HC, it is usually not confined to the VS and often involves the anterolateral LV free wall, but it rarely involves the posterior portion of the LV free wall (through which the M-mode beam passes).

The value of systolic anterior motion (SAM) of the anterior mitral leaflet as a diagnostic marker for HC has been questioned because of its reported occurrence in other cardiac diseases. To determine the true specificity of SAM for HC, Maron and associates[13] from Bethesda, Maryland, and Washington, D.C., examined 721 echoes from patients with a wide variety of cardiac diseases for the presence or absence of SAM under basal conditions. SAM was present in only 22 (3%) of the 721 patients, a specificity of 97%. It was most common in patients with TGA (11 of 51 [21%]). Excluding the TGA patients, the prevalence of SAM was only 1.6% (specificity, 98%) or 11 patients, 8 of

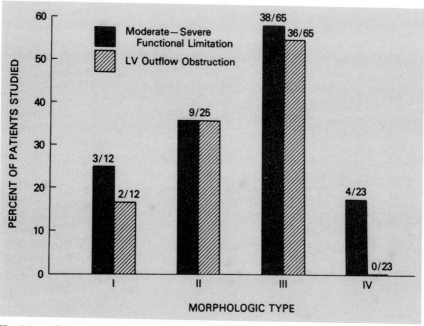

Fig. 6-6.   Relation of distribution of hypertrophy to presence of moderate to severe functional limitation (functional class III) or LV outflow tract obstruction under basal conditions.

whom had ventricular septa thicker than the LV free walls. Thus, the specificity of SAM in the absence of a ventricular septum thicker than the LV free wall, i.e., absence of asymmetric septal hypertrophy (ASH) was 99%. Although SAM is not pathognomonic of HC, it was an uncommon finding in a large population of patients with a variety of cardiac conditions other than HC and, when present, SAM is usually associated with ASH.

Shah and associates[14] from Los Angeles, California, evaluated 35 patients with HC and 10 normal subjects by 2-D echo, utilizing the apical 4-chamber and apical long-axis views. Of the 35 patients, 19 had systolic anterior motion (SAM) of the anterior mitral valve. The mitral leaflets were imaged throughout the cardiac cycle. The normal subjects and the 16 patients with HC without SAM demonstrated mitral valve coaptation that seemed to involve the distal tip of the anterior leaflet. In contrast, patients with HC with SAM had abnormal coaptation, so that the posterior leaflet coapted with a mid-portion of the anterior leaflet, leaving a distal "residual" portion of anterior leaflet in the left ventricle during systole. A sharp angulation of this distal leaflet in mid-systole toward the ventricular septum is believed to represent SAM. They speculated that abnormal mitral leaflet coaptation was necessary for development of SAM, which correlates with the presence of LV outflow gradients in HC.

Improved cineangiographic technique for diagnosis

Green and associates[15] from Birmingham, Alabama, studied 7 patients with HC and 1 with discrete subaortic stenosis by axial left ventriculography (caudocranial left anterior oblique view). In addition to the angiographic findings described on conventional views, the mitral valve, ventricular septum, and posterior LV wall were better profiled than with conventional views and, thus, better evaluated. Systolic anterior motion of the anterior leaflet of the mitral valve was readily identifiable, which is usually not the case in nonangled views. From this experience, the authors strongly recommended that caudocranial left ventriculography be the procedure of choice in patients suspected of LV outflow tract abnormalities and that biventricular angiography be abandoned for diagnostic purposes.

Effect of negative intrathoracic pressure on left ventricular outflow tract obstruction

Changes in LV afterload can have a dramatic effect on the pressure gradient in patients with HC. A decreased afterload, as produced by administration of amyl nitrite or nitroglycerin or by the Valsalva maneuver, significantly increases the LV outflow obstruction. Conversely, an increase in LV afterload by vasoactive agents, such as methoxamine, phenylephrine, angiotensin, and norepinephrine, decreases the gradient and the associated MR. Previous studies have suggested that such changes in ventricular afterload alter the degree of LV outflow obstruction in HC by altering ejection velocity and, hence, the degree to which the anterior mitral leaflet is drawn into the outflow tract by the Venturi mechanism. Inspiration and the Muller maneuver also have been suggested to increase LV afterload by increasing the negativity of intrathoracic pressure which, in turn, increases the LV transmural pressure. Because pharmacologic or physiologic increases in LV afterload decrease or abolish the pressure gradient in HC, these patients represent a unique opportunity to test the hypothesis that increases in the negativity of intrathoracic pressure increase LV afterload by increasing LV transmural pressure.

To study the effect of respiration and negative intrathoracic pressure on the LV outflow tract gradient in patients with HC, Buda and associates[16] from Toronto, Canada, studied 9 patients by use of various respiratory maneuvers during cardiac catheterization. Deep inspiration decreased the LV outflow tract gradient from 60 ± 11 to 34 ± 6 mmHg ($p < 0.01$) and decreased the LV ejection time (corrected for heart rate) from 0.42 ± 0.01 to 0.38 ± 0.01 s ($p < 0.001$) (Fig. 6-7). The Müller maneuver decreased the LV outflow tract gradient from 69 ± 13 to 7 ± 13 mmHg ($p < 0.001$) and decreased the corrected LV ejection time from 0.42 ± 0.02 to 0.34 ± 0.01 s ($p < 0.01$). Echo also showed a reduction or abolition of the systolic anterior motion of the anterior mitral leaflet and auscultatory and phonocardiographic studies disclosed a decrease or abolition of the apical systolic murmur. These findings indicate that negative intrathoracic pressure reduces the LV outflow tract gradient in HC. These authors believe that the negative in-

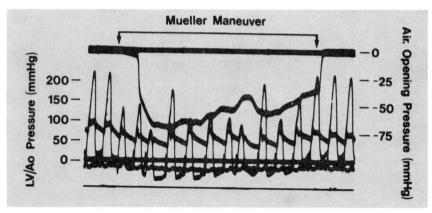

Fig. 6-7. Simultaneous LV inflow and aortic (Ao) pressure tracings showing effect of Müller maneuver on LV outflow tract gradient in patient with HC. The calibration of LV and Ao pressures is on the left and the calibration of airway (Air.) opening pressure (negative intrathoracic pressure) generated by the Müller maneuver is on the right. The onset and offset of the Müller maneuver are indicated by arrows. Because of length of tubing measuring airway opening pressure (negative intrathoracic pressure), there is a delay in onset and offset of this pressure decline in these recordings. The LV outflow tract gradient decreased immediately with application of the Müller maneuver. This reduction in outflow tract gradient persisted throughout the Müller maneuver; however, the gradient increased in 2 postextrasystolic beats but failed to reach control values. Reproduced with permission from Buda et al.[16]

trathoracic pressure produced these changes by increasing LV afterload through an increase in LV transmural pressure. These observations provide an explanation for the decrease in pressure gradient that occurs on inspiration in patients with HC.

HLA-DRW4 antigen linkage

In 1979, Matsumori and associates from Kyoto, Japan, found no significant association between HLA-A and HLA-B antigens in HC, but they did find a given HLA haplotype in relatives of the affected family members of patients with HC. Apparently, the HLA-DR antigens are associated with certain diseases in which there is no or only minimal association with specific HLA-A and HLA-B. In 1981, Matsumori and associates[17] from Kyoto, Japan, and Los Angeles, California, determined HLA-A, HLA-B, HLA-C, and HLA-DR specificities in 33 Japanese patients with HC. HLA-DRW4 was found in 11 (73%) of 15 patients with obstructive HC and in 6 (33%) of 18 patients with nonobstructive HC, and in 33% of 144 normal controls. Thus, these authors found that the obstructive form of HC was associated with genes in the HLA-DR region, and immunogenetic factors linked to HLA appeared to play a role in the pathogenesis of this condition. The study by Matsumori and associates is the first attempt at demonstration of HLA-DR antigen in HC. That these authors from Japan found no association between HLA-A or HLA-B locus antigens and HC is not surprising, since HLA antigen frequencies vary among different ethnic groups. The lack of an association also has been reported in a group of normotensive European white patients with HC. The previously reported study of patients in the southeastern USA by Darsee[18] suggested that there was a linkage between the gene for HC and the genes for the histocompatibility complex. Linkage is proved by studying patients and their families and does not necessarily imply an association with specific antigens. When a linkage disequilibrium has been established, it means that genes for 2 different phenotypes are very close to each other on the same chromosome. With regard to the HLA complex, the proof of linkage often means that an association with specific HLA antigens can only be detected in 1 family, and that other HLA antigens may be associated in a second family. The work of Matsumori and associates has provided the missing piece of the puzzle. In the Japanese patients studied, HC with outflow tract obstruction was associated with 1 of the HLA-D locus antigens. A careful study of the respective first-degree family members would likely corroborate the results of linkage studies reported in American patients. It is now clear that the genes in the HLA-DR region are the most important with regard to establishing an association between a disease and the histocompatibility complex. Current investigations are now concentrating on the HLA-DR region in lieu of the HLA-A and HLA-B loci that were studied extensively for years. The observation by Matsumori and associates that an association with HLA-DRW4 was present only for the obstructive form of HC lends further evidence to the hypothesis that at least 2 different forms of the disease occur. Thus, it may become important to define the disease called HC on the basis of its genetic pattern, and not by the more commonly utilized clinical phenotypes.

Association with lentiginosis

HC has been described in association with several anomalies of neural crest tissue, such as pheochromocytoma, tuberous sclerosis, and neurofibromatosis. These associations, together with the hemodynamic changes induced by catecholamines, led to speculation that the cause of HC might lie in a disturbance of the sympathetic nerve supply to the heart. A less well-known neuroectodermal association is that of HC with lentiginosis, a disorder of the pigmentary elements of the skin, and this association was described initially in 1968. The syndrome, which Moynahan and Polani called "cardiomyopathic lentiginosis," occurred in children, was dominantly inherited, was associated with sensorineural deafness, genital hypoplasia, and psychic and somatic infantilism.

St. John Sutton and associates[19] from Rochester, Minnesota, described 11 patients, 10 male, with HC and lentiginosis. In contrast to the patients reported by Moynahan and Polani, deafness, psychic, sexual and somatic infantilism were either rare or absent in their patients, mainly adults, and detailed clinical and echo family studies revealed no evidence of dominant inheritance. Of the 9 patients who underwent cardiac catheterization, all had LV outflow obstruction with LV-systemic artery peak systolic gradients at rest ranging from 27–150 mmHg, and 3 patients in addition had an RV outflow tract gradient at rest >100 mmHg. Ten of the 11 patients were severely symptomatic and 7 underwent successful septotomy-septectomy with marked symptomatic improvement.

Pre-excitation patterns

ECGs of patients with HC often show patterns suggestive of ventricular pre-excitation. Ventricular mapping studies, however, have suggested that delta waves may not imply ventricular pre-excitation in these patients. To further elucidate the meaning of delta waves in HC, Cosio and associates[20] from Madrid, Spain, performed electrophysiologic studies in 2 patients with HC. One had a short P-R interval and a wide QRS with initial slurring in the right precordial leads and a deep Q wave in leads I, aV_L, and V_6. On the electrophysiologic study, basal A-H was 35 ms, H-V 35 ms, and QRS 130 ms. With atrial pacing, A-H increased to 80 ms at 250 beats/min, H-V and QRS duration did not change, basal initial slurring persisted, and the Q wave became positive, forming a new delta wave. The second patient had a normal P-R and a wide QRS suggestive of right BBB and left anterior hemiblock, but with initial slurring (delta waves) in leads II, III, aV_F, and V_1–V_6. The electrophysiologic study showed a basal A-H interval of 95 ms, H-V of 60 ms, and QRS of 140 ms. With atrial pacing, A-H did not change, H-V increased to 80 ms at 180 beats/min, and QRS widened to 155 ms with increased slurring. At an atrial rate of 200 beats/min, 2:1 H-V block occurred in the absence of A-H-Wenckebach block. Intravenous ajmaline increased H-V and QRS duration in both patients, increasing initial slurring in proportion to QRS widening.

The ECG suggested the WPW syndrome in the first patient and Mahaim pre-excitation in the second. Because of the abnormal behavior of the A-H interval, a partial or total bypass of the AV node is possible in both. Ventricular pre-excitation was ruled out in patient #1 by the normal H-V interval and the lack of change in H-V and QRS duration in the face of A-H prolongation, and in patient #2 by the prolonged H-V interval, which increased further as QRS widened with atrial pacing. The persistence of the delta waves after ajmaline also argues against pre-excitation. These findings suggest that, in HC, delta waves may be due to abnormalities in ventricular excitation not related to anomalous AV connections, and that diagnosis of pre-excitation cannot be reliably made on surface ECGs in HC.

Ambulatory ECG monitoring

The prevalence and prognostic significance of ventricular arrhythmias identified on 24-hour ambulatory ECG monitoring was prospectively assessed in 99 patients with HC by Maron and associates[21] from Bethesda, Maryland. In the absence of antiarrhythmic therapy, high-grade ventricular arrhythmias (grade 3 and above) occurred in 66% of the patients, including 19% with episodes of asymptomatic VT. Clinical outcome was assessed 3 years after the initial 24-hour ambulatory ECG. Of the 84 patients who did not undergo septotomy-septectomy operations, 6 had cardiac arrest, 1 had progressive, eventually fatal CHF, and the other 77 have survived without a cardiac catastrophe (Fig. 6-8). The prevalence rate of cardiac arrest during the follow-up period was the same (3%) (1 of 37) in patients with high-grade arrhythmias as in those with no or low-grade arrhythmias (1 of 29) (Fig. 6-9). The occurrence of cardiac arrest was significantly more common in patients with asymptomatic VT of brief duration on 24-hour ECG (4 [24%] of 17) than in patients without VT (2 [3%] of 66) (p < 0.02). Thus, high-grade ventricular arrhythmias are commonly found on continuous 24-hour ECG monitoring in patients with HC and, although cardiac arrest is relatively uncommon in patients with high-grade ventricular arrhythmias, other than VT, (annual mortality rate = 1%), the finding of VT on 24-hour ECG identifies a subgroup of patients at high risk for sudden death (annual mortality rate = 9%). These findings suggest that 24-hour ECG monitoring should be performed in all patients with HC, and that it may be reasonable to initiate antiarrhythmic therapy if VT is identified.

McKenna and associates[22] from London, England, performed 72-hour ambulatory ECG monitoring in 86 unselected patients with HC to examine the association between arrhythmia and subsequent prognosis. During monitoring, 23 patients had at least 1 episode of supraventricular tachycardia and 24 had VT, of whom 10 had more than 3 episodes (Fig. 6-10). The patients were then followed from 1–4 years (mean, 2.6) and 7 patients died suddenly: 5 of them had had multiform and paired VPC and VT. These arrhythmias were significantly associated with sudden death, whereas supraventricular arrhythmias were not. The patients who died suddenly were

Fig. 6-8.   Flow diagram showing clinical outcome in 99 patients undergoing 24-hour ambulatory ECG monitoring.

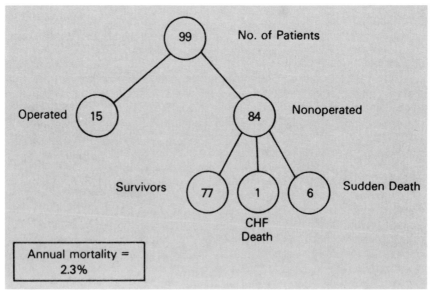

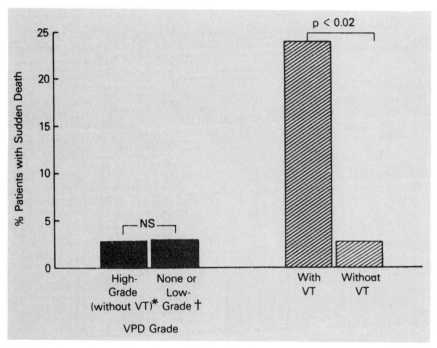

Fig. 6-9. Comparisons of prevalence of sudden death (or cardiac arrest) in patients with or without high-grade ventricular arrhythmias other than ventricular tachycardia (VT) and in patients with or without VT. NS = not significant. VPD = ventricular premature depolarization. *Arrhythmia grades 3 and 4a; † grades 0, 1 and 2.

older (mean age, 58 years), had more symptoms than did the survivors (4 of the 7 had severe functional limitation), and 3 had a family history of HC and sudden death.

McKenna and associates[23] also compared in 19 patients with HC complicated by refractory arrhythmias the therapeutic effects of amiodarone and verapamil. Although verapamil did not reduce the frequency of arrhythmia, amiodarone abolished VT in 10 of 13 patients and significantly reduced the number of VPC. In addition, sinus rhythm was restored by amiodarone in 3 of 5 patients with chronic AF.

Medical treatment and effects

PRACTOLOL, PROPRANOLOL, DIGITALIS

Storstein and Amlie[24] from Oslo, Norway performed a double-blind, randomized, cross-over study in 10 patients with HC to compare the effects of strophanthin (0.5 mg), practolol (10 mg), and propranolol (4 mg) on exercise tolerance with those of a placebo. Exercise was performed with graded submaximal bicycle ergometry. A postural test was performed with and

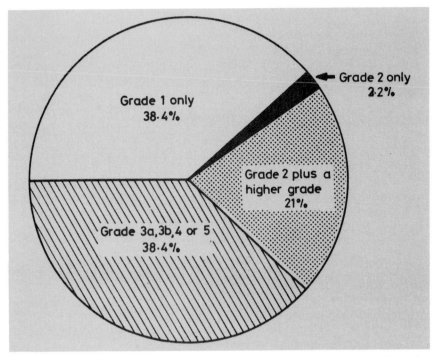

Fig. 6-10. Prevalence of ventricular arrhythmia grades in 86 patients with hypertrophic cardiomyopathy. Reproduced with permission from McKenna et al.[22]

without a drug. The response to 6 minutes standing was similar after placebo and digitalis, with a mean increase in heart rate of 18 beats/min. A significantly diminished increase in heart rate on standing was seen after beta blockers. No change in BP response was observed. Practolol and propranolol significantly reduced heart rate at rest and during and after exercise, as compared with placebo or strophanthin. No change in BP was observed between medications. Total work was not increased by any drug for the group as a whole, but marked intra-individual responses to drugs were observed. Two brothers had similar reactions to drugs. One patient with left BBB tolerated both strophanthin and beta blockers. A fall in BP on increasing work load was seen in 2 patients, both after practolol and after propranolol. Thus, the response to drugs in HC is "individual" and probably dependent on complex pathophysiological mechanisms. Furthermore, digitalis is usually well tolerated without any adverse reactions, and may be of benefit in individual patients with HC.

VERAPAMIL

For many years, beta adrenergic receptor blocking drugs have been the primary pharmacologic agents for treating symptomatic patients with HC.

Although this therapy is often effective, not all patients respond adequately to it and many patients experience unpleasant effects. Recent studies have demonstrated that administration of verapamil to patients with HC reduces LV outflow obstruction, increases exercise capacity, and reduces symptoms, and angiographic, ECG, and echo data have suggested that verapamil reduces LV muscle mass or ventricular septal thickness. To determine the efficacy of long-term therapy with verapamil in patients with HC, Rosing and associates[25] from Bethesda, Maryland, began treating 78 patients with the drug in the hospital; 62 (79%) were in NY Heart Association class III or IV, despite earlier treatment with beta receptor blocking drugs. A total of 42 (54%) of the 78 patients evaluated and 42 (63%) of the 68 discharged from the hospital experienced sustained symptomatic improvement 3–30 months (median, 14) after initiation of verapamil therapy (Fig. 6-11). Of these 42 patients in improved condition, 25 had improvement by at least 1 NY Heart Association functional class, 14 improved by less than 1 functional class, 2 felt better taking verapamil than propranolol and, in 1 patient, verapamil controlled asymptomatic VT. Of the 53 patients who had obstructive HC and were considered candidates for operation, 25 (47%) had sufficient improvement to forgo operation. In patients remaining on verapamil therapy, the duration of treadmill exercise performed 5 days after the start of verapamil therapy increased by 3.1 ± 0.6 min ($53 \pm 10\%$, $p < 0.001$) from the value obtained with no medication. A further increase of 2.3 ± 0.6 min ($25 \pm 7\%$,

Fig. 6-11. Change in functional class of 42 patients who described their style of living as improved with verapamil and thus have continued taking the medication. Upsloping lines connecting same functional class indicate persons who described a decrease in symptoms, but whose functional class remained unchanged. The 2 patients who were still in functional class III and had no change in severity of symptoms stated that they felt "better" with verapamil and chose to continue the medication. The patient who was in functional class I began therapy with verapamil because it decreased the incidence of VT.

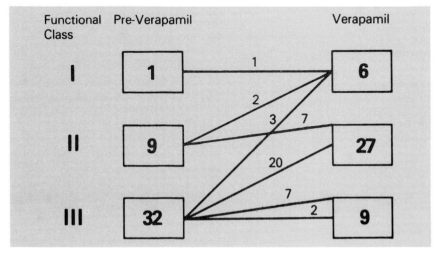

p < 0.0025) over the initial value with verapamil was recorded on the patients' last visit (median, 12 months after the start of therapy). Echo measurements of wall thicknesses and left atrial dimension demonstrated no significant changes during 1 year of verapamil treatment in 31 patients.

Administration of verapamil was associated with adverse hemodynamic effects in 9 patients (12%) and adverse electrophysiologic effects in 10 (13%). Three patients died (with pulmonary edema) and 6 had to have treatment terminated. These results indicate an important role for long-term verapamil therapy in the treatment of HC, but patients must be carefully selected and followed closely for the development of adverse hemodynamic or electrophysiologic effects. The major factor predisposing to verapamil-induced death is based on the sensitivity of patients with the obstructive form of HC to hypotension; a decrease in systemic pressure can increase obstruction to LV outflow by both decreasing afterload and reflexly increasing sympathetic stimulation to the heart.[26] The result is systemic hypotension with persistently high LV pressures. These high intraventricular pressures would make the LV particularly vulnerable to the decrease in coronary pressure that occurs as a result of the systemic hypotension. Thus, primary arrhythmic death or increased LV filling pressures and pulmonary edema might be precipitated. Epstein and Rosing[26] emphasized that serious complications with verapamil probably occur rarely in patients with HC, but their incidence may be further reduced by careful selection of patients with HC for treatment. They suggest that verapamil is probably contraindicated in patients with HC who have: 1) high pulmonary capillary wedge pressures in the presence of obstruction to LV outflow; 2) a history of paroxysmal nocturnal dyspnea or orthopnea in the presence of obstruction to LV outflow; 3) sick sinus syndrome without an implanted pacemaker, and 4) significant AV junctional disease without an implanted pacemaker. Additionally, these authors suggested that the drug should be given only when other alternatives are unavailable and only with extreme caution to patients with: 1) high pulmonary wedge pressures in the absence of obstruction to LV outflow; 2) a history of paroxysmal nocturnal dyspnea or orthopnea in the absence of obstruction to LV outflow, and 3) low systolic BP, particularly in the presence of LV outflow obstruction. The drug can probably be given, but with caution, to patients with 1) systolic hypertension and marked obstruction to LV outflow and 2) moderate prolongation of the P-R interval.

Verapamil improves exercise capacity in patients with HC, but its mechanisms of action are unknown. Bonow and associates[27] from Bethesda, Maryland, examined the effects of oral verapamil (320–480 mg/day) on resting LV systolic and diastolic function in patients with HC. High-temporal-resolution time-activity curves from gated technetium-99m RNA were analyzed before and after verapamil therapy in 40 patients, of whom 16 also were studied during propranolol therapy (80–960 mg/day). All but 1 patient had normal or supranormal systolic function, but 70% had evidence of diastolic dysfunction, defined as peak LV filling rate (PFR) < 2.5 end-diastolic volumes (EDV)/s or time to PFR > 180 ms. Verapamil did not change LV EF, peak ejection rate or ejection time, but did increase PFR (control, 3.3 ± 1.0 EDV/s; verapamil, 4.1 ± 1.1 EDV/s) and reduce time to PFR (control,

187 ± 56 ms; verapamil, 159 ± 34 ms). Only 30% of patients had evidence of diastolic dysfunction during verapamil. In contrast, propranolol did not change LV EF, PFR, or time to PFR, but did prolong ejection time and reduce peak ejection rate. Thus, LV diastolic filling is abnormal in a high percentage of patients with HC, and verapamil normalizes or improves these abnormalities without altering systolic function. This mechanism may contribute to the clinical improvement of many HC patients during verapamil therapy.

Operative treatment

Morrow and associates (see *Cardiology 1981*) from Bethesda, Maryland, have performed since 1960 partial ventricular septectomy and septotomy in >300 patients with HC. The operative mortality has averaged about 8% during the entire 21-year experience of Morrow. The resting LV outflow peak systolic pressure gradient in the survivors was nearly always abolished by 6 months postoperatively. Of the >300 patients, 8 have had MVR, with or without associated partial septectomy-septotomy.

Jeffery and associates[28] from Milwaukee, Wisconsin, described the results of operations in 20 patients aged 16–76 with HC who underwent operation at their institution from 1966 to 1980. All 20 patients were in NY Heart Association functional class III or IV preoperatively and 17 had overt CHF. Of the 20 patients, 19 preoperatively had resting systolic gradients from 25–152 mmHg (mean, 78) between left ventricle and a systemic artery. Sixteen patients had a septotomy alone, 3 had septotomy plus MVR, and 1 had MVR only. MVR was carried out because of associated severe MR. Of the 20 patients, 1 died in the early postoperative period and, during a mean follow-up of 6 years, 6 others died, at least 5 from cardiac-related disorders. At least in the early stages, 18 of the 19 survivors were improved to functional class I or II. The surprising feature of this study is the lack of relief of the LV outflow obstruction in a number of the patients, both intraoperatively and late postoperatively. MVR in 4 of the 20 patients may be out of the ordinary, but probably the influence of Cooley stimulated this procedure in 1 or more of the 4 patients. The procedure consisted of an incision into the ventricular septum no more than 5 mm in depth and extending from the apex up to the base of the aortic valve cusps. No myocardium was removed from the ventricular septum. Thus, of 20 patients operated on in a 14-year period, at least 7 are dead, at least 2 of those 7 had MVR, and at least 1 of them died from consequences of the presence of the prosthesis. Other groups have had better operative results than reported in this series.

Myocardial cell disorganization

It has been well demonstrated by both qualitative and quantitative histologic analysis that marked disorganization of cardiac muscle cells in the ventricular septum is a highly specific and sensitive anatomic hallmark of HC. Qualitative histologic studies also have shown that cellular disorganization also may be present in the LV free wall in patients with HC, but quantitative studies of the extent of cellular disorganization in the LV free wall have not been performed. Such was done, however, in a study performed by Maron and associates[29] from Bethesda, Maryland, who studied by quantitative analysis the LV free wall, as well as the ventricular septum, in 52 patients with HC. Cellular disorganization in the ventricular septum was both common and extensive (mean area of septal tissue section disorganized, 35 ± 4%). Disorganization was also substantial (24 ± 3%) in the LV free wall of these patients, although less marked than in the ventricular septum (p < 0.05) (Fig. 6-12). Anterior LV free wall disorganization was particularly extensive (32 ± 4%) and did not differ significantly from that present in the ventricular septum. Marked cardiac muscle cell disorganization (≥5% of the tissue section) was diffusely distributed in the ventricular septum and LV free wall in 33 (63%) of the 52 patients.

Particularly marked LV free wall and combined free wall and septal disorganization was present in 14 patients without functional limitation in whom sudden death occurred early (≤25 years of age) in life and was the initial manifestation of cardiac disease. In contrast, although identified in the LV free wall in 47% of patients with other congenital or acquired heart diseases or normal hearts, myocardial cell disorganization usually was limited in extent (mean area of section disorganized, 2 ± 0.5%) (Figs. 6-13 and 6-14). Hence, cellular disorganization is widely distributed throughout both the ventricular septum and LV free wall in HC, and this pattern suggests that HC is a diffuse cardiomyopathic process.

Maron and Roberts[30] reviewed several years' work on the frequency of muscle cell disorganization in patients with HC, in other congenital malformations of the heart, and in otherwise normal hearts, including those of fe-

Fig. 6-12. Extent of cardiac muscle cell disorganization in ventricular septum and in LV free wall of 52 patients with hypertrophic cardiomyopathy. Reproduced with permission from Maron et al.[29]

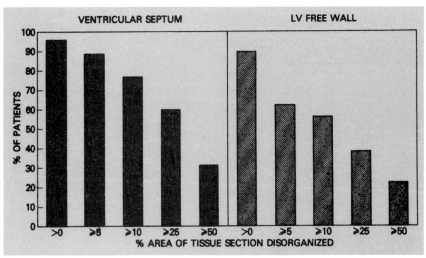

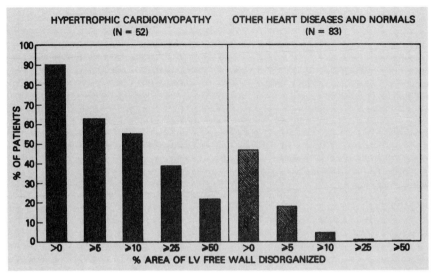

Fig. 6-13. Extent of LV free wall disorganization in 52 patients with hypertrophic cardiomyopathy and in 83 controls. Comparisons of respective bars from patients with hypertrophic cardiomyopathy and control patients each achieved high statistical significance (p < 0.001). Reproduced with permission from Maron et al.[29]

tuses, infants, and adults. The presence of abnormally arranged cardiac muscle cells in the septum is not pathognomonic or unique to patients with HC. However, disorganization is characteristically common and widespread in the septum of such patients and it is possible to reliably distinguish at necropsy patients with HC from patients with other cardiac diseases (or normal hearts) based on the extent of cellular disorganization in the septum. Quantitative histologic studies have demonstrated that marked disorganization (≥5% of a septal tissue section) is both a highly sensitive (89%) and specific (93%) histologic marker for HC, whereas disorganization involving <5% of a section makes this diagnosis unlikely. The extensive nature of the bizarre distortion of septal architecture in patients with HC is illustrated by the fact that the mean area of tissue section disorganized in 78 patients was 32%, compared with about 1% in 360 patients with a variety of other congenital or acquired heart diseases or normal hearts. Furthermore, marked septal disorganization is commonly present in patients showing a variety of clinical, hemodynamic, and morphologic manifestations of HC, including those with and those without obstruction to LV outflow. Septal disorganization probably represents a primary (congenital) derangement of myocardial architecture because marked cellular disorganization is characteristic of infants with HC (and is absent in the normal developing heart). The high frequency with which marked cellular disorganization and genetic transmission of the disease occur suggests that cardiac muscle cell disorganization may be a morphologic manifestation of an underlying genetic defect in HC. Finally, it is possible that the foci of disorganized myocardial cells in

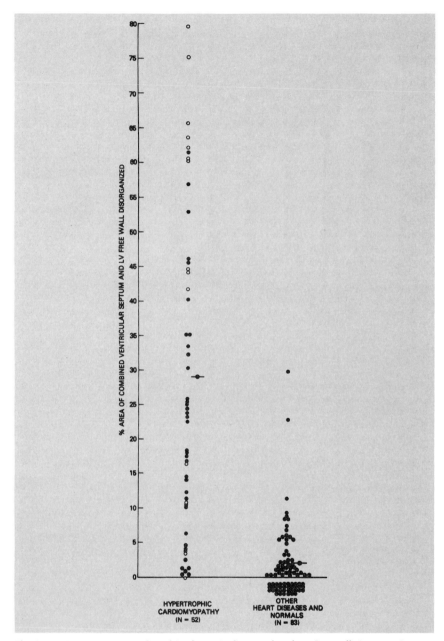

Fig. 6-14. Percentage area of combined ventricular septal and LV free wall tissue sections oc-
cupied by disorganized cardiac muscle cells in 52 patients with hypertrophic cardiomyopathy
and in 83 control patients. Patients 25 years of age or younger in whom sudden death was the
initial manifestation of hypertrophic cardiomyopathy are indicated by open symbols. Mean
values are indicated by the symbol Θ. Reproduced with permission from Maron et al.[29]

the LV wall of patients with HC provide a substrate for malignant ventricular ectopy and may be responsible, at least in part, for the occurrence of premature sudden death in such patients.

Speculation about pathogenesis

Perloff[31] from Los Angeles, California, summarized a number of hypotheses and speculations regarding pathogenesis of HC. He focused chiefly on the catecholamine hypothesis. The 2 anatomic hallmarks of genetic HC are extensive ventricular septal cellular disarray and asymmetric septal hypertrophy. HC may have its origin *in utero*—in failure of regression of disproportionate septal thickness present in normal human embryonic and fetal hearts. Faulty interaction between the adrenergic stimulus (norepinephrine) and myocardial adrenergic receptor sites may play a fundamental role in initiating myocardial cellular disarray. The timing of the autonomic derangement may prove crucial, with the highest yield in immature hearts that still harbor disproportionate septal thickness and are susceptible to the development of marked cellular disorganization. The presence *in utero* of abnormal septal cellular disarray may be responsible for failure of regression of embryonic and fetal disproportionate septal thickness, setting the stage for subsequent progression to the clinically overt disease.

CARDIAC AMYLOIDOSIS

Echo features

The M-mode echo features of cardiac amyloidosis are now well established, but few studies have described both 2-D and M-mode echo features in patients with CHF and biopsy-proven amyloidosis. Siqueira-Filho and associates[32] from Rochester, Minnesota, studied by echo 28 patients with cardiac amyloidosis: 26 by M-mode and 13 by 2-D. All 28 had CHF and biopsy-proven amyloidosis. The M-mode features were the following: 1) normal LV dimensions in 100%; 2) thickened ventricular septum in 88%, LV free wall in 77%, and RV free wall in 79%; 3) decreased thickening of the ventricular septum in 96% and of the LV free wall in 65%; 4) reduced LV global function in 62%; 5) left atrial dilation in 50%, and 6) pericardial effusion in 58%. Two-D echo provided additional features: 1) thickened papillary muscles (in 5 of 13); 2) thickened valves (4 of 13); 3) better appreciation of thickened RV wall, and 4) a characteristic "granular sparkling appearance" of the thickened cardiac walls. The latter was believed to be secondary to amyloid deposition and was noted in 12 of the 13 patients. Thus, M-mode echo is helpful in the recognition of this restrictive type of cardiac disease. The authors considered the "granular sparkling appearance" in the thickened cardiac walls by 2-D echo in patients with unexplained CHF to be virtually diagnostic of cardiac amyloidosis. In 7 patients the ventricular septum was thicker than the LV free wall by a ratio of >1.3. (The ventricular septum was thicker than the LV free wall in 4 of 50 patients with cardiac amyloid studied at necropsy by one of us (WCR).)

Differentiation from constrictive pericardial disease by left ventricular filling

The differentiation of restrictive amyloid heart disease from constrictive pericarditis is often a difficult diagnostic problem that, in occasional patients, is not settled until thoracotomy. To differentiate these 2 entities, Tyberg and associates[33] from New Haven, Connecticut, evaluated LV filling with use of digitized left ventriculograms in 4 patients with restrictive amyloid cardiomyopathy, in 7 patients with constrictive pericardial disease, and in 7 normal control subjects. Left ventriculographic silhouettes were digitized and LV volumes were calculated by computer at 16 ms intervals. Curves of LV volume and LV filling rate were constructed for each patient and also for each group. Patients with restrictive cardiac amyloidosis had no plateau in the diastolic LV filling volume curve and their LV filling rate was slower than normal during the first half of diastole. Patients with constrictive pericardial disease had a sudden and premature plateau in the diastolic LV volume filling curve. In addition, the LV filling rate was faster than normal during the first half of diastole. Statistical analysis of LV filling rate in the patients with amyloid, those with constrictive pericardial disease, and controls showed significant differences during the first half of diastole; those with amyloid had $45 \pm 4\%$, those with pericardial constriction had $85 \pm 4\%$, and normal subjects had $65 \pm 5\%$ of LV filling completed at 50% of diastole ($p < 0.05$). Thus, a significantly different profile of diastolic LV filling volume and LV filling rate occurs during the first half of diastole in patients with amyloid and those with pericardial constriction.

Digoxin sensitivity

Patients with amyloid heart disease are allegedly sensitive to digitalis and this sensitivity may cause abrupt changes in cardiac rhythm or even sudden death. To better understand why digitalis preparations can affect the amyloid-laden heart, Rubinow and associates[34] from Boston, Massachusetts, carried out an in vitro study to assess the interaction of isolated amyloid fibrils and digoxin, and in particular, to determine whether isolated amyloid fibrils bind digoxin. Digoxin (5 mg/ml) was added to 10 mg and 20 mg pellets of purified primary and secondary amyloid fibrils, a normal human liver and heart homogenate, and a homogenate from the heart of a patient with amyloid heart disease who had not received digitalis. After centrifugation, the supernatants were recovered and assayed for digoxin concentrations. Aliquots from the sediments were studied for the presence of digoxin, using rabbit antidigoxin antiserum and an indirect immunofluorescence technique. The results showed that $0.11-0.13$ ng/ml digoxin bound per milligram of fibrils and could not be separated by repeated washings, elution with citrate, or changes in the pH of the buffer (Fig. 6-15). Immunofluorescence studies demonstrated diffusely bright immunofluorescence with the fibril preparation and the amyloid heart homogenate when reacted with digoxin and di-

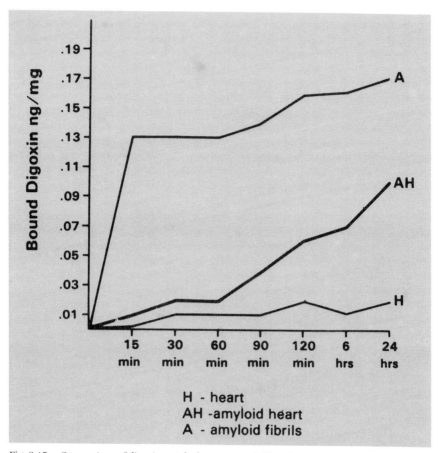

Fig. 6-15. Comparison of digoxin uptake by a nonamyloidotic heart homogenate (H), an amyloidotic heart homogenate (AH) and isolated amyloid fibrils (A). Reproduced with permission from Rubinow et al.[34]

goxin-specific antiserum. These studies demonstrate that isolated amyloid fibrils bind digoxin and suggest that this interaction may play some role in the sensitivity to digitalis that has been observed in some patients with amyloid heart disease.

TOXIC CARDIOMYOPATHY

Doxorubicin cardiomyopathy

In 84 patients (101 endocardial biopsies) receiving doxorubicin (DXR), Bristow and associates[35] from Stanford, California, measured the degree of morphologic damage via ultrastructural examination of endomyocardial biopsies and the degree of performance abnormalities via right-sided cardiac catheterization. Morphologic damage was variable, but was proportional to the total cumulative DXR dose between 100 and 600 mg/m². Performance abnormalities correlated weakly with dose and exhibited a curvilinear relationship. Catheterization abnormalities correlated well with morphologic damage (r = 0.57–0.78) in a subgroup of patients in whom exercise hemodynamics were measured, and this relationship also exhibited a curvilinear, threshold configuration. DXR myocardial damage is proportional to the degree of cytotoxic insult (DXR dose) while myocardial function is preserved until a critical dose or degree of damage is reached, after which myocardial performance deteriorates rapidly.

Shuman and associates[36] from Baltimore, Maryland, recorded serial ECGs, phonocardiograms and echoes in a prospective study of 45 patients who received DXR. QRS voltage, systolic time intervals (STI), echo EF, and rate of ventricular circumferential fiber shortening (V_{cf}) were compared as indicators of DXR cardiotoxicity. Seven patients (16%) developed a decline in LV function. Four of these 7 patients developed symptoms and signs of CHF. The pre-ejection period/LV ejection time (PEP/LV ET) was earliest to change and was the least specific of the noninvasive parameters. The EF was the most specific parameter in predicting clinical cardiotoxicity. In every patient with CHF, significant changes in EF, V_{cf}, and PEP/LV ET preceded the onset of symptoms, suggesting that measurement of the EF and STI will allow early prediction and avoidance of CHF. A fall in the EF ≥ 10% may represent sufficient grounds for discontinuing DXR.

Cyclophosphamide cardiomyopathy

Gottdiener and associates[37] from Bethesda, Maryland, assessed the cardiac effects of chemotherapeutic regimens using high doses of cyclophosphamide (180 mg/kg for 4 days) in 32 patients with hematologic malignant neoplasms. LV systolic function, determined by the fractional shortening by echo, declined substantially 5–16 days after the initiation of cyclophosphamide therapy. Although pericardial effusion by echo occurred in 33% of the patients studied, ECG voltage decreased 5–14 days after beginning cyclophosphamide therapy, even in those patients without pericardial effusion. CHF occurred in 9 patients (28%) within 3 weeks of cyclophosphamide administration and 6 (19%) of them died of CHF. Pericardial tamponade occurred in 6 patients (19%), including 5 who died of CHF. Histopathologic and electron microscopic findings showed endothelial injury and a hemorrhagic myopericarditis. Thus, cyclophosphamide in this high dose is associated with a toxic, often fatal, pericardiomyopathy. Depression of ECG voltage and systolic LV function do not necessarily predict clinical cardiac deterioration.

Gottdiener and associates[38] also used RNA to evaluate 32 patients who sustained long-term remission of soft tissue sarcoma after adjuvant therapy with a cumulative doxorubicin (DXR) dose of 480–550 mg/m² body surface area. LV EF at rest was below normal (>45%) in 8 of 32 patients. The abnormal response of EF to exercise identified an additional 12 patients with diminished LV functional reserve. EF, determined at rest or during exercise, did not differ between patients studied 1–9 months (mean, 5) and those studied 21–43 months (mean, 30) after completing DXR treatment. Sequential studies in 13 patients, 6–15 months after initial post-DXR evaluation, also showed persistent depression of average EF at rest and with exercise, with the continued deterioration of LV function in 6 patients. Thus, LV dysfunction, evident in >50% of asymptomatic patients even long after "acceptable" cumulative doses of DXR, may persist for years.

ENDOMYOCARDIAL FIBROSIS WITH OR WITHOUT EOSINOPHILIA

Relation of eosinophilia and microfilariasis to African endomyocardial fibrosis

One of the most common cardiac conditions in Africa, particularly central Africa, is the condition now called endomyocardial fibrosis, which was first described in 1948 by Davies from Kampala, Uganda. At that time, he noted a few eosinophils in the endomyocardium of the right and left ventricles and mentioned that some patients had mild eosinophilia. Subsequently, and even before that time, Löffler noted severe endocardial fibrosis in 2 patients with extremely elevated blood eosinophil counts. It has been suggested in recent years that undiagnosed severe eosinophilia predates the endomyocardial fibrosis observed in the African patients. To confirm or deny this concept, Andy and associates[39] from Ile-Ife, Nigeria, studied over a 2-year period 44 patients who had an eosinophil count above the 97th centile. Of these 44 patients, 13 developed clinical features of cardiac constriction with TR, and a diagnosis of endomyocardial fibrosis was made. Microfilariasis was believed to be the most likely cause of the raised total eosinophil count in these 13 patients. In all patients, the raised eosinophil count returned to normal after treatment with diethylcarbamazine. Thus, microfilaria-induced eosinophilia, when high, is frequently associated with heart disease that appears to be chronic endomyocardial fibrosis many months after the eosinophil count has returned to normal. This paper provides the clue that the African heart disease called endomyocardial fibrosis is virtually identical with Löffler's fibroplastic parietal endocarditis with eosinophilia.

Operative treatment

Dubost and associates[40] from Paris, France, performed the first endocardiectomy in 1971 and, since then, have operated on 19 other patients with this entity, endomyocardial fibrosis (EMF). There were 13 males and 7 females, aged 12–58 years. Thirteen were white and 7 were black. Nine initially had right-sided CHF, 5 left-sided, and 6 biventricular CHF. The operative technique included excision and replacement of 1 or both AV valves, and resection of RV or LV mural endocardium or both. There were 3 operative deaths; 7 had complete AV dissociation. Four died 1–7 years postoperatively.

Hemodynamic and angiographic studies were performed in 4 patients post-operatively and none had evidence of constriction. All patients were improved: 2 patients were in class I, 9 in class II, and 2 in class III.

Ikaheimo and associates[41] from Oulu, Finland, described a woman with EMF in severe CHF who, after MVR and removal of thrombotic tissue from the LV cavity, became asymptomatic until 14 months later, when she suddenly thrombosed the mitral prosthesis.

Davies and associates[42] from London, England, performed RV mural endocardial resection and combined tricuspid valve replacement and MVR in 1 patient and MVR in another patient with EMF and eosinophilia. Both had severe CHF with biventricular endocardial fibrosis, MR, and TR. Both were symptomatically improved by operation and that improvement was maintained over a 16-month period.

Graham and associates[43] from Houston, Texas, and Riyadh, Saudi Arabia, described TVR, MVR, and limited resection of the thickened mural endocardial RV fibrotic tissue in a man with EMF and severe CHF. By 1 month postoperatively, the patient was doing well.

ENDOMYOCARDIAL BIOPSY IN CARDIOMYOPATHY

There has been debate concerning the usefulness of biopsying ventricular myocardium during life in patients with various forms of cardiac disease, particularly cardiomyopathy. Baandrup and Olsen[44] from London, England, examined histologically 361 biopsies from 201 patients with suspected cardiomyopathy. All biopsies were obtained either with a small Konno-Sakakibara bioptome or the King's College Hospital instrument. The site of the biopsy was the RV aspect of the ventricular septum in 163 patients (264 biopsies), the left ventricle in 20 patients (48 biopsies), and both ventricles in 17 patients (49 biopsies). Of these biopsies, 16% were of such poor quality that morphologic analysis was meaningless. The mean size of the biopsies was 0.8 mm² and an average of 1.4 mm² of tissue was available per patient. Histologic examination of the biopsies proved useful in sorting out the patients with HC, but the findings in the patients with dilated cardiomyopathy were non-specific. If only histologic examinations are to be performed on biopsies of heart muscle during life, the biopsy will rarely be useful diagnostically. The exceptions are in patients with iron or amyloid in the heart and, rarely, for such things as cardiac sarcoid.

Baandrup and associates[45] from London, England, attempted to ascertain whether the morphology of the myocardium obtained by biopsy in patients with dilated cardiomyopathy could predict the functional state of the myocardium, as expressed by the LV EF, LV end-diastolic pressure, duration of symptoms of cardiac dysfunction, and prognosis. Of 125 patients studied, no correlation was found between quantitative, morphologic assessment of the myocardium by biopsy and duration of symptoms of cardiac dysfunction or subsequent course or the hemodynamic variables. Thus, the severity of dilated cardiomyopathy and its prognosis cannot be assessed from histologic changes.

References

1. BRANDENBURG RO, CHAZOV E, CHERIAN G, FALASE AO, GROSGOGEAT Y, KAWAI C, LOOGEN F, JUDEZ VM, ORINIUS E, GOODWIN JF, OLSEN EGJ, OAKLEY CM, PISA Z: Report of the WHO/ISFC task force on definition and classification of cardiomyopathies. Circulation 64:437A–438A, Aug 1981.

2. FUSTER V, GERSH BJ, GIULIANI ER, TAJIK AJ, BRANDENBURG RO, FRYE RL: The natural history of idiopathic dilated cardiomyopathy. Am J Cardiol 47:525–531, March 1981.

3. AMORIM DS, HEER K, JENNER D, RICHARDSON P, DARGIE HJ, BROWN M, OLSEN EGJ, GOODWIN JF: Is there autonomic impairment in congestive (dilated) cardiomyopathy? Lancet 1:525–527, March 1981.

4. IKRAM H, FITZPATRICK D: Double-blind trial of chronic oral beta blockade in congestive cardiomyopathy. Lancet 2:490–492, Sept 1981.

5. HASSELL LA, FOWLES RE, STINSON EB: Patients with congestive cardiomyopathy as cardiac transplant recipients. Indications for and results of cardiac transplantation and comparison with patients with coronary artery disease. Am J Cardiol 47:1205–1209, June 1981.

6. MATTHEWS EC, GARDIN JM, HENRY WL, DEL NEGRO AA, FLETCHER RD, SNOW JA, EPSTEIN SE: Echocardiographic abnormalities in chronic alcoholics with and without overt congestive heart failure. Am J Cardiol 47:570–578, March 1981.

7. STEINBERG JD, HAYDEN MT: Prevalence of clinically occult cardiomyopathy in chronic alcoholism. Am Heart J 101:461–464, Apr 1981.

8. KING M, IMAMITCHI H, MORIGUTCHI M, KAWAMURA K, TAKATSU T: Cardiovascular status in asymptomatic alcoholics, with reference to the level of ethanol consumption. Br Heart J 46:545–551, Nov 1981.

9. KAELBER CT, BARBORIAK J, eds: Symposium on alcohol and cardiovascular diseases. Circulation (Part II): III-1—III-84, Sept 1981.

10. McKENNA W, DEANFIELD J, FARUQUI A, ENGLAND D, OAKLEY C, GOODWIN J: Prognosis in hypertrophic cardiomyopathy: role of age and clinical, electrocardiographic and hemodynamic features. Am J Cardiol 47:532–538, March 1981.

11. MARON BJ, GOTTDIENER JS, BONOW RO, EPSTEIN SE: Hypertrophic cardiomyopathy with unusual locations of left ventricular hypertrophy undetectable by M-mode echocardiography. Identification by wide-angle two-dimensional echocardiography. Circulation 63:409–418, Feb 1981.

12. MARON BJ, GOTTDIENER JS, EPSTEIN SE: Patterns and significance of distribution of left ventricular hypertrophy in hypertrophic cardiomyopathy. Am J Cardiol 48:418–428. Sept 1981.

13. MARON BJ, GOTTDIENER JS, LOWELL WP: Specificity of systolic anterior motion of anterior mitral leaflet for hypertrophic cardiomyopathy. Prevalence in large population of patients with other cardiac diseases. Br Heart J 45:206–212, Feb 1981.

14. SHAH PM, TAYLOR RD, WONG M: Abnormal mitral valve coaptation in hypertrophic obstructive cardiomyopathy: proposed role in systolic anterior motion of mitral valve. Am J Cardiol 48:258–262, Aug 1981.

15. GREEN CE, ELLIOTT LP, COGHLAN HC: Improved cineangiographic evaluation of hypertrophic cardiomyopathy by caudocranial left anterior oblique view. Am Heart J 102:1015–1021, Dec 1981.

16. BUDA AJ, MACKENZIE GW, WIGLE ED: Effect of negative intrathoracic pressure on left ventricular outflow tract obstruction in muscular subaortic stenosis. Circulation 63:875–881, Apr 1981.

17. MATSUMORI A, KAWAI C, WAKABAYASHI A, TERASAKI PI, PARK MS, SAKURAMI T, UENO Y: HLA-DRW4 antigen linkage in patients with hypertrophic obstructive cardiomyopathy. Am Heart J 101:14–16, Jan 1981.

18. DARSEE JR: The hypertrophic heart syndromes: a glance at the chromosome. Am Heart J 101:124–126, Jan 1981.

19. ST. JOHN SUTTON MG, TAJIK AJ, GIULIANI ER, GORDON H, SU WPD: Hypertrophic obstructive cardiomyopathy and lentiginosis: a little known neural ectodermal syndrome. Am J Cardiol 47:214–217, Feb 1981.

20. COSIO FG, SANCHEZ A, VIDAL JM, IGLESIAS J, GARCIA-MARTINEZ J: Preexcitation patterns in hypertrophic cardiomyopathy. Am Heart J 101:233–234, Feb 1981.

21. MARON BJ, SAVAGE DD, WOLFSON JK, EPSTEIN SE: Prognostic significance of 24 hour ambulatory electrocardiographic monitoring in patients with hypertrophic cardiomyopathy: a prospective study. Am J Cardiol 48:252–257, Aug 1981.

22. MCKENNA WJ, ENGLAND D, DOI YL, DEANFIELD JE, OAKLEY C, GOODWIN JF: Arrhythmia in hypertrophic cardiomyopathy: I: influence on prognosis. Br Heart J 46:168–172, Aug 1981.

23. MCKENNA WJ, HARRIS L, PEREZ G, KRIKLER DM, OAKLEY C, GOODWIN JF: Arrhythmia in hypertrophic cardiomyopathy: II: comparison of amiodarone and verapamil in treatment. Br Heart J 46:173–178, Aug 1981.

24. STORSTEIN L, AMLIE JP: The effect of practolol, propranolol and strophanthin compared with placebo on exercise tolerance and a postural test in patients with hypertrophic cardiomyopathy. Eur Heart J 2:289–296, Aug 1981.

25. ROSING DR, CONDIT JR, MARON BJ, KENT KM, LEON MB, BONOW RO, LIPSON LC, EPSTEIN SE: Verapamil therapy: new approach to the pharmacologic treatment of hypertrophic cardiomyopathy: effects of long-term administration. Am J Cardiol 48:545–553, Sept 1981.

26. EPSTEIN SE, ROSING DR: Verapamil: its potential for causing serious complications in patients with hypertrophic cardiomyopathy. Circulation 64:437–441, Sept 1981.

27. BONOW RO, ROSING DR, BACHARACH SL, GREEN MV, KENT KM, LIPSON LC, MARON BJ, LEON MB, EPSTEIN SE: Effects of verapamil on left ventricular systolic function and diastolic filling in patients with hypertrophic cardiomyopathy. Circulation 64:787–796, Oct 1981.

28. JEFFERY DL, SIGNORINI W, FLEMMA RJ, LEPLEY D JR, MULLEN DC: Left ventricular myotomy: physiologic approach to surgical therapy for IHSS. Chest 80:550–556, Nov 1981.

29. MARON BJ, ANAN TJ, ROBERTS WC: Quantitative analysis of the distribution of cardiac muscle cell disorganization in the left ventricular wall of patients with hypertrophic cardiomyopathy. Circulation 63:882–894, Apr 1981.

30. MARON BJ, ROBERTS WC: Hypertrophic cardiomyopathy and cardiac muscle cell disorganization revisited: relation between the two and significance. Am Heart J 101:95–110, July 1981.

31. PERLOFF JK: Pathogenesis of hypertrophic cardiomyopathy: hypotheses and speculations. Am Heart J 101:219–226, Feb 1981.

32. SIQUEIRA-FILHO AG, CUNHA CLP, TAJIK AJ, SEWARD JB, SCHATTENBERG TT, GIULIANI ER: M-mode and two-dimensional echocardiographic features in cardiac amyloidosis. Circulation 63:188–196, Jan 1981.

33. TYBERG TI, GOODYER AVN, HURST VW, ALEXANDER J, LANGOU RA: Left ventricular filling in differentiating restrictive amyloid cardiomyopathy and constrictive pericarditis. Am J Cardiol 47:791–796, Apr 1981.

34. RUBINOW A, SKINNER M, COHEN AS: Digoxin sensitivity in amyloid cardiomyopathy. Circulation 63:1285–1288, June 1981.

35. BRISTOW MR, MASON JW, BILLINGHAM ME, DANIELS JR: Dose-effect and structure-function relationships in doxorubicin cardiomyopathy. Am Heart J 102:709–718, Oct 1981.

36. SHUMAN RD, ETTINGER DS, ABELOFF MD, FORTUIN NJ: Comparative analysis of noninvasive cardiac parameters of the detection and evaluation of adriamycin cardiotoxicity. Johns Hopkins Med J 149:57–63, Aug 1981.

37. GOTTDIENER JS, APPELBAUM FR, FEERANS VJ, DEISSEROTH A, ZIEGLER J: Cardiotoxicity associated with high-dose cyclophosphamide therapy. Arch Intern Med 141:758–763, May 1981.

38. GOTTDIENER JS, MATHISEN DH, BORER JS, BONOW RO, MYERS EC, BARR LH, SCHWARTZ DE, BA-

CHARACH SL, GREEN MV, ROSENBERG SA: Doxorubicin cardiotoxicity: assessment of late left ventricular dysfunction by radionuclide cineangiography. Ann Intern Med 94(part 1): 430–435, Apr 1981.

39. ANDY JJ, BISHARA FF, SOYINKA OO: Relation of severe eosinophilia and microfilariasis to chronic African endomyocardial fibrosis. Br Heart J 45:672–680, June 1981.

40. DUBOST C, PRIGENT C, GERBAUX A, MAURICE P, PASSELECQ J, RULLIERE J, CARPENTIER A, DELOCHE A: Surgical treatment of constrictive fibrous endocarditis. J Thorac Cardiovasc Surg 82:585–591, Oct 1981.

41. IKAHEIMO MJ, KARKOLA PJ, TAKKUNEN JT: Surgical treatment of Loffler's eosinophilic endocarditis. Br Heart J 45:729–732, June 1981.

42. DAVIES J, SAPSFORD R, BROOKSBY I, OLSEN EGJ, SPRY CJF, OAKLEY CM, GOODWIN JF: Successful surgical treatment of two patients with eosinophilic endomyocardial disease. Br Heart J 46: 438–445, Oct 1981.

43. GRAHAM JM, LAWRIE GM, FETEIH NM, DEBAKEY ME: Management of endomyocardial fibrosis: successful surgical treatment of biventricular involvement and consideration of the superiority of operative intervention. Am Heart J 102:771–775, Oct 1981.

44. BAANDRUP U, OLSEN EGJ: Critical analysis of endomyocardial biopsies from patients suspected of having cardiomyopathy. I: morphological and morphometric aspects. Br Heart J 45:475–486, May 1981.

45. BAANDRUP U, FLORIO RA, REHAHN M, RICHARDSON PJ, OLSEN EGJ: Critical analysis of endomyocardial biopsies from patients suspected of having cardiomyopathy. II: comparison of histology and clinical/hemodynamic information. Br Heart J 45:487–493, May 1981.

Congenital Heart Disease

AORTIC ISTHMIC COARCTATION

Operative repair in infants

Operative correction of aortic isthmic coarctation in infants often takes place under urgent and less-than-ideal circumstances. Kamau and associates[1] from Denver, Colorado, operated on 34 infants with aortic coarctation during a 4-year period: 11 were <2 weeks old; 9 were 2–4 weeks old, 8 were 4–8 weeks old, and 6 were 2–6 months old. Associated cardiovascular anomalies were common, particularly patent DA and VSD. The operations in 23 (67%) were performed on an emergency basis. CHF, acidosis, systemic hypertension, cardiogenic shock, or cardiac arrest were indications for the emergency operation. One patient died early and 1 later. In 15 with an adequate-sized aortic isthmus, primary repair was performed with direct suturing. Patch-graft angioplasty was performed in 19: left subclavian artery in 9; left common carotid in 1, and Dacron pericardial patch in 9. Reoperation was required in 2 patients for recurrent or residual coarctation. A number of other operations were required later, particularly closure of VSD. The low operative mortality in these patients can be ascribed to aggressive medical therapy, emergency catheterization, emergency operation, avoidance of systemic hypothermia, and adequate relief of the aortic coarctation. Emergency coarctectomy and repair is the treatment of choice for infants with aortic coarctation and CHF.

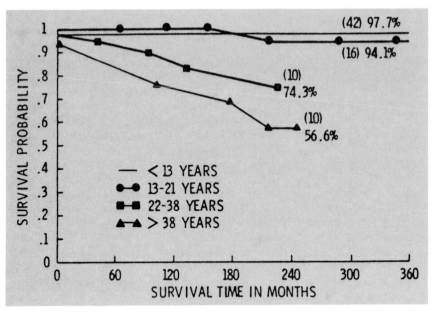

Fig. 7-1. Kaplan-Meier curves of survival probability according to age at operation by quartiles. Percentage specified is survival probability. Number in parentheses represents number of patients followed-up through last interval. Reproduced with permission from Lawrie et al.[2]

Operative repair after age 1 year

Lawrie and associates[2] from Houston, Texas, described their findings in 190 consecutive patients over 1 year of age (mean, 25 years) who underwent surgical correction of aortic isthmic coarctation during a 30-year period. Of the 190 patients, 130 were male and 60 were female. The mean preoperative BP was 160 mmHg systolic (range, 94–300), and diastolic 90 mmHg (range, 50–160). Dacron grafts were used in 65%. Follow-up was obtained at a mean interval of 85 months (range, 1–360). Postoperatively, the mean BP was 133 mmHg (range, 90–195) systolic and 80 mmHg diastolic (range, 50–120). Of the 190 patients, 80% were either normotensive or had mild hypertension after operation. The best BP response was obtained in patients under 13 years of age at the time of operation. Survival was related to age at operation (Fig. 7-1), and each curve was significantly different from the others. Late survival was worse in patients operated on after age 21 years, but patients operated on during adolescence, despite some mild residual hypertension, had an excellent long-term prognosis.

Reoperation

Beekman and associates[3] from Ann Arbor, Michigan, analyzed 21 patients who underwent reoperation between 1957 and 1980 at their medical center; this number represented 8% of all of their patients undergoing aortic isthmic resection. The incidence rate of reoperation was 38% for children < age 3 years and 1.5% for children ≥3 years of age at initial repair. Before reoperation, 14 of the 21 patients were symptomatic, 19 had systolic hypertension in the upper limbs, and 20 had a documented coarctation pressure gradient at rest (mean, 42 mmHg). Surgical techniques used at reoperation were patch aortoplasty in 12 patients, graft interposition in 4, end-to-end anastomosis in 3, and end-to-side left subclavian to descending aorta bypass graft in 2. There was 1 operative death. The 20 survivors were followed a mean of 4.3 years. Significant symptomatic improvement occurred (p < 0.001). Upper limb hypertension also lessened significantly (p < 0.001): 15 patients were no longer hypertensive and 3 had a lesser degree of hypertension. The coarctation pressure gradient at rest decreased significantly (p < 0.001): 13 patients had no residual gradient and 7 had a gradient ≤20 mmHg (Fig. 7-2). Graded treadmill exercise testing performed in 5 patients after reoperation documented upper limb hypertension in 4 and a marked increase in the coarctation gradient with exercise in 3. Thus, the frequency of reoperation is significantly increased in patients who are < age 3

Fig. 7-2.   Coarctation pressure gradient at rest before and after reoperation (REOP) for coarctation (p < 0.001).

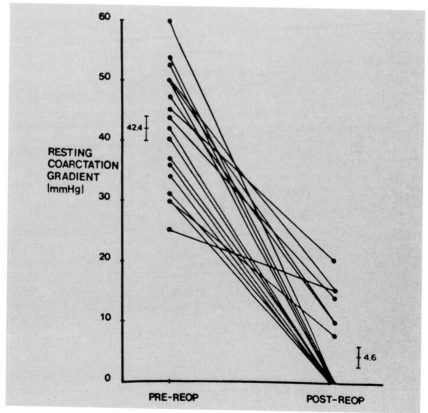

years at initial coarctation repair. Reoperation, however, is a safe and effective procedure. It has a low mortality rate (5%), relieves symptoms, and decreases both hypertension and the coarctation pressure gradient. Patch aortoplasty appears to be the operative procedure of choice. Moderate-to-severe hemodynamic abnormalities, however, may persist during exercise after reoperation.

AORTIC ARCH INTERRUPTION

Operative correction before age 6 months

Most babies with aortic arch interruption become symptomatic in the first month of life. Utilizing the technique of Trusler and Izukawa, reported as a single-stage repair in 1975, Bailey and associates[4] from Loma Linda, California, described 5 neonates, 2–19 days old, with severe CHF in whom the interrupted aortic arch was operatively corrected. Through a transverse bilateral thoracotomy and deep hypothermic circulatory arrest, the entire thoracic aorta was mobilized, the patent DA was ligated close to its attachment on the PA side, and the residual ductal tissue was excised. An end-to-side anastomosis between descending thoracic aorta and ascending aorta was accomplished without undue tension. The associated VSD was closed by a patch. Two patients who were moribund upon arrival in the operating room died. The other 3 survived operation; each has been restudied and found to have good anatomic repair without residual intracardiac shunts. One had a peak systolic pressure gradient of 8 mmHg at the level of the aortic anastomosis.

Moulton and Bowman[5] from New York City and Baltimore, Maryland, repaired type B aortic arch interruption in 8 patients aged 3 days–5 months and weighing 2.1–3.4 kg. In 6 patients, utilizing deep hypothermia and circulatory arrest, the patent DA was closed, the aortic arch was anastomosed to the descending aorta, and the foramen ovale and VSD were closed. In 5 patients, all arch arteries were preserved and no prosthetic material was utilized. One patient died 48 hours postoperatively and the other 7 survived >30 days. Three patients are alive 3–6 years after repair. Repeat cardiac catheterization demonstrated adequate growth of the anastomosis and no residual gradients. Thus, aortic arch interruption in infants and young children can be completely corrected early in life.

CONGENITAL OBSTRUCTION TO LEFT VENTRICULAR OUTFLOW

Usefulness of M-mode echo in diagnosis of congenital aortic valve stenosis

Kececioglu-Draelos and Goldberg[6] from Tucson, Arizona, subjected some of the indices believed to suggest congenital AS to a blinded test in which

M-mode echoes from 28 children with AS were intermixed with records of 90 normal children. They did not test wall thickness in systole and diastole and poststenotic dilation, but they did test eccentricity index, cuspal thickness, multiple diastolic cuspal lines, and found that none of these criteria was sensitive or selective for diagnosing AS by M-mode echo. It is as yet unclear whether 2-D echo will be any more accurate in diagnosis of AS or bicuspid aortic valve when subjected to this kind of randomized controlled investigation.

Operative treatment of congenital aortic valve stenosis and results

Dobell and associates[7] from Montreal, Canada, analyzed 50 patients with congenital AS treated operatively during a 16-year period: 12 were < age 1 year; 17, aged 1–9 years, and 21, aged 10–15 years. Preoperatively, 29 were symptomatic. Of 40 with ECGs, 29 had LV hypertrophy (with a stain pattern in 20) and 11 had normal ECGs. Operation in each was performed with cardiopulmonary bypass and moderate hypothermia. Nine different configurations of aortic valves were seen at operation (Fig. 7-3), the most common being bicuspid (31 patients). Operation consisted of incision of fused commissures almost to the "anulus." Postoperative gradients in the operating room ranged from 0–90 mmHg (mean, 26). Seven patients died in the im-

Fig. 7-3. Types of congenital valvular AS in 50 patients. Numbers of patients are in parentheses. Note that very little could be done with valves *G* and *I*. Reproduced with permission from Dobell et al.[7]

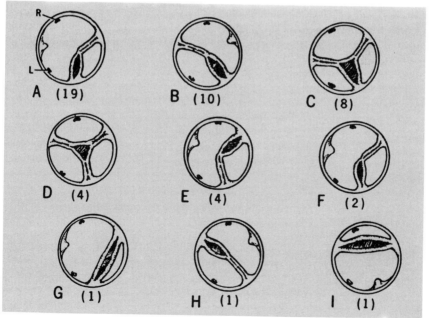

mediate perioperative period and 6 of them were <2 months of age with CHF. Follow-up for a minimum of 8 years in 25 operative survivors operated on from 1964 to 1972 disclosed 1 late death (infective endocarditis) and 4 excellent results; 5 patients underwent AVR and 3 underwent a second valvotomy; 2 had moderate AR and 10 had residual or recurrent moderate AS. There were no late deaths from residual AS. Because of problems with prosthetic and bioprosthetic valves in the pediatric age group, valvotomy is the treatment of choice despite the palliative nature of the operation and the virtual certainty of a second operation.

Left ventricular apicoaortic conduits for complicated left ventricular outflow obstruction in children and young adults

The apicoaortic conduit has been used to alleviate significant LV outflow obstruction when conventional reconstruction is not possible. Ergin and associates[8] from New York City described 6 patients aged 8–20 years who underwent this operation. All had severe LV hypertrophy with preoperative peak systolic pressure gradients of 84 ± 17 mmHg and a LV end-diastolic pressure of 20 ± 7 mmHg. Conduits were placed retroperitoneally with a distal anastomosis to the infrarenal aorta, and the porcine bioprosthesis was positioned in the left upper quadrant. Intraoperatively, the mean gradient was 13 ± 8 mmHg and, after an average follow-up of 18 months, all patients were in functional class I. Cardiac catheterization in 4 patients about 12 months postoperatively disclosed a mean LV conduit gradient of 2.5 mmHg, average LV end-diastolic pressure of 5.5 mmHg, and an EF of 0.77. This approach is effective in relieving complex LV outflow obstruction that cannot be relieved by conventional operations.

Operations for aortic valve atresia

Aortic valve atresia (AVA) is the most common cause of death in the first week of life and a difficult anomaly to treat successfully by surgery. Unlike the case with many forms of congenital heart disease, neonates with AVA are usually well developed. Norwood and associates[9] from Boston, Massachusetts, analyzed 16 infants (5 girls, 11 boys) ranging in age from 1–180 days (median, 4) who were operated on as part of a staged repair for AVA. All had hypoplastic left ventricles and ascending aortas. Mitral atresia also was present in 9. Except for 3 infants, all presented in the first week of life with cyanosis, tachypnea, and decreased peripheral pulses, and most had metabolic acidosis. The initial therapy was to infuse prostaglandin E_1 to maintain patency of the DA. Chest roentgenograms showed cardiac enlargement and vascular congestion. Physiologic correction would attempt to separate pulmonary and systemic circulations, but use the developed right ventricle as the systemic pumping chamber. The latest operation consisted of a direct anastomosis of the pulmonary trunk to the ascending aorta, ligation of the patent DA, establishment of pulmonary blood flow with a central shunt via a tube from the newly constructed ascending aorta to the confluence of the pulmonary trunk, and then creation of a large intraatrial communication, all done through a median sternotomy. Of the 16 infants undergoing the first stage palliation, 8 died. From 6–9 months after the first stage palliation, 3 patients had a modified Fontan repair that partitions atrial flow and transports blood from the right atrium directly to the right PA, using the right ventricle as the systemic pumping chamber. This is bold and imaginative surgery. The experience to date has been poor, but certainly better than anything else yet devised.

CONGENITAL OBSTRUCTION TO LEFT VENTRICULAR INFLOW

Congenital mitral stenosis assessed by echo

Cardiac catheterization permits identification of MS, but it cannot define the precise nature of the MS, nor does the addition of angiocardiography consistently allow exact recognition of supra-, valvular or sub-valvular abnormality or the structure of the chordae or the number of papillary muscles. M-mode echo defines the problem through a unidimensional assessment of limitation of opening of the usually thickened valve, but this technique fails to find some that are abnormal. Digitizing the M-mode study gives information during the rapid LV filling period and on the change between minimum dimension to mitral valve opening and on isovolumic relaxation. Smallhorn and associates[10] from London, England, studied 9 patients, aged 3 months–15 years, with significant congenital MS. Six were recognized clinically and 3 were not. In the 2 patients with a supravalvular membrane studied by 2-D echo, the supravalvular membrane was not displayed. However, in 9 patients, the parasternal long-axis view permitted assessment of anular size, which was normal in all. Nine had dense echoes from thickened leaflets. Ten had reduced valve excursion. In the short-axis view, the mitral orifice was visualized at a lower level than normally, and the number of papillary muscles was judged to be 2 in 6 children and 1 in 4. Operation or necropsy confirmed the accuracy of echo diagnosis in 8 patients. Thus, 2-D echo adds additional accuracy to in vivo and often preoperative recognition of the structure and function of the mitral apparatus in congenital MS.

Cor triatriatum: diagnosis and operative management

Cor triatriatum is a rare congenital cardiac anomaly consisting of an abnormal partition of the left atrium by a fibromuscular "membrane" that divides the atrium into an upper chamber, receiving the pulmonary veins, and a lower chamber that connects to the atrial appendage and to the mitral valve. The upper and lower chambers communicate through a stenotic "membrane." The hemodynamic consequence is pulmonary venous obstruction. Richardson and associates[11] from Iowa City, Iowa, and Pittsburgh, Pennsylvania, over a 23-year period treated 21 patients with this anomaly. Their age at the time of treatment ranged from 1 day–13 years (mean, 26 months); 12 (57%) were < 12 months old at diagnosis. Operation was carried out in 14 patients (67%), in 13 of whom the cor triatriatum was an isolated lesion. Proper diagnosis was made preoperatively in 7 and intraoperatively in 6; proper diagnosis in the other patient was not made until necropsy. Nine patients (64%) had operation via the atrial septum, which was entered from the right atrium, and 4 survived; 5 had operation via the left atrium, and 4 survived. All 14 had operations on cardiopulmonary bypass, with excision of the partitioning "membrane." Seven of the 8 survivors are alive and followed an average of 41 months. The authors recommend that, for infants, a right atrial approach be used, and for larger children, the left atrial approach.

CARDIAC VALVE REPLACEMENT IN CHILDREN

Durability of porcine bioprostheses

Calcification of porcine bioprostheses is greater in children than in adults. Dunn[12] from Philadelphia, Pennsylvania, evaluated long-term durability of porcine bioprostheses in 227 late survivors <21 years of age. The native valves replaced were aortic in 47, mitral in 67, tricuspid in 14, pulmonic in 14; additionally, bioprostheses were evaluated in 77 pulmonary and in 8 apicoaortic conduits. The data, collected from 12 pediatric cardiac surgical centers, were calculated on an actuarial basis and presented in life-table curves. Twenty (10%) porcine bioprostheses were known to have degenerated. At 5 years, 40% of the aortic, 40% of the mitral, 100% of the tricuspid, 100% of the pulmonic, and 89% of the pulmonic conduit bioprostheses remained functional. At that point, 5 (11%) of 47 aortic and 10 (16%) of 61 mitral bioprostheses were dysfunctional. Calcification and dysfunction occurred significantly faster ($p < 0.05$) in the younger children than in the older children, and in those bioprostheses located in left-sided or systemic positions than in those in right-sided positions (Figs. 7-4 and 7-5). These data substantiate previous data about bioprostheses in children, i.e., their tendency to calcify early, particularly the left-sided bioprostheses.

Mitral or aortic valve replacement or both

Williams and associates[13] from Toronto, Canada, reviewed results of cardiac valve replacement in 92 children operated upon from 1963–1980. Tissue valves were used in 53 and mechanical valves in 36. No major differences in the actuarial incidence of major complications between the 2 groups over a similar time period were noted. AVR was done in 39 patients aged 7–19 years (mean, 14), and MVR in 50, aged 8 months–17 years (mean, 8 years) and both MVR and AVR in 3, aged 11–17 years. All 39 who underwent AVR survived operation and were followed from 1 month to 12 years. None died late and two-thirds were asymptomatic. Complications occurred in 13 patients: reoperation in 7; complete heart block in 3; acute bacterial endocarditis in 2, and cerebral embolus in 1. Of the 50 patients with MVR, 16 (32%)

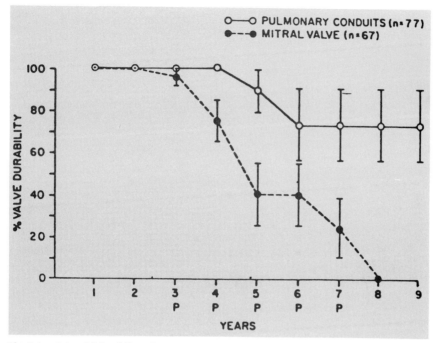

Fig. 7-4. Actuarial durability of porcine valves in pulmonary conduits compared with those in mitral position (group 5-vs-group 2). Bars represent 1 standard deviation. At 3, 4, 5, 6, and 7 years, the p value represents a significant difference (p < 0.05). Reproduced with permission from Dunn.[12]

patients died in the operative period; of the patients > age 10 years, the operative mortality was 10%, significantly less than the 45% mortality rate in the younger children. Of the 34 surviving children, 9 died later. Actuarial survival after MVR was 45% at 9 years. Four patients had reoperations, 4 had complete heart block, 3 had brain damage, and 1 had a systemic embolus.

Thus, late survival for children undergoing AVR is markedly different from that for children having MVR. This difference is attributable to the state

TABLE 7-1. *Mitral valve prostheses or bioprostheses in children.*

			%/PATIENT/YEAR			
GROUP	# PTS	MEAN FOLLOW-UP (yrs)	TE	IE	PD	DEATH
Mechanical valves	74	6.3	1.7	0.85	0.85	1.3
Porcine bioprostheses	13	3.3	0	2.3	16.3	1.4
Dura mater	23	1.9	2.3	—	6.3	2.3

IE = infective endocarditis. PD = prosthetic or bioprosthetic degeneration. TE = thromboembolism.

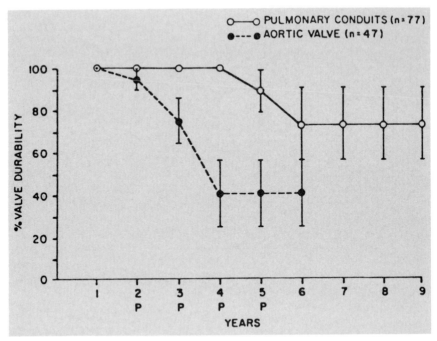

Fig. 7-5. Actuarial durability of porcine valves in pulmonary conduits compared with those in aortic position (group 5-vs-group 1). Bars represent 1 standard deviation. At 2, 3, 4, and 5 years, the p value represents a significant difference (p < 0.05). Reproduced with permission from Dunn.[12]

of the myocardium, age, body size, and the necessity for associated procedures. This experience indicates that cardiac valve replacement in children is a palliative procedure and that late complications are frequent and difficult to manage. Every attempt should be made to repair the child's native valve(s) so that prosthetic replacement is delayed as long as possible.

Attie and associates[14] from Mexico City, Mexico, analyzed 110 children aged 6–15 years in whom MVR was performed because of rheumatic heart disease (Table 7-1). The bioprostheses utilized had significant durability problems. The authors concluded that mechanical prostheses had the best results in children, despite the necessity for anticoagulation therapy when they were used.

EBSTEIN'S ANOMALY

In the elderly

Although the average survival with Ebstein's anomaly when isolated (except for a defect in the atrial septum) is about 25 years, at least 7 patients

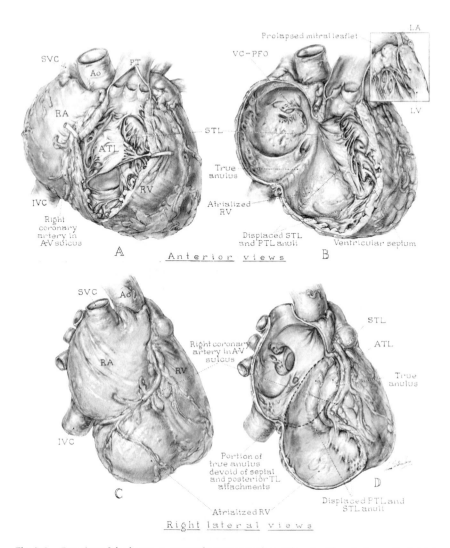

Fig. 7-6. Drawing of the heart. *A*, View of anterior surface of heart with anterior wall of right ventricle (RV) opened to show elongated anterior tricuspid valve leaflet (ATL) attached at true anulus. Ao = aorta. AV = atrioventricular. IVC = inferior vena cava. PT = pulmonary trunk. RA = right atrium. STL = septal tricuspid leaflet. SVC = superior vena cava. *B*, View of heart with anterior walls of RA and RV removed to show posterior and septal portions of true anulus devoid of leaflet attachments with basal portions of the STL and posterior tricuspid leaflet (PTL) attached to body of RV. Caudal to true anulus and cephalad to attachments of the STL and PTL is atrialized portion of RV. Shown in *inset* is portion of LV and left atrium (LA). The posterior leaflet of mitral valve prolapsed mildly into the LA. VC-PFO = valvular competent patient foramen ovale. *C*, View of right lateral surface of the heart showing the dilated RA and posteriorly protruding atrialized portion of RV. *D*, View of heart with right lateral wall removed showing basal attachment of ATL to true anulus (*dashed line*), but that of PTL and STL displaced caudally into body of RV. Reproduced with permission from Cabin et al.[15]

surviving ⩾70 years have been reported. Cabin and associates[15] from Bethesda, Maryland, described a 72-year-old man with Ebstein's anomaly who had been asymptomatic until age 68, when symptoms appeared. He died 4 years later as a consequence of CAD. This is the first patient reported, to the authors' knowledge, with Ebstein's anomaly in whom death was attributable to athersclerotic CAD. The authors found previous reports of 63 patients with Ebstein's anomaly who survived past 1 month of age and in whom the cause of death was determined: 16 (25%) died as a consequence of a cardiac operation; 13 (21%) from chronic CHF; 12 (19%) presumably from arrhythmia because death was sudden; 6 (10%) from paradoxic embolus or brain abscess; 5 (8%) from complications of cardiac catheterization, and 11 (17%) from noncardiac causes. Thus, prolonged symptom-free survival with an anatomically severe form of Ebstein's anomaly such as was present in the patient de-

Fig. 7-7.   Length of life and frequency of true atrial septal defect or patent foramen ovale (ASD) in 121 previously reported necropsy patients with Ebstein's anomaly of the tricuspid valve. Reproduced with permission from Cabin et al.[15]

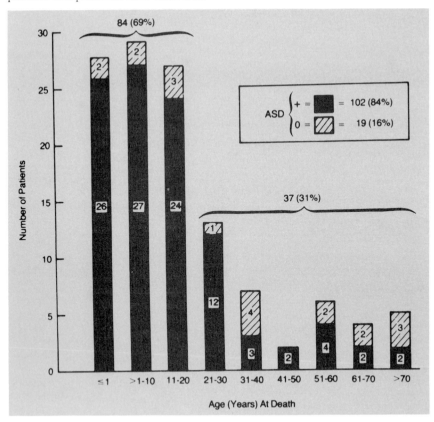

scribed by Cabin and associates is possible (Fig. 7-6). The presence of ASD or valvular incompetent patent foramen ovale generally affects survival adversely.

Of 121 previously reported necropsy patients with Ebstein's anomaly for whom age at death and the status of the atrial septa were described, 28 (23%) died during the first year of life and 84 (69%) by age 20 (Fig. 7-7). The mean age of the 93 patients surviving past the first year of life was 26 years. To determine anatomic factors that might affect prognosis, they examined the relationship, if any, of survival to presence of ASD or patent foramen ovale or other congenital cardiovascular anomalies in the 121 necropsy patients. Of the 28 patients dying in the first year of life, 26 (93%) had an ASD or patent foramen ovale; 5 (18%), a VSD (in combination with ASD or patent foramen ovale in 4), and 6 (21%), pulmonic valve atresia or stenosis. Of the 93 patients surviving the first year of life, 76 (82%) had an ASD or patent foramen ovale, and 17 (18%) did not; 3 (3%) had a VSD (in combination with ASD or patent foramen ovale in 2), and 4 (4%) had pulmonic valve atresia or stenosis. The mean age at death of those surviving the first year of life with an ASD or patent foramen ovale was 20 years, as compared with 41 years for those with an intact atrial septum (p < 0.001). Thus, although there are exceptions, the presence of an ASD or patent foramen ovale overall appears to affect survival adversely.

CORONARY ARTERY ANOMALIES

Origin of the left coronary artery from the pulmonary trunk: operative management

There is disagreement concerning the proper operative management of *infants* with CHF due to anomalous origin of the left coronary artery from the pulmonary trunk. Driscoll and associates[16] from Houston, Texas, described treatment in 23 patients who had CHF before age 6 months: 8 had operations in the first year of life and 15 at later times (mean, 7.5 years). Evidence of myocardial infarction was obtained by ECG in 4 of the 8 undergoing operation in the first year and in 8 of 15 having later operations. The mean EF in the later group averaged 36%. The cardiothoracic ratio by chest roentgenogram was 0.74 in the early operative group, and 0.66 in the later operative group. Of the 8 early operative patients, 2 survived and are alive an average of 2.5 years later: 13 of the 15 later operated patients survived and are alive an average age of 14 years. Surgical management included direct implantation of the left coronary artery in the aorta in 3; aortocoronary bypass (saphenous vein) in 3; ligation of left coronary artery in 2, and subclavian artery-coronary artery bypass in 1. Thus, operative treatment in the first year of life of patients with anomalous origin of the left coronary artery from the pulmonary trunk with depressed LV function is poor. Delay in operative intervention was recommended until after 18 months of age.

Left subclavian-left coronary artery anastomosis for anomalous origin of the left coronary artery from the left main pulmonary artery

Stephenson and associates[17] from Philadelphia, Pennsylvania, in 6 patients, aged 2–76 months, with this anomaly described the results of anastomosing the left subclavian artery to the left coronary artery via a left thoracotomy without cardiopulmonary bypass. In all 6 patients, the left coronary artery was ligated at its origin from the left main PA. Preoperatively, 5 had CHF and ischemic abnormalities on ECG. All 6 had significant cardiomegaly by chest roentgenogram. The LV EF averaged 46%. One patient died after operation; the other 5 were alive 8–92 months postoperatively. Four of the 5 anastomoses were patent at postoperative cardiac catheterization. The postoperative ECG was normal and showed fewer T-wave changes in all patients, and the heart size by chest roentgenogram had decreased to normal. The EF increased by 12% in 4 of the 5 patients. This operation can be performed at an early age and, with the techniques borrowed from coronary revascularization surgery, a 2-coronary system can be developed. The anastomosis has growth potential and results in reversal of LV ischemic changes and improvement in LV contractility.

Coronary arterial fistula: operative management

Congenital coronary arterial fistulas are being recognized with increasing frequency with the widespread use of selective coronary arteriography. Lowe and associates[18] from Durham, North Carolina, identified 28 patients between 1960 and 1981 with this anomaly and found 258 previously reported patients, making a total of 286 patients for review: 55 were symptomatic at presentation. The main clinical manifestation was a continuous precordial murmur. The right coronary artery was most often involved (56%) and its fistula most commonly communicated with a chamber of the right side of the heart: right ventricle (39%), right atrium (33%), or PA (20%). Left coronary arterial fistulas were much less common and usually also drained into the right ventricle or right atrium. Surgical correction was recommended to prevent CHF, angina, infective endocarditis, AMI, pulmonary hypertension, and coronary arterial aneurysm with subsequent rupture or embolism. Operative technique included opening the recipient cardiac chamber while on cardiopulmonary bypass and closing off fistula tracts or, in patients with an easily dissected single communication, simple suture obliteration, often without cardiopulmonary bypass. There were no operative or late deaths in the patients who were operated on at Durham and there have been no recurrent fistulas during a mean follow-up of 10 years. The risk of operative correction appears to be considerably less than that inherent in developing potentially fatal complications, even in asymptomatic patients. Of the 22 patients treated surgically at Durham, 14 underwent suture obliteration and did not require bypass and 6 (27%) required bypass to close multiple tracts. Two patients required bypass to insert a saphenous vein graft because obliteration of the fistula had jeopardized coronary flow.

Aortic origin of conus coronary artery

The conus coronary artery has been reported to arise independently from the aorta in approximately 45% of hearts. Edwards and associates[19] from Minneapolis and Rochester, Minnesota, examined 305 hearts at necropsy to determine the origin of the conus coronary artery and variations in patterns of origin with respect to age. Three patterns were recognized (Fig. 7-8): 1) the conus artery arising from the aorta independently of the right coronary artery; 2) conus artery and the right coronary artery arising from a common ostium, and 3) conus artery arising from the right coronary artery which arose normally from the right aortic sinus. The relative incidence of the 3 patterns varied with age. Pattern 1 was recognized in 14%–24% of hearts from patients < age 2 years, whereas in older patients it occurred in 41%–63%. These data suggest that aortic origin of the conus arterial ostium may appear in some individuals between 2 and 4 years of age, and they support the concept that some coronary arterial patterns are not fully established at the time of birth.

Fig. 7-8. Variations in patterns of conus arterial origin, viewed externally (*A, C, E*) and internally (*B, D, F*). A, B: pattern 1. Independent origins of the conus and right coronary (RCA) arteries from the aorta (Ao). C, D: pattern 2. Common origin of conus artery and RCA. E, F: pattern 3. Only the right coronary artery arises from the right aortic sinus. LAD = left anterior descending coronary artery. LC = left coronary ostium. LCX = left circumflex coronary artery. LV = left ventricle. MV = anterior leaflet of mitral valve. RC = right coronary ostium. Reproduced with permission from Edwards.[19]

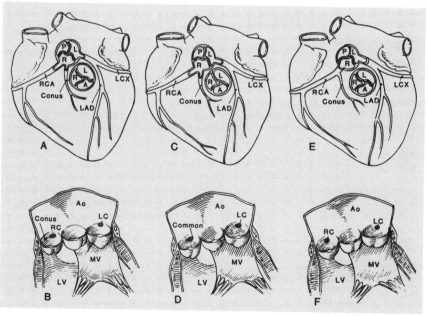

ATRIAL SEPTAL DEFECT

Results of operation in patients >60 years of age

ASD is one of the most common forms of congenital heart disease in adults. Data are somewhat unclear as to the long-term follow-up of patients after repair of ASD in late adulthood. St. John Sutton and associates[20] from Rochester, Minnesota, reviewed 66 patients > age 60 years (mean, 65 years) in whom an ASD was operatively closed between 1955 and 1977. Of the 66 patients, 47 (71%) were women and 19 (29%) were men. Four were in functional class I, 18 in class II, 20 in class III, and 24 in class IV. Only 2 had normal-sized hearts and 64 had increased (cardiothoracic ratio >0.5) heart sizes. Thirty patients (45%) were in sinus rhythm, 34 (52%) had chronic atrial fibrillation, 1 had atrial flutter and 1 had AV block. Right-axis deviation was present in 35 (53%), 37 (56%) had complete right BBB, and 4 (6%) had LV hypertrophy. Seventeen patients had peak systolic PA pressure <40 mmHg, 21 from 40–60 mmHg, and 18 > 60 mmHg. Direct suture closure was done in 47 and a Dacron patch was utilized in 19. Eight of the latter 19 had a sinus venosus type ASD with anomalous pulmonary venous connection. Of the 4 patients who died, all had additional surgical procedures: aortocoronary bypass in 2; tricuspid valve anuloplasty in 1, and tricuspid valve replacement in 1. After operation, the patients were followed 2–20 years (mean, 7). Fourteen died later, a mean of 7 years after operation: 8 from stroke; 3 from CHF, and 3 from miscellaneous causes. Marked symptomatic improvement occurred in all patients regardless of the preoperative PA pressure, pulmonary vascular resistance, or functional class. Actuarial survival curves showed that longevity at 5 and 20 years was significantly increased (p < 0.01) for patients treated operatively, as compared with that predicted for age-matched patients treated medically. Thus, operative closure of ASD in patients >60 years of age produces symptomatic improvement in nearly 95% and the operative mortality is not increased by the presence of CHF or PA hypertension. Operation appears to increase longevity significantly and, therefore, operative closure of ASD for older patients is indicated, except for those with severe associated disease or severe elevation of pulmonary vascular resistance.

Right ventricular function in ASD in adults

Most patients with isolated ASD undergo elective surgical repair during childhood or early adult life before either symptoms or complications develop. In contrast, older adults with an uncorrected ASD frequently have symptoms and pre- and postoperative complications, particularly atrial arrhythmias and right-sided CHF. Although these symptoms and complications are generally attributed to chronic RV volume overload, RV systolic function has not previously been systematically studied. Liberthson and associates[21] from Boston, Massachusetts, assessed RV function with gated cardiac blood pool scanning in 20 adult patients with ASD. All patients had scans both before and 6 or more months after operative closure of the defect. Clinical findings, pre- and postoperative course, and cardiac catheterization data were correlated with scan findings. In all 20 patients, the right ventricle was dilated preoperatively. In 9 patients (aged 18–42 years [mean, 25]), RV wall motion was normal preoperatively. All 9 were asymptomatic and had normal sinus rhythm. Their pulmonary-to-systemic flow ratio ranged from 2:1–5:1, PA systolic pressure from 18–30 mmHg, and RV end-diastolic pressure from 0–8 mmHg. After repair of the ASD, all 9 remained asymptomatic, RV size decreased dramatically, and wall motion was normal.

In the remaining 11 patients (aged 35–63 years [mean, 52]), there was moderate-to-severe preoperative RV hypokinesia. All had preoperative symptoms (NY Heart Association functional class II and III); 6 had atrial fibrillation and 5 had sinus rhythm, 7 had CHF. Pulmonary-to-systemic flow ratio ranged from 1.7:1–5.0:1, PA pressure from 26–70 mmHg, and RV end-diastolic pressure from 4–16 mmHg. Symptoms were lessened and RV size and function improved postoperatively in these 11 patients. Unlike those with normal preoperative RV wall motion, however, only 1 of the 11 had normal postoperative RV function and became asymptomatic.

Left ventricular function in ASD in adults

Bonow and associates[22] from Bethesda, Maryland, offer some comforting data about LV function in patients with unoperated or postoperative ASD. They performed RNA cineangiography at rest and during exercise to estimate LV functional reserve in 11 adults aged 16–59 years with ASD. Five patients were asymptomatic; 3 were severely symptomatic and 3 mildly symptomatic. On M-mode echo, septal motion was paradoxical in 10 and flat in 1.

LV diastolic dimension was reduced below normal. Pulmonary-to-systemic flow ratios were 1.6–2.4, except in 2 with high values (4.3 and 5.3). The PA pressure was elevated in 3 patients. Ten had secundum and 1 a primum ASD, and all had patch closure of the defect. Preoperatively on RNA cineangiography, all patients had normal function at rest, but on exercise it was abnormal in 7: no increase in LV EF in 4 and a decrease in the other 3 ≤ the lower limit of normal (55%). These 3 were the severely symptomatic patients and 2 were the patients with the highest qP/qS. Six months postoperatively, all shunts had been abolished, all patients were asymptomatic, only 1 still had pulmonary hypertension (although less than before surgery), and all had normal LV diastolic dimension on 2-D echo. On RNA study, all had normal LV EF at rest and on exercise. Thus, in ASD with a large left -to- right shunt, diminution in LV functional reserve is related to the RV volume load, and operative closure of ASD favorably alters the mechanical factors and reverses the apparent LV dysfunction, which is secondary rather than intrinsic.

Mitral valve abnormalities associated with secundum type ASD

In a review of 498 consecutive patients with secundum ASD seen between 1950–1979, Liberthson and associates[23] from Boston, Massachusetts, found a 0.4% incidence of severe MVP in 213 patients < age 21 years, 2% in 187 patients aged 21–49 years, and 15% in 98 patients ⩾ age 50 years. They could not find an obvious reason for MR; gross and microscopic examination of the removed valve and papillary muscle gave no clues to pathogenesis or cause. Thus, although its mechanism is not understood, MR is common in older patients with ASD.

Few morphologic studies of the mitral valve have been carried out in necropsy patients with secundum-type ASD. Accordingly, Davies[24] from London, England, examined the mitral valves in 16 adult (ages not given) hearts with unclosed secundum-type ASD, and in 15 he found thickening of the posterior one-half of the anterior mitral leaflet and fusion and fibrous thickening of chordae attached to this portion of anterior mitral leaflet. Histologic examination showed the thickening to consist entirely of fibrous tissue. Davies speculated that the morphologic mitral abnormalities were from abnormal leaflet motion with resultant leaflet trauma, rather than a primary valvular abnormality.

Angiography in AV canal defect

Soto and associates[25] from Birmingham, Alabama, continue to point out the advantages of axial angiocardiographic views to delineate the anatomy of congenital heart defects. In few anomalies is the need for anatomic detail greater than in AV canal defect. They studied 20 patients: 5 with 2 AV valves and 15 with a common AV valve. They could not tell with certainty the free-floating valve from the 1 with a tethered anterior leaflet. The ASD and the ventricular septum were well demonstrated. The deformation, in the 4-chamber and elongated right anterior oblique projections of the LV angiograms, of the normally straight contour, extending from the noncoronary aortic cusp to the crux cordis, was considered the best angiographic sign of AV canal. They identified an abnormal ratio between inlet and outlet portions of the ventricular septum in all patients. Thus, the axial views contribute more than frontal-lateral views to delineating the anatomy of AV canal defects.

Late results of repair of partial AV canal

Goldfaden and associates[26] from Bethesda, Maryland, analyzed results from 44 patients who had primary repair of partial or incomplete AV canal. The mean age of the 44 patients at operation was 12 years (range 1–68); 22 were female and 22 were male. Of the 44 patients, 39 (89%) survived operation. The average follow-up was 11 years; the longest, 25 years. All 44 patients had an ostium primum-type ASD with a cleft in the anterior mitral leaflet. Repair included patch closure of the ASD and direct suture closure of the mitral cleft. All 5 operative deaths occurred before 1965. Only 3 (8%) had significant arrhythmias at the time of discharge from the hospital. Postoperative cardiac catheterization was performed in 35 patients (90%) an average of 11 months after operation: the mean PA wedge pressure was normal (<12 mmHg) in 80%; 7 patients had MR, mild in 5, and severe in 2; 1 patient had left -to- right shunting at the atrial level. Of the 39 operative survivors, 3 died late with an actuarial survival at 13 years of 88 ± 6%. Three patients, however, needed a second operation for dehiscence on the atrial patch in 1 and for MR in 2. The estimated survival free of late reoperation was 82 ± 6%. Late arrhythmias or conduction disturbances occurred in 4 patients: 2 had complete heart block 5 and 9 years after operation (with permanent pacemakers) and 1 patient had fatal cardiac arrest. Thus, 7 of the initial 39 operative survivors had significant arrhythmias, a cumulative incidence in the follow-up period of 32%. Actuarial survival free of any late complication, including late death, serious arrhythmias, or MR was 54 ± 10% at 13 years. Thus, late complications are frequent after repair of incomplete AV canal.

Fixed subaortic stenosis after repair of partial AV canal

In patients with partial AV canal, a cleft is nearly always present in the anterior mitral leaflet and anomalous chordae tendineae attach to the apex of the cleft in the anterior mitral leaflet and course to the crest of the ventricular septum just beneath the aortic valve. It was predicted by Taussig nearly 3 decades ago that some patients with partial AV canal might have obstruction to LV outflow, but hemodynamic demonstration of such rarely has been recorded. Of 99 patients with partial AV canal followed over a long period, Taylor and Somerville[27] from London, England, found 3 patients who developed fixed subaortic stenosis after closure of the ostium primum ASD and repair of the cleft in the anterior mitral leaflet. The narrowing of the LV outflow tract was demonstrated angiographically to be present in both ventricular systole and diastole. Excluding their 10-year-old child who developed LV outflow tract obstruction after MVR and closure of the ostium primum defect, the other 2 children were aged 4 and 3 years at the time of closure of the ostium primum defect and suturing of the cleft in the anterior mitral leaflet. Both patients had small peak systolic pressure gradients between left ventricle and aorta before operation (15 and 21 mmHg). For the child with the 15 mmHg gradient before operation, this gradient had increased 4 years later to 60 mmHg and reoperation was performed, but the LV outflow tract gradient later increased to 80 mmHg. In the child whose preoperative LV outflow tract gradient was 21 mmHg, it had increased 11 years later to 120 mmHg. At reoperation, the surgeon found subvalvular fixed LV outflow tract obstruction very similar to that observed in patients with discrete subaortic stenosis.

The authors emphasized that development of LV outflow tract obstruction after repair of partial AV canal is potentially or actually disastrous and that these patients should be examined with care postoperatively for LV outflow tract obstruction as well as, of course, for MR. Operative resection of the LV outflow tract lesion is hazardous. The authors advised that the LV outflow tract region be examined at operation when the anterior mitral leaflet is sutured and the primum defect is closed. The authors speculated that, when MR was corrected at operation and the ASD closed, forward flow was increased, resulting in increased turbulence in the already narrowed subaortic region. This increased turbulence might stimulate the deposition of fibrous tissue which, in turn, would cause progressive narrowing.

This is an important paper and, unfortunately, this complication is liable to be recognized more and more frequently in the coming years. It would be a good idea to have simultaneous measurements of the LV and aortic pressures preoperatively before repair of partial AV canal so that if even small gradients are observed preoperatively the anomalous chordae tendineae from anterior mitral leaflet to the crest of the ventricular septum might be severed in those patients.

Surgical anatomy of the conduction tissues in AV canal

Thiene and associates[28] in a multicentered study (Padova, Leiden, Liverpool, and London) pooled their specimens of AV canal to portray the anatomy of the conducting tissues so as to help surgeons prevent iatrogenic complete heart block. Of the 16 specimens, 6 came as a result of cardiac surgery, 5 with surgically induced heart block. Whether the AV canal was complete or partial, the conduction system coursed the same way. In addition to the normal triangle of Koch, a second nodal triangle related to the posterior atrial wall. This later triangle was the guide to the penetrating bundle. The AV node was most at risk when the sinus septum was absent. When sutures were placed in the apex of the nodal triangle or deeply through the posterior nodal crest, damage occurred to the penetrating and nonbranching bundles, respectively. To avoid this, the patch should be placed well posterior to the nodal triangle and in the coronary sinus, if necessary, or posterior to the ostium of the coronary sinus.

VENTRICULAR SEPTAL DEFECT

Frequency and course in an unselected population of children

Dickinson and associates[29] from Liverpool, England, took advantage of their Liverpool Registry of Congenital Malformations to obtain cardiologic data on VSD. Cases were registered in the neonatal period or when the diagnosis was recognized in childhood or at necropsy. Between 1960 and 1969, there were 163,692 registered births and, among them, 1,120 were registered as having congenital heart disease. Of this latter group, 294 were registered as having VSD, alone or in association with other cardiac lesions, but VSD was the major anomaly. Diagnosis of VSD was based on necropsy in 48, on cardiac catheterization or open heart surgery in 56, and on clinical features (chiefly auscultation by an experienced physician on more than 1 occasion) in 190. Excluded were conditions such as TF, AV canal and VSD associated with coarctation of the aorta. Although VSD was registered in 385 patients at birth, sufficient data to satisfy their criteria was available in 91%. Major noncardiac malformations were observed in 6 babies (20%); Down's syndrome was the most common (20 patients) followed by gastrointestinal, urological, and skeletal anomalies, all found in more than 11 infants.

Of the patients with VSD, 73% presented with discovery of a precordial murmur in a symptom-free state, and 21% (6 infants) presented in CHF. At necropsy, VSD was found in 7 stillborn infants and in 10 who died without clinical diagnosis of VSD. Of the 55 deaths (19%), 7 were stillborn. Of the other 48, 26 (54%) occurred by 3 months of age and 8 (17%) between 3 and 12 months. Of the 14 deaths (29%) over age 1 year, 6 followed operation. In 24 of the 55 who died, heart disease was not the cause of death; instead, the cause was prematurity or a major noncardiac malformation. Only 24 deaths (8%) in the liveborn could be attributed to the VSD.

Open heart surgery was done in 35 children aged 5–11 years: 7 had had previous PA banding, and 2 others had only the band; 2 of these 9 died. After open repair, 6 hospital deaths and 1 late death occurred. Only 1 episode of bacterial endocarditis occurred in 2,253 patient-years of follow-up. AR, however, developed in 5 (27%): 3 has closure of the VSD and 1 had, in addition, AVR. RV infundibular stenosis, with a pressure gradient >20 mmHg, was found in 13%. Spontaneous closure was recorded in 90 patients (31%), a rate of 40/1,000 patient-years. Patients with Down's syndrome were excluded. Actuarial analysis of the rate of closure over the first 10 years indicated a stepwise, steady trend of 3% per year. They noted spontaneous closure up to age 16 years, but few patients were followed that long. Spontaneous closure occurred in 37% of the 202 asymptomatic patients and in 21% of the symptomatic patients. Only 25% of their patients with VSD developed symptoms, about 70% had a VSD that was small or became small or disappeared in childhood, and about 15% required operation.

Factors affecting echo imaging of VSD

Canale and associates[30] from Tucson, Arizona, analyzed the factors permitting imaging of VSD and allowing estimation of its size. They studied 36 patients, aged 7 days–20 years, with VSD proven by catheterization and angiography, and they reviewed the 28 false-positive images out of 250 two-D echo studies of patients proved not to have VSD. Twenty patients had an isolated VSD (group 1) and 16 had other defects (group 2). Group 1 was subdivided according to the size of the shunt through VSD: large shunt qP/qS >2:1 or smaller shunts, and group 2, according to angiographic evidence of large or small VSD. Group 3 had no VSD. The 3 major views used on 2-D echo were the subcostal 4-chamber view and the parasternal long-axis view. Overall sensitivity for these 3 views was 42%, 69% and 53%, respectively, while specificity was 99%, 92% and 98%, respectively. They described the T artifact as looking like the letter "T" on either or both sides of the imaged septum and probably due to scattered reflections off the first and last echo interface of a true VSD. If they included imaging the "T" artifact, the broadening of septal edges around the defect, the sensitivity increased to 88% and specificity to 100%. The smallest VSD imaged was 2 mm in diameter and the largest, 23 mm. The size was larger in diastole than systole. For group 1 the VSD/aortic root ratio helped separate patients with large shunts from those with small shunts, as did VSD (mm)/body weight (kg). In group 2, the 4-chamber view most often showed echo dropout because of the VSD, but this view also yielded a moderate number of false positives.

Use of multiple views increased sensitivity and specificity, for no false positive VSD (group 3) was imaged in more than 1 view. Thus, to best quantify VSD size and to avoid false-positive diagnoses, multiple views should be employed in looking for the T artifact, and the marked changes in size of the VSD occurring between systole and diastole should be remembered.

Acute effects of nitroprusside in infants with large VSD

Beekman and associates[31] from Ann Arbor, Michigan, reported the use of vasodilator therapy in 5 infants with large VSD with CHF. Babies with large VSD and CHF have increased pulmonary blood flow, and the congested lungs account for the dyspnea and pulmonary complications. The question asked was whether vasodilator therapy in this situation favored forward LV flow or whether it preferentially favored pulmonary flow, in which case the effect would be deleterious. Pulmonary vasodilation in excess of systemic, of course, would increase rather than decrease the excessive pulmonary flow. If both circulations were affected similarly, no benefit would be expected.

Nitroprusside was administered to 5 infants aged 10 days to 6 months with VSD and CHF, and hemodynamic measurements of pulmonary-to-systemic flows were made before nitroprusside at 0.5 μg/kg and after each interval increase of 0.5 μg/kg every 5 minutes until aortic systolic pressure dropped 15% or a maximum dose of 1 μg/kg/min had been reached. Flows and resistances were calculated by the Fick principle from oxygen data. Nitroprusside had an adverse effect: the pulmonary-to-systemic flow increased in all (from 2.2 ± 0.2 to 3.4 ± 0.2) as a result of a marked decrease in systemic flow and no change in pulmonary flow. Thus, if the excessive pulmonary flow cannot be decreased, first acutely and then chronically, vasodilator therapy does not have a therapeutic role in these infants.

AORTOPULMONARY DEFECTS

Determination of time of ductal closure in normal newborns by pulsed Doppler echo

If the DA closes prematurely, the fetus dies. If the premature baby's DA opens and he is in respiratory distress, medical and sometimes surgical care is needed. If the full-term infant's DA is open after the first week of life, then it is abnormal and probably will require operative closure, soon if the DA permits a large left-to-right shunt and produces a cardiopulmonary burden. Patients with certain cyanotic malformations associated with obstruction to pulmonary flow, such as TF, benefit, of course, by persistent patency of the DA or by creation of an artificial DA.

The behavior of the normal DA is, therefore, of interest. How long does it stay open? Information from postmortem studies and from cardiac catheterization suggest that functional closure occurs at 10–15 hours after birth.

Gentile and associates[32] from Seattle, Washington, studied this question in 50 normal newborns by using the pulsed Doppler and M-mode echo to detect evidence of flow. They recorded a diastolic ductal jet in the PA from the parasternal approach and/or continuous turbulent flow into the right PA from the suprasternal approach. The babies were examined, usually within 8 hours after birth and twice daily, until no evidence of ductal flow was recorded. The DA was patent in all babies examined at 8 hours. By 24 hours, 42% had no ductal flow evident; by 40 hours, 78%; by 48 hours, 90%; and by 96 hours, 100%. None had evidence by M-mode echo of significant left-to-right shunting on any examination. In 28%, either a continuous or a nonspecific systolic precordial murmur was heard before the DA closed. Thus, this sensitive noninvasive technique showed that functional DA closure occurs by 4 days of age (and by 1 day in almost half the babies) and that a left-to-right shunt via the DA after 4 days is abnormal.

Patent ductus arteriosus and indomethacin or prostaglandin E_1

As neonatologists began to salvage small premature infants of low birth weight through use of respirators and other supportive measures, a new problem surfaced. The DA opened and, in some, caused a large left-to-right shunt and symptoms of CHF or of respirator-dependency. Surgeons successfully closed the DA that was responsible for the symptoms. Ever since Friedman and associates in La Jolla, California, and Heymann and associates in San Francisco, California, independently in 1976 reported their preliminary experience with use of indomethacin, a prostaglandin synthetase inhibitor, to close persistently patent DA, however, a choice of medical or of surgical management of the problem has been available. This choice has posed a problem, for there are risks each way and the proper choice has not been clear. A national cooperative study is underway, but those results have not been reported.

Yeh and associates[33] from Chicago, Illinois, performed a double-blind controlled study in which indomethacin was administered intravenously (to overcome the problem of incomplete absorption) in 55 premature infants with a significant DA; 27 received a placebo and 28 received indomethacin, all at a mean age of 9 days. They devised a scoring system to evaluate cardiopulmonary function and used clinical and echo criteria to judge success or failure 24 hours after the last dose. Surgery was performed for failure after 3 doses. Below or at 28 weeks of gestational age, 50% of the infants had a patent DA, but only 15% at 29–37 weeks. Of the infants <1,000 g at birth, 49% had a patent DA, whereas of those weighing 2,000–2,040 g, only 16% had a patent DA. The overall frequency of patent DA if the birth weight was ≤ 2,040 g was 20%. The success rate in the indomethacin group was 89% (25/28) and in the placebo, 22% (6/27). No differences were found with respect to survival rate, duration of hospitalization, or frequency of bronchopulmonary dysplasia, necrotizing enterocolitis, or sepsis. Adverse effects of indomethacin were a transient fall in urine output and in serum sodium concentration and a rise in serum potassium. Success from 1 dose was 50% and from 3 doses, 89%. Only 1 baby treated with indomethacin was operated on for patent DA, whereas 7 of 27 who received placebo had surgery. Thus, intravenous indomethacin looks favorable in this circumstance.

Yanagi and associates[34] from Chicago, Illinois, established clinical and echo criteria for diagnosis of symptomatic patent DA in preterm infants on ventilatory support and for decision about improvement or no improvement. The study covered a 24-month period and was divided into 2 phases. In Phase 1, agent or placebo was administered at 24-hour intervals for 3 doses if no improvement occurred, and in Phase 2, every 8 hours. Freshly prepared material was given by orogastric tube. Infants who failed to respond underwent operative closure of the patent DA within 3 days of the last dose. Before randomization, infants were treated with fluid restriction, digitalization (over 16 hours), and furosemide (in 2 doses, 12 hours apart for 1 day). Of 277 infants with respiratory distress syndrome on ventilator support, 69 (25%) had symptomatic patent DA, 33 in Phase 1 and 36 in Phase 2. Medical management failed in 64% in Phase 1 and in 67% in Phase 2. Of the 45 eligible for study, 1 died before study, 4 before completing the study, and 1 was withdrawn at the parents' request. Although in Phase 1, 6 of 8 indomethacin-treated infants improved, as compared with 4 of 9 controls, the results were not statistically significant. In Phase 2 a statistically significant difference was found, favoring indomethacin: 11 of 13 indomethacin -vs- 1 of 9 controls. The total duration of ventilator support did not differ in Phase 1, but was statistically shorter in Phase 2 indomethacin-treated infants: 54 days -vs- 15 days. Side effects, which occurred only in Phase 2, were transient reduction in renal function or gastrointestinal bleeding.

To identify factors affecting the efficacy of indomethacin in closing symptomatic patent DA, Brash and associates[35] from Nashville, Tennessee, studied the pharmacokinetics of intravenous indomethacin in 35 premature infants with symptomatic patent DA. Most responded to indomethacin with ductal constriction. Indomethacin infusions that were ineffective (7 doses in 6 patients) were associated with significantly faster clearance, a shorter half-life, and lower plasma levels. Six infants later had reopening of the ductus. All 6 received indomethacin in the first postnatal week; they could not be distinguished from infants with permanent closure on the basis of indomethacin kinetics, but they were of low gestational age. There was a 20-fold variation in plasma indomethacin levels 24 hours after a dose. In view of this variation and the relation between plasma levels and ductal constriction, the authors suggested that measurement of the plasma indomethacin level could be of value in infants with no response to a first dose.

From Rochester, New York, Merritt and associates[36] tested the hypothesis that intervention to close a patent DA in premature infants with respirator distress might be preferable to delayed efforts at closure after the infant had deteriorated and was in cardioventilatory decompensation. When evidence of a significant patent DA was confirmed by clinical, echo and, in some instances, aortographic criteria, infants were assigned randomly to early treatment with indomethacin or to medical management with fluid restriction, furosemide, and then indomethacin or surgery. End points in analysis were death or bronchopulmonary dysplasia (BPD). Early treatment consisted of intravenous indomethacin (0.2 mg/kg), with the dose repeated up to 3 times at 24-hour intervals if patent DA persisted. BPD was diagnosed radiographically without knowledge of the treatment group. The results showed that BPD was less frequent and that survival was increased in infants undergoing early patent DA intervention. BPD was present in 2 of 20 infants treated early, as compared with 8 of 12 managed medically. One infant in each group underwent surgical ligation because of persisting symptoms. Four infants died in the medically treated group and 1 in the early-treatment group. A single course was used in 10 of 12 treated early and 2 courses in 3; one infant had late reopening of the patent DA. Of the control (medical treatment) babies, 11 of 13 eventually received indomethacin after CHF had developed. Early treatment was at 49 hours of age; medical treatment in the controls was at 167 hours. Thus, preterm infants in respiratory distress appear improved by early treatment with indomethacin. Although it does not eliminate the need in all such babies for surgical closure of patent DA, early treatment carries a statistically significant decrease in BPD and death.

Lewis and associates[37,38] from Los Angeles, Boston, San Francisco, and Kalamazoo reported side effects from PGE_1 in 492 infants with critical congenital heart disease treated in 56 USA centers. They found that 43% had at least 1 intercurrent medical event, equally in the cyanotic and acyanotic groups, but only half were related to PGE_1 and most required minor adjustment in management. Cardiovascular events were the most common (18%), and were more frequent in the cyanotic group and in small infants weighing ≤2 kg. Cutaneous vasodilation was the chief event and its frequency was lessened by use of intravenous, rather than intraarterial, administration of PGE_1. Other events included rhythm disturbance (7%) and hypotension (3%–5%). The frequency of central nervous system events was 16%. They occurred especially in acidotic DA in infants whose survival depends on this channel for providing PA flow when that is deficient because of pulmonic stenosis or atresia, or systemic flow when that is severely impaired. This intraveneous therapy has changed a situation of crisis in a hypoxic, acidotic infant with impending shock or death into a controlled, stabilized situation where necessary cardiac catheterization and other diagnostic studies and operation can be carried out under optimal conditions. When used accordingly for short-term benefit, PGE_1 is a great addition to the pediatric cardiologic armamentarium. The drug must be used with care, however, since it has side effects.

Ligation in premature infants

Brandt and associates[39] described results of ligation of patent DA in 66 preterm infants weighing 700–2700 g. All had respiratory distress and none died at operation. Fifteen infants, however, died 1–120 days postoperatively, primarily from bleeding abnormalities and marked prematurity. At late follow-up of 51 survivors, 1 had died. Of the 51 late survivors, 17 (33%) had bronchopulmonary dysplasia.

Operative treatment in older children and adults

John and associates[40] from India described results in operations for patent DA in 131 patients aged 14–44 years (mean, 22). The 131 represented 22% of 600 patients with patent DA operated on in a 12-year period. In 50 patients, chest roentgenograms showed classic features of an extracardiac shunt and PA hypertension. Hemodynamic studies were done in 62 patients: the pulmonary-to-systemic flow ratio was 1.5:1 in 50% and more than 3.3:1 in 33%; the shunt was bidirectional in 5 patients and the PA pressure was elevated in 50 of the 62 patients. The patent DA was usually approached via a left thoracotomy. Total cardiopulmonary bypass with femoral aortic cannulations and venous ventricular outflow cannulation was utilized in 3 patients and a transaortic closure of the large DA was accomplished with a Dacron patch. Two of the 3 had had calcific deposits evident on chest roentgenograms. Five (3%) of 131 patients died within 30 days of operation and the survivors were followed 1–12 years postoperatively. Three died late: 1 from progressive PA hypertension and PA thrombi; another from AR and LV failure, and a third from lung disease. Thus, most adults with patent DA can be operated on without the use of cardiopulmonary bypass, and calcified patent DA are rare. Factors militating against success are LV failure, severe PA hypertension, and right-to-left shunting.

Aortopulmonary septal defect: operative treatment and results

Incomplete fusion of the conotruncal ridge in the distal aortopulmonary septum results in a defect between the ascending aorta and the pulmonary trunk, an aortopulmonary window. Doty and associates[41] from Iowa City, Iowa, and Moscow, USSR, analyzed 25 patients with malseptation of the aortopulmonary trunk in whom operations were done between 1960 and 1979. Of the 25 patients, 24 were aged 4 months–12 years, and the remaining patient was 48 years old; 19 were male and 6 were female. Cardiac catheterization, performed in 24 patients preoperatively, identified 2 anatomic types: type I (21 patients), the classic defect in close proximity to the left coronary artery, and type II (4 patients) located distally in the ascending aorta and opening into the origin of the right main PA. Hemodynamics showed a large left-to-right shunt with a mean pulmonary-to-systemic flow ratio of 3.0:1, elevated PA pressures (mean, 86 mmHg), and increased pulmonary vascular resistance.

Operative therapy consisted of ligation of the aortopulmonary connection in 8 patients (3 died), and direct repair using cardiopulmonary bypass in 17 (the transaortic approach was used in 16 [2 deaths], and the transpulmonary in 1 [1 death]). The defect was closed by direct suture in 2 patients and by prosthetic patch in 15. Patch closure was satisfactory for most patients with the type I defect. Type II defects required angioplasty to insure that the drainage of the right main PA or the flow from the pulmonary trunk was satisfactory. Deep hypothermic circulatory arrest might be used in repair of the more complicated type defects. Prosthetic patch closure of the defect is the treatment of choice and should be approached transaortically.

VENTRICULAR SEPTAL DEFECT WITH OBSTRUCTION TO RIGHT VENTRICULAR OUTFLOW

Best angiographic demonstration

The group from Birmingham, Alabama, have led the way in having *in vivo* display of anatomic details in congenital cardiac anomalies, especially those of surgical significance. Soto and associates[42] compared postmortem findings with axial cineangiography methods in 12 patients with TF and found that the *long-axis* and *elongated right anterior oblique* views of the right ventriculogram, combined with standard views, permitted accurate definition of the cardiac and great vessel anatomy.

Development of the pulmonary vascular bed in VSD associated with complete or incomplete obstruction to right ventricular outflow

Rabinovitch and associates[43] from Boston, Massachusetts, investigated the pulmonary vascular bed in 12 necropsy patients with TF and in 5 with pulmonic valve atresia. The 17 patients ranged in age from 2 days to 31 years. Of the 17 patients, 6 were unoperated, 6 had undergone open repair only, 4 had had both palliative and reparative operations, and 1 had had only a palliative shunt. Marked PA hypertension had been documented in 2 patients: a 17-year-old patient with TF with late acquisition of pulmonic valve atresia and 2 shunt procedures, and an 18-year-old patient born with pulmonic valve atresia, with insertion of RV outflow patch at age 9 and AVR at age 18. The 2 patients and a 26-year-old patient with a Potts anastomosis at age 3 years had pulmonary plexiform lesions.

These workers identified 3 types of systemic collateral arteries, distinguished by their origin, and each characterized by its type of "anastomosis" with a PA: 1) bronchial arterial collaterals arising from bronchial arteries within the lung; 2) direct aortic collaterals arising from the descending aorta and entering the hilum to supply a lobe or segment with distribution like a PA, and 3) indirect aortic collaterals arising from major branches of the aorta (internal mammary or subclavian) and anastomosing with central pulmonary arteries. Only bronchial arteries were found in TF. Intraacinar PAs were usually smaller than normal. Lung volume was small for age in 8 patients and total alveolar number was reduced in 13, but alveolar size was increased in all but 2. Thus, alveolar and vascular growth appears to be impaired in TF (with either pulmonic valve stenosis or atresia) and repair before age 2 years might favorably influence this growth.

Systemic pulmonary circulation in pulmonic valve atresia with VSD

One of the fascinating aspects of pulmonic valve atresia with VSD is the pattern of pulmonary supply. Most patients surviving considerable periods have their pulmonary circulation provided by arteries arising from the descending thoracic aortic. Thiene and associates[44] from Padua, Italy, described at necropsy the hearts of 25 patients with pulmonic valve atresia with VSD. In 22, the pulmonary trunk was present and located anteriorly and left-sided, and in the remaining 3 patients the pulmonary trunk could not be found, even by histologic analysis of the cardiac base (Figs. 7-9 and 7-10). The pulmonary circulation was exclusively supplied by the DA in 13 patients; in the 11 patients in whom the DA was absent, the pulmonary arterial circulation was supplied entirely by systemic collateral arteries arising from the descending thoracic aorta. In the 1 patient in whom the left lung was supplied by the DA, the right lung was supplied by 2 large systemic collateral arteries. This study demonstrates that, in patients with pulmonic valve atresia and VSD, the DA is frequently absent and the lungs are entirely supplied by systemic collateral arteries, that systemic collateral arteries and a DA do not coexist in supplying the same lung but, indeed, are inversely related, and that peripheral pulmonary vessels function in gas exchange regardless of the anatomic source of blood supply.

Late operative results of repair of tetralogy of Fallot

Hamilton and associates[45] from Liverpool, England, analyzed early and late results in 175 consecutive patients, operated on in 1969–1976, when aged 5 months–18 years (mean, 6 years). In the early experience, they were more conservative about not opening the pulmonary "anulus" and they ac-

Fig. 7-9. Schematic representations of pulmonary atresia with VSD and identifiable pulmonary trunk. *A*, ductus-dependent pulmonary circulation (12 cases). *B*, pulmonary circulation dependent upon systemic collateral arteries without ductus arteriosus (9 cases). *C*, left lung supplied by left ductus arteriosus and right lung supplied by systemic collateral arteries (1 case). The aortic arch is depicted as left-sided for simplification. Reproduced with permission from Thiene et al.[44]

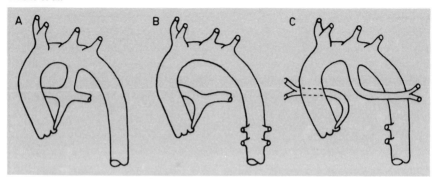

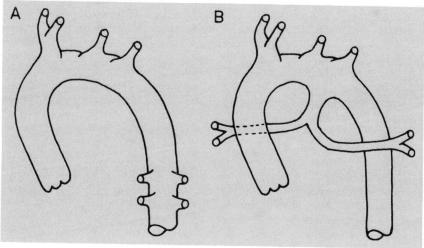

Fig. 7-10.   Schematic representation of cases without identifiable pulmonary trunk. *A*, pulmonary arterial supply dependent upon systemic collateral arteries (2 cases). *B*, confluent pulmonary arteries supplied by left ductus arteriosus (1 case). Reproduced with permission from Thiene et al.[44]

cepted a ratio of RV/LV systolic peak pressure of 0.8 at the end of the operation. Later, they viewed such a ratio as the indication for a second period of cardiopulmonary bypass and for transanular relief of the RV outflow obstruction. Both early and late mortality were related to this ratio. The overall mortality was 8%, and in patients >2 years old, 5%. In those <2 years, the mortality dropped over the 8 years from 3%–15%. In 137 patients without a previous shunt, the mortality was 7%, whereas in 38 with a prior shunt, it was 11%. The late mortality was 1% in a mean follow-up period of 7 years. Only 26 had symptoms; the other 133 were asymptomatic and normally active. Complete heart block was present in 3, two of whom had pacemakers. Reoperation was performed successfully in 5 patients.

Systemic ventricular function in tetralogy of Fallot, VSD, and complete transposition after repair in infancy

Dysfunction of the systemic ventricle at rest and at exercise has been reported in older patients with TF, VSD, and TGA, but it is not known if repair of these anomalies in infancy can prevent ventricular dysfunction. Borow and associates[46] from Boston, Massachusetts, utilized work-function curves relating systemic ventricular end-diastolic pressure to minute work index (MWI) to assess ventricular performance in 8 patients with TF, 5 with VSD, and 9 with TGA. All had undergone repair when they were <18 months of age. Of the 9 patients with TGA, 4 had Mustard's repair and 5 had Senning's repair. When studied a minimum of 13 months after operation, all had satisfactory anatomic results. Results also were compared with 7 control subjects who had either normal hearts or mild pulmonic stenosis. All patients had normal systemic ventricular hemodynamics at rest; a work-function curve for each patient was generated by use of a methoxamine infusion to increase afterload and measurement of end-diastolic pressure, mean ventricular systolic pressure, and cardiac index. Heart rate was maintained within a narrow range for each patient.

The systemic ventricle of the TGA patients responded to the afterload stress with a smaller increase in MWI than in patients with TF (p < 0.05), VSD (p < 0.01) or the control group (p < 0.01). This difference in MWI for the TGA patients occurred despite an increase in systemic ventricular end-diastolic pressure for all groups. The net result was a highly significant difference in the mean slope of work-function curves for the TGA patients, as compared with TF (p < 0.02), VSD (p < 0.01), or the control group (p < 0.01). There was no difference in the mean slope for the TF, VSD, and control groups. This afterload stress test at an early postoperative follow-up identified preclinical systemic ventricular dysfunction in TGA patients that were not evident in age-matched TF and VSD patients. With the development of alternative surgical procedures to repair TGA, it will be of interest to learn if these findings persist with procedures that use the left ventricle as the systemic ventricle.

Response to supine exercise after operative correction of tetralogy of Fallot after early childhood

Rocchini[47] from Ann Arbor, Michigan, studied 15 patients who had had a severe form of TF repaired from 1 to 12 years earlier when >8 years of age. Eight, who had extensive patching of the RV outflow tract, had residual pulmonic regurgitation and 7 with a Dacron conduit and Hancock valve did not. All postoperative patients were asymptomatic. Graded treadmill exercise testing before cardiac catheterization showed decreased endurance in all and development of VPC in 6. None had residual shunts and all postoperative patients had resting RV systolic pressure <60 mmHg, but RV systolic pressure and outflow gradient increased in all groups on supine exercise, while stroke index was lower in the postoperative patients. In postoperative patients, in contrast to those with mild pulmonic stenosis, the RV end-diastolic and PA wedge pressure increased on exercise. Thus, these asymptomatic patients who had excellent operative repair had both RV and LV compliance abnormalities. The mild pulmonic stenosis was not considered the cause of the abnormality on exercise in the postoperative patients, and the presence or absence of pulmonary regurgitation made no significant difference. Rocchini suggested that the severity of the tetralogy and the age (>8 years) at operation may have affected the results.

Lung function in tetralogy of Fallot after intracardiac repair

Wessel and associates[48] from Chicago, Illinios, studied lung function as it relates to palliative or reparative surgery for TF in 123 patients, 54 of whom had undergone primary intracardiac repair. They found a strong association of abnormal lung volumes and poor surgical results, especially pulmonic re-gurgitation or cardiomegaly with residual defects. They found primary in-tracardiac repair with excellent results to be the best guarantee against post-operative restrictive lung volume.

Patch reconstruction of the right ventricular outflow tract with "pulmonic valve" insertion

Relief of RV outflow tract obstruction with a transanular patch and its attendant pulmonic regurgitation is generally well tolerated. In some pa-tients, however, a transanular patch is not well tolerated and may cause RV dysfunction. These patients include those who have increased pulmonary vascular resistance, distal PA stenosis, single PA or aneurysmal dilation of a PA. Also, some patients who undergo repair of TF may have RV distention and failure secondary to residual RV outflow tract obstruction that may be associated with TR. Laks and associates[49] from New Haven, Connecticut, used a "pulmonic valve" beneath a RV outflow patch, rather than a valved conduit, in 12 patients (aged 18 months–17 years) so that they could insert a larger porcine valve and avoid anastomotic narrowing or conduit com-pression beneath the sternum: 7 had TF; 3, absent pulmonic valve, and 2, pulmonic valve atresia. No early complications or deaths occurred at a mean follow-up of 28 months. Repeat cardiac catheterization disclosed that the preoperative RV-PA peak systolic pressure gradient had been reduced from 58 ± 25 mmHg to 12 ± 7 mmHg at rest and it was located at the valve level. The gradient increased with exercise to 31 ± 9 mmHg. These results suggest that RV outflow reconstruction with a porcine valve insertion can be per-formed with reasonably good hemodynamic results. It allows insertion of a larger porcine valve, avoids pulmonic regurgitation, and prevents com-pression of the external conduit behind the sternum.

COMPLETE TRANSPOSITION OF THE GREAT ARTERIES

Management of hypoxemia after balloon atrial septostomy

Henry and associates[50] from St. Louis, Missouri, reviewed a 5-year experi-ence with 43 patients with d-TGA who underwent balloon atrial septostomy (BAS) at first cardiac catheterization, 33 being in their first week of life (22 in the first 2 days). They analyzed the outcome of survival to elective surgery between 6 and 12 months of age in relation to associated lesions of small or large patent DA or VSD, to degree of hypoxemia, and to use of prostaglandin E_1 in 4 infants to dilate the DA. They found improvement in paO_2 on PGE_1 infusion and decline on withdrawal. Because of severe hypoxemia after BAS, palliative surgery was carried out in 9 patients (21%): Blalock-Hanlon sep-tectomy in 3 (2 deaths) and Blalock-Taussig shunt in 5 (0 deaths). Five died before reparative surgery took place and 7 died at operation or postopera-tively. Thus, 72% of the original group survived to the time of analysis 2–56 months later. The early mortality with the Mustard operation was 9% (23 patients) and 15% (13 patients) with the Senning operation, and the mortality was higher in those with prior palliation operations.

Among factors contributing to improved survival, they credited cyanosis in the first hours of life that led to early referral to a pediatric cardiac center for prompt diagnostic studies and therapeutic BAS. Furthermore, they advocated conservative medical supervision for the next few months, even though arterial oxygen levels might be "unsatisfactory", in preference to doing a palliative Blalock-Hanlon operation or premature open repair. They advised 2–4 days of PGE₁ infusion if acidosis accompanied the hypoxia in the first days after BAS.

Factors influencing survival after balloon atrial septostomy

Among the most dramatic turnarounds in modern pediatric cardiology and cardiac surgery have been the conversion from an early mortality rate of about 90% by the first birthday for the untreated infant with TGA to a salvage rate of about 95% by 1 year for the infant treated early after birth by balloon atrial septostomy (BAS) and in the first year of life by physiologic rerouting of venous return to compensate for the transposed great arteries. Leanage and associates[51] from London, England, found, however, that some TGA patients died before reaching the second 6 months of life. To discover why, they analyzed 144 patients with TGA seen since 1966 and utilized a modified log rank survival test with multivariate capability. They found the following to be related, largely independently, to a statistically significant excess mortality: PA hypertension; the presence and size of a VSD or persistent patent DA; relative anemia; absence of LV outflow tract obstruction; low arterial oxygen saturation; AS and aortic coarctation, and BAS between 1 and 4 weeks of life. Next they calculated the predictive value of the above factors that could be determined either at balloon septostomy or by cardiac catheterization at 3 months of age. They found that they could predict outcome accurately in 76% of the patients. By offering early surgery to those at greater risk, the overall mortality rate should be further reduced.

Results of Rastelli procedure for TGA, VSD, and left ventricular outflow obstruction

The combination of TGA, VSD, and LV outflow tract obstruction fortunately is uncommon. Rastelli introduced a procedure for treatment of patients with this combination utilizing a diversion of the LV outflow to the aorta by occluding the proximal pulmonary trunk and creating a conduit within the right ventricle that would carry blood through the ventricular septum into the aorta. RV flow was carried to the distal pulmonary trunk by means of an external conduit. Moulton and associates[52] from London, England, reviewed 41 children in whom the Rastelli operation had been done from 1971–1978 for this combination of anomalies. The homograft valve Dacron tube was the conduit used. The patients ranged in age at operation from 27 months–15 years (mean, 8 years). All were cyanotic at operation with arterial saturations from 55%–88% (mean, 78). Previous palliative operations had been done in 33. The operative procedure included positioning the conduit to the left of the aorta after hypothermic ischemic arrest. A large interventricular patch was used to direct blood from the left ventricle through the VSD into the aorta. The pulmonary trunk was ligated proximally, the pulmonary trunk distal to the ligature was opened, and the conduit was trimmed so that the valve was as close to the pulmonary trunk as possible. Four (10%) of the 41 patients undergoing the procedure died in the hospital, but none of the last 13 patients operated on (since January 1977) died. Seven patients died later. Two patients developed RV aneurysms associated with residual VSD and another 2 had residual VSD. The overall survival at 8 years was 58%.

Obstructed right-sided porcine valved extracardiac conduits

Use of valved extracardiac conduits has revolutionized repair of complex congenital cardiac anomalies including TGV, truncus arteriosus, and pulmonic atresia with VSD. Agarwal and associates[53] from Rochester, Minnesota, described findings in 13 patients in whom a right-sided porcine valved extracardiac conduit had become obstructed. The 13 patients were from a group of 308 patients who received these conduits from 1972–1977. The period that the conduit had been in place in the 13 patients averaged 50 months. Four were asymptomatic, 8 had exertional dyspnea, and 1 had dizziness. As the conduit became obstructed, the intensity of the precordial murmur increased in 11, cyanosis worsened or reappeared in 2, and CHF appeared in 1. The peak RV-PA systolic pressure gradient averaged 87 mmHg. Catheter pullback localized the obstruction to the proximal portion of the conduit in 5, to the level of the bioprosthesis in 9, and to the distal portion of the conduit or to the main right or left PA in 6. The bioprosthesis only was obstructed in 5, the conduit alone in 4, and both in 4. Bioprosthetic changes included thrombosis, commissural fusion, calcification, cuspal tears, cuspal fusion to the wall of the conduit and infective endocarditis (1 patient). Fibrous tissue, usually quite thick, lined the interior of the conduit. Thus, obstruction remains a major problem with conduits inserted in this position.

Mustard operation

Aziz and associates[54] from Chicago, Illinois, described 2-D echo, hemodynamic, and angiographic observations in 17 children, 6 months–9 years after the Mustard operation performed in the first year of life (in all but 2) for TGA. Of the 17 patients, 7 (group I) had normal hemodynamics without structural abnormality. Of the other 10, 1 (group II), had stenosis of the superior vena caval segment, and 3 (group III) had significant narrowing of the isthmic segment of the pulmonary venous atrium, and each of them had a mid-diastolic murmur at the lower right sternal border. Group IV included 6 patients with TR and moderate-to-marked cardiomegaly radiologically. All had a dilated pulmonary venous atrium on 2-D echo, the tricuspid valve was abnormally horizontal in 5 and, in the sixth patient, the septal leaflet was immobile, having been incorporated into the closure of a coexisting VSD. In contrast to the other 3 groups with intact ventricular septa, 5 of the 6 patients in group IV had a VSD.

To understand the high frequency of TR, they studied 20 specimens of d-TGA, with or without cardiac surgery, and without a VSD, and 7 (35%) had anatomic abnormalities of the tricuspid valve. In contrast, of 20 specimens with a VSD, 12 (60%) had abnormal tricuspid valve. Of 10 hearts with obstruction of LV outflow, with or without VSD, 4 had abnormalities of the tricuspid valve. Common to all was attachment of the medial leaflet by papillary muscles either to the septum or septal band. The medial and posterior leaflets often were not clearly separated (were "mitralized"), and occasionally the medial and anterior leaflets were fused or the anterior leaflet was divided into 2 leaflets. Thus, 2-D echo can reliably detect structural abnormalities of the surgically revised atria after the Mustard operation, TR is probably related to pre-, intra-, and postoperative factors, and associated VSD makes it likely that the tricuspid valve will be abnormal.

Ninomiya and associates[55] from Toronto, Canada, compared 2-D echo with cineangiocardiograms in 24 patients who, 1–12 years earlier, had undergone a Mustard operation for d-TGA. They found an excellent correlation ($r = 0.98$) of the 2 methods. For 2-D measurements, they used the apical 4-chamber and the parasternal short-axis views. Endocardial outlines and calibration grids were traced and the tracings were digitized. RV volumes were calculated according to a formula after the volume of 20 equal slices parallel to the long axis of the heart had been calculated. EF was calculated from end-systolic and end-diastolic volumes and was "of acceptable accuracy," although they could not accurately estimate RV volume from the echo data.

From Detroit, Michigan, Arciniegas and associates[56] reported results of using the intraarterial baffle (thin Dacron fabric) operation (Mustard) from 1971–1979 in 120 consecutive patients with d-TGA aged 29 days–17 years (mean, 28 months). The ventricular septum was intact in 82 patients: 22 had a large VSD and LV outflow obstruction with peak systolic pressure gradients >50 mmHg, and 8 had an intact ventricular septum with severe LV outflow obstruction. The perioperative mortality was 5%, 26%, 28% and 12%, respectively. The late postoperative mortality for all groups was 7.5%. Late cardiac arrhythmias occurred in 33 patients (41%), but sinus rhythm was present in all patients after direct, high SVC cannulation was instituted. Although the late survivors were acyanotic and well, late postoperative hemodynamic and angiographic evaluation in 61 patients disclosed severe SVC obstruction in 12 (20%) and pulmonary venous obstruction in 4 (6%). Thus, the Mustard operation dramatically improves the survival rate and quality of life after correction of d-TGA.

Piccoli and associates[57] from Liverpool, England, analyzed 80 patients with TGA without significant VSD or LV outflow obstruction. The patients were in age 42 days–12 years (mean, 15 months), and in weight, 3.2–38 kg. Balloon atrial septostomy had produced significant increases of arterial oxygen saturation. Deep hypothermia and circulatory arrest were employed. A pericardial baffle was used to partition the right atrium. There were 2 operative deaths and 3 late deaths. At a mean follow-up of 4.5 years, 74% of the patients were symptom free. Conduction disturbances involving either sino-atrial or AV conduction were present in 5 and 6 patients, 7 of whom required reoperation. "Primary" RV failure occurred in 1 patient. The high morbidity rate suggests that there is a better method for correcting TGA.

Rastelli operation (intraventricular baffle)

From 1970–1978, Pitlick and associates[58] from Stanford, California, treated 30 patients, 14 with d-TGA and 16 with double-outlet right ventricle (DORV) with the Rastelli procedure. Using a knitted Teflon patch, they directed LV blood through the VSD and out the aorta. In all 14 patients with d-TGA and in 4 with DORV, a RV conduit was used between right ventricle and pulmonary trunk. The conduit was unvalved in 4, and had a porcine aortic valve in 14. Seven patients died in the early postoperative period, 2 with d-TGA, 5 with DORV: patients <3 years of age and those weighing <10 kg had a higher operative mortality than did the older and heavier patients (p < 0.05). Of the remaining 23 patients, 6 died later, and the other 17 were acyanotic and had improved exercise tolerance and marked weight gain, as compared with the preoperative status. Postoperative catheterization data were obtained in 16 survivors: 8 had peak LV-aortic systolic pressure gradients >30 mmHg; 6 patients had residual left-to-right shunts, and several had obstructive pulmonary vascular disease. Thus, this operation should be avoided in patients weighing <10 kg and palliative procedures to increase pulmonary blood flow should be done in them. Mid-childhood was recommended as the optimum time for operative repair with an intraventricular baffle. For patients with DORV and subpulmonic VSD, they recommend an intraatrial baffle and closure of the VSD.

Jatene operation (great artery switch)

Freedom and associates[59] from Toronto, Canada, presented data on the anatomic correction in 8 patients with d-TGA. Indications for surgery were hypoxic CHF and PA hypertension. Careful mobilization of the distal aorta, proximal pulmonary trunk, and proximal coronary arteries prevented twisting and kinking of the coronary arteries. The VSD was closed via the pulmonic valve. Postoperatively, arterial oxygen saturations were normal and none had hemodynamic evidence of great vessel obstruction or arterial kinking. These authors believe that anatomic correction with coronary arterial implantation has a role in carefully selected patients but, for the most part, they do not suggest its use in patients with an "unprepared" left ventricle; most patients with an intact ventricular septum or only a small VSD should have atrial partitioning (Mustard operation) at the present time.

Williams and associates[60] from Toronto, Canada, investigated the feasibility of arterial repair of TGA in patients who were not ideal candidates for the Mustard or Rastelli operations. Each of the 8 patients (aged 10 days–15 years) selected had systemic LV pressures without fixed LV outflow tract stenosis. Two patients had intact ventricular septa and 6 had VSD. Repair was performed using hypothermic cardiopulmonary bypass in 5 and hypothermic circulatory arrest in 3. The 2 great arteries were divided, transferred, and anastomosed directly. Transferring the coronary arteries to the pulmonary trunk did not cause major problems. Six children survived and were well 6–30 months later. All 6 survivors were in sinus rhythm and had normal pulmonary vasculature with decreased cardiac sizes roentgenographically. AR was detected in 5 of 6 children, but was not significant. RV outflow stenosis occurred in 2 patients, VSD in 1, and right coronary arterial stenosis in 1. LV function was normal in 4 and unchanged in 1. Thus, this procedure in carefully selected patients provides good results and avoids many complications of the intraatrial baffle operations.

CORRECTED TRANSPOSITION

2-D echo features

Using side-by-side photographs of the sector scan (in long-axis, short-axis, apical 4-chamber, parasternal, and subcostal views) with photograph or diagram of the anatomic specimen, Hagler and associates[61] from Rochester, Minnesota, depicted the diagnostic features that enabled them to recognize the condition and any associated malformations (such as Ebstein's anomaly or straddling AV valves) and to determine ventricular situs and morphology in 27 patients aged 2 months–58 years. In AV and ventriculoarterial discordance, they described the AV valve as more superiorly oriented and fish-mouthed in diastole with 2 papillary muscles and fine ventricular architecture in ellipsoidal shape as characteristic of the LV morphology. They recognized the coarsely trabeculated RV interior with its more inferiorly located, triangular-shaped AV valve. Muscular discontinuity of AV and semilunar valve (SV) characterized the RV anatomy and AV-SV continuity, that of the left ventricle.

Operative treatment of associated defects and results

AV discordance (congenitally *corrected transposition*) has a number of associated intracardiac anomalies that have been difficult to treat without a high late morbidity. Williams and associates[62] from Toronto, Canada, reviewed their 19-year experience with 35 patients with AV discordance: 18 patients had VSD with pulmonic stenosis (PS); 6 had VSD with TR; 5 had isolated TR, and 6 had isolated VSD. Three died in the perioperative period and 6 later. At a mean follow-up of 4.4 years, the overall mortality was 26%. All 18 patients with VSD and PS survived operation, but 3 died later; of the 6 with VSD and TR, 1 died in the perioperative period and 2 later; of the 5 with isolated TR, all survived, and of the 6 with isolated VSD, 2 died in the perioperative period and none 2–20 years later. Of the 35 patients, 12 had tricuspid valve operations, and they were older, on average, than the 23 patients without AV valve operations. Complete heart block was present preoperatively in 5 patients (14%). During intracardiac repair, an additional 13 patients developed heart block in association with closure of the VSD. Permanent cardiac pacemakers were utilized in 14 patients, but heart block did not have an adverse effect on mortality. Thus, the operative risk for repair of these associated anomalies is high and the late results are only fair. Conduction problems and TR are common and difficult to treat.

UNIVENTRICULAR HEART

Septation procedure

The univentricular heart is one of the most challenging congenital defects requiring surgical repair. Feldt and associates[63] from Rochester, Minnesota, analyzed 45 patients with univentricular heart and 2 AV valves in whom "correction" was carried out with an intraventricular patch dividing the ventricular chamber into 2 ventricles. Of the 45 patients, 21 (47%) died during hospitalization after operation and 8 others (18%) died later. Of the 16 survivors, 12 had fair-to-good results and 4 had poor results. Two factors were significantly related to increased survival: 1) no previous history of CHF, and 2) no previous palliative procedure. Multivariate analysis revealed a small subgroup in 11 patients with a survival rate of 82%; they had a subaortic chamber to the left, never CHF, never a palliative operation, never profound polycythemia, and were between 5 and 15 years of age at operation. Presently, the Fontan procedure (RA-to-PA shunt) is employed by these authors for patients with univentricular hearts and low PA pressures. Nearly half of the patients with univentricular heart, however, are not qualified for a Fontan procedure and this group should be considered for the septation procedure because of the poor long-term outlook for patients without operation.

PERSISTENT TRUNCUS ARTERIOSUS

Operation under 1 year of age

Musumeci and associates[64] from Liverpool, England, operated on 13 symptomatic infants with type I or II truncus arteriosus (TA) between January 1974 and November 1980. Death occurs in >60% of newborns with TA before 6 months of age and in >80% by 12 months of age. Pulmonary vascular obstructive disease develops and may render a third of the survivors inoperable by 4 years of age. Two surgical approaches have been utilized: banding of the pulmonary trunk was done in 10 of the 13 infants when they were 14 days–12 months old and weighed 2.1–7.9 kg; 4 died early postoperatively and a fifth, a few months later of intractable CHF. Of the 5 long-term survivors, 1 had "debanding" and open repair at 4 years with a Hancock bioprosthesis: truncal valve regurgitation, trivial initially, had worsened and that valve was replaced, with survival 3 years later. A second survivor developed marked stenosis of the right PA and, at 5 years, underwent debanding with enlargement of this PA and placement of an aortic root homograft in the PA. A third child, not yet reoperated, has diminished PA flow from tight pulmonic stenosis and has moderate truncal regurgitation. A fourth child, not yet reoperated, has decreased PA flow due to high pulmonary vascular resistance and is inoperable. In the second surgical approach, the other 3 patients underwent primary repair. At 4 months, a Hancock prosthesis was used in 1 but, by age 5 years, it had become severely obstructed. The child survives 2 months after replacement of the conduit by an aortic homograft. Such a conduit was used satisfactorily in the 2 most recent patients, operated on at 6 and 8 months, respectively.

ARRHYTHMIAS IN INFANTS AND CHILDREN

Frequency and significance of arrhythmias in infants

To determine the frequency and significance of arrhythmias in newborn infants, Southall and associates[65] in London, England, performed ECGs on 3,383 apparently healthy newborn infants aged 1–56 days (mean, 3). Those found on standard ECG to have arrhythmia or pre-excitation underwent continuous 24-hour ECG monitoring, as did 134 randomly selected newborns (controls). Babies with arrhythmia and 65 without were examined clinically and by ECG, some by 24-hour monitoring, and at 2–6-week intervals through 12 weeks of age or longer.

Of the 3,383 babies, 1% had a disorder of rhythm or conduction, which had disappeared in most (23 [85%] of 27) by 3 months and in virtually all by 12 months. In 26 babies, the neonatal arrhythmia consisted of atrial or ventricular premature complexes, but 1 infant had atrial flutter, 2 had multifocal atrial tachycardia, and 2 had supraventricular tachycardia. Three received digoxin and lost the arrhythmia; 1 improved on propranolol and the arrhythmia in the fifth subsided spontaneously. Three infants with multiple VPC had paroxysmal VT and they were not treated. Two babies had WPW that disappeared. One had persistent complete right BBB. Twelve infants had short episodes of bradycardia with rates <100/min and, on 24-hour recording, 3 showed even more marked slowing (≤60/min). Thus, the frequency of disturbances of rhythm and conduction in apparently healthy newborn infants is about 1%, and usually the disturbance disappears by the third month.

Supraventricular tachycardia

Epstein and Benditt[66] from Davis, California, and Minneapolis, Minnesota, described the 5–20 year (mean, 10) follow-up of 6 children with supraventricular tachycardia (SVT) lasting >1 year and refractory to the usual antiarrhythmic therapy. Although only 2 had symptoms of cardiac dysfunction, 2 continued to have chronic and 1 intermittent SVT and 2 returned to normal sinus rhythm spontaneously. The mechanism of the SVT was not elicited.

Garson and Gillette[67] from Houston, Texas, reviewed clinical and electrophysiologic findings in 103 children, aged 2 days–17 years, with SVT studied between 1969 and 1979: 37 had reentry without a bypass tract (25 AV node); 51 had reentry with a bypass tract (28 manifest WPW, 18 concealed, 5 Lown-Ganong-Levine), and 15 had an ectopic focus (11 atrial, 4 junctional). Arrhythmias appeared in a variety of clinical situations, had different potential for pharmacologic or surgical cure, and had different prognoses long-term. Atrial ectopic focus was 1 of the 2 least satisfactory to treat, for it either did not revert or it recurred, and the second was junctional ectopic focus tachycardia, for therapy was unsuccessful. They concluded that digoxin was the most satisfactory of the pharmacologic agents, and that electrophysiologic studies should be carried out in children unresponsive to digoxin.

Porter and associates[68] from Houston, Texas, studied 13 patients, aged 6 weeks–16 years, with recurrent SVT refractory to digoxin and/or propranolol. After electrophysiologic studies, verapamil (0.1 mg/kg) was given intravenously (i.v.) in 30 seconds while the arrhythmia was occurring. In the 5 patients with little or no response, a second dose was given and, in 1 patient, a third dose. Normal sinus rhythm appeared immediately after verapamil in 5 with AV nodal reentrant tachycardia and in 2 with an accessory pathway. Of 4 patients with ectopic atrial tachycardia, the arrhythmia stopped in 2 and continued in the other 2. The 2 patients with junctional ectopic tachycardia had an unfavorable hypotensive response to verapamil. Oral verapamil was used in 7 patients who had responded to the drug given i.v. In 4 it was successful in preventing recurrence and it caused no ill effects for up to 2 years. Three had AV nodal reentry and 1 a Kent bundle. In none did programmable stimuli induce arrhythmia while they continued to receive the verapamil i.v. In 3 patients, the drug was discontinued for lack of response in 2 and for aggressive behavior in 1. Verapamil i.v. was cautiously recommended to convert reentrant SVT dependent on nodal conduction and orally to prevent recurrence in those patients in whom the arrhythmia could not be induced by programmed stimulation while the patient was receiving verapamil i.v.

Sapire and associates[69] from Philadelphia, Pennsylvania, and Galveston, Texas, treated 6 children, aged 3 months–11 years, with verapamil because of SVT resistant to therapy or because of complications of therapy: 3 had congenital heart disease (2 were early postoperative); 2 had WPW syndrome; 3 had ectopic SVT, and 1 had atrial flutter. They gave verapamil i.v. (0.15–0.25 mg/kg). (They now prefer the lower dose.) Of 4 patients so treated, 3 successfully converted to normal rhythm, 1 patient responded to oral verapamil only, and 1 (the patient with atrial flutter) did not respond. Those who did respond to therapy i.v. usually had return of SVT within a few hours, so they were maintained with good relief on oral therapy at a dose estimated from response to the drug i.v. and from knowledge that 80% of the agent is rapidly removed by the liver at first pass. They recommend 40 mg every 8 hours as an effective starting dose, but the dose they used in maintenance was 80 mg every 6 or 8 hours. They found no adverse effects from oral therapy for periods up to 42 months. Because of verapamil's slowing effect on conduction through the AV node, they recommended its use in reentrant tachycardia and because of its blocking the slow inward calcium current and abolishing phase 4 automaticity, they advocated its use in ectopic (automatic) tachycardia.

Ventricular tachycardia

Vetter and associates[70] from Philadelphia, Pennsylvania, studied 7 otherwise normal children (6 boys) with VT and found that it had an automatic more often than a reentrant mechanism and a RV more often than a LV origin. The VT was first observed at ages 5–18 years and each had documented at least 4 episodes of spontaneous VT of more than 5 beats in duration and sometimes sustained for days. Findings by physical examination, ECG, hemodynamic, and angiographic studies were otherwise normal. The absence of structural heart disease and the left bundle-branch pattern of the VT (4 patients) characterized this disorder in children and contrasted with the opposite findings in adults. On electrophysiologic study, the VT could be reproducibly initiated in 2 children and terminated in 1 in the basal state. In the others, initiation of VT required rapid ventricular pacing, single ventricular stimuli and rapid pacing, or single ventricular stimulus after lidocaine. Tachycardia could not be induced in 4. The VT could be terminated in 1 patient by single VPC or by rapid ventricular pacing, in another by a single VPC after lidocaine had been administered, and in a third, reproducibly only after phenytoin. In the remaining 4, VT could not be terminated by electrical stimulation, either before or after antiarrhythmic drugs. Thus, they appeared to have automatic rather than reentrant VT. Endocardial mapping defined the RV outflow tract as the point of origin of the VT in those with left bundle-branch pattern.

Rocchini and associates[71] from Ann Arbor, Michigan, studied 38 children with VT, 21 (55%) of whom had a cardiovascular abnormality, especially MVP (5 patients), repaired TF (4 patients), "myocarditis" (3 patients), and prolonged Q-T syndrome (3 patients). The remaining 6 had other forms of congenital heart disease and 17 patients had no cardiac disease. The mean follow-up was 3.2 years with and 3.9 years without cardiac disease. In 3 patients, cardiac disease was fatal (not the arrhythmia) and none of the 17 without cardiac disease died. Symptoms due to VT occurred in 17 of 21 with, and in 6 of 17 without, heart disease. Five of 17 symptomatic children with heart disease had nonfatal cardiac arrest (cardioversion). Both the presence of heart disease and the rapidity of the VT produced symptoms. Symptomatic patients had a faster rate (220 ± 28 beats/min) than the asymptomatic ones (134 ± 12 beats/min). All symptomatic patients and 1 asymptomatic patient had a rate >150 beats/min. Exercise testing increased the arrhythmia in 8 of 11 symptomatic children and, in the asymptomatic patients, it either abolished (4 patients) or decreased (5 patients) the arrhythmia; in 4 asymptomatic patients with brief runs of VT, it abolished the arrhythmia.

Electrophysiologic data on 7 indicated that atrial pacing failed to provoke VT, but in 1 with spontaneous VT, overdrive pacing suppressed the tachyarrhythmia and in 3, i.v. procainamide or phenytoin abolished it. A wide spectrum of antiarrhythmic agents was tried. Therapy abolished symptoms and VT and reduced the ventricular arrhythmia in all 23 symptomatic patients, but failed to abolish it in 2 of 5 asymptomatic patients. In patients after repair of TF, phenytoin was the antiarrhythmic agent of choice, and they maintain most patients with and without cardiac disease on therapy.

Operative treatment of tachycardia unassociated with accessory connections

When medical means for converting a life-threatening tachyarrhythmia and maintaining normal sinus mechanism fail, surgical ablation is available after preoperative electrophysiologic studies and intraoperative mapping. Division of identified accessory pathways has become a well-established therapy in these circumstances. Gillette and colleagues[72] from Houston, Texas, described 5 patients aged 9 months–16 years with tachyarrhythmias unresponsive to medication and unassociated with accessory connections: 1 had ventricular reentrant tachyarrhythmia due to a small (0.5 cm) tumor at the apex of the left ventricle found and excised at operation; 1 had right atrial, and 2 had left atrial automatic tachycardia that responded to cryoablation of the abnormal focus, and 1 had AV junctional automatic ectopic tachycardia and underwent incision and ligation of the bundle of His and then, when the arrhythmia recurred 2 weeks later, cryodestruction of the His bundle along with pacemaker insertion to counteract the complete heart block that ensued. All were asymptomatic and on no medication postoperatively.

Review of tachyarrhythmias

Gillette[73] from Houston, Texas, reviewed findings from noninvasive and invasive studies in children with tachyarrhythmias. The 3 most important advances in treatment include use of *verapamil* for reentrant supraventricular tachycardia (SVT); of *propranolol* (up to 16 mg/kg/day in 4 doses) for refractory tachyarrhythmia due to AV nodal reentry and atrial automatic focus tachyarrhythmia, and of *phenytoin* for ventricular arrhythmias. In addition, surgical treatment of children with refractory arrhythmia due to WPW, automatic focus SVT, and VT offers good chance of relief. Pacemaker treatment of tachyarrhythmias is another possibility in the form of patient-activated overdrive suppression and also automatic overdrive pacemakers. Gillette believes that it is now possible to diagnose and to treat effectively practically every type of SVT and VT in children who have relatively normal hearts except for the arrhythmia.

PEDIATRIC ECHOCARDIOGRAPHY

Identification of congenital cardiac malformations by echo in midtrimester fetus

Allan and associates[74] from London, England, performed echo in 21 patients scheduled to undergo midtrimester termination of pregnancy and compared their findings with the anatomic specimens. The gestational ages were 16–27 weeks. They validated the accuracy of the technique in 18 normal hearts and in both hearts with anomalies, but they had 1 false positive. The last was suspected to have a VSD, but the septum was intact. They accurately recognized ASD and aortic isthmic coarctation. They considered 20–27 weeks of gestation to be the optimal time for fetal echo because at this time the fetal lungs are collapsed and do not interfere with imaging. This technique has great potential. To parents who have lost an infant from congenital heart disease, it can be very reassuring in the next pregnancy to know midway through that the fetal heart appears normal.

Suprasternal notch 2-D echo for diagnosing congenital heart disease

Snider and Silverman[75] from San Francisco, California, focused on the suprasternal notch view of the 2-D echo in 1,033 children with congenital heart disease to evaluate the information yielded by long-axis and short-axis views. Technically satisfactory studies were obtained in 93%. In 279, the structures were normal. The suprasternal notch view provided a window for evaluating the aortic arch, PAs, and brachiocephalic vessels in cooperative patients who could have their necks hyperextended and could tolerate a small transducer with minimal mechanical motion. This view permitted evaluation of some abnormalities not observed in other views, and, therefore, is a useful complement to 2-D precordial and subxiphoid views.

Usefulness in identifying persistent pulmonary hypertension in infants

One recently recognized and still poorly understood cause of severe cyanosis and early death in newborns is the condition known as *persistent fetal circulation*, as Gersony called it, or *persistent pulmonary hypertension of the newborn* (PPHN) as Valdes-Cruz calls it. In a prospective study, Valdes-Cruz and associates[76] from New York City employed a technique that she helped develop for the early diagnosis and assessment of response to treatment in this condition. Five years earlier, she reported the use of contrast echo for detection of right-to-left shunting at the level of the foramen ovale and DA, and she used this technique to verify the site of shunting and its course while also measuring some indicators of RV and LV dimensions and performance on M-mode echo obtained in 4 time-periods through 36 hours of age. The study was carried out prospectively and longitudinally with assignments made at 36 hours to 1 of 4 groups based on clinical course with need for and response to inspired oxygen (FiO_2). Group I contained 115 normal full-term infants; group II, 16 with mild-to-moderate pulmonary disease; group III, 25 with severe pulmonary disease requiring higher FiO_2, and group IV, 10 infants with PPHN. In the 10 with PPHN, right-to-left shunting was through the foramen ovale only, so she suggested that premature closure of the DA might play a role in the entity. The babies in group IV differed from those in the other 3 groups by showing simultaneous prolongation of both RV and LV preejection periods, isometric contraction times, and reduction in ventricular ejection times. These observations suggest that the problem may be due, in part, to depressed RV and LV function. The abnormalities were present before clinical deterioration, hypoxia and acidosis, so they may have some predictive value as well as importance for confirmation of diagnosis and assessment of effects of treatment.

MISCELLANEOUS TOPICS IN PEDIATRIC CARDIOLOGY

Frozen section of lung biopsy as a diagnostic aid in congenital heart disease

Pulmonary vascular resistance (PVR) complicates congenital cardiovascular defects, so that certain patients may not be candidates for corrective surgery and irreversible changes in PVR preclude favorable results after many defects have been repaired. Rabinovitch and associates[77] from Boston, Massachusetts, believe that the PVR measured at preoperative catheterization is a one-time observation and that it is important to have an alternative way to assess the pulmonary circulation. Through a morphometric analysis of lung tissue obtained by biopsy, they determined the type of severity of abnormalities of structure and growth of the PAs that reflect increased PA blood flow, pressure, and resistance. In patients in whom hemodynamic data could not be obtained, this technique also has been useful in deciding whether or not to perform a palliative or corrective operation. Eight patients with congenital heart defects had quantitative pulmonary morphometric analysis carried out. In 2, the PA had never been entered; 4 had moderate-to-severe elevation of the PVR, and 2 had mild elevation of PA pressure, but were being considered for a Fontan procedure (right atrial-PA shunt). The lung was biopsied and the obtained tissue was inflated and fixed with hot glutaraldehyde. From cryostat sections, arterial concentration was assessed relative to alveolar concentration and the degree of arterial vascularity was assessed by wall thickness and extension of muscle. On the basis of the morphologic assessment, 6 patients underwent corrective surgery and 2 underwent a palliative procedure. Assessment of PA obstruction by lung biopsy with frozen section proved helpful in deciding between a palliative and a surgical procedure.

Usefulness of quantitative analysis of the pulmonary wedge angiogram in congenital heart disease

Rabinovitch and associates[78] from Boston, Massachusetts, performed 93 PA wedge angiograms in 85 children with congenital heart defects undergoing preoperative evaluation (70 patients) or after surgical repair (15 patients). The cardiac lesions were VSD in 39, AV canal in 14, d-TGA in 9, and patent DA in 4. They related angiographic evidence of rate of tapering, background haze, and pulmonary circulatory time to hemodynamic data of PA pressure, flow, and resistance. In 27 patients, lung biopsy was obtained at surgery after wedge angiography. The wedge angiography utilized an inflated balloon-tipped, wedged catheter and the injection was made proximally, permitting evaluation of an entire segment of lung. Deflation after the injection permitted assessment of arterial and venous phases. They found that the rate of tapering assessed angiographically correlated well with the severity of structural changes on biopsy and with pulmonary vascular resistance measured at cardiac catheterization. Patients who persisted in too rapid tapering postoperatively had more severe changes on their biopsy. Although resting hemodynamics showed normal measurements after operation, complete regression of severe peripheral structural changes may not occur. This has been repeatedly demonstrated in long-term postoperative follow-up studies. Thus, quantitative assessment of the PA wedge angiogram correlates with hemodynamic assessment and offers valid information on the structural state of the peripheral pulmonary vascular bed.

Radiation exposure during cardiac catheterization

Cardiac catheterization with angiocardiography obviously is a valuable presurgical procedure. Because of the radiation exposure, Gersony and Bierman[79] from New York City and Boston, Massachusetts, counsel against its indiscriminate use, in particular in the evaluation of patients with mild congenital heart disease, for the diagnosis can usually be made by careful auscultation aided by ECG, chest radiograph, and echo. Furthermore, for patients believed to have an abnormality of surgical significance, M-mode and 2-D echo before cardiac catheterization provides considerable information about cardiac structure and function and this information can minimize fluoroscopy time at catheterization and can even aid in catheter placement without fluoroscopy. Postoperative cardiac catheterization is recommended only if that study has a good chance of helping in decisions for future management or in defining the long-term consequences of recently developed operations.

Martin and associates[80] from New York City, utilizing thermoluminescent dosimetry, measured the radiation exposure to the skin, thyroid gland, and gonads in 50 consecutive pediatric patients undergoing cardiac catheterization and angiocardiography via cinephotofluorography. The average exposures were 17.1 R to the skin, 2.3 R to the thyroid gland, and 0.1 R to the gonads. Fluoroscopy accounted for approximately 80% of the skin and thyroid exposure and cinephotofluorography for 20%–25%. Occasional primary-beam irradiation was the major contributor of gonad exposure. Internal scatter of the incident X-ray beam was primarily responsible for the thyroid exposure. The average gonadal exposure was 0.1 R. Thyroid exposure was greater and, in a previous study when cut film was used, averaged 7.7 R, as compared with 2.3 R now with cinephotofluorography. Studies indicate that the frequency of thyroid cancer is 1.6–9.3 cases per million per year per rad. If these children have a normal life span, the risk of developing thyroid cancer is about 0.7/1,000. The national incidence is 5% of that, namely 0.04/1,000. (It may be of some comfort to know that radiation-induced thyroid cancer has a low mortality of 3%–4%.) These investigators recommend minimizing thyroid and gonadal exposure by lead-rubber shielding, careful positioning of the incident fluoroscope beam, and proper collimation of all

X-ray beams, and calibration of X-ray equipment. They consider cinephoto-fluorography to be preferable to serial filming because of smaller film sizes and increased efficiency of the detector.

Waldman and associates[81] from San Diego, California, determined radiation exposure to children during the various aspects of cardiac catheterization. By use of lithium fluoride thermoluminescent dosimeters, radiation exposure was measured during precatheterization chest roentgenography, fluoroscopy (hemodynamic assessment phase of catheterization), and cineangiography in 30 infants and children, aged 3 days–21 years. Dosimeters were placed over the eyes, thyroid gland, anterior chest, posterior chest, abdomen, lower back and gonads. The average absorbed chest doses were 24.5 mR during chest roentgenography, 5,810 mR during catheterization fluoroscopy, and 1,592 mR during cineangiography. During the entire catheterization, the average doses were 26 mR to the eyes, 431 mR to the thyroid area, 150 mR to the abdomen, and 11 mR to the gonads. Thus, radiation exposure during cardiac catheterization in children is low to the eyes and gonads, but high to the chest and thyroid area. To decrease radiation dosage, they suggested low pulse-rate fluoroscopy, substitution of contrast echo for cineangiography, large-plate abdominal/gonadal shielding, a selective shield for the thyroid area, and a very small field during catheter manipulation. Obviously, minimum radiation consistent with accurate diagnosis is optimal. Erroneous or incomplete diagnosis is more dangerous, however, than radiation-related hazards.

Asplenia syndrome: immunologic assessment

Susceptibility to infection and death from sepsis are frequent in patients born without spleens and with complex cyanotic congenital heart disease. Cyanotic infants with levocardia and situs inversus or visceral heterotaxy should be suspect for asplenia plus the combination of pulmonic stenosis or atresia, malposition of the great arteries, defects of atrial and ventricular septa, and anomalies of systemic and pulmonary venous return. Biggar and associates[82] reported an immunologic study in 8 such patients who survived the first 2 years of life and had not been septic. All received daily penicillin prophylactically. Five had undergone palliative operations. Diagnosis of asplenia was established by the presence of Howell-Jolly bodies in the peripheral blood and by the absence of a spleen on scanning. Immunologic studies revealed normal serum I_gG and I_gA levels, but isolated I_gM deficiency in 1 and I_gE deficiency in 2. All had normal C3 and serum complement activity. When 7 children were immunized with dodecavalent pneumococcal vaccine, 4 failed to have a 2-fold or greater antibody response. The authors advised penicillin prophylaxis and parental education to try to reduce the frequency of sepsis.

Uhl's disease in twins

Uhl's anomaly, a rare developmental disorder of RV myocardium frequently associated with RV pump failure and ventricular arrhythmias and in the presence of an anatomically normal tricuspid valve, was first described in 1952 in an infant who died in CHF. Almost half of the 49 subsequently reported patients survived to adulthood. Hoback and associates[83] reported the occurrence of this anomaly in identical twin brothers, both of whom died suddenly in their late 30's (from documented ventricular fibrillation in 1). Earlier, M-mode and 2-D echo and RNA studies documented RV volume overload with poor function and delayed transit times. The authors stated that the noninvasive studies should suffice to make the diagnosis of Uhl's anomaly without cardiac catheterization.

Cardiac malformations in the fetal alcohol syndrome

The fetal alcohol syndrome was described in 1968 and, since then, more than 700 patients have been reported. Sandor and associates[84] from Vancouver, Canada, analyzed cardiac findings in 76 patients exposed to the teratogen of heavy maternal alcohol intake. In addition to characteristic facies and developmental and growth retardation, 41% had cardiac malformations when examined between birth and 18 years. The most common anomaly was VSD (26 patients), alone or together with pulmonic stenosis, aortic coarctation, AR, and ASD. Thirteen patients underwent cardiovascular operations.

MISCELLANEOUS TOPICS IN PEDIATRIC CARDIAC SURGERY

Aortic arch anomalies: types and operative treatment

A variety of aortic arch anomalies may produce tracheoesophageal compression and, occasionally, superior venal cava (SVC) compression. Aortic arch anomalies resulting in tracheoesophageal compression were treated in 42 patients during a 30-year period in Iowa City, Iowa, and the results were reported by Richardson and associates[85]: 19 (45%) had a right aortic arch with a left ligamentum arteriosum; 17 (40%) had double aortic arch, and 6 (15%) had an aberrant right subclavian artery. The diagnosis was accurately made by esophagram in 38 (90%) patients and by aortography in 4. Each had left thoracotomy and division of the constricting ring. Though postoperative respiratory complications were common, surgical treatment resulted in only 2 deaths (5%), and 1 patient died late. All survivors were relieved of their symptoms at a mean follow-up of 94 months. This series extends back to 1950 and significant improvements in respiratory therapy have occurred subsequently, so that in the absence of other severe congenital anomalies, the risk of operation should now be <1%.

Intracardiac surgery in infants under age 3 months

Primary repair of complex congenital cardiac malformations in infants is now commonplace. Kirklin and associates[86,87] from Birmingham, Alabama, reviewed their experience with 170 patients undergoing 174 *open* intracardiac operations from 1967–1980 to determine the risk factors for postoperative mortality. Operations in the first 2 months of life had a mortality of 43%, as compared with a 22% mortality for patients in the same age group undergoing closed operations. The mortality rate was considerably lower later in their experience (p < 0.0001). A poor preoperative condition (acidosis or shock) increased the mortality rate to 87%, as compared with 22% in patients with only moderate or severe symptoms, but without recent deterioration. The presence of major associated intracardiac anomalies increased the hospital mortality and was highest in infants <1 month of age. The longer the period of cardiopulmonary bypass, the higher the hospital mortality. Infants undergoing total circulatory arrest had a lower mortality than those maintained on cardiopulmonary bypass for the entire operation. Most (72%) deaths occurred from low cardiac output. Ischemic arrest was directly related to the probability of cardiac death unless cardioplegia was used. Thirteen percent of deaths were associated with acute respiratory failure. The latest mortality rates in patients without acute preoperative deterioration was about 7%.

They also analyzed their 142 infants <3 months of age who left the operating room alive after intracardiac operations from 1967–1980. The probability of postoperative in-hospital cardiac death from acute postoperative CHF, the most common mode of death, was found by multivariate logistic analysis to be significantly related only to the strength of the pedal pulses, the pedal skin temperature, and the cardiac index for the first 5 postoperative hours. When the cardiac index was not analyzed, and when cold cardioplegic myocardial preservation methods were used, only pedal pulses and pedal skin temperature were significant predictors of hospital death. The BP and heart rate were not related to hospital death. Oliguria occurred in 23% of the patients and was related primarily to inadequate cardiac output. It, too, was associated with an increased probability of hospital death.

Infradiaphragmatic total anomalous pulmonary venous connection: operative treatment

Total anomalous pulmonary venous connection (TAPVC) is a rare congenital malformation, particularly when the pulmonary venous blood enters a common descending vein and joins the portal vein or inferior vena cava (infradiaphragmatic). Pulmonary edema and severe cyanosis occur early and infants usually require urgent treatment in the first few days of life. Since 1971, 20 infants with this anomaly were treated operatively by Bove and associates.[88] The mean weight was 3.0 kg and the age range was 1–90 days. The mean preoperative P_{O_2} was 36 mmHg, all patients had pulmonary edema, and all had a persistent patent DA. During deep hypothermic circulatory arrest, the common pulmonary vein in all patients was anastomosed to the left atrium, the descending vein was ligated in 11, divided in 4, and left open in 5. ASD was closed with a patch in 6 and sutured in 14. Eight (40%) died in the perioperative period. Acidosis on admission was significantly greater among nonsurvivors (mean pH, 7.29) than among survivors (mean pH, 7.37). The 12 survivors were asymptomatic 4–96 months after operation and none required a cardiac drug. Six had postoperative catheterization that showed normal pressures and no shunt in each. The mortality in patients with infradiaphragmatic TAPVC appears to depend on the status of the blood pH; if the patient is not acidotic, the chance for operative survival and long-term cure appears good.

Glenn shunt: long-term results

From 1958 to about 1968, the Glenn shunt (anastomosis of the superior vena cava to right main PA) was the standard procedure for RV bypass. Its limitations included increasing cyanosis from venous collaterals, ventilation-perfusion abnormalities, decreased blood flow to the opposite lung, and the development of pulmonary arteriovenous fistulas. Pennington and associates[89] from St. Louis, Missouri, evaluated 50 patients who had undergone a Glenn shunt during an 18-year period for tricuspid atresia and other cyanotic cardiovascular defects. Fifteen patients died in the perioperative period and 13 of them were <4 months old. Results were poor in patients with Ebstein's anomaly, truncus arteriosus, TGA, and complex defects *other than* tricuspid atresia and single ventricle. The other 35 patients were followed 1–15 years (mean, 7). Of 25 patients with tricuspid atresia, 6 died early and 2 later. Eleven patients underwent additional operative procedures because of an increase in cyanosis, 4 patients without other shunts underwent a Fontan procedure, and 6 patients are alive after the Glenn shunt without other operative procedures. Minimal evidence existed that there was intrapulmonary shunting. Late deterioration due to venous collaterals and decreased blood flow to the opposite lung necessitated Blalock-Taussig shunts in 6 and a Fontan procedure in 10. All survived the Fontan procedure. Thus, the Glenn shunt does not necessarily result in pulmonary abnormalities, and, therefore, it may be indicated as a staged procedure in a few selected patients before the Fontan procedure.

Effect of physical training on exercise performance after repair of congenital heart disease

Goldberg and associates[90] from New Haven, Connecticut, and New York City performed exercise testing in adolescents several years (mean, 8.1 years) after successful cardiac surgery for TF (16 patients) or VSD (10 patients) performed at a mean age of 5.8 years. Using a bicycle ergometer with work-load increased and heart rate and oxygen consumption measured until exhaustion, they found that 65% scored below average. They then embarked on a 6-week home-training program using an exercise bicycle for about 45 minutes of submaximal exercise every other day for 6 weeks, with prescribed workload increases after the first and second weeks. The heart rates were 150–170 beats/min. Compliance was remarkably good: 88% completed 16 of the possible 21 sessions and 69% completed 18 or more. Post-training testing showed significantly decreased oxygen consumption and heart rate at each work load, indicating improved aerobic efficiency. Exercise obviously should be encouraged after cardiac surgery for these anomalies, without fear of an arrhythmia.

Comparison of prostaglandin E_1 resistance after open heart operations

Rubis and associates[91] from Philadelphia, Pennsylvania, compared the effects of prostaglandin E_1 (PGE$_1$) (0.1–1.0 μg/g/min) with these of nitroprusside (0.5–8.7 μg/g/min) in 26 children aged 3–16 years (mean, 6) in reducing PA pressure and resistance and systemic artery (SA) pressure and resistance: 5 patients had ASD; 10, VSD; 3, TF, and 8, other anomalies. Side effects prevented treatment with PGE$_1$ in 5 patients. The drugs were infused into a central venous catheter until the mean PA or mean SA pressure decreased at least 10%. Results were available for 21 patients. The mean SA pressure after PGE$_1$ fell an average of 12 ± 5.6 mmHg (p < 0.05). The decrease in mean PA pressure (3 ± 7.1 mmHg) was not significant. There was a significant fall (p < 0.02) in systemic vascular resistance index, but an insignificant average decrease in pulmonary vascular resistance (1 ± 3.2). The average heart rate increased significantly (6 ± 9.3 beats/min [p < 0.02]). When the children were evaluated by subgroups for age and preoperative pulmonary blood flow, there was no real difference in drug response. Fourteen children also received nitroprusside 30–45 minutes after PGE$_1$ had been discontinued. Changes in control were similar to those in the group of 21 receiving PGE$_1$: 14 patients had an average fall of 11 ± 7.2 mmHg in mean SA pressure and a mean fall of 6 ± 4.7 mmHg in mean PA pressure. The systemic vascular index and pulmonary vascular index fell 5 ± 3.8 and 1 ± 1.6, respectively. Cardiac index increased 0.2 ± 0.33 liters/min/M². There was no statistically significant difference between drugs, although nitroprusside appeared to cause a more uniform hemodynamic response than did PGE$_1$ among children and was not limited by side effects as was PGE$_1$.

References

1. KAMAU P, MILES V, TOEWS W, KELMINSON L, FRIESEN R, LOCKHART C, BUTTERFIELD J, HERNANDEZ J, HAWES CR, PAPPAS G: Surgical repair of coarctation of the aorta in infants less than six months of age: including the question of pulmonary artery banding. J Thorac Cardiovasc Surg 81:171–179, Feb 1981.

2. LAWRIE GM, DEBAKEY ME, MORRIS GC JR, CRAWFORD ES, WAGNER WF, GLAESER DH: Late repair of coarctation of the descending thoracic aorta in 190 patients. Arch Surg 116:1557–1580, Dec 1981.

3. BEEKMAN RH, ROCCHINI AP, BEHRENDT DM, ROSENTHAL A: Reoperation for coarctation of the aorta. Am J Cardiol 48:1108–1114, Dec 1981.

4. BAILEY LL, JACOBSON JG, DOROSHOW RW, MERRITT WH, PETRY EL: Anatomic correction of interrupted aortic arch complex in neonates. Surgery 89:553–557, May 1981.

5. MOULTON AL, BOWMAN FO JR: Primary definitive repair of type B interrupted aortic arch, ventricular septal defect, and patent ductus arteriosus. J Thorac Cardiovasc Surg 82:501–510, Oct 1981.

6. KECECIOGLU-DRAELOS Z, GOLDBERG SJ: Role of M-mode echocardiography in congenital aortic stenosis. Am J Cardiol 47:1267–1727, June 1981.

7. DOBELL ARC, BLOSS RS, GIBBONS JE, COLLINS GF: Congenital valvular aortic stenosis: surgical management and long-term results. J Thorac Cardiovasc Surg 81:916–920, June 1981.

8. ERGIN MA, COOPER R, LACORTE M, GOLINKO R, GRIEPP RB: Experience with left ventricular apicoaortic conduits for complicated left ventricular outflow obstruction in children and young adults. Ann Thor Surg 32:369–376, Oct 1981.

9. NORWOOD WI, LANG P, CASTANEDA AR, CAMPBELL DN: Experience with operations for hypoplastic left heart syndrome. J Thorac Cardiovasc Surg 82:511–519, Oct 1981.

10. SMALLHORN J, TOMMASINI G, DEANFIELD J, DOUGLAS J, GIBSON D, MACARTNEY F: Congenital mitral stenosis: anatomical and functional assessment by echocardiography. Br Heart J 45:527–534, May 1981.

11. RICHARDSON JV, DOTY DB, SIEWERS RD, ZUBERBUHLER JR: Cor triatriatum (subdivided left atrium). J Thorac Cardiovasc Surg 81:232–238, Feb 1981.

12. DUNN JM: Porcine valve durability in children. Ann Thor Surg 32:357–368, Oct 1981.

13. WILLIAMS WG, POLLOCK JC, GEISS DM, TRUSLER GA, FOWLER RS: Experience with aortic and mitral valve replacement in children. J Thorac Cardiovasc Surg 81:326–333, March 1981.

14. ATTIE F, KURI J, ZANONIANI C, RENTERIA V, BUENDIA A, OVSEYEVITZ J, LOPEZ-SORIANO F, GARCIA-CORNEJO M, MARTINEZ-RIOS MA: Mitral valve replacement in children with rheumatic heart disease. Circulation 64:812–817, Oct 1981.

15. CABIN HS, WOOD TP, SMITH JO, ROBERTS WC: Ebstein's anomaly in the elderly. Chest 80:212–214, Aug 1981.

16. DRISCOLL DJ, NIHILL MR, MULLINS CE, COOLEY DA, McNAMARA DG: Management of symptomatic infants with anomalous origin of the left coronary artery from the pulmonary artery. Am J Cardiol 47:642–648, March 1981.

17. STEPHENSON LW, EDMUNDS LH JR, FRIEDMAN S, MEIJBOOM E, GEWITZ M, WEINBERG P: Subclavian-left coronary artery anastomosis (Meyer operation) for anomalous origin of the left coronary artery from the pulmonary artery. Circulation 64:130–133, Aug 1981.

18. LOWE JE, OLDHAM HN JR, SABISTON DC JR: Surgical management of congenital coronary artery fistulas. Ann Surg 194:373–380, Oct 1981.

19. EDWARDS BS, EDWARDS WD, EDWARDS JE: Aortic origin of conus coronary artery: evidence of postnatal coronary development. Br Heart J 45:555–558, May 1981.

20. ST. JOHN SUTTON MG, TAJIK AJ, McGOON DC: Atrial septal defect in patients ages 60 years or older: operative results and long-term postoperative follow-up. Circulation 64:402–409, Aug 1981.

21. LIBERTHSON RR, BOUCHER CA, STRAUSS HW, DINSMORE RE, McKUSICK KA, POHOST GM: Right ventricular function in adult atrial septal defect: preoperative and postoperative assessment and clinical implications. Am J Cardiol 47:56–60, Jan 1981.

22. BONOW RO, BORER JS, ROSING DR, BACHARACH SL, GREEN MV, KENT KM: Left ventricular functional reserve in adult patients with atrial septal defect: pre- and postoperative studies. Circulation 63:1315–1322, June 1981.

23. LIBERTHSON RR, BOUCHER CA, FALLON JT, BUCKLEY MJ: Severe mitral regurgitation: a common occurrence in the aging patient with secundum atrial septal defect. Clin Cardiol 4:229–232, Sept/Oct 1981.

24. DAVIES MJ: Mitral valve in secundum atrial septal defects. Br Heart J 46:126–128, Aug 1981.

25. SOTO B, BARGERON LM JR, PACIFICO AD, VANINI V, KIRKLIN JW: Angiography of atrioventricular canal defects. Am J Cardiol 48:492–499, Sept 1981.

26. GOLDFADEN DM, JONES M, MORROW AG: Long-term results of repair of incomplete persistent atrioventricular canal. J Thorac Cardiovasc Surg 82:669–673, Nov 1981.

27. TAYLOR NC, SOMERVILLE J: Fixed subaortic stenosis after repair of ostium primum defects. Br Heart J 45:689–697, June 1981.

28. THIENE G, WENINK ACG, FRESCURA C, WILKINSON JL, GALLUCCI V, HO SY, MAZZUCCO A, ANDERSON

RH: Surgical anatomy and pathology of the conduction tissues in atrioventricular defects. J Thorac Cardiovasc Surg 82:928–937, Dec 1981.

29. DICKINSON DF, ARNOLD R, WILKINSON JL: Ventricular septal defect in children born in Liverpool 1960 to 1969: evaluation of natural course and surgical implications in an unselected population. Br Heart J 46:47–54, July 1981.

30. CANALE JM, SAHN DJ, ALLEN HD, GOLDBERG SJ, VALDES-CRUZ LM, OVITT TW: Factors affecting real-time, cross-sectional echocardiographic imaging of perimembranous ventricular septal defects. Circulation 63:689–697, March 1981.

31. BEEKMAN RH, ROCCHINI AP, ROSENTHAL A: Hemodynamic effects of nitroprusside in infants with a large ventricular septal defect. Circulation 64:553–558, Sept 1981.

32. GENTILE R, STEVENSON G, DOOLEY T, FRANKLIN D, KAWABORI I, PEARLMAN A.: Pulsed Doppler echocardiographic determination of time of ductal closure in normal newborn infants. J Pediatr 98:443–448, March 1981.

33. YEH TF, LUKEN JA, THALJI A, RAVAL D, CARR I, PILDES RS: Intravenous indomethacin therapy in premature infants with persistent patent ductus arteriosus: a double-blind controlled study. J Pediatr 98:137–145, January 1981.

34. YANAGI RM, WILSON A, NEWFELD EA, AZIZ KU, HUNT CE: Indomethacin treatment for symptomatic patent ductus arteriosus: a double-blind control study. Pediatrics 67:647–652, May 1981.

35. BRASH AR, HICKEY DE, GRAHAM TP, STAHLMAN MT, OATES JA, COTTON RB: Pharmacokinetics of indomethacin in the neonate: relation of plasma indomethacin levels to response of the ducts arteriosus. N Engl J Med 305:67–72, July 1981.

36. MERRITT TA, HARRIS JP, ROGHMANN K, WOOD B, CAMPANELLA V, ALEXSON C, MANNING J, SHAPIRO DL: Early closure of the patent ductus arteriosus in very low-birth-weight infants: a controlled trial. J Pediatr 99:281–286, Aug 1981.

37. LEWIS AB, FREED MD, HEYMANN MA, ROEHL SL, KENSEY RC: Side effects of therapy with prostaglandin E$_1$ in infants with critical congenital heart disease. Circulation 64:893–898, Nov 1981.

38. FREED MD, HEYMANN MA, LEWIS AB, ROEHL SL, KENSEY: Prostaglandin E$_1$ in infants with ductus arteriosus-dependent congenital heart disease. Circulation 64:899–905, Nov 1981.

39. BRANDT B III, MARVIN WJ, EHRENHAFT JL, HEINTZ S, DOTY DB: Ligation of patent ductus arteriosus in premature infants. Ann Thorac Surg 32:167–172, Aug 1981.

40. JOHN S, MURALIDHARAN S, JAIRAJ PS, MANI GK, BABUTHAMAN, KRISHNASWAMY S, SUKUMAR IP, CHERIAN G: The adult ductus: review of surgical experience with 131 patients. J Thorac Cardiovasc Surg 82:314–319, Aug 1981.

41. DOTY DB, RICHARDSON JV, FALKOVSKY GE, GORDONOVA MI, BURAKOVSKY VI: Aortopulmonary septal defect: hemodynamics, angiography, and operation. Ann Thorac Surg 32:244–250, Sept 1981.

42. SOTO B, PACIFICO AD, CEBALLOS R, BARGERON LM JR: Tetralogy of Fallot: an angiographic-pathologic correlative study. Circulation 64:558–566, Sept 1981.

43. RABINOVITCH M, HERRERA-DELEON V, CASTANEDA AR, REID L: Growth and development of the pulmonary vascular bed in patients with tetralogy of Fallot with or without pulmonary atresia. Circulation 64:1234–1249, Dec 1981.

44. THIENE G, FRESCURA C, BORTOLOTTI U, DEL MASCHIO A, VALENTE M: The systemic pulmonary circulation in pulmonary atresia with ventricular septal defect: concept of reciprocal development of the fourth and sixth aortic arches. Am Heart J 101:339–344, March 1981.

45. HAMILTON DI, DE EUSANIO G, PICCOLI GP, DICKINSON DF: Eight years' experience with intracardiac repair of tetralogy of Fallot: early and late results in 175 consecutive patients. Br Heart J 46:144–151, Aug 1981.

46. BOROW KM, KEANE JF, CASTANEDA AR, FREED MD: Systemic ventricular function in patients with tetralogy of Fallot ventricular septal defect and transposition of the great arteries repaired during infancy. Circulation 64:878–885, Nov 1981.

47. ROCCHINI AP: Hemodynamic abnormalities in response to supine exercise in patients after operative correction of tetrad of Fallot after early childhood. Am J Cardiol 48:325–330, Aug 1981.

48. WESSEL HU, WEINER MD, PAUL MH, BASTANIER CK: Lung function in tetralogy of Fallot after intracardiac repair. J Thorac Cardiovasc Surg 82:616–628, Oct 1981.

49. LAKS H, HELLENBRAND WE, KLEINMAN CS, STANSEL HC JR, TALNER NS: Patch reconstruction of the right ventricular outflow tract with pulmonary valve insertion. Circulation 64(Suppl II):154–161, Aug 1981.

50. HENRY CG, GOLDRING D, HARTMAN AF, WELDON CS, STRAUSS AR: Treatment of d-transposition of the great arteries: management of hypoxemia after balloon atrial septostomy. Am J Cardiol 47:299–306, Feb 1981.

51. LEANAGE R, AGNETTI A, GRAHAM G, TAYLOR J, MACARTNEY FJ: Factors influencing survival after balloon atrial septostomy for complete transposition of great arteries. Br Heart J 45:559–572, May 1981.

52. MOULTON AL, DELEVAL MR, MACARTNEY FJ, TAYLOR JFN, STARK J: Rastelli procedure for transposition of the great arteries, ventricular septal defect, and left ventricular outflow tract obstruction. Br Heart J 45:20–28, Jan 1981.

53. AGARWAL KC, EDWARDS WD, FELDT RH, DANIELSON GK, PUGA FJ, McGOON DC: Clinicopathological correlates of obstructed right-sided porcine-valved extracardiac conduits. J Thorac Cardiovasc Surg 81:591–601, Apr 1981.

54. AZIZ KU, PAUL MH, BHARATI S, COLE RB, MUSTER AJ, LEV M, IDRISS FS: Two dimensional echocardiographic evaluation of Mustard operation for d-transposition of the great arteries. Am J Cardiol 47:654–664, March 1981.

55. NINOMIYA K, DUNCAN WJ, COOK DH, OLLEY PM, ROWE RD: Right ventricular ejection fraction and volumes after Mustard repair: correlation of two dimensional echocardiograms and cineangiograms. Am J Cardiol 48:317–324, June 1981.

56. ARCINIEGAS E, FAROOKI ZQ, HAKIMI M, PERRY BL, GREEN EW: Results of the Mustard operation for dextrotransposition of the great arteries. J Thorac Cardiovasc Surg 81:580–587, Apr 1981.

57. PICCOLI GP, WILIKINSON JL, ARNOLD R, MUSUMECI F, HAMILTON DI: Appraisal of the Mustard procedure for the physiological correction of "simple" transposition of the great arteries. J Thorac Cardiovasc Surg 82:436–446, Sept 1981.

58. PITLICK P, FRENCH J, GUTHANER D, SHUMWAY N, BAUM D: Results of intraventricular baffle procedure for ventricular septal defect and double outlet right ventricle or d-transposition of the great arteries. Am J Cardiol 47:307–314, Feb 1981.

59. FREEDOM RM, CULHAM JAG, OLLEY PM, ROWE RD, WILLIAMS WG, TRUSLER GA: Anatomic correction of transposition of the great arteries: pre- and postoperative cardiac catheterization, with angiocardiography in five patients. Circulation 63:905–914, Apr 1981.

60. WILLIAMS WG, FREEDOM RM, CULHAM G, DUNCAN WJ, OLLEY PM, ROWE RD, TRUSLER GA: Early experience with arterial repair of transposition. Ann Thorac Surg 32:8–15, July 1981.

61. HAGLER DJ, TAJIK AJ, SEWARD JB, EDWARDS WD, MAIR DD, RITTER DG: Atrioventricular and ventriculoarterial discordance (corrected transposition of the great arteries). Wide-angle two-dimensional echocardiographic assessment of ventricular morphology. Mayo Clin Proc 56:591–600, Oct 1981.

62. WILLIAMS WG, SURI R, SHINDO G, FREEDOM RM, MORCH JE, TRUSLER GA: Repair of major intracardiac anomalies associated with atrioventricular discordance. Ann Thorac Surg 31:527–531, June 1981.

63. FELDT RH, MAIR DD, DANIELSON GK, WALLACE RB, McGOON DC: Current status of the septation procedure for univentricular heart. J Thorac Cardiovasc Surg 82:93–97, July 1981.

64. MUSUMECI F, PICCOLI GP, DICKINSON DF, HAMILTON DI: Surgical experience with persistent truncus arteriosus in symptomatic infants under one year of age: report of 13 consecutive cases. Br Heart J 46:179–185, Aug 1981.

65. SOUTHAL DP, JOHNSON AM, SHINEBOURNE EA, JOHNSTON PGB, VULLIAMY DG: Frequency and outcome of disorders of cardiac rhythm and conduction in a population of newborn infants. Pediatrics 68:58–66, July 1981.

66. EPSTEIN ML, BENDITT DG: Long-term evaluation of persistent supraventricular tachycardia in children: clinical and electrocardiographic features. Am Heart J 102:80–84, July 1981.

67. GARSON A JR, GILLETTE PC: Electrophysiologic studies of supraventricular tachycardia in children. I. clinical-electrophysiologic correlations. Am Heart J 102:233–250, Aug 1981.

68. PORTER C-BJ, GILLETTE PC, GARSON A JR, HESSLEIN PS, KARPAWICH PP, MCNAMARA DG: Effects of verapamil on supraventricular tachycardia in children. Am J Cardiol 48:487–491, Sept 1981.

69. SAPIRE DW, O'RIORDAN AC, BLACK IFS: Safety and efficacy of short- and long-term verapamil therapy in children with tachycardia. Am J Cardiol 48:1091–1097, Dec 1981.

70. VETTER VL, JOSEPHSON ME, HOROWITZ LN: Idiopathic recurrent sustained ventricular tachycardia in children and adolescents. Am J Cardiol 47:315–322, Feb 1981.

71. ROCCHINI AP, CHUN PO, DICK M: Ventricular tachycardia in children. Am J Cardiol 47:1091–1097, May 1981.

72. GILLETTE PC, GARSON A JR, HESSLEIN PS, KARPAWICH PP, TIERNEY RC, COOLEY DA, MCNAMARA DG: Successful surgical treatment of atrial, junctional, and ventricular tachycardia unassociated with accessory connections in infants and children. Am Heart J 102:984–991, Dec 1981.

73. GILLETTE PC: Advances in the diagnosis and treatment of tachydysrhythmias in children. Am Heart J 102:111–120, July 1981.

74. ALLAN LD, TYNAN M, CAMPBELL S, ANDERSON RH: Identification of congenital cardiac malformations by echocardiography in midtrimester fetus. Br Heart J 46:358–362, Oct 1981.

75. SNIDER AR, SILVERMAN NJ: Suprasternal notch echocardiography: a two-dimensional technique for evaluating congenital heart disease. Circulation 63:165–173, Jan 1981.

76. VALDES-CRUZ LM, DUDELL GG, FERRARA A: Utility of M-mode echocardiography for early identification of infants with persistent pulmonary hypertension of the newborn. Pediatrics 68:515–525, Oct 1981.

77. RABINOVITCH M, CASTANEDA AR, REID L: Lung biopsy with frozen section as a diagnostic aid in patients with congenital heart defects. Am J Cardiol 47:77–84, Jan 1981.

78. RABINOVITCH M, KEANE JF, FELLOWS KE, CASTANEDA AR, REID L: Quantitative analysis of the pulmonary wedge angiogram in congenital heart defects: correlation with hemodynamic data and morphometric findings in lung biopsy tissue. Circulation 63:152–164, Jan 1981.

79. GERSONY WM, BIERMAN FZ: Cardiac catheterization in the pediatric patient. Pediatrics 67:738–740, May 1981.

80. MARTIN EC, OLSON AP, STEEG CN, CASARELLA WJ: Radiation exposure to the pediatric patient during cardiac catheterization and angiocardiography: emphasis on the thyroid gland. Circulation 64:153–158, July 1981.

81. WALDMAN JD, RUMMERFIELD PS, GILPIN EA, KIRKPATRICK SE: Radiation exposure to the child during cardiac catheterization. Circulation 64:158–163, July 1981.

82. BIGGAR WD, RAMIREZ RA, ROSE V: Congenital asplenia: Immunologic assessment and a clinical review of eight surviving patients. Pediatrics 67:548–551, Apr 1981.

83. HOBACK J, ADICOFF A, FROM AHL, SMITH M, SHAFER R, CHESLER E: A report of Uhl's disease in identical adult twins: evaluation of right ventricular dysfunction with echocardiography and nuclear angiography. Chest 79:306–310, March 1981.

84. SANDOR GGS, SMITH DF, MACLEOD PM: Cardiac malformations in the fetal alcohol syndrome. J Pediatr 98:771–773, May 1981.

85. RICHARDSON JV, DOTY DB, ROSSI NP, EHRENHAFT JL: Operation for aortic arch anomalies. Ann Thorac Surg 31:426–432, May 1981.

86. KIRKLIN JK, BLACKSTONE EH, KIRKLIN JW, MCKAY R, PACIFICO AD, BARGERON LM JR: Intracardiac

surgery in infants under age 3 months: incremental risk factors for hospital mortality. Am J Card 48:500–506, Sept 1981.

87. KIRKLIN JK, BLACKSTONE EH, KIRKLIN JW, McKAY R, PACIFICO AD, BARGERON LM JR: Intracardiac surgery in infants under age 3 months: predictors of postoperative inhospital cardiac death. Am J Card 48:507–512, Sept 1981.

88. BOVE EL, DE LEVAL MR, TAYLOR JFN, MACARTNEY FJ, SZARNICKI RJ, STARK J: Infradiaphragmatic total anomalous pulmonary venous drainage: surgical treatment and long-term results. Ann Thorac Surg 31:544–549, June 1981.

89. PENNINGTON DG, NOURI S, HO J, SECKER-WALKER R, PATEL B, SIVAKOFF M, WILLMAN VL: Glenn shunt: long-term results and current role in congenital heart operations. Ann Thorac Surg 31:532–539, June 1981.

90. GOLDBERG B, FRIPP RR, LISTER G, LOKE J, NICHOLAS JA, TALNER NS: Effect of physical training on exercise performance of children following surgical repair of congenital heart disease. Pediatrics 68:691–699, Nov 1981.

91. RUBIS LJ, STEPHENSON LW, JOHNSTON MR, NAGARAJ S, EDMUNDS LH JR: Comparison of effects of prostaglandin E_1 and nitroprusside on pulmonary vascular resistance in children after open-heart surgery. Ann Thorac Surg 32:563–570, Dec 1981.

8

Drugs for Congestive Heart Failure

VASODILATOR THERAPY: GENERAL ASPECTS

Colucci and associates[1] from Boston, Massachusetts, reviewed the role of vasodilators in the treatment of patients with severe CHF and increased systemic vascular resistance. The potential mechanisms of attenuation of vasodilator effect are outlined in Table 8-1.

The use of vasodilators in the treatment of CHF spans a relatively brief period. Parenteral agents first received attention in 1971. Despite a proliferation of reports, there continues to be a paucity of long-term controlled (or uncontrolled) studies from which to assess critically the relevance of the phenomenon of vasodilator tolerance to clinical practice. Thus, there is only a single controlled trial of long-term nitrate therapy and preliminary reports of controlled long-term trials of hydralazine. Controlled studies of converting enzyme inhibitor have not yet appeared. In a number of studies, a marked attenuation of the hemodynamic effects of the alpha adrenergic antagonist *prazosin* has been shown. Controlled long-term studies have demonstrated a beneficial long-term clinical effect of this agent.

Much of the clinical experience with vasodilator drugs was derived in patients with angina pectoris or systemic hypertension. The response of patients with CHF differs from that of patients with other types of disease and, therefore, much of this experience with vasodilators may not be directly ap-

TABLE 8-1. *Potential mechanisms of attenuation of vasodilator effects.*

INCREASED SYMPATHETIC NERVOUS SYSTEM ACTIVITY
  Increased central nervous system-mediated sympathetic activity (norepinephrine)
  Increased peripheral neuron norepinephrine release or decreased uptake
  Increased adrenal medullary activity (epinephrine)
INCREASED RENIN-ANGIOTENSIN-ALDOSTERONE SYSTEM ACTIVITY
  Increased renin release
  Increased angiotensin production
    increased aldosterone secretion
    increased vasoconstriction
  Decreased aldosterone metabolism
INCREASED VASCULAR SMOOTH MUSCLE CELL REACTIVITY
  Increased number and/or affinity of receptors for vasoconstrictor substances (i.e., alpha
    adrenergic agonists, angiotensin II)
  Decreased number and/or affinity of receptors for vasodilator substances (i.e., beta adrenergic
    agonists, prostaglandins)
  Increased intrinsic smooth muscle cell contractility
  Increased smooth muscle cell sodium content (hyperkalemia, digitalis glycosides)

---

plicable to patients with CHF. Nevertheless, this previous experience serves as a useful departure point for a consideration of the relevance of vasodilator attenuation in the therapy of CHF.

In Table 8-2, several vasodilators used in the treatment of CHF are categorized according to their major pharmacologic mechanism of action. Although the drugs within each class may differ considerably with regard to route of administration, duration of action, and site of action (i.e., arterial, venous, or mixed), this classification is useful because it is likely that drugs within each group will elicit similar compensatory mechanisms.

Conti[2] from Gainesville, Florida, introduced an excellent symposium on the use of vasodilators in patients with CHF. This review, which includes papers by Cohn[3] from Minneapolis, Minnesota, Chatterjee and associates[4] from San Francisco, California, Rouleau and associates[5] from Montreal, Canada, and Awan and associates[6] from Davis and Sacramento, California, discussed the effectiveness of vasodilator therapy, with particular attention to new data on the use of *prazosin*. Exactly where vasodilators fit in the scheme of management of CHF is still not entirely clear. Current medical management, of course, generally consists of an investigation of the etiology of the CHF and treatment with salt restriction, diuretics, and digitalis. Additionally, an attempt is made to reduce cardiac workload by weight reduction and control of systemic hypertension and by altering afterload (preload and impedance). Vasodilators contribute both to the control of systemic hypertension and to unloading of the heart.

Although *hydralazine* provokes myocardial ischemic events in patients with systemic hypertension without CHF by producing reflex tachycardia, the frequency of and mechanisms underlying ischemic events when this drug is administered as a vasodilator agent to patients with CHF is unknown. Ac-

TABLE 8-2. *Pharmacologic classes of vasodilators used in the treatment of heart failure.*

DIRECT SMOOTH MUSCLE RELAXERS
    Nitrates
    Nitroprusside
    Hydralazine
    Minoxidil
ALPHA ADRENERGIC ANTAGONISTS
    Phentolamine
    Phenoxybenzamine
    Prazosin
    Trimazosin
RENIN-ANGIOTENSIN SYSTEM ANTAGONISTS
    Converting enzyme inhibitors (e.g., captopril)
    Competitive antagonists (e.g., saralasin)
BETA ADRENERGIC AGONISTS
    Isoproterenol
    Pirbuterol
    Terbutaline
    Salbutamol

---

cordingly, Packer and associates[7] from New York City analyzed responses to hydralazine in 52 consecutive patients with severe chronic CHF secondary to CAD. Twelve patients (23%) had 16 ischemic events during the initial administration of hydralazine (angina at rest in 12, AMI in 4); these generally occurred in the absence of significant tachycardia and hypotension. In contrast, of the 35 patients (of the 52) who received *nitroprusside* (8 of whom had ischemic events with hydralazine), this drug provoked ischemia in only 1, although it resulted in greater decreases in systemic arterial pressure than occurred with hydralazine. In patients with an ischemic event only with hydralazine, LV filling pressure decreased 15 mmHg with nitroprusside, but only 4 mmHg with hydralazine (p < 0.01). Provocation of ischemia with hydralazine may, therefore, be due to the relative preservation of elevated LV preload with this drug, since ischemic events are not common with nitroprusside despite greater decreases in systemic pressures.

Breathlessness and fatigue limit the capacity of patients with chronic CHF to participate in physical activities. As a result, patients with CHF tend to gauge quality of life in terms of symptom-free activities they can undertake. Physicians attempt to alleviate these limiting symptoms and increase the exercise capacity of patients with CHF by therapeutic interventions. In recent years, a variety of systemic vasodilators and inotropic agents have been introduced to aid digitalis and diuretics in improving cardiac performance in these patients. Although the pumping function of the heart is enhanced at rest, clarification is required as to whether exercise tolerance also is improved. Weber and associates[8] from Philadelphia, Pennsylvania, reviewed clinical experience with a number of systemic vasodilators and positive inotropic agents, with attention focused on the influence of these drugs on exercise performance in CHF patients. This experience includes salutary investigations of: 1) 28-week double-blind study of *hydralazine* -vs- placebo in 19 patients with CHF; 2) 52-week double-blind, crossover study of *trimazosin* (alpha blockade) -vs- placebo in 27 patients with CHF of varying severity, and 3) open study of *amrinone* (positive inotropic agent) in 12 patients with CHF.

PRAZOSIN

In contrast to hydralazine, which acts predominantly on arteriolar resistance vessels, and to nitrates, which act principally on venous vessels, prazosin (PZ) owing to its postsynaptic alpha adrenoreceptor blocking property, has a strong effect on both systemic venous capacitance and arteriolar resistance vessels. Therefore, reductions of aortic impedance and cardiac preload should result from use of PZ. PZ is available in oral form and does not have the untoward side effects reported with hydralazine therapy. Contrary to a number of studies that had demonstrated the same beneficial effect of PZ in chronic CHF by means of noninvasive examination, rapid attenuation of the acute salutary action of PZ has recently been contended. Consequently, the value of PZ for chronic CHF treatment has been questioned by some workers. Bertel and associates[9] from Basel, Switzerland, investigated the long-term effects of PZ on hemodynamics and symptoms in patients with severe CHF resistant to the conventional treatment with digitalis and diuretics. Twelve CHF patients (New York Heart Association class III and IV) resistant to conventional CHF therapy were treated with PZ (3–20 mg/day). In 11 patients, oral PZ treatment was well tolerated; the agent was discontinued in the remaining patient because of orthostatic dizziness. After 4 weeks of PZ, total systemic vascular resistance decreased from 2,245 to 1,603 dynes-sec-cm^{-5}, mean BP declined from 100 to 90 mmHg, pulmonary capillary wedge pressure decreased from 29 to 25 mmHg, and cardiac index increased from 1.92 to 2.30 liters/min/M^2. The increase of stroke volume index correlated with the fall in peripheral vascular resistance and the decline in pulmonary capillary wedge pressure. In parallel, exercise tolerance increased signicantly: 4 patients improved from functional class IV to II, 4 from class IV to III, and 1 from class III to II, while 2 patients were unchanged. In the 8 patients followed for 6 months, it was objectively shown by serial cardiac catheterization that the beneficial hemodynamic effects of ambulatory PZ were maintained throughout this expansive observation period. Thus, PZ is a valuable vasodilator for long-term treatment in otherwise refractory CHF when the agent is given in sufficient (individualized) dosage.

Prazosin has balanced effects on systemic arteries and veins similar to nitroprusside and, when administered orally, acutely improves cardiac output and LV filling pressure. A few reports of apparent "tachyphylaxis" to PZ have created some doubts about its chronic efficacy. To investigate the long-term hemodynamic effects of PZ in severe CHF, Feldman and associates[10] from Stanford, California, gave PZ for 3 months to 13 advanced CHF patients. Following the first PZ dose, cardiac output (CO) rose from 3.2 to 4.3 liters/min, PA diastolic pressure decreased from 23 to 18 mmHg, mean systemic arterial BP decreased from 85 to 76 mmHg, and heart rate did not change. At the end of a 48–72-hour titration to an optimal PZ regimen, significant beneficial effects of CO (3.2 to 4.5 liters/min) and on PA diastolic pressure (24 to 18 mmHg) were still observed. The patients were restudied by cardiac catheterization after 3 months of PZ treatment. In contrast to the few reports of rapid development of tolerance to PZ, observed were continued salutary effects on CO (3.0 to 3.8 liters/min) and PA diastolic pressure (23 to 18 mmHg), without significant change in mean arterial pressure (81 to 78 mmHg). Systemic vascular resistance in the untreated state correlated with the percentage PZ-induced change in CO. Finally, excessive lowering of PA diastolic pressure appeared to blunt the beneficial CO rise in some CHF patients.

To evaluate whether long-term administration of PZ in the ambulatory therapy of chronic refractory CHF results in gradual attenuation of its marked salutary peripheral circulatory relaxing actions, 16 patients with CHF due to CAD receiving chronic PZ (16 mg daily) were assessed for the development of vasodilator tolerance for 12 months by Awan and associates[11] from Davis and Sacramento, California. In 6 patients, such tolerance was documented after 7 months, but was readily surmountable, thereby allowing continuation of effective chronic PZ therapy. Each of the 6 tolerance patients underwent 4 forearm plethysmographic studies: before chronic PZ (Study I; 4.0 mg study dose): after 7 months of PZ (Study II; 4.0 mg); repeated following 1 additional week on higher effective PZ dose of 32 mg daily (Study III; 8.4 mg); and following 2 weeks of PZ withdrawal (Study IV; 4.0 mg). The PZ study dose increased forearm blood flow and decreased forearm vascular resistance and venous tone in Studies I, III and IV; these variables were unchanged by PZ in Study II. Despite vasodilator tolerance to the initial daily dosage at 7 months (Study II), symptomatic effectiveness and improved cardiac performance were sustained throughout the entire 12 months of chronic PZ therapy by increasing dosage (Study III) and/or brief interruption of the vasodilator (Study IV); New York Heart Association class IV pre-PZ symptoms improved to class 2.7 at 3 months, to class 2.4 at 6 months, and to class 2.5 at 12 months chronic PZ. Thus, chronic PZ tolerance occurred in approximately one-third of CHF patients after several months of chronic PZ therapy, and chronic PZ symptomatic efficacy can be maintained in such CHF patients by overcoming tolerance with higher effective PZ dosage or brief discontinuation of PZ.

Awan and associates[12] from Davis and Sacramento, California, also evaluated the cardiocirculatory actions of PZ orally by cardiac catheterization, forearm plethysmography, echo, treadmill exercise, and symptoms in patients with advanced long-standing CHF. Prazosin orally (2–7 mg) reduced forearm venous tone and decreased forearm vascular resistance. Concomitantly, mean systemic arterial pressure declined, LV filling pressure decreased, and cardiac index (CI) was raised. These effects of a single dose of PZ on LV function were rapid in onset, maximal at 1 hour, and sustained for the entire 6 hours of observation. After 2 weeks of outpatient therapy with 2 to 7 mg PZ 4 times daily, echo LV end-diastolic dimension decreased and the duration on treadmill exercise increased. Symptoms (dyspnea, fatigue, angina) were diminished throughout the course of PZ therapy, and NY Heart Association functional class improved from III to II. Thus, PZ possesses sustained nitroprusside-like balanced dilator actions on the systemic arterial and venous beds that are effectively translated into beneficial hemodynamics of augmenting lowered cardiac output and relieving excessive LV filling pressure. Delayed vasodilator tolerance, occurring in 30% of patients, is prevented by prior use of aldosterone antagonists and is easily treated. Subacute hemodynamic suppression of beneficial PZ vasodilator actions is transient and does not preclude successful sustained PZ therapy of severe chronic CHF.

To investigate the mechanism of pharmacodynamic tolerance reported to occur during PZ therapy of chronic CHF, Stein and associates[13] from Indianapolis, Indiana, measured plasma norepinephrine, plasma epinephrine, plasma renin activity (PRA) and plasma aldosterone, and hemodynamics in 8 patients with chronic CHF, NY Heart Association functional classes III and IV, before and during 10 weeks of PZ therapy. Initially, PZ therapy produced significant hemodynamic improvement, but no significant changes in norepinephrine, epinephrine, PRA, or aldosterone. During ambulatory therapy, fluid retention developed in 4 patients, and 3 of them had symptoms or clinical evidence of CHF for which they required an increase in diuretic or PZ therapy. Plasma norepinephrine levels for the whole group were significantly higher after 4 weeks of therapy ($p < 0.01$). Repeat inpatient studies after 10 weeks showed a persistent hemodynamic response to PZ in 7 patients. One patient demonstrated complete hemodynamic tolerance, whereas 3 others showed partial tolerance. In these 4 patients, the cardiac output increased only to 3.8 ± 1.2 liters/min as compared with 5.0 ± 2.1 liters/min during initial PZ therapy. Plasma norepinephrine increased further and levels were significantly higher for the whole group than before PZ therapy ($p < 0.05$). No significant changes in epinephrine, PRA, or aldosterone were demonstrated. This increase in plasma norepinephrine suggests that the sympathetic nervous system could be involved in the pharmacodynamic tolerance to PZ therapy in CHF.

Stein and associates[14] from Indianapolis, Indiana, also evaluated the acute and chronic effects of prazosin (PZ) treatment in 11 patients with chronic CHF (New York Heart Association functional classes III and IV). Before treatment, the mean systemic arterial pressure averaged 100 ± 15 mmHg; LV filling pressure, 29 ± 11 mmHg; and systemic vascular resistance, 2372 ± 1121 dynes-sec-cm^{-5}. PZ administration resulted in hemodynamic improvement in all but 1 patient, with significant lowering of the mean arterial pressure, LV filling pressure, and systemic vascular resistance. Nine patients completed a 10-week course of ambulatory treatment. Five patients remained improved, while 4 developed significant fluid retention, including 2 with obvious CHF. The CHF was controlled by increasing diuretic and/or PZ treatment. After 10 weeks, all 9 patients had advanced to New York Heart Association functional class II. Repeat hemodynamic measurements disclosed complete hemodynamic tolerance in 1 patient, whereas 3 other patients showed partial tolerance with a lower cardiac output response to PZ.

The 9 patients, however, still showed significant lowering of the mean arterial pressure, LV filling pressure, and systemic vascular resistance. Although pharmacodynamic tolerance occurred in 4 of 9 patients, beneficial clinical and hemodynamic effects were demonstrated in most patients after 10 weeks of PZ treatment.

Although the effect of systemic vasodilator therapy on LV function in CHF has been extensively evaluated, little is known about its effect on pulmonary vascular resistance (PVR) and RV function. Colucci and associates[15] from Boston, Massachusetts, studied the effects of the alpha adrenergic agonist PZ on RV function, as determined by RNA ventriculographic technique that assessed RV and LV EF simultaneously. In 11 patients treated for 2 months with PZ, RV EF increased from 0.28 ± 0.04 to 0.44 ± 0.07 (p < 0.01). In 10 patients who received a single dose of PZ 48 hours after withdrawal of prior PZ therapy, RV EF increased from 0.29 ± 0.05 to 0.38 ± 0.06 (p < 0.01). These studies suggest that PZ has beneficial effects on RV function, both immediately and long-term, in patents with severe CHF. Although the mechanism of this effect is not known, possibilities include a direct effect of PZ on the pulmonary vasculature, a secondary reduction in RV afterload due to improved LV performance, and a withdrawal of reflex-mediated pulmonary vasoconstriction due to improved LV performance.

PROSTAGLANDIN E_1

The optimal utility of nitroprusside during the acute phase of active ischemia post-AMI requires clarification because of potential adverse effects on myocardial energetics, and the possibility of increasing thiocyanate levels represents a potential concern during prolonged administration of nitroprusside infusions. Therefore, it is imperative that safe anti-ischemic pharmacologic agents with beneficial vasorelaxant actions be developed to provide effective ventricular unloading in acute and chronic CAD patients having severe CHF post-AMI. The naturally occurring prostaglandins are recognized to possess marked vasodilator and platelet disaggregatory properties. Thus, in CAD patients with potentially active myocardial ischemia, the prostaglandins may provide a unique physiologic approach to therapy of acute and chronic severe ischemic CHF, allowing improvement of cardiac function with concomitant relief of impaired myocardial energetics. Accordingly, Awan and associates[16] from Davis and Sacramento, California, evaluated the cardiocirculatory actions of prostaglandin E_1 by cardiac catheterization and forearm plethysmography in 9 patients with severe CHF from CAD refractory to digitalis and diuretics. The infusions of prostaglandin E_1 were brief (69 ± 5 min), did not alter heart rate, and produced modest declines in mean systemic BP (from 85 to 76 mmHg) and LV filling pressure (from 19 to 15 mmHg). Simultaneously, prostaglandin E_1 raised cardiac index (from 1.9 to 2.5 liters/min/M^2), elevated stroke work index (from 28 to 35 ml/beat/M^2) and increased stroke work index (from 26 to 30 g·m/M^2). Additionally, total systemic vascular resistance decreased (from 1862 to 1282 dynes-sec-cm^{-5})

and double product of LV aerobic index of HR·systolic BP diminished (from 9492 to 8278 units). Concomitantly, forearm vascular resistance fell, forearm blood flow rose, and forearm venous tone remained unchanged. Thus, prostaglandin E_1 is a potent systemic arteriolar dilator with marked beneficial effects on cardiac function in chronic CAD patients having severe ischemic LV failure refractory to conventional therapy.

CAPTOPRIL

Recent evidence suggests that the renin-angiotensin-aldosterone system may be activated in chronic CHF, and that decrease of angiotensin II generation by converting enzyme blockade with intravenous *teprotide* improves cardiac function by peripheral vasodilation. Thereby, angiotensin-converting enzyme (ACE) inhibition appears to enhance cardiac performance in a manner similar to other potent systemic vasodilators such as *nitroprusside, prazosin,* and combined *hydralazine-nitrates.* Because overactivity of the renin axis may perpetuate CHF by increasing circulating angiotensin II, which may disturb peripheral circulatory dynamics and cause secondary hyperaldosteronism, leading to fluid retention and possible attenuation of the response to vasodilator therapy, a more physiologic approach to the relief of chronic CHF than standard vasodilators may be the utilization of an oral angiotensin II-converting enzyme inhibitor in the ambulatory therapy of CHF. Awan and associates[17] from Davis and Sacramento, California, evaluated the therapeutic effectiveness of oral ACE inhibition with captopril in chronic normotensive CHF. Acute cardiocirculatory actions were determined by cardiac catheterization and forearm plethysmography, and ambulatory effects were assessed by echo, RNA, treadmill exercise, and clinical symptoms in 10 patients with severe CHF. Captopril (90 mg) produced marked (peak 1 hour) and sustained (5 hours) decrease of LV filling pressure (23–15 mmHg), decline of systemic vascular resistance, and increase in cardiac index (2.0–4.1 liters/min/M^2), while mean BP declined mildly (87–80 mmHg) without heart rate change. Both forearm venous tone and vascular resistance decreased considerably. After 1 week of ambulatory therapy (90 mg, 3 times daily), RNA EF and echo shortening fraction increased, and exercise duration (341–453 s) and New York Heart Association functional class improved (3.6–2.2). Thus, ACE-induced vasodilation by oral captopril improves cardiac performance and clinical status in refractory CHF.

To determine whether temporary cessation of captopril therapy compromises cardiac performance, Maslowski and associates[18] from Christchurch, New Zealand, measured hemodynamic, hormonal, and electrolyte indices for 2 days before, and 4 days after discontinuation of long-term captopril therapy in 5 patients with CHF. Captopril withdrawal resulted in a 4-fold rise in plasma angiotensin II, higher levels of noradrenaline, and a 13.5-mmHg increase in mean arterial pressure. Despite these changes, cardiac output at rest and during exercise was well maintained, and right-sided heart pressures were unaltered. Although plasma aldosterone levels increased 3-fold, neither sodium retention nor potassium depletion occurred. Cortisol levels rose in parallel with angiotensin II levels. These results indicate that, in the short term, cardiac performance is not impaired and electrolyte balance is not adversely affected by the abrupt withdrawal of captopril.

PIRBUTEROL

Sharma and associates[19] from Minneapolis, Minnesota, gave a single oral dose (5–30 mg) pirbuterol, a new sympathomimetic drug, to 14 patients with refractory CHF, and obtained hemodynamic measurements and plasma pirbuterol levels at control and then serially for 6 hours after drug administration. Ten patients received 20–30 mg pirbuterol, the optimal dose range. In this group, cardiac index was significantly increased (1.9 to 2.6 liters/min/M²). PA wedge pressures fell significantly (24 to 20 mmHg). Decreases also occurred in mean PA pressure, aortic diastolic pressure, and systemic and pulmonary vascular resistances. Systolic and mean aortic pressures and heart rate showed no significant change from control. Hemodynamic effects persisted for 5 hours. Pirbuterol was clinically well tolerated. Although its mechanism of action is unclear, both inotropic and vasodilator effects are highly likely. Thus, pirbuterol orally has marked and prolonged salutary hemodynamic effects and offers promise in CHF treatment.

Canepa-Anson and associates[20] from London, Hillingdon, and Birmingham, England, studied the effects of pirbuterol in 41 patients with severe CHF (New York Heart Association functional class III or IV). Single-dose studies were carried out in 12 patients to determine the magnitude and time-course of the effects of pirbuterol. Six patients received orally a single dose of 10 mg, and 6 received 20 mg. Measurements were made half-hourly from control for 6 hours. Incremental-dose studies involving 3 sequential doses given at 1.5-hour intervals were carried out in 29 patients to determine the dose-response relationship. Nine patients received a low-dose regimen (pirbuterol, 7.5, 7.5, and 15 mg orally), and 20 received a high-dose regimen (pirbuterol, 10, 10, and 20 mg). Measurements were made every 1.5 hours from control for 6 hours. Blood samples for pirbuterol concentration were taken hourly in the single-dose studies and every 1.5 hours in the incremental-dose studies. Single-dose studies showed that acute administration of pirbuterol improved hemodynamic performance without changes in heart rate or BP. Control values were cardiac index (CI) 2.0 liters/min/M², stroke index (SI) 21 ml/m², LV filling pressure 28 mmHg, and systemic vascular resistance (SVR) 1870 dynes-sec-cm⁻⁵. The onset of action was rapid, and significant effects were found within 0.5 hours and persisted to 5.5 hours. Mean peak changes were: CI, +45%; SI, +45%; LV filling pressure, −28%, and SVR, −27%. Incremental-dose studies showed that increasing dose produced an increase in plasma pirbuterol concentrations and CI. The 20 mg dose was found to be optimal. Because pirbuterol is effective, well tolerated, and combines vasodilator and positive inotropic actions, it may have advantages over other drugs in the treatment of chronic CHF.

Although it has been shown that the initial administration of pirbuterol to patients with CHF increases cardiac output and reduces systemic vascular resistance and pulmonary capillary wedge pressure, it is not known whether the drug exerts these effects through direct myocardial stimulation, a decrease in systemic vascular resistance, or both. To determine whether the initial effect of pirbuterol on LV function would be sustained during long-term therapy, Colucci and associates[21] from Boston, Massachusetts, evaluated LV EF and cardiac index in 12 patients before administering pirbuterol, after the first dose of the drug, and after 1 week and 1 month of administration. The drug's initial effect was a 35% increase in cardiac index, but no significant change in heart rate or mean arterial pressure. After 1 month of therapy, the mean cardiac index and EF had returned to baseline values, and no clinical effect was evident in most patients. This apparent tolerance was not accompanied by changes in heart rate, BP, or body weight, and it occurred in the presence of therapeutic drug levels during long-term therapy. The density of beta adrenergic receptors on lymphocytes from patients treated with pirbuterol was significantly depressed, as compared with that of patients with CHF of comparable severity but not treated with pirbuterol. The authors concluded that tolerance to the hemodynamic and clinical effects of pirbuterol develops during long-term administration and that this tolerance may be related to a decrease in myocardial or vascular beta adrenergic receptors or both.

Awan and associates[22] from Davis and Sacramento, California, evaluated the temporal cardiocirculatory responses to pirbuterol (0.4 mg/kg), by cardiac catheterization and limb plethysmography, in 10 CAD patients with severe CHF refractory to digitalis and diuretics. Pirbuterol considerably improved LV dysfunction during the 6-hour period of hemodynamic monitoring: control lowered cardiac index (CI) of 1.7 liters/min/M^2 rose to 2.6 at 1 hour, 2.4 at 3 hours, and was 2.2 at 6 hours; control excessive LV filling pressure of 24 mmHg fell to 19 at 1 hour, 18 at 3 hours and 22 at 6 hours. Concomitantly, peak heart rate (HR) increment (6 beats/min) was minimal, mean arterial BP decrement was only 10 mmHg, total systemic vascular resistance (SVR) declined, forearm venodilation occurred, and rate·pressure product of myocardial oxygen consumption was unaltered. Further, hemodynamic actions of pirbuterol were compared with intravenously administered *dobutamine* in 9 patients with CHF. Both agents produced similar effects of LV pump function: CI was markedly augmented from 1.8 to 2.6 liters/min/M^2 by dobutamine and from 1.8 to 2.9 liters/min/M^2 by pirbuterol, and stroke work index was increased from 19 to 27 g·m/m^2 by dobutamine and from 20 to 29 g·m/m^2 by pirbuterol. Although dobutamine did not change mean arterial pressure and LV filling pressure, pirbuterol modestly diminished AP from 83 to 75 mmHg and moderately decreased LV filling pressure from 23 to 18 mmHg. Dobutamine reduced total SVR 22%, whereas pirbuterol reduced total SVR 42%. During extended ambulatory therapy (0.4 mg/kg 3 times daily) with pirbuterol orally, scintigraphic LV EF rose from 0.25 to 0.29. Concomitantly, treadmill exercise duration increased from 267 to 366 seconds, and New York Heart Association functional class improved from 3.5 to 2.4. Thus, oral pirbuterol has dobutamine-like beneficial hemodynamic effects on LV pump function, but causes a greater fall in total SVR consistent with the combined inotropic and peripheral vasodilator actions of this oral beta receptor agonist. Salutary hemodynamic responses to pirbuterol orally were maintained for 6 hours after a single dose. Further, during sustained ambulatory pirbuterol therapy, substantial augmentation of LV function and exercise capacity was observed and resulted in marked amelioration of CHF symptomatology.

TERBUTALINE

The relatively new cardioselective beta adrenergic receptor agonist, terbutaline sulfate, when given subcutaneously has marked peripheral circulatory effects, and causes some cardiac beta$_1$ adrenergic receptor stimulation. These cardiovascular influences include salutary reductions in biventricular end-diastolic volume and peripheral vascular resistance, and increases in RV and LV EF. Slutsky[23] from San Diego, California, evaluated the acute cardiocirculatory effects of inhaled terbutaline in 13 CHF patients. Terbutaline (0.5 mg), was given via inhalation by nebulizer. Data were obtained before and 10 and 30 minutes after inhalation, by right-sided cardiac catheterization and by gated equilibrium RNA. All patients responded with increased cardiac output (3.5 to 4.3 liters/min) and stroke volume (40 to 49 ml) without change in heart rate. Decreases occurred in peripheral vascular resistance (1924 to 1443 dynes-sec-cm^{-5}), LV filling pressure (21 to 15 mmHg) and systemic arterial oxygen tension (81 to 72 mmHg). Both LV and RV EF rose (0.24 to 0.38 and 0.36 to 0.51, respectively) with concomitant declines in biventricular end-diastolic volumes. All these variables changed rapidly at 10 minutes post-inhalation and returned to control levels by 30 minutes after the agent had been administered. Thus, moderate inhaled doses of terbutaline produced prompt potent, and transient salutary hemodynamic effects due to its peripheral vasodilator and cardiotonic properties, without untoward arrhythmogenic or angina-provoking influences.

PRENALTEROL

There is a continued need for effective pharmacologic agents for beneficial therapeutic management of CAD patients with severe CHF following AMI. Although dopamine and dobutamine have well-recognized salutary actions in the management of severe low-output cardiac pump failure, the lack of an oral formulation of either of these agents restricts the application of these drugs to hospitalized patients with refractory CHF. Prenalterol is a new selective beta$_1$ receptor agonist with the known property of augmenting cardiac contractility. In contrast to dopamine and dobutamine, this drug is available both in parenteral and oral forms, thereby permitting prolonged oral therapy in patients responding to the parenteral preparation. Awan and associates[24] from Davis and Sacramento, California, evaluated the hemodynamic efficacy of prenalterol by cardiac catheterization in 9 patients with refractory CHF due to chronic CAD. Prenalterol, (4.8 mg intravenously, markedly augmented cardiac index (1.9–2.6 liters/min/M²) and substantially elevated stroke work index (24–30 ml/beat/M²). Additionally, prenalterol raised stroke work index (21–28 g·m/M²) and decreased total systemic vascular resistance (1,702 to 1,260 dynes-sec-cm⁻⁵). Concomitantly, heart rate, mean BP and LV filling pressure were unaltered. The heart rate-systolic BP product of myocardial oxygen consumption was unchanged and precipitation of cardiac arrhythmia or myocardial ischemia was not observed. Thus, prenalterol produced considerable improvement of depressed cardiocirculatory performance without untoward effects and, therefore appears to be a valuable new cardiotonic in the clinical management of severe low-output ventricular dysfunction due to CAD.

Waagstein and associates[25] from Umea, Sweden, studied the hemodynamic effects of 75 to 225μg/kg prenalterol intravenously at rest and during exercise in 8 patients with chronic CHF after AMI, valvular surgery, and dilated cardiomyopathy. All were New York Heart Association functional class III and IV CHF and were receiving digitalis and diuretics. With prenalterol, at rest, LV filling pressure fell (17 to 12 mmHg), cardiac index (CI) rose (2.1 to 2.9 liters/min/M²), heart rate (HR) increased mildly, systemic vascular resistance (SVR) declined moderately, and peripheral arterial pressure was unchanged. During prenalterol, exercise compared with control, LV filling pressure rise was less and CI, HR, and SVR responses were similar; dyspnea and angina were reduced in most patients. The 8 patients were then given prenalterol orally (30 to 200 mg/day) and placebo for 6 days each, with comparative evaluation by echo, systolic time intervals, exercise testing, and continuous ECG monitoring. With prenalterol orally, 5 of 8 patients improved symptomatically, EF increased (0.44 to 0.53), and systolic time interval of pre-ejection period shortened (by 10 ms) without change in resting HR or systemic arterial BP. The incidence of VPC was not increased. Compared with placebo, prenalterol orally increased exercise capacity 10%. Thus, prenalterol may be of value for long-term CHF treatment, in addition to conventional therapy.

AMRINONE AND DOBUTAMINE

Amrinone, a new inotropic agent, has been shown to be beneficial in patients with CHF, but its hemodynamic effects have not been compared with those of other currently useful catecholamines. Klein and associates[26] from New York City compared the effects of intravenously administered dobutamine and amrinone in 8 patients with severe chronic CHF. Dobutamine was infused until a maximal increase in cardiac index was reached or undesirable effects were produced. This dose was then continued for 8 hours.

After a return of hemodynamic values to baseline level, amrinone was infused at a rate of 40 μg/kg/min for 1 hour and then 10 μg/kg/min for 24 hours. Both drugs significantly improved cardiac index while simultaneously decreasing systemic vascular resistance and right atrial and pulmonary wedge pressures ($p < 0.05$). Initially no differences could be found between the drugs. With prolonged infusion, however, amrinone produced a sustained improvement, whereas dobutamine showed decreased effectiveness. Thus, amrinone is comparable in effect with the optimal dose of dobutamine and would appear to an extremely promising drug in the acute treatment of severe CHF.

DIURESIS

Several studies have reported that diuresis and phlebotomy increase cardiac output in some patients with CHF. These observations have been used as evidence that the failing left ventricle functions at times on the descending limb of Starling's ventricular function curve. According to this hypothesis, diuresis and phlebotomy improve cardiac output by reducing preload and shifting the left ventricle up the descending limb of Starling's curve. Others, however, have observed that reducing LV filling pressures in patients with CHF by mechanically impeding venous return decreases, rather than increases, the cardiac output. Additionally, administration of diuretics to patients with AMI and CHF has produced no change in cardiac output. Wilson and associates[27] from Philadelphia, Pennsylvania re-examined the effects of diuresis on performance of the failing left ventricle, and the effect of diuresis on echo LV dimensions to determine to what extent diuretic-induced alterations in LV performance were related to changes in LV size, i.e., preload. Diuresis increased stroke volume (43 ± 23 ml to 50 ± 18 ml [$p < 0.05$]), but decreased pulmonary wedge pressure (28 ± 3 mmHg to 19 ± 5 mmHg [$p < 0.01$]), mean BP (100 ± 14 mmHg to 88 ± 10 mmHg [$p < 0.01$]) and systemic vascular resistance ($2,059 \pm 622$ dynes-sec-cm^{-5} to $1,783 \pm 556$ dynes-sec-cm^{-5} [$p < 0.05$]). Echo LV diastolic dimension was not changed by diuresis (6.0 ± 0.8 cm to 6.0 ± 0.8 cm). Percent change in stroke volume correlated with systemic vascular resistance ($p < 0.05$) and with LV diastolic dimension ($p < 0.05$), but not with pulmonary wedge pressure or right atrial pressure. Thus, diuresis improved performance of the failing ventricle and reduced afterload, but it did not alter LV diastolic dimension, an index of preload. These data suggest that diuresis improves LV function by decreasing afterload.

References

---

1. COLUCCI WS, WILLIAMS GH, ALEXANDER RW, BRAUNWALD E: Mechanisms and implications of vasodilator tolerance in the treatment of congestive heart failure. Am J Med 71:89–99, July 1981.

2. CONTI R: Introduction. Symposium on congestive heart failure. Am J Med 71:131–134, July 1981.

3. COHN JN: Physiologic basis of vasodilator therapy for heart failure. Am J Med 71:135–139, July 1981.

4. CHATTERJEE K, RUBIN SA, PORTS TA, PARMLEY WW: Influence of oral prazosin therapy on exercise hemodynamics in patients with severe chronic heart failure. Am J Med 71:140–146, July 1981.

5. ROULEAU J, WARNICA JW, BURGESS JH: Prazosin and congestive heart failure: short- and long-term therapy. Am J Med 71:147–152, July 1981.

6. AWAN NA, NEEDHAM KE, EVENSON MK, AMSTERDAM EE, MASON DT: Therapeutic application of prazosin in chronic refractory congestive heart failure. Am J Med 71:153–160, July 1981.

7. PACKER M, MELLER J, MEDINE N, YUSHAK M, GORLIN R: Provocation of myocardial ischemic events during initiation of vasodilator therapy for severe chronic heart failure: clinical and hemodynamic evaluation of 52 consecutive patients with ischemic cardiomyopathy. Am J Cardiol 48:939–946, Nov 1981.

8. WEBER KT, ANDREWS V, KINASEWITZ GT, JANICKI JS, FISHMAN AP: Vasodilator and inotropic agents in treatment of chronic cardiac failure: clinical experience and response in exercise performance. Am Heart J 102(Suppl 2):569–577, Sept 1981.

9. BERTEL O, BURKART F, BUHLER FR: Sustained effectiveness of chronic prazosin therapy in severe chronic congestive heart failure. Am Heart J 101:529–533, May 1981.

10. FELDMAN RC, BALL RM, WINCHESTER MA, JAILLON P, KATES RE, HARRISON DC: Beneficial hemodynamic response to chronic prazosin therapy in congestive heart failure. Am Heart J 102:534–540, May 1981.

11. AWAN NA, LEE G, DEMARIA AN, MASON DT: Ambulatory prazosin treatment of chronic congestive heart failure: development of late tolerance reversible by higher dosage and interrupted substitution therapy. Am Heart J 101:541–547, May 1981.

12. AWAN NA, EVENSON MK, NEEDHAM KE, MASON DT: Management of refractory congestive heart failure with prazosin. Am Heart J 102(Suppl 2):626–634, Sept 1981.

13. STEIN L, HENRY DP, WEINBERGER MH: Increase in plasma norepinephrine during prazosin therapy for chronic congestive heart failure. Am J Med 70:825–832, Apr 1981.

14. STEIN L, FOSTER PR, FRIEDMAN AW, STATZA J, MCHENRY PL: Acute and chronic haemodynamic effects of prazosin in left ventricular failure. Br J 45:186–92, Feb 1981.

15. COLUCCI WS, HOLMAN BL, WYNNE J, CARABELLO B, MALACOFF R, GROSSMAN W, BRAUNWALD E: Improved right ventricular function and reduced pulmonary vascular resistance during prazosin therapy of congestive heart failure. Am J Med 71:75–80, July 1981.

16. AWAN NA, EVENSON MK, NEEDHAM KE, BEATTIE JM, AMSTERDAM EA, MASON DT: Cardiocirculatory and myocardial energetic effects of prostaglandin E_1 in severe left ventricular failure due to chronic coronary heart disease. Am Heart J 102:703–709, Oct 1981.

17. AWAN NA, EVENSON MK, NEEDHAM KE, WIN A, MASON DT: Efficacy of oral angiotensin-converting enzyme inhibition with captopril therapy in severe chronic normotensive congestive heart failure. Am Heart J 101:22–31, Jan 1981.

18. MASLOWSKI AH, NICHOLLS MG, IKRAM H, ESPINER EA, TURNER JG: Hemodynamic, hormonal, and electrolyte responses to withdrawal of long-term captopril treatment for heart failure. Lancet 2:959–961, Oct 1981.

19. SHARMA B, HOBACK J, FRANCIS GS, HODGES M, ASINGER RW, COHN JN, TAYLOR CR: Pirbuterol: a new oral sympathomimetic amine for the treatment of congestive heart failure. Am Heart J 102(Suppl 2)533–541, Sept 1981.

20. CANEPA-ANSON R, DAWSON JR, KUAN P, WARNES CA, POOLE-WILSON PA, REUBEN SR, SUTTON GC: Single-dose and dose-response studies with oral pirbuterol, a new beta agonist in chronic heart failure. Am Heart J 102(Suppl 2):578–583, Sept 1981.

21. COLUCCI WS, ALEXANDER RW, WILLIAMS GH, RUDE RE, HOLMAN BL, KONSTAM MA, WYNNE J, MUDGE GH, BRAUNWALD E: Decreased lymphocyte beta-adrenergic-receptor density in pa-

tients with heart failure and tolerance to the beta-adrenergic agonist pirbuterol. N Engl J Med 305:185–190, July 1981.

22. AWAN NA, NEEDHAM K, EVENSON MK, HERMANOVICH J, JOYE JA, DEMARIA AN, MASON DT: Therapeutic efficacy of oral pirbuterol in severe chronic congestive heart failure: acute hemodynamic and long-term ambulatory evaluation. Am Heart J 102(Suppl 2):555–563, Sept 1981.

23. SLUTSKY R: Hemodynamic effects of inhaled terbulazine in congestive heart failure patients without lung disease: beneficial cardiotonic and vasodilator beta-agonist properties evaluated by ventricular catheterization and radionuclide angiography. Am Heart J 101:556–560, May 1981.

24. AWAN NA, NEEDHAM KE, EVENSON MK WIN A, MASON DT: Hemodynamic actions of prenalterol in severe congestive heart failure due to chronic coronary disease. Am Heart J 101:158–161, Feb 1981.

25. WAAGSTEIN F, REIZ S, ARINIEGO R, HJALMARSON A: Clinical results with prenalterol in patients with heart failure. Am Heart J 102(Suppl 2):548–554, Sept 1981.

26. KLEIN NA, SISKIND SJ, FRISHMAN WH, SONNENBLICK EH, LEJEMTEL TH: Hemodynamic comparison of intravenous amrinone and dobutamine in patients with chronic congestive heart failure. Am J Cardiol 48:170–175, July 1981.

27. WILSON JR, REICHEK N, DUNKMAN WB, GOLDBERG S: Effect of diuresis on the performance of the failing left ventricle in man. Am J Med 70:234–239, Feb 1981.

9

Miscellaneous Topics

ELECTROCARDIOGRAPHIC TOPICS

Simplified esophageal ECG using bipolar recording leads

The common technique for esophageal ECG in the bedside diagnosis of arrhythmias involves connecting a unipolar recording lead positioned in the esophagus to the V_1 terminal of a standard ECG machine. This technique improves discrimination of the P wave, as compared with the P wave in standard surface ECG leads, but requires patience, experience, and skill from the operator. The P wave obtained with a unipolar recording lead is generally smaller than the associated QRS complex and may be difficult to identify during rapid ventricular rhythms. Bipolar recording leads in the esophagus have been used with specialized electronic equipment in several research projects. Bipolar recording leads have not, however, been applied in clinical settings to ascertain the atrial rate, atrial rhythm, and AV relation during arrhythmias. Hammill and Pritchett[1] from Durham, North Carolina, evaluated in 15 patients a technique that uses bipolar recording leads and standard ECG equipment for bedside diagnosis of arrhythmias. Of the 22 cardiac rhythms evaluated in 15 patients, the unipolar lead recorded a P wave that was smaller than the QRS complex (0.83 ± 0.47 mV and 1.28 ± 0.79 mV, respectively, [$p < 0.01$]) and was obscured when the 2 depolarizations were nearly simultaneous. The bipolar lead recorded a P wave that was larger than the QRS complex (0.93 ± 0.62 mV and 0.33 ± 0.3 mV, respectively, [$p < 0.001$]) and was never obscured. The unipolar lead recorded a P -to-QRS ratio that was smaller than that recorded by the bipolar lead (0.8 ± 0.5

and 3.3 ± 1.8, respectively, [p < 0.001]). A bipolar esophageal lead can be recorded simply at the bedside using a standard ECG machine and is superior to the conventional unipolar lead.

Differentiation of left ventricular hypertrophy (secondary to AS) from lateral wall ischemia

Beach and associates[2] from Aberdeen, Scotland, described ECG features in 41 patients with AS in whom the peak systolic gradient between left ventricle and systemic artery ranged from 45–170 mmHg (mean, 90). Their ages were 26–69 years (mean, 54); 21 were men and 20 were women. Significant coronary narrowing was excluded in 39 of the 41 patients. Apparently none of the 41 patients had dysfunction of the mitral valve. The ECG findings in 41 patients with AS were compared with those in 20 patients with lateral wall healed AMI without clinical evidence of LV hypertrophy. Nine of the 41 patients with AS had repolarization abnormalities in the lateral leads without the standard voltage criteria of LV hypertrophy. The repolarization pattern of AS usually could be distinguished from that of CAD by the presence of 1 or more of the following 5 features: depression of the J point; asymmetry of the T wave with rapid return to baseline; terminal positivity of the T wave ("over-shoot"); T inversion in $V_6 > 3$ mm, and T inversion in $V_6 > V_4$.

Effect of aging on ECG

As the population over the age of 70 increases, objective, noninvasive methods of assessing the presence or absence and the severity of heart disease assume an ever-increasing importance. This is particularly true because the history in the elderly person is frequently unreliable, physical examination is often difficult, and clinical expressions of heart disease are often attenuated by decreased physical demands. Thus, the ECG in the elderly person receives additional importance. Fisch[3] from Indianapolis, Indiana, reviewed the frequency of ECG abnormalities in persons > age 65 years and compared them with the frequency of abnormalities in persons without clinical evidence of heart disease < age 25 years. A summation of these observations is tabulated in Table 9-1. Fisch concluded that the increasing incidence of abnormal ECGs with aging, a parallel increase in the frequency of heart disease, and a high statistical correlation between abnormal ECG and clinical heart disease indicate that the specific ECG abnormalities that correlate positively with evidence of clinical heart disease are independent markers of heart disease. Fisch found, for example, that the frequency of abnormal ECGs in patients >65 years of age was 57%, whereas the frequency of abnormal ECGS in persons <25 without clinical evidence of heart disease was approximately 1%.

Previous cross-sectional population studies have shown age differences in ECG wave patterns, including lower wave amplitudes and a leftward shift of the frontal-plane axis in older people. Cross-sectional results may be due to cohort differences and the data imply only that these changes actually occur in persons as they age. To determine ECG changes with aging in the same persons, Bachman and associates[4] from Boston, Massachusetts, obtained

TABLE 9-1. *Frequency of ECG abnormalities in patients >65 years compared to persons <age 25 years (from Fisch[3]).*

ECG ABNORMALITY	%	
	<25 YRS*	>65 YRS**
Left axis deviation	1.4	51
Right axis deviation	0.1	1
Prolonged P-R interval	0.3	9
Right BBB	0	5
Left BBB	0.1	3
ST-T changes	0	16
Atrial premature complexes	0.7	10
VPC	0.8	6
Atrial fibrillation	0.1	8
LV hypertrophy	2.1	8

* Based on study of 776 patients without clinical evidence of heart disease admitted to an institution for the acutely disturbed. ** Based on a pooled sample of 2,482 ECGs, 57% of which were abnormal.

ECGs 10 years apart in 440 healthy men of the Normative Aging Study, who were 23–66 years old at first examination. At this first examination, R- and S-wave amplitudes were smaller and frontal-plane axis measurements were shifted to the left in older men. Longitudinal changes in these same variables were consistent with the cross-sectional results. In addition, the P-R and Q-T interval durations were longer, the QRS duration was shorter and the T-wave amplitude was smaller at the second examination. The longitudinal rate of change of S-wave amplitude varied among age groups, decreasing more in younger men. Thus, some previously described cross-sectional age differences truly represent longitudinal age trends in ECG patterns.

ECHOCARDIOGRAPHIC TOPICS

Standardized anatomic nomenclature

Edwards and associates[5] from Rochester, Minnesota, described various methods for examination of the heart at autopsy and emphasized the value of tomographic sections. The concept of regional analysis of the heart with a standardized system of nomenclature was offered for both the pathologist and the clinician.

Left ventricular function with ejection fraction <50% and normal valves

Wilson and associates[6] from Philadelphia, Pennsylvania, examined the relation between echo and hemodynamic findings in 48 patients with normal cardiac valves and LV EF <50%. Pulmonary wedge pressure (PWP) correlated with the PR-AC interval and with left atrial dimension, but not with LV diastolic dimension. A PR-AC interval ≤60 ms was observed in 26 (90%) of 29 patients with a PWP ≥14 mmHg -vs- 1 of 10 patients with PWP <14 mmHg. The correlation between PWP and PR-AC interval was substantially better in patients with a PR interval ≤200 ms than in patients with a PR interval >200 ms. The PR-AC interval also correlated with the EF. A left atrial dimension ≥4.0 cm was observed in 29 (83%) of 35 patients with a PWP ≥14 mmHg -vs- 0 of 9 patients with a PWP <14 mmHg. Stroke volume (SV) correlated with aortic root excursion and with SV calculated from formulas based on mitral valve motion or aortic valve motion. No echo formula provided valid estimates of cardiac output. M-mode echo provides a relatively useful noninvasive method of assessing LV filling pressure in patients with reduced EF and no valvular disease.

Comparison of anatomic, echo and ECG findings in left ventricular hypertrophy

Anatomic, echo and ECG findings of LV hypertrophy were compared in 34 subjects by Reichek and Devereux from New York City.[7] Echo LV mass correlated well with postmortem LV weight (r = 0.96) and accurately diagnosed LV hypertrophy (sensitivity, 93%; specificity, 95%). In contrast, Romhilt-Estes (R-E) point score and Sokolow-Lyon (S-L) voltage criteria for ECG LV hypertrophy were insensitive (50% and 21%, respectively), but specific (both 95%). R-E correlated weakly with LV weight (r = 0.64), but S-L did not. Echo LV mass was then compared with R-E and S-L in an unselected clinical series of 100 subjects, in 28 subjects with severe AS and in 14 with severe AR. Results in the clinical series were comparable to those in the necropsy series. In the AS and AR groups, with a high prevalence of LV hypertrophy, the low sensitivity of R-E point score and S-L criteria led to poor overall results. Analysis of individual ECG variables showed that most voltage information is contained in leads aV_L and V_1. Correction of voltage for distance from the left ventricle did not substantially improve results. Individual nonvoltage criteria were each nearly as sensitive as R-E point score. Thus, the ECG is specific but insensitive in recognition of LV hypertrophy. Moreover, when the prevalence of true LV hypertrophy is less than 10%, more false-positive than true-positive diagnoses will be obtained. M-mode echo LV mass is superior to ECG criteria for clinical diagnosis of LV hypertrophy.

Effect of left ventricular size on distance from mitral E point to ventricular septum

Increased mitral valve E point to ventricular septal separation (EPSS) is widely used as an echo index of depressed LV EF, yet LV size has not been examined as an independent variable potentially affecting EPSS. Accordingly, Child and associates[8] from Los Angeles, California, studied the relationship between EPSS and functionally normal or depressed LV, with or without increased end-diastolic dimensions (EDD). Twenty normal controls had EPSS 3.2 ± 2.2 mm (mean ± SD); EDD, 47 ± 5 mm; EPSS/EDD ("normalized" EPSS), 0.07 ± 0.04, and fractional shortening (FS%), 38 ± 6%. Nine patients with pure, chronic MR had dilated LV (EDD = 65 ± 7 mm) with normal LV function (FS%, 41 ± 5%; angiographic EF, 62 ± 9%); 8 patients had dilated cardiomyopathy (EDD, 69 ± 8 mm) with decreased LV function (FS%, 16 ± 7%; angiographic EF, 32 ± 8%); and 8 patients with cardiac amyloid had nondilated left ventricles (EDD, 42 ± 5 mm) with decreased LV function (FS%, 19 ± 6%; angiographic EF, 35 ± 7%). Mitral E point to ventricular septal separation and EPSS/EDD accurately separated individuals with normal and abnormal LV function irrespective of LV size (p < 0.00001). Increased internal dimensions per se did not affect EPSS unless depressed LV function coexisted. Thus, EPSS is a valid predictor of depressed ejection phase indices independent of LV size.

Quantitation of left ventricular area, volume and mass by 2-D echo

The reliability of 2-D echo quantitation of LV section area, volume and mass was assessed in vitro in 13 postmortem human hearts (LV weight 115—454 g) by Helak and Reichek[9] from Philadelphia, Pennsylvania. The pathologic diagnoses included: 2 normal; 5 CAD with AMI and/or aneurysm; 3 valvular heart disease; 2 cardiomyopathy, and 1 LV hypertrophy. Hearts were divided into 6—24 short-axis slices (n, 123) and imaged in a tank filled with mineral oil, then the images were planimetered. Calibrated photographs and actual LV weight served as reference standards. Estimates of section LV cavity volume and myocardial volume were derived by multiplying the appropriate area by section thickness. Section LV mass was obtained by multiplying the myocardial volume by myocardial density. Total LV cavity volume and myocardial mass were derived by using Simpson's rule and a short-axis area-apical-length method. In absolute terms, 2-D echo underestimated LV cavity area, but accurately estimated LV myocardial area. Excellent correlations were obtained between 2-D echo and photographic standards for section cavity area, and volume. Area-length estimates of total LV cavity volume also correlated well with reference standards. Similarly, section LV myocardial area correlated well with photographic myocardial area, and 2-D echo and photographic estimates of section LV mass correlated well with actual LV weight. Consequently, total LV mass obtained with Simpson's rule or the area-length method was highly reliable. Thus, 2-D echo provides reliable estimates of LV volume and mass using the short-axis Simpson's rule of area-length methods and appropriate regression corrections. The area-length method is simple enough to permit clinical application.

Reproducibility of echo measurements

Wong and associates[10] from Los Angeles, California, analyzed the variables of heart size, body position, and transducer angle affecting the reproducibility of LV internal dimensions as measured by M-mode echo. Echoes were recorded in 24 subjects as the thorax was incrementally rotated and tilted. Transducer angle was noted from a 3-plane level attached to the probe. Constants were the technician, transducer placement, and the interpreter. Heart rates varied insignificantly; respirations were held. Groups A and B were defined by their initial LV internal dimensions at end-diastole ($LVID_d$): mean 49 ± 6 mm and 73 ± 9 mm, respectively. With body position constant, the measurement error between duplicate recordings of $LVID_d$ was ± 1.2 mm in group A and ± 4.5 mm in group B (p < 0.001). Transducer angle varied 12° between duplicate recordings in both groups. As the position of the thorax changed, the transducer followed, maintaining approximately the same incline with the chest wall. In both groups, errors for combined $LVID_d$ recorded with rotation and tilt, respectively, were unchanged from the duplication error. Thus, when the spatial orientation between the transducer and heart is held constant, it is the size of the heart that determines the reproducibility of the measurement of LV internal dimensions.

Pietro and associates[11] from Boston, Massachusetts, determined serial reproducibility on standard M-mode and 2-D-guided M-mode records for 10 normal volunteers and 20 patients. Overall intraobserver variability in the normal group was $518 \pm 2\%$ (M-mode) and $3.1 \pm 0.8\%$ (2-D and M-mode), and in the patient group $3.1 \pm 0.6\%$ (M-mode) and $4.7 \pm 0.6\%$ (M-mode) (p = ns). Variability on serial examination, however, was 2-fold to 3-fold greater. In the normal group, reproducibility varied by $11 \pm 2\%$ (M-mode) and $9 \pm 1\%$ (2-D, M-mode), while in the patient group, it was $9 \pm 1\%$ (M-mode) and $9 \pm 1\%$ (2-D, M-mode). The lowest serial variability achieved was for the diastolic LV dimension on serial M-mode examination (4%); the largest variability pertained to measurement of the ventricular septum (14%). Other structures had intermediate variation in reproducibility. Thus, establishing performance variability for an echo laboratory is an important part of the interpretation of serial records.

Real-time computerization of 2-D echo

A principal limitation of conventional 2-D echo is the lack of direct acquisition in computerization of images. To overcome this difficulty, Garcia and associates[12] from Los Angeles, California, delineated the development of an interface system that couples a standard medical imaging computer to the video output of commercially available 2-D echo machines and their videotape recorders. Importantly, acquisition in this new system is real time, and the computer digitizes and stores the 2-D echo video images on magnetic disks at a rate of 30 frames/second. This milestone development in cardiac ultrasound technique delineates the computerized system for real-time acquisition, enhanced processing, analysis, and display of cross-sectional images of the LV derived by 2-D echo. The new methodology combines a standard imaging computer system with the video output of current 2-D echo units using a 128×128 or 64×64 matrix window and stores the real-time 30 frames/second digitized images on a magnetic disk. Computerized beat-to-beat and frame-by-frame processing employs space-time smoothing and automatic detection of endocardial interfaces by standard threshold and second-derivative techniques. Multiple views are displayed in real time with 256 levels of gray and color. The methodology was used to analyze and graphically display frame -by- frame changes throughout the cardiac cycle. In addition, regional wall motion and thickness were analyzed in 12 sectors of individual cross-sections, using a standardized angular subdivision originating at the center of area and indexed by an external reference point. An algorithm was developed to correct cross-sectional interface definition from the commonly used trailing-to-leading edge to the more valid lead-to-leading outline technique. Computerized analysis of spatial and temporal variations of cardiac contraction were demonstrated in several clinical and experimental applications, including bicycle exercise testing, investigation of AMI, and assessment of interventions. This initial evaluation indicates that the new real-time computerized digital acquisition and data analysis represents a major advancement toward quantification of LV function using noninvasive 2-D echo technique.

Doppler ultrasound detection of intracardiac and great vessel flow patterns

Ultrasonic contrast techniques allow tracking of blood flow in patients with cardiac malformations. One problem often encountered in M-mode contrast methodology, however, is inability to generate adequate microbubbles for recordings. Since echo Doppler should be more sensitive for detection of microbubbles, the results of 75 saline injections were studied at heart catheterization in 16 patients by the simultaneous recording of contrast M-mode and echo Doppler sounds by Goldberg and associates[13] from Tucson, Arizona. For the first part of this investigation, an ATL 500 system was utilized. The M-mode of this system provided information identical to that of the Smith Kline 20A machine. Records were evaluated without identification of the patient. In all instances in which microbubbles were not expected on the basis of flow patterns, none were detected by Doppler. One error occurred for M-mode. Contrast in the direction of flow was visualized in 50 of 55 injections by echo Doppler. In these, a frequency dispersion was present, but even more striking was a marked rise in the time-interval histographic input-signal strength indicator. Only 40 of 55 simultaneous M-mode echoes showed a contrast effect. Doppler microbubble detection was usually represented by a much stronger signal than was M-mode contrast. This investigation demonstrates that range-gated Doppler is an effective method for detecting microbubbles.

USEFULNESS IN STROKE

Greenland and associates[14] from Minneapolis, Minnesota, assessed the use of echo in the evaluation of stroke by recording M-mode and 2-D echoes in 100 consecutive hospitalized patients. Of the 95 persons satisfactorily imaged with 2-D echo, 47 lacked clinical and routine laboratory evidence of heart disease; no potential embolic source or other finding that altered therapy was diagnosed by echo. In the remaining 48 patients with clinical or routine laboratory evidence of heart disease, 2 with LV thrombus as a potential embolic source were identified by 2-D echo. M-mode echo failed to detect the thrombus in either patient. No patient with left atrial thrombi, MS, cardiac tumor or valvular vegetations was identified. One patient had possible MVP. Thus, echo in patients lacking other available evidence of heart disease is unlikely to yield findings that alter the clinical approach to patients with stroke; echo has greater clinical utility in stroke patients with clinically evident heart disease.

COMPUTER ENHANCEMENT OF LEFT VENTRICULAR CONTRAST ANGIOGRAPHY

For the past several years, contrast ventriculography has served as the standard by which cardiac performance is assessed in the cardiac catheterization laboratory. Because of the invasive nature of the procedure and the quantities of angiographic contrast required, application of the technique is limited. Peripheral injection of radiopaque contrast material, although less traumatic, does not produce an adequate diagnostic image of the LV because the high contrast of adjacent and overlying structures limits detectability of the low-contrast image of the diluted radiopaque material. This limitation might be minimized by applying technology originally developed for improving the optical quality of celestial photographs. Thus, digital image subtraction could eliminate the static high-contrast structures, permitting possible subsequent contrast enhancement to make low-contrast ventricular border outlines readily visible. Vas and associates[15] from Los Angeles, California, investigated the feasibility of currently available image-enhancement technology for delineating the LV following peripheral venous injection of contrast material at fluoroscopic dose rates in 10 dogs and in 8 patients. The technique employs a fast analog -to- digital conversion system capable of digitizing video frames on line. By averaging into digital-image memory the first 30 video frames and then subtracting each incoming frame from this memory, most of the background was eliminated, thereby leaving only the contrast-filled LV. Since the technique employs conventional fluoroscopic exposure rates rather than cineangiography, there was marked reduction in X-ray exposure. An in vitro study using the Rando whole-body phantom demonstrated that a 5 mm object with 2% contrast could be imaged within the complex chest anatomy with an incident exposure rate of only 30 mR/sec, using digital subtraction after contrast enhancement. In vivo studies were performed to assess the relative accuracy of LV border definition using this new technique in comparison with the enhanced images in 8 patients. The mean difference in planimetered area of the 2 cardiac silhouettes was 13 mm². In 4 patients, both direct and peripheral venous LV angiograms were obtained. There was a small (2%−7%) systematic difference between calculated end-diastolic and end-systolic LV volume, with peripheral venous volumes being invariably smaller. Differences in calculated EF were of smaller magnitude; the maximum absolute difference in EF was 2%. This technique appears applicable to angiographic studies involving either cardiac or peripheral vascular injection of contrast material, and it allows high-quality images to be obtained at approximately 7-fold reduction in radiation dose (5 mA, 65 to 85 kv).

HEART IN ATHLETES

Cyclists

Bekaert and associates[16] from Ghent, Belgium, investigated cardiac dimensions and LV function by noninvasive methods in 14 professional road-race cyclists and in 11 age-matched sedentary control subjects. The ECG findings were in agreement with previous studies in endurance athletes and the vectocardiographic data showed anterior displacement of the electrical forces. Echo dimensions at end-diastole showed higher values in the cyclists for LV internal diameter, LV free wall thickness, and ventricular septal thickness. Derived values for LV volume and LV mass also were much higher in the cyclists. A significant correlation was found between maximal oxygen consumption and end-diastolic LV diameter.

Oarsmen

Previous echo studies have shown that athlete's hearts differ in chamber size and wall thickness from those of sedentary control subjects. Several studies also have shown changes in echo dimensions after short periods of training. Relations between echo variables and maximum oxygen intake in trained athletes have not been described. Accordingly, Wieling and associates[17] from Amsterdam, the Netherlands, studied 9 freshmen and 14 senior oarsmen undergraduates during 7 months of training and compared them with 17 age- and sex-matched sedentary control subjects by standard M-mode echo and maximum oxygen uptake. At the start of the season, the senior oarsmen had a greater AV end-diastolic dimension and a thicker ventricular septum (VS) and LV free wall than did control subjects and freshmen oarsmen. The latter 2 groups did not differ from each other. During the training period, a slight and gradual increase in LV end-diastolic dimension and thickness of the VS and LV free wall occurred in the freshmen. In seniors, only LV end-diastolic dimension increased significantly. Maximal oxygen uptake increased in the fourth and seventh months during the period of intensive rowing. No relation was noted between echo variables and maximal oxygen uptake. Thus, a combination of heavy dynamic and static exercise can lead to significant changes in both LV wall thickness and chamber size within months. Echo variables measured at rest cannot be used as suitable indices of performance capacity.

Marathon runners

It is not unusual for a person engaged in strenuous endurance training to have below-normal hematocrits and hemoglobins, and low or marginally low hematocrit readings are particularly common in long-distance runners. The clinical significance of so-called "sports anemia," as related to its impact on long-distance running performance, has not been studied. Accordingly, Dressendorfer and associates[18] from Davis, California, and Honolulu, Hawaii, measured red blood cell (RBC) counts, blood hemoglobin concentrations, and related hematologic factors in 12 male marathon runners during a 20-day, 312-mile road race. The RBC count decreased significantly from 5.17 to 4.36 million per cu mm and the hemoglobin levels from 16.0 to 13.4 g/dl. Although runners became marginally anemic during the race, their running speeds were not significantly changed. There were no abnormal clinical signs other than rare instances of hematuria. This study indicates that a sudden increase in long-distance running mileage above the regular training level may cause "sports anemia," a functional pseudoanemia that usually does not impair endurance performance.

Elevated serum creatine kinase isoenzyme MB (CK-MB) level is regarded as a sensitive and specific marker for myocardial injury. Siegel and associates[19] from Boston, Massachusetts, measured the serum CK-MB level in male marathon runners during training and after competition. Mean serum CK-MB, measured by a quantitative electrophoretic technique (normal, <5 IU/L), showed borderline elevation during training, with peaks 24 hours after competition. Mean CK-MB in 64 serum samples from 35 runners after competition was 130 IU/L or 8.3% of total CK activity. Levels of CK-MB averaging 26 times the upper limits of normal would usually be considered indicative of massive myocardial necrosis. Myocardial scintigraphy with technetium 99m-pyrophosphate was performed after competition in 12 randomly selected runners with a mean post-race serum CK-MB level of 160 IU/L or 13%. Infarct-avid ("hot-spot") scintigraphy, appropriately timed to detect underlying myocardial abnormalities, was within normal limits in all subjects. Normal results of infarct-avid scintigraphy coincident with marked serum CK-MB elevations strongly suggests that CK-MB arises from a noncardiac or skeletal muscle source in these runners.

IDIOPATHIC HYPERKINETIC HEART SYNDROME

Anxiety, cardiac overactivity and hypercontractility, and favorable response to beta blockade characterize the idiopathic hyperkinetic heart syndrome. (IHHS). Its natural history is unknown. It has been suggested that it evolves toward hypertrophic cardiomyopathy. Fiorentini and associates[20] from Milan, Italy, investigated 14 patients with IHHS by intravascular and echo methods each year for 5 years. During this period, 7 were maintained untreated (group I) and 7 received propranolol (group II). The thickness of the ventricular septum and LV free wall by echo, and the ratio between the

2, were within normal limits in the control state and remained so for the duration of follow-up, both in the treated (persistent circulatory normalization was documented) and in the untreated patients (cardiac hypokinesis was unchanged or somewhat increased). Substitution of a placebo for propranolol in group II at the end of follow-up caused a prompt recurrence of the overactivity of the heart. Thus, it appears that transition toward hypertrophic cardiomyopathy is not a feature of IHHS, that propranolol does not produce an irreversible circulatory adjustment, and that it is unlikely that a reciprocal potentiation between anxiety and cardiac overactivity perpetuates the disorder.

In 1959, Gorlin and associates (*J Clin Invest* 38:2144, 1959) described 8 patients in whom the cardiac output was elevated and other specific cardiac abnormalities were found and they termed this condition the hyperkinetic heart syndrome. The syndrome was later more fully described and the basic hemodynamic abnormality of increased LV ejection rate was characterized. Despite many subsequent studies, no information on the natural history and progression of this condition has been reported. Accordingly, Gillum and associates[21] from Boston, Massachusetts, followed-up on 19 of the originally reported 24 patients with the IHHS. These patients were followed from 11–25 years. One patient died of severe MS; of the remaining 18 patients, 9 had complete physical examination and ECG. Only 1 was symptomatic at the time of re-examination. Precordial murmurs, originally present in 8 of 9 patients, were present in only 5 of 9 at re-examination. A hyperkinetic circulation was found in only 2 patients at follow-up. Systolic systemic hypertension, present in 7 at the original examination, was present in only 4 at follow-up. ECG abnormalities, usually LV hypertrophy, regressed in most. Persistent elevation of the cardiac index and systolic ejection rate were present at repeat catheterizations in the single symptomatic patient who had CHF. Thus, uncomplicated IHHS has an excellent long-term prognosis.

PERICARDIAL HEART DISEASE

Tamponade in unoperated patients

Guberman and associates[22] from Cincinnati, Ohio, reviewed observations in 56 patients with cardiac tamponade seen by the members of the cardiology division at the University of Cincinnati from 1963 to 1980. A paradoxic arterial pulse was critical in diagnosis, because most patients did not have a small quiet heart, and BP was often well maintained. Of the 55 patients, 52 had enlarged cardiac silhouettes by chest roentgenogram; heart sounds were diminished in 19 patients; arterial systolic BP was ≥100 mmHg in 35, and arterial pulse pressure was ≥40 mmHg in 27. Echo in 23 patients showed abnormally increased RV dimensions and decreased LV dimensions during inspiration, except in 1 patient with LV dysfunction. The causes of cardiac tamponade were metastatic tumor in 18 patients, idiopathic pericarditis in 8, and uremia in 5; 5 cases of tamponade occurred after heparin administration in AMI. Myxedema and dissecting aortic aneurysm each caused tamponade in 2 patients. Pericardiocentesis relieved tamponade initially in 40 of 46 patients; however, 2 suffered fatal complications. Pericardial resection was done in 18, including 12 of these 46.

Pericardial metastases detected by echo

Although echo is recognized as a very sensitive method of diagnosing pericardial effusion, the echo has not been considered very sensitive in sorting out the cause of pericardial effusions. Among 69 patients with pericardial effusion studied by echo by Chandraratna and Aronow[23] from Long Beach, California, the etiology of the pericardial effusion in 9 was invasion of the pericardia by malignant neoplasm. In 7 of the 9 patients with pericardial metastases, irregular cauliflower-like masses protruding from the visceral or parietal pericardia into the echo-free space of the pericardial effusion was noted by 2-D echo. These masses had a to-and-fro motion within the pericardial space during ventricular systole. Six of the 9 patients had dense linear echoes connecting the visceral and parietal pericardia, and these were interpreted as malignant adhesions. Thus, cross-sectional echo may be useful in detecting pericardial metastases as well as pericardial effusions.

Echo mimicking of pericardial effusion

Echo is a sensitive technique for the detection of pericardial effusion, but the abnormal echo patterns seen with effusions are not entirely specific for that diagnosis. Come and associates[24] from Boston, Massachusetts, and Baltimore, Maryland, described 4 patients in whom anatomic structures, a coronary artery -to- coronary sinus fistula (1 patient), and tumors metastatic to pericardium (3 patients), produced posterior and, in 2 patients, anterior spaces compatible with pericardial fluid. Echo patterns mimicking pericardial effusion have previously been reported in patients with anatomic abnormalities such as mitral anular calcium, pleural effusions, left atrial enlargement, anterior mediastinal or pericardial tumors, foramen of Morgagni hernia, and LV pseudoaneurysm. It appears that structures of fluid or tissue density, interposed between the heart and the air-filled lung, can produce echo patterns simulating pericardial effusion.

Pneumococcal pericarditis

In a pre-antibiotic era, pericarditis was often encountered as a complication of untreated pneumococcal disease. The use of antimicrobial therapy against Streptococcus pneumoniae obviously has decreased the incidence of pericarditis and also decreased the recognition of this entity when it does occur. Berk and associates[25] from Boston, Massachusetts, reviewed clinical and laboratory features in 6 patients with pericarditis caused by Streptococcus pneumoniae. The diagnosis of pneumococcal pericarditis was delayed or missed entirely during life in all 6 patients. The frequent absence of pericardial friction rubs and cardiomegaly on chest roentgenograms contributed to the difficulty in recognizing this illness. Although ECG and physical examination usually disclosed abnormalities, they were not sufficiently specific to suggest pericarditis.

Morphologic features of operatively excised parietal pericardia

Mambo[26] from Saskatoon, Canada, reexamined histologic sections of parietal pericardium excised at thoracotomy in 35 patients who were operated on primarily because of pericardial effusion (19 patients), pericardial constriction (12 patients), or pericardial cysts (4 patients). Of the 19 patients with predominant effusion, histologic study of the excised parietal pericardium showed only nonspecific fibrous changes in 8, tuberculous granulomatous inflammation in 4, purulent inflammation in 4, neoplasms in 4, and siderotic deposits in 4. Of the 12 patients with clinical evidence of constriction, calcific deposits were the predominant histologic finding in 8, and none had granulomas, 2 had nonspecific fibrous thickening, and 2 had granulomatous inflammation of presumed tuberculous origin. Of the 35 patients, pericardial disease was an incidental finding in 13 (37%). Of the 35 patients, 22 presented with symptoms of primary pericardial disease and the other 13 presented with symptoms unrelated to the pericardium. Two of the latter 13 patients had pericardial disease discovered at operation for the purpose of performing aortocoronary bypass. Of the 35 patients, partial or complete parietal pericardiectomy was carried out in 25, pericardial windows were created in 6 patients, and 4 had pericardial cysts removed. This paper is simply 1 of many in recent years that show that most patients with myocardial constriction from pericardial disease do not have a specific histologic diagnosis made from the excised tissues.

Postpericardiotomy syndrome in adults

Engle and associates[27] from New York City studied adults undergoing intrapericardial surgery and compared the findings with concurrent results in children and with a clinical study in adults 20 years earlier. The postpericardiotomy syndrome (PPS) occurred in 28% of 119 children, in 18% of 142 adults studied in 1978 and 1979, and in 17% of 115 adults studied from 1958−63. Major changes in the adult surgery over the 2 decades were the younger age of the adults then (16% > age 50 years, as opposed to 74% now) and the types of surgery done then (congenital heart disease in 34%, valvular heart disease with valvotomy in 66%) -vs- now (congenital heart disease in 2%, valve replacement in 37%, and aortocoronary bypass grafting in 53%). The remainder had a combination of valve replacement and aortocoronary bypass. Infants < age 2 years rarely had PPS (3.5% incidence) whereas the incidence in adolescents was about 35%. In adults < age 40 years, the incidence was about the same as in children, but declined as age increased: to 20%, for ages 40−59 years; 14%, for ages 60−70 years, and 10% in the elderly. Antiheart antibody, determined by an immunofluorescent technique, and antiviral antibodies to a battery of 8 common viral agents, were determined on sera preoperatively, and on the tenth day, in third week postoperatively, and additionally if the patient had the syndrome clinically. Just as in the children, all with PPS developed antiheart antibody (AHA) in high titer, whereas those with no syndrome had no detectable titer (54%) or slight elevation (28%). Furthermore, a 4-fold or greater rise in antiviral antibody occurred in 68% of those with PPS, but in only 5% of those with negative or intermediate AHA.

Thus, this common postoperative complication is an autoimmune phenomenon, probably triggered by a recent viral illness. If the viral infection is acquired in the hospital around the time of surgery or intensive care, precautions to minimize exposure to viral agents might reduce the incidence of PPS.

Pericardial effusion and tamponade late after open heart operations

For a variety of reasons, late pericardial tamponade, effusion, or constriction may occur after open heart surgery. Clinical and laboratory findings in 28 patients with late pericardial effusions following open heart surgery in 596 patients were reported by Borkon and associates[28] from Baltimore, Maryland. Eleven patients were asymptomatic; 17 were symptomatic, 9 with and 8 without cardiac tamponade. Pericardiocentesis was not done in any of the asymptomatic patients, but it was done in 13 of the 17 symptomatic patients, including all 8 in whom tamponade developed an average of 13 days postoperatively. Most patients were diagnosed by M-mode echo and chest roentgenograms. Warfarin administration was implicated as the cause of the effusions in most patients. None died. Effective drainage was accomplished in all 28 patients.

Ofori-Krakye and colleagues[29] from New Haven, Connecticut, reported cardiac tamponade after cardiac surgery in 10 of 1,200 patients. This group had a slightly longer lag phase, and clinical hemodynamic compromise appeared from 15–180 days (mean, 49) postoperatively. Pericardiocentesis was successful in 9 patients and a pericardiectomy was required in 1.

Rice and associates[30] from Chicago, Illinois, reported 5 patients with constrictive pericarditis secondary to open heart surgery from 10 weeks–6 years after cardiac operation. Each had pericardiectomy. In 4 of the 5 patients, the postpericardiotomy syndrome had developed after the original cardiac procedure.

Thus, although extremely unusual, pericardial effusion, with or without tamponade or constriction, may occur in patients who have had postpericardiotomy syndrome or long-term warfarin therapy. Careful follow-up of patients is required for diagnosis, particularly after postpericardiotomy syndrome.

HEART IN SYSTEMIC DISEASES

Mucocutaneous lymph node syndrome

The mucocutaneous lymph node syndrome (MLNS) (Kawasaki's disease) is a clinical entity consisting of high fever, mucocutaneous involvement, and cervical lymphadenopathy that affects infants and young children. The acute inflammatory features consist of angiitis with involvement of multiple organ systems. It has been suggested that the morphologic changes are indistinguishable from those observed in infantile periarteritis nodosa. Although this syndrome is predominantly found in Japan, it has become increasingly recognized in other countries. Carditis and coronary arterial lesions frequently have been demonstrated in association with MLNS. However, the natural history of carditis and coronary arterial aneurysms is unclear. Furthermore, there are no clinical data that evaluate serially the relation between carditis and coronary aneurysms. Hiraishi and associates[31] from Kanagawa Prefecture, Japan, studied 79 patients with MLNS prospectively. Changes were categorized according to the duration of illness: stage I (1−10 days); stage II (11−20 days); stage III (21−30 days); stage IV (31−60 days), and stage V (61 days−40 months). The presence of myocarditis in stages I and II was suggested in 40 of 79 patients (51%) by ECG, echo, radiographic, and clinical abnormalities. Myocarditis was accompanied by pericarditis in 6 patients and by both endocarditis and pericarditis in 1 patient. These signs of inflammation were resolved by stage III in all but 3 patients with ECG abnormalities. In the active stage, large coronary arterial lesions were suspected only because of an abnormal spherical echo-free space in the region of the coronary arteries on 2-D echo and ECG evidence of deep Q waves in leads II, III, and aVF. One or more coronary aneurysms was noted in 5 patients during stages III, IV, and V. Aneurysm regression demonstrated by angiography did not correlate with echo changes in aneurysm size in 1 patient. Moreover, the occurrence of coronary aneurysm did not correlate with the presence of signs of carditis, because the frequency of carditis was the same in patients with and without aneurysm.

Hurler syndrome

QUANTITATION OF CORONARY NARROWING

Patients with the Hurler syndrome (dwarfism, severe mental retardation, skeletal malformations, hepatosplenomegaly, and corneal opacities) are known to have a variety of cardiovascular lesions that affect the coronary arteries, cardiac valves, mural endocardium, myocardial walls, and aorta. Within the affected cardiac structures are large clear cells (known as Hurler cells), granular cells, acid mucopolysaccharide material, and collagen. Although it is well known that the epicardial coronary arteries may be narrowed in the Hurler syndrome, the extent of the narrowing has not been described. To fill this void, Brosius and Roberts[32] examined each of the 4 major epicardial coronary arteries in 6 patients with the Hurler syndrome in a quantitative manner at necropsy, and described the results of that examination. The amount of cross-sectional area luminal narrowing in each 5 mm segment of each of the 4 major epicardial coronary arteries (right, LM, LAD, and LC) was described at necrospy in 6 children (aged 3−16 years) with the Hurler syndrome. In 5 patients, at least 1 of the 4 major coronary arteries was narrowed 76%−100%, and in 4 of these 5 patients, all 4 major arteries were narrowed to this extent (Fig. 9-1). Of the 24 major coronary arteries in the 6 patients, 17 (71%) were narrowed 76%–100% at some point. A total of 182 segments was examined from the 24 major coronary arteries, and the extent of narrowing was as follows: 96%–100%, 14 (8%); 76%–95%, 61 (34%); 51%–75%, 59 (32%); 26%–50%, 39 (21%), and 0–25%, 9 (5%). When a score from 1–4 was applied to each 5 mm segment according to its category of narrowing (1 = 0–25%; 2 = 26%–50%; 3 = 51%–75%, and 4 = 76%–100%), the 182 segments had a total score of 570 and a mean score of

Fig. 9-1. Bar graph showing percent of 5 mm segments of the 4 major coronary arteries in 5 categories of narrowing in each of the 6 patients with the Hurler syndrome.

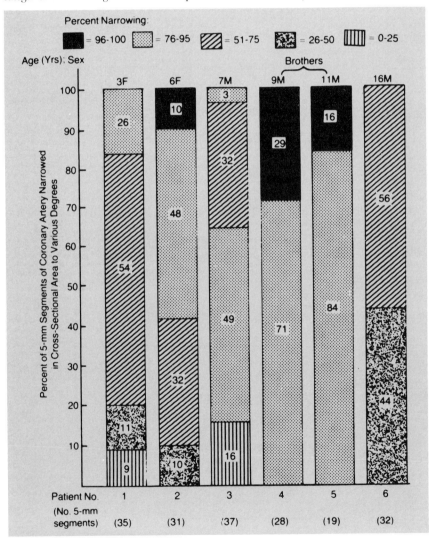

3.2, indicating that each segment was narrowed an average of about 70% in cross-sectional area. Thus, narrowing of the major epicardial coronary arteries at necropsy is usually diffuse and severe in the Hurler syndrome, which is the cause of the most severe coronary narrowing in childhood.

MITRAL VALVE DEFORMITY BY ECHO

Johnson and associates[33] from Lexington, Kentucky, described thickening of the mitral valve leaflets by M-mode echo in 5 children with the Hunter-Hurler syndrome. Three had a murmur of MR.

Takayasu's disease

Occlusive thromboaortopathy (Takayasu's disease), which has a worldwide distribution, is a chronic inflammatory arteriopathy of unknown origin and is prevalent in women. The nature of the disease gives rise to 4 main complications, namely, Takayasu's hypotensive ischemic retinopathy, secondary hypertension, AR, and aortic or arterial aneurysm. Coronary arterial lesions rarely are associated with this disease. These cardiovascular disorders vary and the prognosis for survival and physical activity differs with the individual patient. Thus, an adequate classification representative of the clinical features of this disease and predictive of the prognosis has long been required. It has been suggested that the prognosis of patients with severe single or multiple complications is poorer than that of patients without or with only mild complications. Ishikawa[34] from Kyoto, Japan, described the course, complications, and survival of 81 patients with Takayasu's disease who were followed after its diagnosis had been established. Of the 81 patients, 9 were men and they were followed prospectively for 7.4 ± 5.8 years after the established diagnosis. These patients were classified according to the presence and severity of the 4 major complications present when the diagnosis was established: no complications (group 1); mild single complication (group IIa) and severe single complication (group IIb), or multiple complications (group III). When the data were analyzed by the life-table method, severe events attributed to Takayasu's disease, as well as death, were used as end points. Seven of the 81 patients were treated surgically; 2 of the 7 died and 1 had severe events postoperatively. In the remaining 74 female patients, the 10-year cumulative eventless survival rate after diagnosis in combined groups I and IIa (44 patients) and in combined groups IIb and III (30 patients) was 97 ± 3% (mean ± SEM) and 59 ± 11%, respectively (p < 0.002). These data are useful for predicting death or severe events, or both, and provide basic information regarding possible elective surgery for patients with this intractable disease.

Systemic lupus erythematosus

QUANTITATION OF CORONARY NARROWING

Involvement of the heart in systemic lupus erythematosus (SLE) is well established and, in patients not treated with corticosteroids, the pericardium, endocardium, and myocardium are affected. After institution of corticosteroid therapy, systemic hypertension with resulting LV hypertrophy became a frequent occurrence in patients with SLE. Additionally, many patients with SLE treated with corticosteroids clinically have had manifestations of CAD and, at necropsy, narrowing of 1 or more major epicardial coronary arteries. The extent of the coronary narrowing in patients with SLE, however, has not been described in detail. To fill this deficiency, Haider and Roberts[35] from Bethesda, Maryland, studied quantitatively at necropsy the 4 major epicardial coronary arteries in 22 young adult patients with SLE. The degrees of cross-sectional area luminal narrowing by atherosclerotic plaques of each 5 mm segment of each of the 4 major (right, LM, LAD, and LC) epicardial coronary arteries in 22 necropsy patients (age 16–37 years, 21 women) with SLE was determined, and the findings were compared with those in 13 control subjects. Of 623 coronary segments in the patients with SLE, 80 (13%) were narrowed 76%–100% (controls, 0% of 431 segments); 125 (20%), 51%–75% (controls, 6%); 273 (44%), 26%–50% (controls, 63%) and 145 (23%), 0%–25% (controls, 31%) (Fig. 9-2). Of the 22 patients with SLE, 10 had 1 or more of the 4 major coronary arteries narrowed 75%–100% in cross-sectional area, and 12 patients had lesser degrees of narrowing, similar to that in the 13 control subjects. The 10 patients with SLE and severe coronary narrowing, when compared with the 12 patients with SLE and no severe (<75%) coronary narrowing, had significantly higher: 1) mean values of total serum cholesterol (382 -vs- 290 mg/dl); 2) mean systolic/diastolic systemic arterial pressures (175/119 mmHg -vs- 151/93 mmHg); 3) frequencies of mitral valvular disease (7 of 10 patients -vs- 0 of 12 patients), and 4) frequencies of pericardial adhesions (7 of 10 patients -vs- 3 of 12 patients).

Scleroderma

ARRHYTHMIAS AND CONDUCTION DISTURBANCES

Disorders of rhythm and conduction are characteristic of the cardiac involvement in progressive systemic sclerosis (PSS), but their overall frequency in this condition is not well established. Clements and associates[36] from Los Angeles, California, analyzed 46 ambulatory patients with PSS, performing 24-hour continuous ECGs (Holter monitor) in them. Conduction disturbances (sinus node dysfunction, first-degree heart block, pre-excitation), supraventricular arrhythmias (supraventricular tachycardia, atrial fibrillation, premature contractions of atrial or junctional origin) and ventricular arrhythmias (VT, multifocal VPC) were observed on Holter monitoring in 26 subjects. Although these arrhythmias and conduction disorders were predictably observed in patients who complained of palpitations or syncope, or who had an ECG that showed first-degree heart block, ventricular bigeminy, left anterior superior hemiblock, prolonged P wave, right- or left-axis deviation, RV or LV hypertrophy, pathologic Q waves or low voltage, they were often found in patients who lacked other clinical evidences of heart disease. Arrhythmias and conduction disturbances were not significantly more frequent among patients with cardiomegaly or interstitial change on chest roentgenogram nor were they related to the presence or severity of abnormal lung

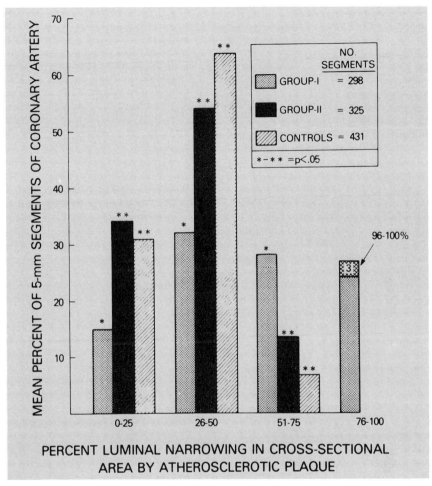

Fig. 9-2. Percent of 5 mm segments of all 4 major epicardial coronary arteries narrowed to various degrees in 22 necropsy patients (group I and group II with systemic lupus erythematosus) and in 13 control subjects.

function. This study suggests that Holter monitoring may be a valuable adjunct in evaluating heart disease in PSS.

Hyperthyroidism

EFFECTS OF THYROID HORMONE ON LEFT VENTRICULAR FUNCTION

That thyroid affects the heart directly has only recently been appreciated. Thyroxine has positive chronotropic effects on myocardial cells in tissue culture and in human myocardium. Cohen and associates[37] from New York City measured systolic time intervals, echo indices of LV contractile function, and serum triidothyronine and thyroxine levels before treatment in 9 patients with hyperthyroidism and again every 2 weeks for 8 weeks after therapy and then every 4 weeks until the subjects were clinically and chemically euthyroid. Six of the 9 patients became transiently hypothyroid. Although the preejection period corrected for heart rate (preejection period index) increased as the patients became euthyroid, the change was not significant. Preejection period index increased dramatically in the patients becoming hypothyroid (p < 0.005). Corrected LV ejection time (LV ejection time index) also increased as the patients became euthyroid (p < 0.001), and increased again with the appearance of hypothyroidism (p < 0.05). There was a linear correlation between velocity of circumferential fiber shortening and serum triiodothyronine level and between velocity of circumferential fiber shortening and serum thyroxine level at all stages of thyroid function. Thus, thyroid hormone definitely enhances LV function in humans, and both excess and deficiency cause predictable reversible changes in myocardial contractile function. Furthermore, echo measurements of velocity of circumferential fiber shortening provide rapid estimates of the chemical status of thyrotoxic patients before and after treatment.

INCREASED CLEARANCE OF PROPRANOLOL

Feely and associates[38] from Dundee, Scotland, studied the pharmacodynamics of oral propranolol during chronic treatment of 6 patients with thyrotoxicosis and again when each was euthyroid. The mean total plasma propranolol steady-state concentration was 42% lower when the patients were thyrotoxic. After treatment of thyrotoxicosis, there was a fall (p < 0.05) in mean oral clearance of both total (4.2 ± 0.6 to 2.7 ± 0.4 liters/min) and free 30 ± 5 to 25 ± 4 liters/min) propranolol, although the half-life of propranolol did not change significantly. The free fraction of propranolol was larger in the thyrotoxic (14 ± 1%) than in the euthyroid (11 ± 1%) state (p < 0.05). These results suggest that the pharmacokinetics of propranolol are significantly altered in thyrotoxicosis.

Chronic hypercalcemia

Roberts and Waller[39] from Bethesda, Maryland, described certain clinical and morphologic cardiac observations in 18 necropsy patients, aged 33–58 years (mean, 45) (14 women), with chronic hypercalcemia (11.6–34.4 mg/dl [mean, 19.4]) from 1–9 years (mean, 5). Primary hyperparathyroidism was present in 9 patients and secondary hyperparathyroidism in the other 9 (of renal origin in 7). Cardiac valve anular and coronary arterial calcific deposits were present in 10 patients (group I) including 4 (mean age, 51 years) with considerable narrowing of 2 or 3 of the 4 major epicardial coronary arteries. None of the other 8 patients (group II) had cardiac valve anular or cuspal calcific deposits; only 2 had coronary calcific deposits, small in each, and none had significant coronary luminal narrowing. Calcium was in the media ("medial calcinosis"), with or without intimal deposition, of the coronary arteries in 5 patients. Comparison of the patients in groups I and II disclosed similar mean ages, durations of hypercalcemia and serum calcium levels, but significantly (p < 0.05) higher mean total serum cholesterol levels (216 -vs- 163 mg/dl) and heart weights (426 -vs- 320 g). This study demonstrates that chronic hypercalcemia is associated with accelerated deposition of calcium in the cardiac anuli and valvular cusps, in the media and intima of the coronary arteries, and in individual myocardial fibers (dystrophic calcification), and that coronary intimal calcification may be associated with or produce luminal narrowing, especially in patients with serum total cholesterol levels >200 mg/dl. Thus, chronic hypercalcemia may be viewed as a "risk factor" to accelerated coronary atherosclerosis.

Diabetes mellitus

HEART RATE CHANGES

Patients with diabetes mellitus (DM) have faster resting heart rates than age- and sex-matched subjects without DM. The cause of the faster heart rates in the patients with DM, however, is unclear. Heart rate, of course, is controlled by both parasympathetic and sympathetic systems, and in normal subjects pharmacological blockade with atropine considerably increases heart rate, whereas additional sympathetic blockade with propranolol decreases the heart rate, but not to pre-blockade levels. Ewing and associates[40] from Edinburgh, Scotland, measured resting heart rates in diabetic patients during repeated autonomic function tests that reflect either parasympathetic or sympathetic integrity. The resting heart rates were measured lying, sitting, and standing in 61 patients with DM with various degrees of cardiovascular reflex abnormalities. Those with parasympathetic abnormalities alone had the highest heart rates, whereas those with both parasympathetic and sympathetic involvement had slightly less rapid heart rates, which were still faster than those in diabetics with normal cardiovascular reflexes. Thirty-eight other diabetics in whom autonomic function tests had been done at least 3 times had a similar pattern of resting heart rate. Twenty-five had unchanged tests; those with parasympathetic involvement alone had the highest heart rates. The other 13 subjects whose autonomic function changed from normal to abnormal showed a sequential increase in heart rate as cardiac parasympathetic damage developed, followed by a fall in heart rate, but not back to normal, as sympathetic damage developed as well. The increased resting heart rates in diabetics may be due to cardiac parasympathetic damage alone or to combined parasympathetic and cardiac sympathetic damage. The sequential heart rate changes support the view that the vagus nerve is affected before the cardiac sympathetic nerves.

Obesity

CHF is common in obese persons, but systemic hypertension, diabetes mellitus, and other cardiac and respiratory diseases also are fairly common in obese patients. Divitiis[41] performed cardiac catheterization in 10 obese persons aged 20–55 years (mean, 36) who weighed 81–183 kg (mean, 124). Their excess poundage ranged from 29–100 kg (mean, 70). None of the 10 persons had diabetes mellitus, systemic hypertension, or signs of cardiac or respiratory failure or associated disease. The cardiac output and stroke volume were high, ventricular end-diastolic and atrial pressures ranged from normal to high and correlated with body weight, signs of volume overloading, and reduced LV compliance. The PA pressure was elevated and correlated well with weight, pulmonary vascular resistance being normal. Mean aortic pressure did not correlate with weight and systemic arterial resistance tended to have a negative correlation. LV function was impaired particularly for the heaviest subjects. These observations show that depressed LV function already is present in relatively young obese people, even if they are free from signs of CHF or associated conditions. The degree of impairment of cardiac function roughly parallels the degree of obesity.

Celiac disease

Pericarditis, of course, is rare in patients with gastrointestinal disorders. It has been described in inflammatory bowel disease, but never before in association with celiac disease. Dawes and Atherton[42] however, from Prescot, England, described 2 patients with celiac disease in whom the presenting feature was recurrent pericarditis. In each, treatment with a gluten-free diet led to clinical and ECG improvement of the pericarditis.

IATROGENIC HEART DISEASE

On a general medical service

Steel and associates[43] from Boston, Massachusetts, found that 36% of 815 consecutive patients on a general medical service of a university hospital had an iatrogenic illness, defined as any illness resulting from a diagnostic procedure or from any form of therapy, and cardiac drugs and procedures led the list (Table 9-2). In 9% of all persons admitted, the incident was considered major in that it threatened life or produced considerable disability. In 2% of the 815 patients, the iatrogenic illness was believed to contribute to the death of the patient. Exposure to drugs was a particularly important factor in determining which patients had complications. Given the increasing number and complexity of diagnostic procedures and therapeutic agents, monitoring of untoward events is essential, and attention should be paid to educational efforts to reduce the risks of iatrogenic illness.

Radiation heart disease

In the early part of this century, the heart was considered a "radio-resistant" organ. With the introduction of megavoltage radiotherapy for treatment of neoplasms, however, it became apparent that the heart could, indeed, be damaged by high-dose radiation. The nature and extent of the damage, however, is debated. To delineate more specifically the types and degrees of cardiac damage by radiotherapy, Brosius and associates[44] from Bethesda, Mary-

TABLE 9-2. *Hospital interventions leading to iatrogenic complications.*

TYPE OF INTERVENTION	COMPLICATIONS	
	#	% MAJOR
DRUGS	208	19
Nitrates	26	15
Digoxin	15	33
Lidocaine	15	13
Aminophylline	15	7
Quinidine/disopyramide/procainamide	13	15
Heparin/warfarin	13	54
Penicillins	10	10
Benzodiazepines	10	0
Antihypertensives	10	30
Propranolol	9	44
Other and multiple	72	15
DIAGNOSTIC AND THERAPEUTIC PROCEDURES	175	28
Cardiac catheterization	45	—
Intravenous therapy	34	—
Urinary tract catheterization	10	—
Other (e.g., arteriography, peritoneal dialysis, use of nasogastric tube, Swan–Ganz catheterization, or hemodialysis)	86	—
MISCELLANEOUS	114	21
Falls	35	—
Other (e.g., transfusion, diet management, transportation, or nursing procedures)	79	—
TOTAL COMPLICATIONS	497	22

land, studied 16 patients aged 15–33 years who received >3,500 rads to the heart 5–144 months before death. All 16 had some radiation-induced damage to the heart: 15 had thickened pericardia (5 of whom had evidence of cardiac tamponade); 8 had increased interstitial myocardial fibrosis, particularly in the right ventricle; 12 had fibrous thickening of the mural endocardium and 13 of the valvular endocardium (Table 9-3). Except for valvular thickening, the changes were more frequent in the right side of the heart than in the left, presumably because of higher radiation doses to the anterior surface of the heart. In 6 of the 16 study patients and in 1 of 10 control subjects, 1 or more major epicardial coronary arteries were narrowed from 76%–100% in cross-sectional area by atherosclerotic plaque, 1 patient had a healed myocardial infarct at necropsy, and 1 died suddenly. In 10 patients and in the 10 control subjects, the 4 major epicardial coronary arteries were examined quantitatively: 6% of the 469 five-mm segments of coronary artery from the patients were narrowed from 76%–100% (controls, 0.2%, [p = 0.06]) and 22% were narrowed from 51%–75% (controls, 12%) (Fig.

TABLE 9-3. *Clinical and necropsy findings in 16 patients with radiation heart disease.*

PATIENT	AGE (yrs)	AGE (yrs) AT Dx	CALCULATED RAD TO HEART ANT	POST	Mo. FROM RAD TO DEATH	CT	TC*	HCT† (%)	HW (g)	PE	TE M	V	RV	IMF VS	LV	# 5 mm S CAs	# 5 mm S >75% XSA	TICA RV	LV
1	15	12	5,202	3,000	34	0	129	43	170	300‡	+	+	+	0	0	...	...	+	0
2	19	16	5,648	3,600	35	0	139	20	270	0	+	+	+	0	0	...	...	0	0
3	24	23	5,842	3,500	22	+	140	39	245	100	0	+	+	+	+	50	0	+	0
4	24	20	5,295	3,600	42	+	120	29	190	260	+	+	+	0	0	54	0	+	0
5	25	22	5,186	3,092	39	0	172	30	290	75	0	+	0	...	0	44	2	0	0
6	25	23	4,100	4,000	11	0	176	37	250	0	+	+	+	+	...	55	0	+	0
7	26	19	4,185	3,000	78	0	146	21	250	200	+	+	0	0	+	...	...	0	0
8	26	24	3,987	3,600	5	0	250	34	290	0	+	+	0	0	0	50	8	0	0
9	27	20	7,047	4,000	53	+	198	...	370	0	+	+	+	...	0	44	0	0	0
10	29	27	4,932	4,200	20	0	168	31	155	0	+	0	0	0	0	42	0	0	0
11	29	17	4,054	4,000	144	0	168	27	240	0	0	0	0	...	0	37	1	0	0
12	29	21	4,341	4,025	84.62§	+	...	27	225	0	+	+	0	0	0	43	12	0	0
13	30	25	5,419	4,495	44	0	187	35	170	0	+	+	0	0	0	...	...	0	0
14	30	27	8,769	4,800	27.2§	+	130	31	...	375	+	0	0	0	0	...	...	0	0
15	33	20	6,600	5,000	137	0	170	45	230	0	0	0	0	0	0	50	5	0	0
16	33	24	8,866	5,000	104	0	308	48	350	0	+	+	+	0	+	13	5	+	+

+ = present; 0 = absent or none; · · · = no data; CA = coronary artery; CT = cardiac tamponade; Hct = hematocrit; HW = heart weight; IMF = interstitial myocardial fibrosis; LV = left ventricle; M = mural; PE = pericardial effusion; RV = right ventricle; S = segments; TC = total serum cholesterol; TE = grossly thickened endocardium; TICA = thickened intramural coronary artery; V = valve; VS = ventricular septum; XSA = cross-sectional area. * Highest recorded value. † Value about 1 month before death. ‡ Number of milliliters. § Received 2 courses of radiotherapy.

9-3). The proximal portion of the arteries in the patients had significantly more narrowing than the distal portions. The arterial plaques in the patients were largely composed of fibrous tissue: the media frequently were replaced by fibrous tissue, and the adventitia were often densely thickened by fibrous tissue. In 5 patients, there was focal thickening (with or without luminal narrowing) of the intramural coronary arteries. Thus, radiation to the heart may produce a wide spectrum of functional and anatomic changes, but particularly damage to the pericardia and the underlying epicardial coronary arteries.

Applefeld and associates[45] from Baltimore, Maryland, described clinical and hemodynamic observations in 7 patients who developed clinical evidence of chronic constrictive pericarditis 51–268 months (mean, 116) after radiotherapy for Hodgkin's disease in 6 patients and for breast carcinoma in 1. Catheterization data in all 7 disclosed typical hemodynamic features of myocardial constriction. Of the 5 patients who had pericardiectomy, only 2 had an excellent functional result, 1 had residual constriction, and 2 died. The authors recommended the following for radiation-induced pericardial disease: in patients who have cardiac tamponade, i.e., dyspnea and hypotension, and an echo-confirmed pericardial effusion, they advised a surgically produced subxiphoid pericardial window. In patients with incapacitating ef-

Fig. 9-3. Percent of 5 mm segments of all 4 major coronary arteries narrowed to various degrees in 10 patients with radiation heart disease and 10 control subjects.

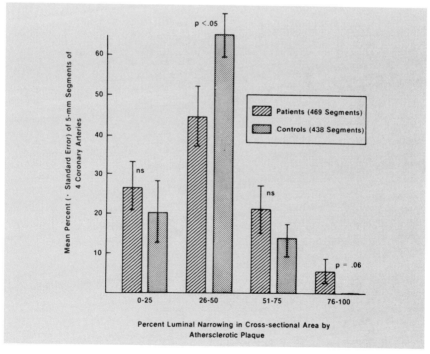

fort dyspnea, fatigue or marked hepatomegaly, they advised pericardiectomy if constrictive pericarditis were confirmed by catheterization. These authors did not advise pericardiectomy solely on the basis of hemodynamic confirmation of constrictive pericarditis or simply for the recurrence of pleural effusions.

An effusive pericarditis appearing during the initial 24–36 months after the completion of mediastinal irradiation and requiring up to an additional 24 months for spontaneous complete resolution has been the most frequent form of radiation-induced pericardial disease. Late appearance ($>$48 months) of radiation-induced chronic pericardial disease has not been commonly recognized. Applefeld and associates[46] recognized radiation-induced chronic pericardial disease in 9 patients (53–124 months; mean, 88) after radiotherapy for Hodgkin's disease. Depending on whether abnormal cardiac hemodynamics occurred before or after a fluid challenge, patients were considered to have either constrictive pericarditis (group 1) or occult constrictive pericarditis (group 2). There were no differences between these groups in various radiotherapy data, the use of chemotherapy, or the interval after treatment when the diagnosis of chronic pericardial disease was made. There were no consistent noninvasive variables to support the diagnosis of radiation-induced chronic pericardial disease before cardiac catheterization. Four patients underwent pericardiectomy. Two of the 4 operated patients had an excellent surgical result; a third patient died 4 months postoperatively of drug-induced granulocytopenia; the fourth patient has persistent visceral constrictive pericarditis 18 months after surgery.

The pericardium is the most frequent location of metastases to the heart and high-dose irradiation to mediastinum also may lead to pericardial disease in patients with cancer. Posner and associates[47] from Boston, Massachusetts, reviewed medical records at their hospital during a 3-month period and found 31 with a variety of malignant neoplasms and associated pericardial disease. Of the 31 patients with pericardial problems, 58% had metastases to pericardia, 32% had "idiopathic pericarditis," and 10% had radiation-induced pericardial disease. Facial swelling, arrhythmias, and pericardial tamponade occurred frequently in the patients with malignant pericardial disease. The patients with "idiopathic pericarditis" were characterized merely by having fever, pericardial friction rub, and improvement with nonsteroidal antiinflammatory drugs. The patients with radiation-induced pericardial disease had effusive-constrictive pericardial disease requiring pericardiectomy. Pericardiocentesis documented the diagnosis of malignant pericardial disease in 85% of the patients, and the other 15% required biopsy for diagnosis. Specific therapy directed at the pericardial disease improved survival in those with malignancies to pericardia and also those with radiation-induced pericardial disease.

INTRACARDIAC MASSES: DETECTION BY ECHO

DePace and associates[48] from Philadelphia, Pennsylvania, analyzed atrial masses in 19 patients: thrombi in 10 patients (all had MS); 7 with myxoma; 1

with a leiomyosarcoma; and, 1 (right atrium) with angiosarcoma. M-mode echo detected 6 of the 7 myxomas, 1 thrombus, and neither of the other tumors. Two-D echo, in contrast, detected the atrial masses in all 19 patients. Thus, 2-D echo appears to be the technique of choice in the detection, localization, and differentiation of intraatrial masses.

Come and associates[49] in 4 patients with large *masses in the left atrium* documented angiographically, morphologically, or both, the left atrium appeared clear of echoes in 2 of 4 studied by M-mode echo (4 patients) and 2-D echo (3 patients). Thus, even large tumors located within the body of LA may not be apparent or may be underestimated in size by currently available ultrasonic techniques. The relatively homogeneous nature of certain masses may, in part, be responsible for the inability to visualize some of them adequately by echo. Of their 4 patients, 2 had thrombi in the body of left atrium and the other 2 had myxomas weighing 70 and 125 g, respectively. The clots weighed 35 and 100 g, respectively.

Riggs and associates[50] from Chicago, Illinois, detected *right atrial masses* by 2-D echo in 5 pediatric patients: hemoangioendothelioma in 1; Wilms' tumor (having extended up the inferior vena cava) in 2; a large vegetation of tricuspid valve within right atrium in 1, and a large thrombus on a catheter in 1. Thus, masses within the right atrium, at least in the pediatric age group, can reliably be evaluated and diagnosed by 2-D echo and false-positive diagnoses are less likely than in evaluation of ventricular cavity masses.

Papillary fibroelastomas are benign tumors of the heart and are most often incidental findings at cardiac operation or necropsy. Rarely, symptoms or even sudden death can occur from little tumors. Shub and associates[51] from Rochester, Minnesota, described cardiac papillary fibroelastomas in 2 patients, diagnosed in each by 2-D echo with the tumors then excised. One patient had been asymptomatic and had a 1 × 1 cm papilloma removed from the mitral valve, the other patient had intermittent chest pains and sweating associated with a 1.5 × 1.0 cm papilloma on the aortic valve. The papilloma located on the mitral valve was excised through an aortotomy, without damage to the underlying mitral leaflet. The papilloma on the aortic valve was located on the noncoronary cusp. It did not protrude into a coronary ostium and it, too, was excised without excision of the underlying valve cusp. Thus, in retrospect, it is doubtful that cardiac operation was warranted in either of these patients.

SYSTEMIC VENOUS, PULMONARY ARTERIAL, AND PULMONARY PARENCHYMAL CONDITIONS

Cost effectiveness in diagnosis of symptomatic deep vein thrombosis

A variety of approaches have been used to make treatment decisions in patients with clinically suspected deep vein thrombosis. Until the past decade, most decisions were based on clinical diagnosis alone, but now an increasing number of studies have demonstrated clinical diagnosis to be nonspecific in this condition. Accordingly, many centers now use objective methods to assess patients with clinically suspected venous thrombosis. Venography is the accepted diagnostic standard, but it is invasive, produces discomfort, and has recently been replaced by less invasive tests. Hull and associates[52] from Hamilton, Canada, analyzed 516 patients with clinically suspected deep vein thrombosis, each of whom was evaluated by 3 diagnostic approaches: physical; venography, and the combination of impedance plethysmography and leg scanning. The cost effectiveness of these studies was analyzed. Clinical diagnosis was cost ineffective. Venography was cost effective, more so when applied as an outpatient investigation. Impedance plethysmography plus leg scanning is a practical, less invasive alternative to outpatient venography. The cost of inpatient diagnosis is likely to remain the major cost and, therefore, emphasis should be placed on outpatient diagnostic procedures.

Superior vena cava syndrome

Parish and associates[53] from Rochester, Minnesota, reviewed the Mayo clinic experience with superior vena cava (SVC) obstruction during the last 20 years. The diagnosis of SVC obstruction was often made at the bedside by typical symptoms, including suffocation, dyspnea, cough and, less commonly, pain, syncope, dysphagia, and hemoptysis. The most important physical findings were the increased collateral veins covering the anterior chest wall and the dilated neck veins with edema of the face, arms, and chest. The chest roentgenogram usually showed widening of the superior mediastinum. Of the 86 cases of SVC obstruction, 67 (78%) were due to malignancy and 19 (22%) to benign causes. The cause of obstruction was usually established by bronchoscopy, open lung biopsy, or biopsy of the superficial lymph node. Of the 6 benign cases resulting from thrombosis of the SVC, 3 were due to the use of central venous catheters.

Nonneoplastic causes of the SVC syndrome include phlebitis, either pyogenic or traumatic, upper respiratory infections, pneumonia, fibrosing mediastinitis, and cardiac disease. Idiopathic SVC thrombosis is infrequent, accounting for <2% of all SVC syndromes. The use of thrombolytic therapy in idiopathic SVC thrombosis has been limited, with only 1 report before that of Herrera and associates[54] from Aurora, Colorado. Although intravenous heparin has been effective in preventing such thrombus propagation, the clot remains, with persistent upper body edema, orthopnea, and venous engorgement. Anastomosis of the azygos vein to the right atrium and emergency thrombectomy have been performed in the past. Thrombolytic therapy, however, dissolves the clot and relieves long-term sequelae. The patient described by Herrera and associates had successful treatment of idiopathic SVC thrombosis with *streptokinase*, which indicates that thrombolytic therapy is the management of choice for this condition.

Infection of pulmonary arterial catheters

There have been several reports of infections following catheterization of the superior vena cava from the subclavian or internal jugular vein and of infection associated with PA catheters. Positive results of catheter tip culture may be the result of contamination during placement or removal of the PA catheter or colonization during transient or persistent bacteremia. Contamination is likely when an isolated organism is cultured from the catheter tip but from no other site, whereas colonization is indicated if an organism cultured from a catheter tip has been cultured previously from some other site. Catheter-related sepsis is suggested by culture of the same pathogenic organism from the PA catheter and the blood without previous isolation from another focus. Michel and associates[55] from Rochester, Minnesota, determined the incidence of catheter contamination or colonization and of catheter-related sepsis associated with placement and management of indwelling PA catheters in critically ill patients.

Bacteriologic cultures were performed on the tips of PA catheters removed from 153 critically ill patients who had required PA catheterization for management of hypovolemic or septicemic shock or for hemodynamic monitoring during mechanical ventilation with positive end-expiratory pressure. Positive results were obtained in 29 (19%). Colonization was probable in 17 patients, and contamination in 12. There were no instances of sepsis definitely attributable to the catheter. Positive catheter-tip culture was associated significantly with known presence of a focus of infection before catheter insertion and with periods >4 days that the catheter remained in place.

Noninvasive tests -vs- angiography in diagnosing pulmonary embolism

The accepted method for diagnosing pulmonary embolism with precision is pulmonary angiography. This test, however, is invasive and expensive and requires specialized equipment and personnel. Therefore, pulmonary angiography is used routinely to diagnose pulmonary embolism in relatively few hospitals. Perfusion lung scans, in contrast, are widely used as aids in diagnosis. The normal lung scan effectively rules out pulmonary embolism and, thus, this test is highly sensitive. In contrast to the sensitivity of this test, however, the specificity of lung scanning has not been clearly defined. Some patients with positive lung scans do not have PA occlusion demonstrated by angiography. The use of ventilation scanning as an adjunct to the perfusion scan has improved the accuracy of noninvasive testing, but again the specificity of the combined tests is unclear. Although noninvasive tests for pulmonary embolism have undefined specificity, many physicians treat patients with anticoagulants on the basis of such information.

Cheely and associates[56] from Chapel Hill, North Carolina, studied 243 patients in whom 248 pulmonary angiograms were performed because of suspected pulmonary embolism. Ventilation and perfusion lung scanning was carried out in 140 of the 243 patients, and in 38 of them the probability of pulmonary embolism was believed to be either high or low. Of 19 patients with subsegmental or nonsegmental perfusion defects that were matched with ventilation defects, none had pulmonary embolism. Conversely, angiography was positive in 17 of 19 patients with multiple segmental or lobar perfusion defects in areas of normal ventilation. Doppler flow examinations of the veins of the legs showed normal flow in 61 (77%) of 79 patients with pulmonary emboli; this test was an insensitive indicator of embolism. No patients died as a result of pulmonary angiography, but serious complications occurred in 2%. Anticoagulation with either heparin or warfarin in 83 patients was associated with bleeding in 25, two of whom died as a consequence of the bleeding.

The results of this study demonstrate that pulmonary embolism can be diagnosed with high likelihood if ventilation-perfusion lung scanning shows multiple segmental or lobar perfusion defects that ventilate normally. Alternately, pulmonary embolism can effectively be excluded if scanning is normal or shows nonsegmental or subsegmental perfusion defects that ventilate abnormally. When the results of the lung scan do not meet these criteria of high or low probability, the diagnosis of pulmonary embolism can only be made with certainty by pulmonary angiography. Since the risk of complications from angiography done by experienced operators is less than the risk of complications from anticoagulant therapy, patients who are not clearly categorized by lung scanning should undergo angiography before long-term treatment is started.

Clinical features of pulmonary embolism without preexisting cardiac or pulmonary disease

Stein and associates[57] from Detroit, Michigan, and Bethesda, Maryland, studied 215 patients with acute pulmonary embolism uncomplicated by preexisting cardiac or pulmonary disease. The patients had been included in the Urokinase Pulmonary Embolism Trial or the Urokinase-Streptokinase Embolism Trial. Presenting syndromes were 1) circulatory collapse with shock (10%) or syncope (9%); 2) pulmonary infarction with hemoptysis (25%) or pleuritic pain and no hemoptysis (41%), and 3) uncomplicated embolism characterized by dyspnea (12%) or nonpleuritic pain, usually with tachypnea (3%), or deep venous thrombosis with tachypnea (0.5%). The most frequent symptoms were dyspnea (84%), pleuritic pain (74%), apprehension (63%), and cough (50%). Hemoptysis occurred in only 28%. Dyspnea, hemoptysis, or pleuritic pain occurred separately or in combination in 94%. All 3 occurred in only 22%. The most frequent signs were tachypnea (respiration rate ≥ 20/min [85%]), tachycardia (heart rate ≥ 100 beats/min [58%]), accentuated pulmonary component of the second heart sound (57%), and rales (56%). Signs of deep venous thrombosis were present in only 41% and a pleural friction rub, in 18%. Either dyspnea or tachypnea occurred in 96%. Dyspnea, tachypnea, or deep venous thrombosis occurred in 99%. As a group, the identified clinical manifestations, although nonspecific, are strongly suggestive of acute pulmonary embolism. Conversely, acute pulmonary embolism rarely was identified in the absence of dyspnea, tachypnea, or deep venous thrombosis.

Left ventricular function in chronic obstructive pulmonary disease

The relationship between RV and LV function in patients with severe chronic obstructive pulmonary disease (COPD) remains unclear. Although subtle abnormalities in LV ejection during early systole have been observed, important LV dysfunction in patients with COPD rarely is clinically apparent. Slutsky and associates[58] from San Diego, California, assessed LV response to supine bicycle exercise in 12 patients with severe COPD (group 3), in 8 patients with both CAD and COPD (group 4), in 10 normals (group 1), and in 10 patients with CAD (group 2) by gated equilibrium RNA. Most individuals in all groups also had pulmonary catheter-obtained measurements of LV filling pressures during exercise. Normal individuals increased their EF during exercise by increasing stroke volume (SV) and reducing end-systolic volume (ESV) without changing end-diastolic volume (EDV); PA and wedge (PAW) pressures were unaltered. CAD patients (group 2) showed no change in EF with increased EDV, ESV, SV, and PAW. COPD patients (group 3) exhibited decreases in EDV, ESV, and SV, accounting for abnormal EF responses in 6 of 12; PAW was unchanged and the marked elevation of PA pressure correlated with reduced EDV. Group 4 patients (CAD plus COPD) had abnormal EF responses with increased EDV and ESV without change in SV. Thus, an abnormal LV function response to exercise in COPD patients may be multifactorial, thereby indicating the possible need for therapeutic modalities in addition to those employed in alleviating pulmonary parenchymal disease. Successful therapy of COPD and cardiac dysfunction may need to include agents that provide reduction of LV myocardial oxygen requirements, in addition to the conventional measures of improving lung ventilation-perfusion relationships, decreasing reversible bronchospasm, and terminating pulmonary infection. Equilibrium RNA and thallium myocardial stress scintigraphy may be of clinical value in determining management of the COPD patient, even in those in whom CAD may not be considered a likely associated disease process.

Hydralazine in cor pulmonale

Oral hydralazine has been shown to be effective in decreasing pulmonary arteriolar resistance and increasing cardiac output in some patients with primary pulmonary hypertension. To determine whether a similar response could be observed in patients with cor pulmonale, Rubin and Peter[59] from Durham, North Carolina, determined the hemodynamic status before and after the oral administration of hydralazine (25 mg, then 50 mg every 6 h for 48 h) in 12 patients at rest and in 8 during upright exercise. After hydralazine, there was an increase in cardiac output at rest (4 to 6 liters/min [$p < 0.001$]), and reductions in arteriovenous oxygen difference (8 to 6 volume % [$p < 0.001$]), mean PA pressure (52 to 44 mmHg [$p < 0.01$]), and pulmonary arteriolar resistance (11 to 6 units [$p < 0.0005$]). Similar hemodynamic changes occurred during exercise, including an increase in PA saturation from 27%–39% ($p < 0.001$) and a decrease in total pulmonary resistance from 13 to 9 units ($p < 0.01$). Results of pulmonary function tests performed before and after hydralazine did not change with drug administration. These findings indicate that the lung vascular bed in some patients with cor pulmonale is capable of responding to hydralazine with a reduction in pulmonary resistance and an increase in cardiac output, both at rest and during exercise.

Pulmonary embolectomy

It is estimated that almost 300,000 patients have PA emboli annually in the USA and that almost half these patients die. Glassford and associates[60] from Nashville, Tennessee, diagnosed PA embolism in 1,416 patients in a 10-year period and found that 219 (15%) died; 116 of these 1,416 patients had PA angiography and 29 of these (25%) died. PA embolectomy was performed in 20 patients, of whom 8 died. These 20 patients ranged in age from 22–77 years; 8 were men and 12 were women. Seven of 10 patients having arteriograms before embolectomy survived, whereas only 5 of 10 without arteriograms before surgery survived. Most patients in the latter category were having active cardiopulmonary resuscitation at the time. The authors believe that appropriate diagnostic studies, including at least a lung scan and, in most patients, pulmonary arteriogram should be done as soon as the diagnosis is suspected. PA embolectomy, once the diagnosis of PA embolus has been established, should be reserved for those whose PA pressure is greatly elevated and in whom more than 50% of the pulmonary vasculature is obstructed, or in whom there is continuing hemodynamic instability.

CARDIAC AND/OR PULMONARY TRANSPLANTATION

Gaudiani and associates[61] from Stanford, California, reported observations in 25 patients who lived ⩾5 years after cardiac replacement between 1968 and 1975. Of the 92 patients operated upon during that period, the long-term survival rate at 5 years was 30%. The average age of the 25 patients (23 males, 2 females) at operation was 40 ± 10 years. The average duration of survival was 6.7 years (5–10.5 years). Hemodynamic and clinical characteristics were followed on an annual basis to assess cardiac function, coronary anatomy, and quality of extended rehabilitation. The LV EF remained constant at 0.59 ± 0.08 one year postoperatively and 0.57 ± 0.09 at the most recent study. Segmental wall motion measured by fluroscopic examination and mid-wall intramyocardial markers also remained normal. Of 21 patients who had coronary angiograms after transplantation, 4 (19%) had developed significant narrowing. Segmental function in the areas served by the stenotic artery in these patients, however, did not consistently decline. The long-term survivors had fewer than 1 unscheduled admission to the hospital per year, 16 (64%) were gainfully employed, and 22 (88%) enjoyed substantial benefit. Thus, cardiac transplantation offers good survival with good quality of life in selected patients with terminal cardiac disease.

Reitz[62] from Stanford, California, described observations in the first 3 patients having combined heart and lung transplantations at his medical center. Patient #1 was a 45-year-old woman with primary pulmonary hypertension; #2, a 30-year-old man with Eisenmenger's syndrome due to a large VSD, and #3, a 29-year-old man with Eisenmenger's syndrome secondary to complete TGA, VSD and patent DA. Immunosuppressive therapy for the first patient was cyclosporin A (10 mg/kg/day) and prednisone (0.2 mg/kg/day) and she is now 6 months post-transplant with good functional capacity and normal hemodynamics by cardiac catheterization. Patient #2 is well 4.5 months later and is presently taking cyclosporin A (7 mg/kg/day) and prednisone (0.2 mg/kg/day). The first patient had 2 documentated episodes of acute cardiac allograft rejection at 10 and 25 days and was treated with methylprednisolone. Patient #2 had no rejection episodes detected. Patient #3 had significant intraoperative complications due to the previous operations (Baffes and Mustard procedures). These complications caused his death 4 days postoperatively. This initial experience of combined heart-lung transplantation is encouraging.

THORACIC AORTIC DISEASE

Aortic dissection

ANATOMY, CONSEQUENCES, CAUSES

This article by Roberts[63] is one of the few in recent years describing certain anatomic features of aortic dissection. It contains 21 illustrations of various anatomic features and tables discussing sites of secondary or reentry tears, complications (Table 9-4), and causes of death. Aortic dissection generally is a catastrophic cardiovascular event that, in most patients, is entirely preventable by proper treatment of systemic hypertension. Exactly how systemic hypertension is involved in the pathogenesis of aortic dissection is unclear, but it is clear that aortic dissection would virtually vanish if systemic hypertension disappeared. Patients with congenitally bicuspid aortic valves (with or without associated aortic isthmic coarctation), however, have an increased frequency of aortic dissection, as compared with individuals with 3-cuspid aortic valves, irrespective of the presence or absence of systemic hypertension. Most dissections involve the entire aorta. Those that stop within the aorta, with or without a reentry site, generally do so because of extensive atherosclerotic plaques that may cause atrophy or degeneration of the underlying media, which is where the longitudinal dissection is located. Although there are many exceptions, dissection involving the entire aorta generally indicates relatively mild or absent atherosclerosis. A common and poorly appreciated complication of aortic dissection is stenosis of the lumen of 1 or more major pulmonary arteries (peripheral pulmonic stenosis) due to extension of blood from the common adventitia of the aorta to that of the pulmonary trunk. Narrowing of the lumen of the true channel of the aorta by a compressing hematoma in the false channel (true aortic stenosis) is another unappreciated, but not uncommon, complication of aortic dissection.

CINEANGIOGRAPHY

Angiography in patients with suspected aortic dissection has usually been in the form of biplane roentgenograms. Improvements in cineangio-

TABLE 9-4. *Aortic dissection: complications. Reproduced with permission from Roberts.* [63]

THROUGH-AND-THROUGH RUPTURE OF AORTA WITH EXTRAVASATION OF BLOOD INTO:

  Pericardial sac

  Pleural space

  Mediastinum

  Retroperitoneum

  Wall of pulmonary trunk and/or main right and left pulmonary arteries (because of common adventitia with aorta)

    peripheral pulmonary stenosis

  Atrial and/or ventricular cardiac septum

    atrioventricular conduction defect

  Lung

  Esophagus

PARTIAL OR COMPLETE OBSTRUCTION BY MEDIAL HEMATOMA OF LUMEN OF ARTERY ARISING FROM AORTA

  Coronary

    Sudden death

    Acute myocardial infarction

  Innominate and/or common carotid

    Syncope, confusion, stroke, coma

  Innominate and/or subclavian

    Upper limb gangrene, paralysis

  Intercostal and/or lumbar

    Spinal cord ischemia-paraplegia

  Celiac

  Renal

    Oliguria

  Mesenteric

    Bowel ischemia

  Common iliac

    Lower leg gangrene, paralysis

SEPARATION OF BRANCH OF AORTA FROM AORTA

AORTIC REGURGITATION

OBSTRUCTION OF AORTA ITSELF (TRUE AORTIC STENOSIS)

  By compression of true lumen by medial hematoma

  Intussusception of aorta

---

graphic equipment and techniques, however, prompted Arciniegas and associates[64] from Birmingham, Alabama, to assess and compare the merits of biplane cine- and large-film aortic angiography in the diagnostic evaluation of patients with acute aortic dissection. The authors studied 20 patients with acute aortic dissection within 24 hours of operation, at necropsy, or both. Biplane large-film aortic angiography was performed in 11 patients (group I) and biplane aortic cineangiography in 9 (group II). The morphology of the aortic valve was defined precisely in 5 of 10 patients in group I and in all 9 patients in group II. AR was diagnosed in all patients in both groups in whom it was present. Intimal tears were localized in 5 of 10 patients in group I and in 8 of 9 in group II. Intimal flaps were not identified angiographically in 3 patients in group I and were identified in 4 patients in group II. The presence of retrograde dissection was established in 3 of 8 patients in group I and in 4 of 4 patients in group II. There was no difference between cine- and large-film angiography in the ability to identify a nonclotted false lumen. It is concluded that, in addition to improved diagnostic capabilities, technical advantages make cineangiography a good alternative to large-film angiography in the diagnostic evaluation of patients with acute dissection of the aorta.

COMPUTED TOMOGRAPHY

Moncada and associates[65] from Chicago, Illinois, utilized computed tomography (CT) of the torso combined with simultaneous intravenous injection of contrast medium in 16 patients suspected of having aortic dissection. All patients had subsequent percutaneous aortography within 24 hours of the CT examination. The aorta was normal in 4 patients, 1 had an apparently fusiform aneurysm of the ascending aorta, and 11 patients had aortic dissection (type I in 5, and type III in 6). All 11 patients with aortic dissection had the dissection diagnosed by CT as well as by angiography. Thus, CT appears to be an excellent diagnostic procedure for aortic dissection. Moncada and associates recommend that a CT-enhancement study be the preliminary study in all patients suspected of having aortic dissection. The CT examination, however, has some important limitations, including inability to detect aortic valve dysfunction and failure to provide adequate perspective on involvement by dissection of the branches arising from aorta. Potential benefits of CT, however, include avoidance of the aortogram in some patients, the relative noninvasiveness of the procedure, rapidity and ease of the procedure, and less expense, radiation, contrast media, and discomfort to the patient than with an aortogram.

2-D ECHO

Victor and associates[66] from Philadelphia, Pennsylvania, evaluated the usefulness of 2-D echo in establishing the diagnosis of aortic dissection in 15 patients who later proved to have aortic dissection. Two-D echo detected the "intimal flap" in 12 of the 15 patients and the 3 false-negative studies were in patients with a localized dissection. Of 27 other patients evaluated, who were proved not to have a dissection by other means, 1 was diagnosed as having aortic dissection by 2-D echo. Although these authors found 2-D echo to be quite useful in diagnosing aortic dissection, that has not been the case with a number of other echo investigators.

OPERATIVE TREATMENT

Turley and associates[67] from San Francisco, California, described findings in 21 patients with aortic dissection treated operatively from 1975–1980. The dissection involved the ascending aorta in 10 and the descending thoracic aortic in all 21. Operative technique included resection of the intimal tear and prosthetic graft interposition. Resuspension of the aortic valve was necessary in 3 patients. Cardiopulmonary bypass was utilized in all patients and cardioplegia in the ascending aortic dissection group. In 5 patients, all with chronic dissections, anastomosis was performed to the adventitial layer so there was distal perfusion to the true and false lumens. In 10 patients, obliteration of the false lumen was attempted by directing the flow to the distal lumen only. One patient died in the operative period.

To evaluate the false lumen postoperatively, computed tomography was employed in patients in whom obliteration of the false lumen had been attempted: it was patent in 7 and obliterated in 1. The mechanism of late patency of the false lumen was major vessel run-off. This report demonstrates that there is persistence of perfusion of the false lumen in patients even in whom obliteration has been attempted and that long-term survival is dependent upon resection of the segment of aorta containing the entry site. This fact has been known for a long time, but the new finding by CT scan proving that the false channel stays open is important to our understanding of the "surgical" history of aortic dissection.

Meng and associates[68] from Chicago, Illinois, analyzed 20 consecutive patients with ascending aortic dissection operated upon from 1970–78: 14 were men and 6 were women and their mean age was 45 years. Five of the 20 had the Marfan's syndrome and all who had portions of aorta excised had medial cystic necrosis. All 20 patients were operated on within 48 hours of onset of symptoms. Femoro-femoral bypass was used. Of 8 patients having primary repair, 1 died early and 1 later (stroke). Nine patients had resuspension of the aortic valve and interposition aortic graft: 2 died intraoperatively (ruptured abdominal aneurysm). Three patients had composite valve replacement and aortic graft and none died. This operation is perhaps the most technically demanding of all acquired cardiovascular operations. A wide variety of techniques should be available to the surgeon to permit, if appropriate, primary repair of valve and aorta, interposition graft with valve suspension or, occasionally, composite prosthetic valve and graft replacement.

Traumatic disruption

High-speed accidents often cause traumatic disruption or transection of the aorta. During a 10-year period, Akins and associates[69] from Boston, Massachusetts, treated 44 patients for traumatic disruption of the thoracic aorta. The injury occurred in the proximal thoracic descending aorta in 42, aortic arch in 1, and just above the aortic valve in 1. Aortography was done in 42. Operative repair was carried out in 21 patients within 48 hours, with an operative mortality of 24%; 14 had repair from 2–79 days after the accident, and 2 (14%) died. All 14 had received beta blockade and antihypertensive therapy between the accident and operation. Five patients had operative therapy electively delayed because of severe injury to other organ systems; there were no early or late deaths in this group. Two had immediate operative repair when a delayed diagnosis was made 21–56 days after injury and 2 patients refused surgery. In the 37 patients operated on, left atrial-femoral venous-left heart bypass with pump return to the left femoral artery was used in 23 patients, a heparinized intrathoracic shunt was used in 12, standard cardiopulmonary bypass in 2, and nothing in 1. A Dacron graft was used in 33 patients, primary repair in 3, and 1 patient had primary closure. All 9 operative deaths occurred in a subgroup of 23 patients in whom the modified left heart bypass was used. A number of major and minor complications occurred in these severely injured patients with multiple injury, but the long-term results were generally good.

These data from the 1970s suggest a trend away from left heart bypass and toward the use of shunt surgery. No patient underwent interposition graft without some form of protection to the spinal cord. Although, the mortality was higher with left heart bypass, this was an earlier treated group, and the effects of heparinization required for left heart bypass complicated management.

Soyer and associates[70] from Paris and Rouen, France, treated 34 patients over a 20-year period with traumatic rupture of the thoracic aorta: 14 had acute ruptures and 20 had ruptured false aneurysms. There were 2 deaths in the acute ruptures, and no deaths in the chronic false aneurysm group. Most patients were operated on with femoro-femoral bypass, but in the last several patients these investigators used no shunt but merely rapid cross clamping and anastomosis.

Transverse or descending aortic aneurysm: operative treatment

Arteriosclerotic aneurysms involving the transverse aortic arch are great surgical challenges. Cooley and associates[71] from Houston, Texas, have had perhaps the largest experience in the world with these types of aneurysms and they reported 25 patients repaired with use of hypothermic cardiopulmonary bypass techniques. They first categorized their 25 patients into 4 types: *Type A* was a saccular aneurysm involving only the transverse aorta, and repair consisted of an application of a patch graft; *Type B*, a fusiform aneurysm involving both ascending and transverse aorta, with the descending aorta being relatively normal; *Type C*, the aneurysm extended from the ascending aorta into the proximal portion of the descending aorta; *Type D* involved the entire ascending and descending thoracic aorta. They used 2 forms of support for operations on the arch: 1) deep hypothermic circulatory arrest for about 45 minutes with cerebral cooling; 2) moderate hypothermia with individual perfusion of the carotid arteries. Twenty patients equally distributed between types A–D had deep hypothermic arrest. The overall survival was 50%. In a more recent (Nov 1980–Jan 1981) experience, 5 patients underwent moderate hypothermia and isolated cerebral perfusion, 4 are long-term survivors. This paper presents some innovative surgical techniques for which this group from Houston has been renowned. Analysis of their techniques suggests that the deep hypothermic circulatory arrest is perhaps preferable, since the setup for the isolated cerebral perfusion is considerably more cumbersome and time consuming. If AVR or coronary bypass also is to be done, the more complex perfusion technique would be preferable.

Crawford and Saleh[72] from Houston, Texas, described deep hypothermic circulatory arrest techniques in 8 patients with this lesion, utilizing a variety of exclusion and aneurysmorrhaphy techniques to promote hemostasis and simplify the operation. All patients survived operation and had uncomplicated postoperative courses. The cerebral ischemia time ranged from 25–55 minutes (mean, 36). The mean temperature was about 14°C. These techniques are innovative and impressive. Regardless of the technique used, rapid surgical techniques are required for the salvage of a high percentage of these patients.

In one of the world's largest experiences of aneurysms confined to the thoracic aorta, Crawford and associates[73] from Houston, Texas, reported 148 patients operated upon in a 24-year period (1956–1980). From 1956–1967, 36 patients were treated by femoro-femoral bypass or shunts, with a 6% incidence of paraplegia and a 22% mortality rate; from 1962–1980, 112 patients were treated without shunts or bypass, with an incidence of paraplegia of 1% and a mortality rate of 9%. The current operation consisted of aneurysmal replacement using inclusion technique with cardiac hemodynamics controlled by vasodilators, fluid replacement, and careful anesthetic management. Cardiovascular hemodynamics, blood gases, electrolytes, and plasma osmolarity were monitored frequently to achieve the desirable physiologic response to aortic cross clamping and operation. During the past 4 years, proximal blood pressure has been controlled with nitroprusside and, during this period, 69 patients had a 6% operative mortality with no paraplegia or renal failure. A double-balloon endobronchial tube permitted collapse of the left lung to improve exposure. Radial artery lines and a urinary catheter were employed, and a Swan-Ganz thermodilution catheter into the pulmonary trunk was used to intermittently record pulmonary capillary wedge pressure and cardiac output.

One has to be careful about extrapolating such data for surgeons that do this kind of surgery infrequently. In less experienced hands, shunt procedures are probably indicated, particularly when the operation appears complex. In those with considerable experience, the no-shunt technique works well, provided the ischemic time is brief. Certainly, in patients with acute dissection of the descending thoracic aorta, any form of temporary bypass or shunt is unsuccessful because of the damage to the aorta, and simple cross clamp above and below the dissection, as outlined by Crawford and associates, is preferable.

PHARMACOLOGIC TOPICS

Cholestyramine resin in digitoxin toxicity

Digitoxin has a long half-life and is associated with a substantial incidence of toxicity. It is, of course, partially excreted in the bile and later reabsorbed, thus contributing to its half-life. A nonabsorbable agent that binds digitoxin in the gut should help speed its disappearance from the serum. Cholestyramine resin, an ion-exchange resin used for some patients with hyperlipoproteinemia, appears to be such an agent. Several reports have described such a digitoxin-binding effect in animals. Pieroni and Fisher[74] described a 72-year-old woman with clinical, laboratory, and ECG evidence of digitoxin toxicity. Digitoxin elimination was studied before, during, and after administration of cholestyramine resin. The resin resulted in an accelerated elimination of digitoxin and would appear to be a valuable adjunct to therapy of patients with digitoxin toxicity.

Inhibition of prostacyclin and platelet thromboxane A_2 after low-dose aspirin

To compare the inhibitory effects of aspirin on prostaglandin synthesized by vessel walls and platelets, Preston and associates[75] from Sheffield, England, obtained vein segments from 5 subjects before they were given 150–300 mg aspirin and at various intervals afterward. They then measured prostacyclin (PGI_2) synthesis with a radioimmunoassay for its stable metabolite, 6-keto-prostaglandin $F_{1\alpha}$. Platelet production of thromboxane A_2 was measured with a radioimmunoassay for its stable metabolite, thromboxane B_2. Two hours after aspirin had been given, 81%–100% inhibition of PGI_2 synthesis was demonstrated; 86% inhibition was still evident in 1 subject tested 8 hours after administration. Simultaneously, platelet production of thromboxane B_2 was completely inhibited for more than 24 hours. Thus, there is little difference between the initial inhibitory response of platelet cyclooxygenase and that of vessel-wall cyclooxygenase to these doses of aspirin. The results also indicate that, in male subjects, the prolonged template bleeding time after aspirin is not the consequence of selective inhibition of platelet production of thromboxane.

Nifedipine and left ventricular function after beta blockade

Joshi and associates[76] from Heath Park, Cardiff, studied the acute effects of nifedipine on LV function and hemodynamics at constant heart rates in 12 patients on beta blocker therapy (atenolol, 100 mg orally every 6 h for 24 h). Nifedipine significantly depressed LV peak dP/dt and peak dP/dt P^{-1}. Nifedipine also significantly reduced systemic vascular resistance. This reduction was associated with decreased systolic BP and increased LV stroke output, with nonsignificant increases in EF and mean circumferential shortening velocity. The LV end-diastolic pressure did not change. Thus, nifedipine increases cardiac output in association with arterial dilation, despite evidence of a negative inotropic effect. Such intrinsic negative inotropic effects would normally be masked by compensatory sympathetic activity. Of the 12 patients studied, 8 had CAD with normal LV function and 4 had entirely normal hearts.

Inactivation of digoxin by gut flora and reversal by antibiotic therapy

In approximately 10% of patients given digoxin, substantial conversion of the drug to cardioinactive, reduced metabolites (digoxin reduction products

[DRPs]) occurs. The site and clinical importance of this conversion is unknown. Lindenbaum and associates[77] from New York City gave digoxin daily for 4 weeks to 4 volunteers and measured urinary excretion of DRPs. They found that the urinary excretion of DRP was greatest after a poorly absorbed tablet had been ingested, and least after intravenous administration. Stool cultures from subjects known to make DRPs in vivo ("excretors") converted digoxin to DRPs; cultures from nonexcretors did not. Three excretors were given digoxin tablets for 22–29 days. A 5-day course of erythromycin or tetracycline, administered after a baseline period of 10–17 days, markedly reduced or eliminated DRP excretion in urine and stool. Serum digoxin concentrations rose as much as 2-fold after antibiotics were given. The authors concluded that, in some persons, digoxin is inactivated by gastrointestinal bacteria. Changes in the enteric flora may markedly alter the state of digitalization.

CARDIAC SURGICAL TOPICS

Alteration of coagulation and certain chemistries by open heart surgery without transfusions

Milam and associates[78] from Houston, Texas, determined alterations of coagulation status and certain clinical chemistry laboratory determinations in 75 adults undergoing cardiopulmonary bypass procedures for acquired heart disease. The studies were carried out both during and after operation. No patient received a transfusion of blood or blood components. With hemodilution, the mean hematocrit value dropped from 38% to 28% during the procedure. Fibrin degradation products and euglobulin lysis time were transiently abnormal. Factor V diminished somewhat during the procedure, whereas factors VIII and IX increased after operation. Clottable fibrinogen values decreased slightly, but increased to an abnormally high value at 24 and 48 hours. Mean value of platelet counts decreased from 194,000 to 144,000/μl immediately after operation. Knowledge of expected deviation of coagulation factors and certain clinical chemistry tests after open heart surgery is helpful in evaluating the status of the postoperative patient.

Complement activation during cardiopulmonary bypass

Use of pump-oxygenator systems for heart surgery has been associated with a complex array of postoperative clinical sequelae, including coagulopathies; a systemic inflammation-like reaction characterized by increased capillary permeability, increased accumulation of interstitial fluids, leukocytosis, and fever; and profound organ dysfunction that is particularly manifest in the pulmonary, renal, and central nervous systems. These physiologic effects, which are most dramatic after prolonged extracorporeal circulation, have been collectively termed the "post-perfusion syndrome" or "post-pump syndrome." The striking similarities between these clinical findings and the known biologic activities of the complement-derived anaphylatoxins C3a and C5a suggest that these inflammatory mediators may participate in promoting some of these symptoms. Both C3a and C5a act as spasmogens: they stimulate release of mast cell histamine, contract smooth muscle, and increase vascular permeability. In addition, C5a possesses the unique ability to interact directly with specific high-affinity receptors on peripheral-blood neutrophils. Binding of C5a initiates cellular responses that include chemotaxis, lysosomal enzyme release, superoxide generation, autoaggregation, and increased adherence. The last 2 responses are believed to be responsible for the immediate neutropenia and pulmonary-vascular leukostasis that are produced by intravenous administration of C5a. Similar phenomena have been demonstrated in patients undergoing renal dialysis with dialyzers equipped with cellophane membranes and in patients subjected to nylon-fiber-filtration leukophoresis.

Chenoweth and associates[79] from La Jolla, California, observed complement activation in 15 adults undergoing total cardiopulmonary bypass. Plasma levels of C3a were significantly elevated ($p < 0.0001$) at the beginning of the procedure, and they continued to increase steadily thereafter. At the end of the procedure, C3a levels were more than 5 times higher than preoperative levels. Plasma levels of C5a (a factor that binds avidly to neutrophils) did not change significantly during cardiopulmonary bypass. Instead, there was significant neutrophilia ($p = 0.03$) during bypass, and significant transpulmonary neutropenia ($p = 0.0002$) occurred when cardiopulmonary circulation was reestablished at partial bypass. The neutropenia is consistent with pulmonary-vascular sequestration of C5a-activated granulocytes. Incubation of blood with the nylon-mesh liner of bubble oxygenators, as well as vigorous oxygenation of whole blood, promotes conversion of complement. Thus, complement-derived inflammatory mediators C3a and C5a produced during extracorporeal circulation may contribute to the pathogenesis of "post-pump syndromes."

Prostacyclin administration during cardiopulmonary bypass

In a double-blind trial, Longmore and associates[80] from London, England, gave prostacyclin to 12 of 23 patients undergoing aortocoronary bypass grafting. The treatment group showed a preservation of platelet number and function, with a halving of blood loss in the first 18 hours postoperatively. The heparin-sparing effect of prostacyclin was confirmed, as were the vasodilator effects, which were not troublesome. The values for hemoglobin, hematocrit, and both white blood cell and platelet counts were consistently higher in the prostacyclin-treated group, both during and after bypass. Activated clotting time was significantly longer in the prostacyclin-treated group after administration of heparin, but before bypass.

Ventricular-assist pumping for cardiogenic shock after cardiac operation

Profound refractory CHF remains a major cause of death after cardiac surgery. The intraaortic balloon has been useful as a form of mechanical circulatory assistance in these types of patients when volume augmentation and pharmacologic therapy have been unsuccessful in allowing the patient to be separated from cardiopulmonary bypass. Nevertheless, at least half of these patients die from cardiogenic shock, despite counterpulsation with the intraaortic balloon. Therefore, a form of mechanical circulatory support is needed that is capable of maintaining the systemic circulation and unloading the left ventricle while the myocardium recovers. Pierce and associates[81] from Hershey, Pennsylvania, utilized a ventricular-assist pump to support the circulation in 8 patients who could not be separated from cardiopulmonary bypass after open heart operations. In 5 patients with LV CHF, the systemic circulation was maintained with pumping from the left ventricle or left atrium to the aorta for 7 ± 2 days; 3 of these 7 patients were well 4–17 months after operation. In 2 patients with biventricular failure, RV and LV bypass supported the circulation, but neither patient survived. One other patient had isolated RV failure, and pumping from the right atrium to the PA maintained the pulmonary circulation for 2 days; this patient lived for 18 months. Thus, use of the ventricular-assist pump in these 8 patients provided complete support of the systemic or pulmonary circulation or both. Thus, profoundly depressed ventricular function is potentially reversible if technical problems in employing the pump can be avoided.

UNCATEGORIZABLE

Abdominal binding during cardiopulmonary resuscitation

Earlier studies in dogs showed improved BP and carotid flow with abdominal binding during cardiopulmonary resuscitation (CPR). Chandra and associates[82] from Baltimore, Maryland, assessed the effect of abdominal binding at pressures of 60–110 cm of water during CPR in 10 patients who had cardiac arrest. Abdominal binding for brief periods (30–60 s) raised mean arterial pressure from 54 ± 7 mmHg before binding to 67 ± 8 mmHg after binding. In 6 patients studied who had abdominal binding performed for 4 minutes, this beneficial effect was still apparent at the end of the time period. No abdominal visceral injury was found in 6 patients at necropsy. Thus, abdominal binding is an effective, yet simple, technique for increasing BP during CPR in man, with considerable field-use potential.

Changes in cardiovascular health knowledge with age

Although the acquisition of health knowledge does not ensure healthier behavior, it may be a prerequisite for the success of other efforts aimed at changing behavior. White and Albanese[83] devised a standardized test of cardiovascular health knowledge and administered it to 1,367 students, aged 12–18 years, and 562 adults, aged 20–60 years. Mean scores were: ages 12–14 years, 42 ± 0.7% (SEM); 15–18 years, 49 ± 0.1%; 20–40 years, 69 ± 0.7%, and 40–60 years, 68 ± 0.7% correct. Cardiovascular health knowledge increased linearly in the student population, averaging 3% per year. Increases continued to occur in adults, but plateaued after age 40 years, despite an increasing incidence of cardiovascular disease in this age group. Health knowledge was highly correlated with the highest educational achievement. At all age levels, knowledge of diagnostic tests was highest and knowledge of pathophysiology lowest. A personal or family history of heart disease or history of an elevated serum cholesterol was not a stimulus for increases in health knowledge!

References in cardiologic history

Fye[84] provides 135 references, most during the past 20 years, on history of cardiology. This is a fine list of key books and articles in journals.

The heart man*

There is a road that winds down from Kpayerkolli toward the sea, and in the dry season it is a road of red dust. In West Africa, where the villages are small and scattered in the bush, Kpayerkilli is just one of many such villages, and if you do not go with someone who knows it you will never find it. If you walk there, you will be coated with dust; it will sift into your ears and eyes and cover your clothes.

The road is always full of people, especially children, since there are so many of them. A road means freedom to walk, freedom from poisonous snakes, and from the rough jungle terrain. If you talk to the children on the road, they will shyly say they are glad to meet you, that they are well (even if they are not), and that they are going to school soon. They will not tell you about the Heart Man.

You will see them come to the point where the road goes on and the little path turns off toward their village, and they will run wildly off the road and down the path. When you ask why, they will not tell you. Only when they are older, and when you are their friend, will they tell you. It is not in any book.

The reason they run, they explain, is that there is a Heart Man, from a big city. He comes out to the villages where there are many children. He likes young hearts because they are tender and full of life. He looks for children coming off the road and when he catches one, he takes the heart right out, still beating, for his own use. One little bush-child is gone and nothing can be done, for the Heart Man disappears. That is why the children run so when they come off the road, and they grease their bodies down so that they will be slippery.

What has this to do with us? We are highly educated professionals, not little African children running through the bush. But we are in grave danger from the Heart Man, who is in every culture in a different form. He is after our hearts.

Our road is the superhighway, and we live in the fast lane. We cannot travel there unless we are really moving. We suffer from this pace. Physicians state that lack of time is their number one dissatisfaction. Large numbers of patients, heavy on-call schedules, reading, teaching, and research all take up professional time. There are many things to look at besides the patient. From the patient's viewpoint this may be seen as a loss of compassion, but sometimes it is just life on the highway; we have to look at the laboratory results and scans as we whiz by the patient. Time is a Heart Man after our hearts, and he wants to drive us faster and faster, until we go right past all for which we should stop. This Heart Man also goes after our personal lives, until we neglect ourselves and our families.

We travel down our road repetitively and it can bore and irritate us. We see the chronically ill over and over again; sometimes they are helpless victims, sometimes, with cigarettes and alcohol, they cause their own demise. Our scientific knowledge is impressive, but there are still many things we cannot cure. And it frustrates us to see these patients return again and again. It can harden our hearts and steal them from their true purpose, which is to feel compassion.

Our road has more signs than the one in West Africa does. There are so many signs that they may also distract us.

One sign is the dollar sign—it is a necessary sign, but all too easy to focus on. We feel it is our right to earn money in keeping with our education and experience. No one disputes that our education has monetary value or that we have accrued large debts. But the Heart Man is lurking behind the dollar sign, and he loves to get us and squeeze the good motivation out of us until he has in his hands a greedy little heart.

Another sign is the one-way sign. We endure long years of training, alternately ego-buffeting and ego-building, and we become professionals. Now, we feel that we are different, maybe even better, than others. We may start to see things only one way—our way. But the Heart Man is stealing our heart, and if he is not stopped all that will be left is an empty, self-seeking space.

There is one scene on our road that we too often forget, and that is the scene of an accident. We are unaware that the Heart Man causes the accidents even though we may witness them on our own road. At the scene of the accident we see colleagues who have lost their hearts, and on occasion their lives. Drug abuse, alcoholism, and suicide result in the loss of 700 physicians a year—several entire medical school classes. We travel by and think that it could never happen to us, but it could next time, next year, or next decade.

We need to keep our hearts young and tender and not let demands of time, frustration, love of money, or selfishness steal them from us. We need to acknowledge our vulnerability to the Heart Man who comes in these guises to change our hearts and take them away from us. We need to run away from him when he comes, run hard and fast, until we come at last to our own village.

* The commencement address by David L. Schiederman, MD, at his graduation from the Medical College of Wisconsin.[85]

References

1. HAMMILL SC, PRITCHETT ELC: Simplified esophageal electrocardiography using bipolar recording leads. Ann Intern Med 95:14–18, July 1981.

2. BEACH C, KENMURE ACF, SHORT D: Electrocardiogram of pure left ventricular hypertrophy and its differentiation from lateral ischaemia. Br Heart J 46:285−289, Sept 1981.

3. FISCH C: Electrocardiogram in the aged: an independent marker of heart disease? Am J Med 70:4−6, Jan 1981.

4. BACHMAN S, SPARROW D, SMITH LK: Effect of aging on the electrocardiogram. Am J Cardiol 48:513−516, Sept 1981.

5. EDWARDS WD, TAJIK AJ, SEWARD JB: Standardized nomenclature and anatomic basis for regional tomographic analysis of the heart. Mayo Clin Proc 56:479−497, Aug 1981.

6. WILSON JR, ROBERTSON JF, HOLFORD F, REICHEK N: Evaluation of M-mode echographic estimates of left ventricle function: relationship of selected ultrasonic and hemodynamic parameters. Am Heart J 101:249−254, March 1981.

7. REICHEK N, DEVEREUX RB: Left ventricular hypertrophy: relationship of anatomic, echocardiographic and electrocardiographic findings. Circulation 63:1391−1398, June 1981.

8. CHILD JS, KRIVOKAPICH J, PERLOFF JK: Effect of left ventricular size on mitral E point to ventricular septal separation in assessment of cardiac performance. Am Heart J 101:797−805, June 1981.

9. HELAK JW, REICHEK N: Quantitation of human left ventricular mass and volume by two-dimensional echocardiography: in vitro anatomic validation. Circulation 63:1398−1407, June 1981.

10. WONG M, SHAH PM, TAYLOR RD: Reproducibility of left ventricular internal dimensions with M-mode echocardiography: effects of heart size, body position and transducer angulation. Am J Cardiol 47:1068−1074, May 1981.

11. PIETRO DA, VOELKEL AG, RAY BJ, PARISI AF: Reproducibility of echocardiography: a study evaluating the variability of serial echocardiographic measurements. Chest 79:29−32, Jan 1981.

12. GARCIA E, GUERET P, BENNETT M, CORDAY E, ZWEHL W, MEERBAUM S, CORDAY S, SWAN HJC, BERMAN D: Real time computerization of two-dimensional echocardiography. Am Heart J 101:783−792, June 1981.

13. GOLDBERG SJ, VALDES-CRUZ LM, FELDMAN L, SAHN DJ, ALLEN HD: Range gated Doppler ultrasound detection of contrast echographic microbubbles for cardiac and great vessel blood flow patterns. Am Heart J 101:793−796, June 1981.

14. GREENLAND P, KNOPMAN DS, MIKELL FL, ASINGER RW, ANDERSON DC, GOOD DC: Echocardiography in diagnostic assessment of stroke. Ann Intern Med 95:51−53, July 1981.

15. VAS R, DIAMOND GA, FORRESTER JS, WHITING JS, SWAN HJC: Computer enhancement of direct and venous injected left ventricular contrast angiography. Am Heart J 102:719−728, Oct 1981.

16. BEKAERT I, PANNIER JL, VAN DE WEGHE C, VAN DURME JP, CLEMENT DL, PANNIER R: Non-invasive evaluation of cardiac function in professional cyclists. Br Heart J 45:213−218, Feb 1981.

17. WIELING W, BORGHOLS EAM, HOLLANDER AP, DANNER SA, DUNNING AJ: Echocardiographic dimensions and maximal oxygen uptake in oarsmen during training. Br Heart J 46:190−195, Aug 1981.

18. DRESSENDORFER RH, WADE CE, AMSTERDAM EA: Development of pseudoanemia in marathon runners during a 20-day road race. JAMA 246:1215−1218, Sept 11, 1981.

19. SIEGEL AJ, SILVERMAN LM, HOLMAN BL: Elevated creatine kinase MB isoenzyme levels in marathon runners: normal myocardial scintigrams suggest noncardiac source. JAMA 246:2049−2052, Nov 6, 1981.

20. FIORENTINI C, OLIVARA MT, MORUZZI P, GUAZZI MD: Long-term follow-up of the primary hyperkinetic heart syndrome: an echocardiographic and hemodynamic study. Am J Med 71:221−227, Aug 1981.

21. GILLUM RF, TEICHHOLZ LE, HERMAN MV, GORLIN R: The idiopathic hyperkinetic heart syndrome: clinical course and long-term prognosis. Am Heart J 102:728−734, Oct 1981.

22. GUBERMAN BA, FOWLER NO, ENGEL PJ, GUERON M, ALLEN JM: Cardiac tamponade in medical patients. Circulation 64:633−640, Sept 1981.

23. CHANDRARATNA PAN, ARONOW WS: Detection of pericardial metastases by cross-sectional echocardiography. Circulation 63:197–199, Jan 1981.

24. COME PC, RILEY MR, FORTUIN NJ: Echocardiographic mimicry of pericardial effusion. Am J Cardiol 47:365–370, Feb 1981.

25. BERK SL, RICE PA, REYNHOLDS CA, FINLAND M: Pneumococcal pericarditis: a persisting problem in contemporary diagnosis. Am J Med 70:247–251, Feb 1981.

26. MAMBO NC: Diseases of the pericardium: morphologic study of surgical specimens from 35 patients. Human Pathology 12:978–987, Nov 1981.

27. ENGLE MA, GAY WA JR, MCCABE J, LONGO E, JOHNSON D, SENTERFIT LB, ZABRISKIE JB: Postpericardiotomy syndrome in adults: incidence, autoimmunity and virology. Circulation 64(Suppl II):58–60, Aug 1981.

28. BORKON AM, SCHAFF HV, GARDNER TJ, MERRILL WH, BRAWLEY RK, DONAHOO JS, WATKINS L JR, WEISS JL, GOTT VL: Diagnosis and management of postoperative pericardial effusions and late cardiac tamponade following open-heart surgery. Ann Thorac Surg 31:512–519, June 1981.

29. OFORI-KRAKYE SK, TYBERG TI, GEHA AS, HAMMOND GL, COHEN LS, LANGOU RA: Late cardiac tamponade after open heart surgery: incidence, role of anticoagulants in its pathogenesis and its relationship to the postpericardiotomy syndrome. Circulation 63:1323–1328, June 1981.

30. RICE PL, PIFARRE R, MONTOYA A: Constrictive pericarditis following cardiac surgery. Ann Thorac Surg 31:450–453, May 1981.

31. HIRAISHI S, YASHIRO K, OGUCHI K, KUSANO S, ISHII K, NAKAZAWA K: Clinical course of cardiovascular involvement in the mucocutaneous lymph node syndrome: relations between clinical signs of carditis and development of coronary arterial aneurysm. Am J Cardiol 47:323–330, Feb 1981.

32. BROSIUS FC, ROBERTS WC: Coronary artery disease in the Hurler syndrome. Qualitative and quantitative analysis of the extent of coronary narrowing at necropsy in six children. Am J Cardiol 47:649–653, March 1981.

33. JOHNSON GL, VINE DL, COTTRILL CM, Noonan JA: Echocardiographic mitral valve deformity in the mucopolysaccharidoses. Pediatrics 67:401–406, March 1981.

34. ISHIKAWA K: Survival and morbidity after diagnosis of occlusive thromboaortopathy (Takayasu's disease). Am J Cardiol 47:1026–1032, May 1981.

35. HAIDER YS, ROBERTS WC: Coronary arterial disease in systemic lupus erythematosus: quantification of degrees of narrowing in 22 necropsy patients (21 women) aged 16 to 37 years. Am J Med 70:775–781, Apr 1981.

36. CLEMENTS PJ, FURST DE, CABEEN W, TASHKIN D, PAULUS HE, ROBERTS N: The relationship of arrhythmias and conduction disturbances to other manifestations of cardiopulmonary disease in progressive systemic sclerosis (PSS). Am J Med 71:38–46, July 1981.

37. COHEN MV, SCHULMAN IC, SPENILLO A, SURKS MI: Effects of thyroid hormone on left ventricular function in patients treated for thyrotoxicosis. Am J Cardiol 48:33–48, July 1981.

38. FEELY J, STEVENSON IH, CROOKS J: Increased clearance of propranolol in thyrotoxicosis. Ann Intern Med 94(part 1):472–474, Apr 1981.

39. ROBERTS WC, WALLER BF: Effect of chronic hypercalcemia on the heart: analysis of 18 necropsy patients. Am J Med 71:371–384, Sept 1981.

40. EWING DJ, CAMPBELL IW, CLARKE BF: Heart rate changes in diabetes mellitus. Lancet 1:183–185, Jan 1981.

41. DIVITIIS O, FAZIO S, PETITTO M, MADDALENA G, CONTALDO F, MANCINI M: Obesity and cardiac function. Circulation 64:477–482, Sept 1981.

42. DAWES PT, ATHERTON ST: Coeliac disease presenting as recurrent pericarditis. Lancet 1:1021–1022, May 1981.

43. STEEL K, GERTMAN PM, CRESCENZI C, ANDERSON J: Iatrogenic illness on a general medical service at a university hospital. N Engl J Med 304:638–642, March 1981.

44. BROSIUS FC, WALLER BF, ROBERTS WC: Radiation heart disease. Am J Med 70:519–530, March 1981.

45. APPLEFELD MM, SLAWSON RG, HALL-CRAIGS M, GREEN DC, SINGLETON RT, WIERNIK PH: Delayed pericardial disease after radiotherapy. Am J Cardiol 47:210–213, Feb 1981.

46. APPLEFELD MM, COLE JF, POLLOCK SH, SUTTON FJ, SLAWSON RG, SINGLETON RT, WIERNIK PH: The late appearance of chronic pericardial disease in patients treated by radiotherapy for Hodgkin's disease. Ann Intern Med 94:338–341, March 1981.

47. POSNER MR, COHEN GI, SKARIN AT: Pericardial disease in patients with cancer. The differentiation of malignant from idiopathic and radiation-induced pericarditis. Am J Med 71:407–413, Sept 1981.

48. DEPACE NL, SOULEN RL, IOTLER MN, MINTZ GS: Two dimensional echocardiographic detection of intraatrial masses. Am J Cardiol 48:954–960, Nov 1981.

49. COME PC, RILEY MF, MARKIS JE, MALAGOLD M: Limitations of echocardiographic techniques in evaluation of left atrial masses. Am J Cardiol 48:947–953, Nov 1981.

50. RIGGS T, PAUL MH, DELEON S, ILBAWI M, PAJCIC S: Two dimensional echocardiography in evaluation of right atrial masses: five cases in pediatric patients. Am J Cardiol 48:961–966, Nov 1981.

51. SHUB C, TAJIK AJ, SEWARD JB, EDWARDS WD, PRUITT RD, ORSZULAK TA, PLUTH JR: Cardiac papillary fibroelastomas: two-dimensional echocardiographic recognition. Mayo Clin Proc 56:629–633, Oct 1981.

52. HULL R, HIRSH J, SACKETT DL, STODDART G: Cost effectiveness of clinical diagnosis, venography, and noninvasive testing in patients with symptomatic deep-vein thrombosis. N Engl J Med 304:1561–1567, June 1981.

53. PARISH JM, MARSCHKE RF, DINES DE, LEE RE: Etiologic considerations in superior vena cava syndrome. Mayo Clin Proc 56:407–413, July 1981.

54. HERRERA JL, WILLIS SM, WILLIAMS TH: Successful streptokinase therapy of acute idiopathic superior vena cava thrombosis. Am Heart J 102:1063–1064, Dec 1981.

55. MICHEL L, MARSH HM, McMICHAN JC, SOUTHORN PA, BREWER NS: Infection of pulmonary artery catheters in critically ill patients. JAMA 245:1032–1036, Mar 13, 1981.

56. CHEELY R, MACARTNEY WH, PERRY JR, DELANY DJ, BUSTAD L, WYNIA VH, GRIGGS TR: The role of noninvasive tests versus pulmonary angiography in the diagnosis of pulmonary embolism. Am J Med 70:17–22, Jan 1981.

57. STEIN PD, WILLIS PW, DeMETS DL: History and physical examination in acute pulmonary embolism in patients without preexisting cardiac or pulmonary disease. Am J Cardiol 47:218–223, Feb 1981.

58. SLUTSKY R, HOOPER W, ACKERMAN W, ASHBURN W, GERBER K, MOSER K, KARLINER J: Evaluation of left ventricular function in chronic pulmonary disease by exercise gated equilibrium radionuclide angiography. Am Heart J 101:414–420, Apr 1981.

59. RUBIN LJ, PETER RH: Hemodynamics at rest and during exercise after oral hydralazine in patients with cor pulmonale. Am J Cardiol 47:116–122, Jan 1981.

60. GLASSFORD DM JR, ALFORD WC JR, BURRUS GR, STONEY WS, THOMAS CS JR: Pulmonary embolectomy. Ann Thorac Surg 32:28–32, July 1981.

61. GAUDIANI VA, STINSON EB, ALDERMAN E, HUNT SA, SCHROEDER JS, PERLROTH MG, BIEBER CP, OYER PE, REITZ BA, JAMIESON SW, CHRISTOPHERSON L, SHUMWAY NE: Long-term survival and function after cardiac transplantation. Ann Surg 194:381–385, Oct 1981.

62. REITZ BA: Heart and lung transplantation. Heart Transplantation 1:80–81, 1981.

63. ROBERTS WC: Aortic dissection: anatomy, consequences, and causes. Am Heart J 101:195–214, Feb 1981.

64. ARCINIEGAS JG, SOTO B, LITTLE WC, PAPAPIETRO SE: Cineangiography in the diagnosis of aortic dissection. Am J Cardiol 47:890–894, Apr 1981.

65. MONCADA R, CHURCHILL R, REYNES C, GUNNAR RM, SALINAS M, LOVE L, DEMOS TC, PIFARRE R: Diagnosis of dissecting aortic aneurysm by computed tomography. Lancet 1:238–241, Jan 1981.

66. VICTOR MF, MINTZ GS, KOTLER MN, WILSON AR, SEGAL BL: Two dimensional echocardiographic diagnosis of aortic dissection. Am J Cardiol 48:1155–1159, Dec 1981.

67. Turley K, Ullyot DJ, Godwin JD, Wilson JM, Lipton M, Carlsson E, Ebert PA: Repair of dissection of the thoracic aorta: evaluation of false lumen utilizing computed tomography. J Thorac Cardiovasc Surg 81:61–68, Jan 1981.

68. Meng RL, Najafi M, Javid H, Hunter JA, Goldin MD: Acute ascending aortic dissection: surgical management. Circulation 64:231–234, Aug 1981.

69. Akins CW, Buckley MJ, Daggett W, McIlduff JB, Austen WG: Acute traumatic disruption of the thoracic aorta: a ten-year experience. Ann Thorac Surg 31:305–309, Apr 1981.

70. Soyer R, Brunet A, Piwnica A, Blondeau P, Carpentier A, Donzeau-Gouge P, Bical O, Dubost CH: Traumatic rupture of the thoracic aorta with reference to 34 operated cases. J Cardiovasc Surg 22:103–108, March/April 1981.

71. Cooley DA, Ott DA, Frazier OH, Walker WE: Surgical treatment of aneurysms of the transverse aortic arch: experience with 25 patients using hypothermic techniques. Ann Thorac Surg 32:260–272, Sept 1981.

72. Crawford ES, Saleh SA: Transverse aortic arch aneurysm: improved results of treatment employing new modifications of aortic reconstruction and hypothermic cerebral circulatory arrest. Ann Surg 194:180–188, Aug 1981.

73. Crawford ES, Walker HSJ III, Saleh SA, Normann NA: Graft replacement of aneurysm in descending thoracic aorta: results without bypass or shunting. Surgery 89:73–85, Jan 1981.

74. Pieroni RE, Fisher JG: Use of cholestyramine resin in digitoxin toxicity. JAMA 245:1939–1940. May 15, 1981.

75. Preston FE, Whipps S, Jackson CA, French AJ, Wyld PJ, Stoddard CJ: Inhibition of prostacyclin and platelet thromboxane A_2 after low-dose aspirin. N Engl J Med 304:76–79, Jan 1981.

76. Joshi PI, Dalal JJ, Ruttley MSJ, Sheridan DJ, Henderson AH: Nifedipine and left ventricular function in beta-blocked patients. Am Heart J 45:457–459, Apr 1981.

77. Lindenbaum J, Rund DG, Butler VP, Tse-Eng D, Saha JR: Inactivation of digoxin by the gut flora: reversal by antibiotic therapy. N Engl J Med 305:789–794, Oct 1981.

78. Milam JD, Austin SF, Martin RF, Keats AS, Cooley DA: Alteration of coagulation and selected clinical chemistry parameters in patients undergoing open heart surgery without transfusions. Amer J Clin Path 76:155–162, Aug 1981.

79. Chenoweth DE, Cooper SW, Hugli TE, Stewart RW, Blackstone EH, Kirklin JW: Complement activation during cardiopulmonary bypass. Evidence for generation of C3a and C5a anaphylatoxins. N Engl J Med 304:497–502, Feb 1981.

80. Longmore DB, Bennett JG, Hoyle PM, Smith MA, Gregory A, Osivand T, Jones WA: Prostacyclin administration during cardiopulmonary bypass in man. Lancet 1:800–803, Apr 1981.

81. Pierce WS, Parr GVS, Myers JL, Pae WE Jr, Bull AP, Waldhausen JA: Ventricular-assist pumping in patients with cardiogenic shock after cardiac operations. N Engl J Med 305:1606–1610, Dec 31, 1981.

82. Chandra N, Snyder LD, Weisfeldt ML: Abdominal binding during cardiopulmonary resuscitation in man. JAMA 246:351–353, July 24–31, 1981.

83. White CW, Albanese MA: Changes in cardiovascular health knowledge occurring from childhood to adulthood: a cross-sectional study. Circulation 63:1110–1115, May 1981.

84. Fye WB: History of cardiology. Circulation 64:434–436, Aug 1981.

85. Schiedermayer DL: The heart man. JAMA 246:2852, Dec 18, 1981.

Author Index

Subject Index